Textbook of Medicinal Chemistry

Textbook of Medicinal Chemistry

Edited by **Erica Helmer**

SYRAWOOD
PUBLISHING HOUSE
New York

Published by Syrawood Publishing House,
750 Third Avenue, 9th Floor,
New York, NY 10017, USA
www.syrawoodpublishinghouse.com

Textbook of Medicinal Chemistry
Edited by Erica Helmer

International Standard Book Number: 978-1-68286-316-9 (Hardback)

Printed in China.

Contents

Preface

Medicinal chemistry is an interdisciplinary field that incorporates concepts from various disciplines such as organic chemistry, pharmacology, biochemistry, etc. This book is a compilation of chapters that discuss topics like analytical chemistry, synthesis of chemical compounds, drug design, discovery and composition, etc. It presents researches and case studies by internationally acclaimed scholars. The book would be a comprehensive source of reference for all the students and academicians engaged in this field.

This book is a comprehensive compilation of works of different researchers from varied parts of the world. It includes valuable experiences of the researchers with the sole objective of providing the readers (learners) with a proper knowledge of the concerned field. This book will be beneficial in evoking inspiration and enhancing the knowledge of the interested readers.

In the end, I would like to extend my heartiest thanks to the authors who worked with great determination on their chapters. I also appreciate the publisher's support in the course of the book. I would also like to deeply acknowledge my family who stood by me as a source of inspiration during the project.

Editor

Synthesis and anti-HSV-1 evaluation of new 3*H*-benzo[*b*]pyrazolo[3,4-*h*]-1,6-naphthyridines and 3*H*-pyrido[2,3-*b*]pyrazolo[3,4-*h*]-1,6-naphthyridines

Alice MR Bernardino[1], Alexandre R Azevedo[1], Luiz CS Pinheiro[1], Júlio C Borges[1], Izabel CP Paixão[2], Milene Mesquita[2,3], Thiago ML Souza[2,3] and Maurício S dos Santos[4*]

Abstract

Background: Herpes simplex virus type-1 (HSV-1) is the primary cause of facial lesions (mouth, lips, and eyes) in humans. The widespread use of acyclovir and nucleoside analogues has led to emergence of HSV strains that are resistant to these drugs. Recently, non-nucleoside anti-HSV compounds have received considerable attention. 1,6-Naphthyridines are a class of heterocyclic compounds that exhibit a broad spectrum of biological activities such as inhibitor of HIV-1 integrase, HCMV, FGF receptor-1 tyrosine kinase, and the enzyme acetylcholinesterase. We previously reported the synthesis, SAR studies, and evaluation anti-HSV-1 activity of 3*H*-benzo[*b*]pyrazolo[3,4-*h*]-1,6-naphthyridines. In the course of our search for new 1,6-naphthyridines derivatives with potential activity against HSV-1, we have synthesized and evaluated new 3*H*-benzo[*b*]pyrazolo[3,4-*h*]-1,6-naphthyridines **(1a-k)** and 3*H*-pyrido[2,3-*b*]pyrazolo[3,4-*h*]-1,6-naphthyridines **(2a-c)**.

Results: A known synthetic approach was used for preparing new 3*H*-benzo[*b*]pyrazolo[3,4-*h*]-1,6-naphthyridines **(1a-k)** and 3*H*-pyrido[2,3-*b*]pyrazolo[3,4-*h*]-1,6-naphthyridines **(2a-c)**, starting from ethyl 4-chloro-1-phenyl-1*H*-pyrazolo[3,4-*b*]pyridine-5-carboxylate **(7)**. All compounds were identified by FTIR, ^{1}H NMR, and mass spectrometry. The antiviral effect on HSV-1 virus replication was determined.

Conclusions: The compounds **1d**, **1f**, **1g**, and **1h** exhibited the highest anti-HSV-1 activity. In general, 3*H*-benzo[*b*]pyrazolo[3,4-*h*]-1,6-naphthyridines were more effective inhibitors than their corresponding 3*H*-pyrido[2,3-*b*]pyrazolo[3,4-*h*]-1,6-naphthyridines. The compound **1h** reduced the virus yield in 91% at 50 μM and exhibited a low cytotoxicity (CC_{50} 600 μM).

Keywords: HSV-1, 1,6-naphthyridines, pyrazolonaphthyridines, heterocycles

Background

Herpes simplex virus type-1 (HSV-1) is a large enveloped virus containing double-stranded DNA genomes of approximately 152 kb in size. HSV-1 is the primary cause of facial lesions (mouth, lips, and eyes) in humans [1,2]. Most of clinical anti-herpes virus compounds are nucleoside analogues, such as acyclovir (ACV), which is the most common drug used on treatment of HSV infections [3-5]. However, the widespread use of these compounds has been associated with the emergence of drug-resistant HSV strains [5]. The discovery of new non-nucleoside anti-HSV-1 agents with different mechanisms of action could offer an additional strategy against drug resistance of viruses. Several examples of non-nucleoside inhibitors have been proposed as candidate drugs for the treatment of herpes [3,6-11].

1,6-Naphthyridines are a class of heterocyclic compounds that exhibit a broad spectrum of biological activities such as inhibitor of HIV-1 integrase [12-15], HCMV [16,17], FGF receptor-1 tyrosine kinase [18], and

* Correspondence: mauriciounifei@yahoo.com.br
[4]Departamento de Física e Química, Instituto de Ciências Exatas, Universidade Federal de Itajubá, 37500-903, Itajubá, MG, Brazil
Full list of author information is available at the end of the article

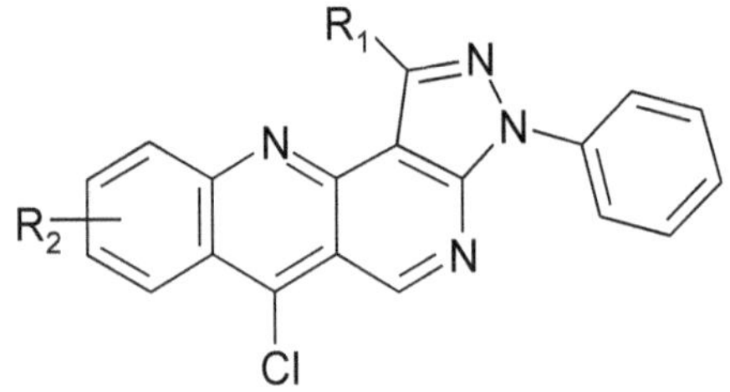

I

R_1	R_2
H	8-OMe
Me	H
Me	10-Cl
Me	8-Cl
Me	10-Me
Me	8-Me

Figure 1 Structure of 3*H*-benzo[*b*]pyrazolo[3,4-*h*]-1,6-naphthyridines I previously evaluated against HSV-1.

the enzyme acetylcholinesterase [19]. Many routes for the syntheses of 1,6-naphthyridines derivatives have previously been reported [20-24].

Recently, our research group reported the synthesis, SAR studies, and evaluation anti-HSV-1 activity of 3*H*-benzo[*b*]pyrazolo[3,4-*h*]-1,6-naphthyridines derivatives **I** (Figure 1) [25]. In the course of our search for new 1,6-naphthyridines derivatives with potential activity against HSV-1, we have synthesized and evaluated new 3*H*-benzo[*b*]pyrazolo[3,4-*h*]-1,6-naphthyridines **(1a-k)** and 3*H*-pyrido[2,3-*b*]pyrazolo[3,4-*h*]-1,6-naphthyridines **(2a-c)** (Scheme 1).

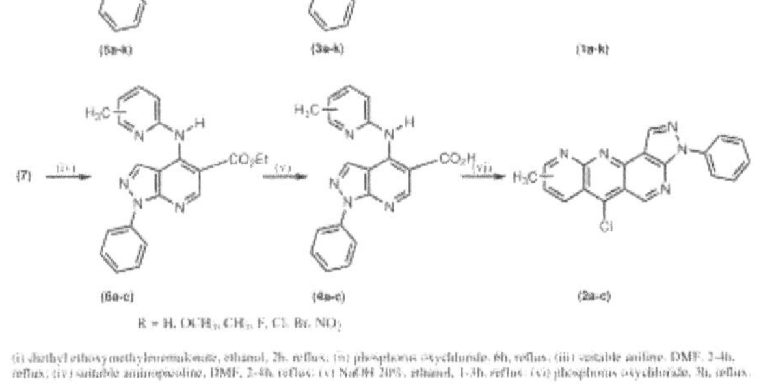

Scheme 1 Synthetic approach used to obtain the 3*H*-benzo[*b*]pyrazolo[3,4-*h*]-1,6-naphthyridine derivatives (1a-k), and new three 3*H*-pyrido[2,3-*b*]pyrazolo[3,4-*h*]-1,6-naphthyridine derivatives (2a-c).

Results and discussion

Chemistry

A known synthetic approach was used for preparing the 3*H*-benzo[*b*]pyrazolo[3,4-*h*]-1,6-naphthyridines **(1a-k)** and 3*H*-pyrido[2,3-*b*]pyrazolo[3,4-*h*]-1,6-naphthyridines **(2a-c)**, starting from ethyl 4-chloro-1-phenyl-1*H*-pyrazolo[3,4-*b*]pyridine-5-carboxylate **(7)** (Scheme 1) [26-28]. In the first step, ethyl α-carboethoxy-β-(5-pyrazolylammonium)acrylate **(8)** was prepared by the condensation between 5-amino-1-phenyl-1*H*-pyrazole **(9)** and diethyl ethoxymethylenemalonate, in ethanol. The cyclization of the acrylate **8** was carried out by refluxing in phosphorus oxychloride to afford 4-chlorol-phenyl-1*H*-pyrazolo[3,4-*b*]pyridine-5-carboxylate **(7)** in 75% yield [26-28]. Nucleophilic displacement of the chlorine atom in compound **7** by aromatic amines gave ethyl 4-(arylamino)-1-phenyl-1*H*-pyrazolo[3,4-*b*]pyridine-5-carboxylates **(5a-k)** in yields 52-82% [26,29]. Similarly, aminopicolines were used to obtain ethyl 4-[(methylpyridin-2-yl)amino]-1-phenyl-1*H*-pyrazolo[3,4-*b*]pyridine-5-carboxylates **(6a-c)** in yields 50-60%. These were achieved by heating at 140°C without solvents for 2-4 h an equimolar mixture of the appropriate aniline or aminopicoline and the compound **7**. However, better results were obtained when these reactions were carried out in solvents such as DMF [25]. Subsequent hydrolysis of the esters **5a-k** and **6a-c** afforded the corresponding 4-(arylamino)-1-phenyl-1*H*-pyrazolo[3,4-*b*]pyridine-5-carboxylic acids **(3a-k)** and 4-[(methylpyridin-2-yl) amino]-1-phenyl-1*H*-pyrazolo[3,4-*b*]pyridine-4-carboxylic acids **(4a-c)**, in high yields, 86-93 and 80-93%, respectively [28]. For producing 3*H*-benzo[*b*]pyrazolo[3,4-*h*]-1,6-naphthyridines **(1a-k)** and 3*H*-pyrido[2,3-*b*]pyrazolo[3,4-*h*]-1,6-naphthyridines **(2a-c)**, the respective carboxylic acids **3a-k** and **4a-c** were cyclized with phosphorus oxychloride at 110°C over a period of 3 h

[25,30]. The tetracyclic compounds **1a-k** and **2a-c** were isolated in 60-70% yield.

Biological evaluation

The targets 3*H*-benzo[*b*]pyrazolo[3,4-*h*]-1,6-naphthyridines (**1a-k**) and 3*H*-pyrido[2,3-*b*]pyrazolo[3,4-*h*]-1,6-naphthyridines (**2a-c**) were evaluated for inhibition of HSV-1 replication in infected Vero cells. Results are shown in Table 1. Compounds **1d**, **1f**, **1g**, and **1h** exhibited the highest anti-HSV-1 activity. Compound **1h** reduced the virus yield in 91% at 50 μM. In general, 3*H*-benzo[*b*]pyrazolo[3,4-*h*]-1,6-naphthyridines (**1a-k**) were more effective inhibitors than their corresponding 3*H*-pyrido[2,3-*b*]pyrazolo[3,4-*h*]-1,6-naphthyridines (**2a-c**).

Compounds with nearly the same antiviral effects were evaluated for cytotoxicity in Vero cells. EC_{50} and the selectivity index (SI) were determined in parallel. Several of the new compounds prevented the cytopathic effect of HSV-1 in Vero cells, at micromolar concentrations, and were minimally toxic to Vero cells resulting in a good SI. The MTT assay indicated that compound **1h** exhibited a low cytotoxicity (CC_{50} 600 μM). Trypan blue and MTT showed similar results (data not shown). ACV results have been included for comparison purposes (Table 2).

Conclusions

In summary, a new series of 3*H*-benzo[*b*]pyrazolo[3,4-*h*]-1,6-naphthyridines (**1a-k**) and 3*H*-pyrido[2,3-*b*]pyrazolo[3,4-*h*]-1,6-naphthyridine (**2a-c**) were synthesized and some of them were potent anti-HSV-1 agents. The compounds **1d**, **1f**, **1g**, and **1h** exhibited the highest anti-HSV-1 activity, being the 3*H*-benzo[*b*]pyrazolo[3,4-*h*]-1,6-naphthyridine derivatives, in general, more effective inhibitors than their corresponding 3*H*-pyrido[2,3-*b*]pyrazolo[3,4-*h*]-1,6-naphthyridines. The compound **1h** reduced the virus yield in 91% at 50 μM and exhibited a low cytotoxicity (CC_{50} 600 μM). The mechanism of antiviral activity of these compounds is under investigation.

Table 1 Anti-HSV-1 activity of 3*H*-benzo[*b*]pyrazolo[3,4-*h*]-1,6-naphthyridines (1a-k) and 3*H*-pyrido[2,3-*b*]pyrazolo[3,4-*h*]-1,6-naphthyridines (2a-c)

Compound	*R*	% of inhibition of virus yield (HSV-1)
1a	H	20,6
1b	9-OCH_3	50,0
1c	9-CH_3	68,0
1d	9-Cl	80,0
1e	8-Cl	60,0
1f	9-NO_2	80,0
1g	8-NO_2	87,0
1h	9-F	91,0
1i	8-F	65,0
1j	9-Br	30,0
1k	8-Br	30,0
2a	7-CH_3	11,0
2b	8-CH_3	ND
2c	9-CH_3	65,0
ACV	-	96.0 ± 1.0

The experimental concentration of 1a-k and 2a-c was 50 μM and for ACV 10 μM.
Results are presented as the mean of triplicate experiments.
ACV has been included for comparison purposes.

Table 2 Anti-HSV-1 activity, cytotoxicity and SI in Vero cells for 6-chloro-3-phenyl-9-fluoro-3*H*-benzo[*b*]pyrazolo[3,4-*h*]-1,6-naphthyridine (1h)

Compounds	*R*	EC_{50}[a] (μM)	CC_{50}[b] (μM)	S.I.[c]
1h	9-F	0,07	600	8571
ACV		1.09 ± 0.25	960 ± 156	880

ACV has been included for comparison purposes.
[a]50% Effective concentration or concentration required to inhibit HSV-1 virus yield.
[b]50% Cytotoxic concentration or concentration required to reduce the viability of host cells by 50%.
[c]Selective index (CC_{50}/EC50).

Experimental

Melting points were determined on a Fisatom 430D and are uncorrected. ^{1}H NMR spectra were recorded on a Varian Unity Plus spectrometer for 300 MHz, with tetramethylsilane as the internal standard. Chemical shifts (δ) are reported in parts per million (ppm) and the coupling constants (J) in Hertz (Hz). Fourier transform infrared absorption spectra were recorded in a Perkin-Elmer Spectrum One FTIR spectrophotometer. The solid samples were measured using potassium bromide (KBr) pellets. Thin-layer chromatography was performed on Uniplates (silica gel). All chemicals were reagent grade. High-resolution mass spectral analysis was recorded using a Finingan MAT 711A.

General procedures for the synthesis of 3*H*-benzo[*b*]pyrazolo[3,4-*h*]-1,6-naphthyridine derivatives (1a-k), and 3*H*-pyrido[2,3-*b*]pyrazolo[3,4-*h*]-1,6-naphthyridine derivatives (2a-c)

The key intermediate ethyl 4-chloro-1-phenyl-1*H*-pyrazolo[3,4-*b*]pyridine-5-carboxylate (**7**) was prepared according to literature [26-28]. An equimolar mixture of 7 (4 mmol) and anilines or aminopicolines in 10 mL DMF was heated under reflux for 2-4 h. The reaction mixture, after cooling, was poured into 50 mL of ice-water. The precipitated was filtered, dried, and recrystallized from a mixture of ethanol and water. The compounds obtained **5a-k** and **6a-c** were reacted with 10 mL NaOH (20%) and 10 mL of ethanol under reflux for 1-3 h. On cooling to room temperature, the mixture was acidified with diluted hydrochloric acid (1:3), and the precipitate was filtered and recrystallized from DMF and water. A mixture of the acids **3a-k** and **4a-c** (1 mmol), and phosphorus oxychloride (5 mL) was heated under reflux for 3 h. The reaction mixture was inverted over crushed ice. In some cases the excess of phosphorus oxychloride was removed under reduced pressure before inverting over crushed ice and neutralized. The new compounds **1a-k** and **2a-c** were isolated in yields 60-70%. The resulting precipitate was collected and purified by flash column chromatography (FC, silica gel). The structures of the compounds were elucidated by FTIR, ^{1}H NMR, and mass spectrometry.

(1a) 6-chloro-3-phenyl-3*H*-benzo[*b*]pyrazolo[3,4-*h*]-1,6-naphthyridine

Yield 70%; mp 259-260°C; IR (KBr, cm^{-1}) ν_{max} C-H 3084, C = C 1596, C = N 1502; ^{1}H NMR (DMSO-d6, 300 MHz) δ 8.92 (1H, s, H-1), 8.40 (1H, d, *J* = 8.1 Hz, H-10), 7.95 (1H, dd; *J* = 8.1 Hz, H-9), 7.70 (1H, dd, *J* = 8.1 Hz, H-8), 7.81 (1H, d, *J* = 8.1 Hz, H-7), 9.40 (1H, s, H-5), 8.33 (2H, d, *J* = 7.5 Hz, H-2', H-6'), 7.50 (2H, t, *J* = 7.5 Hz, H-3', H-5'), 7.52 (1H, t, *J* = 7.5 Hz, H-4'); EI (70eV) *m/z* (%): M$^+$ 330.00761 (100).

(1b) 6-chloro-3-phenyl-9-methoxy-3*H*-benzo[*b*]pyrazolo [3,4-*h*]-1,6-naphthyridine

Yield 68%; mp > 300°C; IR (KBr, cm^{-1}) ν_{max} C-H 3083, C = C 1595, C = N 1504; ^{1}H NMR (DMSO-d6, 300 MHz) δ 8.99 (1H, s, H-1), 7.26 (1H, s, H-10), 7.78-7.56 (5H, m, H-3', H-4', H-5', H7, H-8), 9.36 (1H, s, H-5), 8.31 (2H, d, *J* = 8.0 Hz, H-2', H-6'), 4.07 (3H, s, Ar-OCH_3); EI (70 eV) *m/z* (%): M$^{+\cdot}$ 360.07037 (100).

(1c) 6-chloro-3-phenyl-9-methyl-3*H*-benzo[*b*]pyrazolo [3,4-*h*]-1,6-naphthyridine

Yield 65%; mp > 300°C; IR (KBr, cm^{-1}) ν_{max} C-H 3083, C = C 1595, C = N 1503; ^{1}H NMR (DMSO-d6, 300 MHz) δ 8.99 (1H, s, H-1), 7.79-7.57 (6H, m, H-3', H-4', H-5', H7, H-8, H-10), 9.42 (1H, s, H-5), 8.40 (2H, d, *J* = 8.4 Hz, H-2', H-6'), 1.39 (3H, s, Ar-CH_3); EI (70eV) *m/z* (%): M$^{+\cdot}$ 344.81022 (100).

(1d) 6,9-dichloro-3-phenyl-3*H*-benzo[*b*]pyrazolo[3,4-*h*]-1,6-naphthyridine

Yield 60%; mp > 300°C; IR (KBr, cm^{-1}) ν_{max} C-H 3082, C = C 1598, C = N 1503; ^{1}H NMR (DMSO-d6, 300 MHz) δ 9.08 (1H, s, H-1), 7.99-7.53 (6H, m, H-3', H-4', H-5', H7, H-8, H-10), 9.38 (1H, s, H-5), 8.41 (2H, d, *J* = 8.4 Hz, H-2', H-6'); EI (70 eV) *m/z* (%): M$^{+\cdot}$ 364.01693 (100).

(1e) 6,8-dichloro-3-phenyl-3*H*-benzo[*b*]pyrazolo[3,4-*h*]-1,6-naphthyridine

Yield 68%; mp > 300°C; IR (KBr, cm^{-1}) ν_{max} C-H 3084, C = C 1598, C = N 1503; ^{1}H NMR (DMSO-d6, 300 MHz) δ 8.97 (1H, s, H-1), 7.87 (1H, d, *J* = 8.1 Hz, H-10), 7.89 (1H, d, *J* = 8.1 Hz, H-9), 8.22 (1H, s, H-7), 9.31 (1H, s, H-5), 8.27 (2H, d, *J* = 8.1 Hz, H-2', H-6'), 7.46 (2H, dd, *J* = 7.5 Hz, H-3', H-5'), 7.65 (1H, t, *J* = 7.5 Hz, H-4'); EI (70 eV) *m/z* (%): M$^{+\cdot}$ 364.01789 (100).

(1f) 6-chloro-3-phenyl-9-nitro-3*H*-benzo[*b*]pyrazolo[3,4-*h*]-1,6-naphthyridine

Yield 60%; mp > 300°C; IR (KBr, cm^{-1}) ν_{max} C-H 3084, C = C 1596, C = N 1503; ^{1}H NMR (DMSO-d6, 300 MHz) δ 8.92 (1H, s, H-1), 8.84 (1H, s, H-10), 8.05 (1H, d, *J* = 7.5 Hz, H-8), 8.02 (1H, d, *J* = 7.5 Hz, H-7), 9.40 (1H, s, H-5), 8.31 (2H, d, *J* = 7.5 Hz, H-2', H-6'), 7.52 (2H, dd, *J* = 7.5 Hz, H-3', H-5'), 7.71 (1H, t, *J* = 7.5 Hz, H-4'); EI (70 eV) *m/z* (%): M$^{+\cdot}$ 375.03743 (100).

(1g) 6-chloro-3-phenyl-8-nitro-3*H*-benzo[*b*]pyrazolo[3,4-*h*]-1,6-naphthyridine

Yield 60%; mp 280-281°C; IR (KBr, cm^{-1}) ν_{max} C-H 3100, C = C 1592, C = N 1500; ^{1}H NMR (DMSO-d6, 300 MHz) δ 8.90 (1H, s, H-1), 8.12 (1H, d, *J* = 7.8 Hz, H-10), 8.80 (1H, d, *J* = 7.8 Hz, H-9), 8.89 (1H, s, H-7), 9.42 (1H, s, H-5), 8.30 (2H, d, *J* = 7.5 Hz, H-2', H-6'), 7.51 (2H, dd, *J* = 7.5 Hz, H-3', H-5'), 7.68 (1H, t, *J* = 7.5 Hz, H-4'); EI (70 eV) *m/z* (%): M$^+$. 375.70261 (100).

(1h) 6-chloro-3-phenyl-9-fluoro-3*H*-benzo[*b*]pyrazolo[3,4-*h*]-1,6-naphthyridine

Yield 62%; mp 275-277°C; IR (KBr, cm^{-1}) ν_{max} C-H 3100, ν C = C 1600, ν C = N 1503; ^{1}H NMR (DMSO-d6, 300 MHz) δ 9.34 (1H, s, H-1), 8.45 (1H, s, H-10), 7.83-7.62 (1H, m, H-8), 9.02 (1H, d, *J* = 8.4 Hz, H-7), 9.49 (1H, s, H-5), 8.20 (2H, d, *J* = 7.5 Hz, H-2', H-6'), 7.25 (2H, dd, *J* = 7.5 Hz, H-3', H-5'), 7.41 (1H, t, *J* = 7.5 Hz, H-4'); EI (70 eV) *m/z* (%): M$^+$. 348.04188 (100).

(1i) 6-chloro-3-phenyl-8-fluoro-3*H*-benzo[*b*]pyrazolo[3,4-*h*]-1,6-naphthyridine

Yield 65%; mp 278-279°C; IR (KBr, cm^{-1}) ν_{max} C-H 3051, C = C 1598, C = N 1503; ^{1}H NMR (DMSO-d6, 300 MHz) δ 9.06 (1H, s, H-1), 8.03 (1H, d, *J* = 7.5 Hz, H-10), 8.05 (1H, m, H-9), 8.02 (1H, d, *J* = 8.4 Hz, H-7), 9.37 (1H, s, H-5), 8.32 (2H, d, *J* = 7.5 Hz, H-2', H-6'), 7.51 (1H, t, *J* = 7.5 Hz, H-4'), 7.69 (2H, dd, *J* = 7.5 Hz, H-3', H-5'); EI (70 eV) *m/z* (%): M$^+$. 348.09473 (100).

(1j) 9-bromo-6-chloro-3-phenyl-3*H*-benzo[*b*]pyrazolo[3,4-*h*]-1,6-naphthyridine

Yield 60%; mp > 300°C; IR (KBr, cm^{-1}) ν_{max} C-H 3052, C = C 1593, C = N 1503; ^{1}H NMR (DMSO-d6, 300 MHz) δ 9.05 (1H, s, H-1), 8.09 (1H, s, H-10), 7.90-7.50 (5H, m, H-3', H-4', H-5', H7, H-8), 9.30 (1H, s, H-5), 8.30 (2H, d, *J* = 7.5 Hz, H-2', H-6'); EI (70 eV) *m/z* (%): M$^+$. 409.96178 (100).

(1k) 8-bromo-6-chloro-3-phenyl-3*H*-benzo[*b*]pyrazolo[3,4-*h*]-1,6-naphthyridine

Yield 68%; mp > 300°C; IR (KBr, cm^{-1}) ν_{max} C-H 3085, C = C 1596, C = N 1501; ^1H NMR (DMSO-d6, 300 MHz) δ 8.95 (1H, s, H-1), 7.92-7.52 (5H, m, H-3', H-4', H-5', H7, H-10), 8.42 (1H, d, *J* = 8.4 Hz, H-9), 9.40 (1H, s, H-5), 8.30 (1H, d, *J* = 7.5 Hz, H-2', H-6'); EI (70 eV) *m/z* (%): M^+. 409,67991 (100).

(2a) 6-chloro-3-phenyl-7-methyl-3*H*-pyrido[2,3-*b*]pyrazolo [3,4-*h*]-1,6-naphthyridine

Yield 60%; mp 230-232°C; IR (KBr, cm^{-1}) ν_{max} C-H 3085, C = C 1596, C = N 1501; ^1H NMR (DMSO-d6, 300 MHz) δ 8.72 (1H, s, H-1), 8.26 (1H, d, *J* = 7.5 Hz, H-9), 7.68 (1H, d, *J* = 7.5 Hz, H-8), 9.44 (1H, s, H-5), 8.26 (2H, dd, *J* = 7.5 Hz, H-2', H-6'), 7.50 (1H, t, *J* = 7.5 Hz, H-4'), 7.68 (2H, dd, *J* = 7.5 Hz, H-3', H-5'), 1.37 (3H, s, Ar-CH_3); EI (70eV) *m/z* (%): M^+. 345.74391 (100).

(2b) 6-chloro-3-phenyl-8-methyl-3*H*-pyrido[2,3-*b*]pyrazolo [3,4-*h*]-1,6-naphthyridine

Yield 65%; mp 255-256°C; IR (KBr, cm^{-1}) ν_{max} C-H 3084, C = C 1596, C = N 1502; ^1H NMR (DMSO-d6, 300 MHz) δ 8.72 (1H, s, H-1), 8.92 (1H, s, H-9), 7.91 (1H, s, H-7), 9.58 (1H, s, H-5), 8.42 (2H, d, *J* = 7.5 Hz, H-2', H-6'), 7.59 (1H, t, *J* = 7.5 Hz, H-4'), 7.78 (2H, dd, *J* = 7.5 Hz, H-3', H-5'), 1.42 (3H, s, Ar-CH_3); EI (70 eV) *m/z* (%): M^+. 345.78660 (100).

(2c) 6-chloro-3-phenyl-9-methyl-3*H*-pyrido[2,3-*b*]pyrazolo [3,4-*h*]-1,6-naphthyridine

Yield 62%; mp 247-249°C; IR (KBr, cm^{-1}) ν_{max} C-H 3084, C = C 1596, C = N 1502; ^1H NMR (DMSO-d6, 300 MHz) δ 8.83 (1H, s, H-1), 7.67 (1H, d, *J* = 7.5 Hz, H-8), 7.93 (1H, d, *J* = 7.5 Hz, H-7), 9.41 (1H, s, H-5), 8.39 (2H, d, *J* = 7.5 Hz, H-2', H-6'), 7.56 (1H, t, *J* = 7.5 Hz, H-4'), 7.75 (2H, dd, *J* = 7.5 Hz, H-3', H-5'), 1.39 (3H, s, Ar-CH_3); EI (70 eV) *m/z* (%): M^+. 345.76572 (100).

Biological assays

Compounds were tested as inhibitor of HSV replication in Vero (African green monkey kidney, obtained from the American Type Culture Collection) cells. They were grown in DMEM (Gibco Laboratories) supplemented with 2% heat-inactivated fetal bovine serum (purchased from Fazenda Pig), 8% calf serum (purchased from Centro Pan-Americano de Febre Aftosa), 2.25% sodium bicarbonate, 500 U/mL penicillin, 100 µg/mL streptomycin, and 2.5 µg/mL amphotericin B. HSV-1 (ACR-29 strain) was kindly provided by Marcia Wigg (Universidade Federal do Rio de Janeiro, Brazil) and was routinely propagated in Vero cells. Virus stocks were stored at -70°C until use. ACV was purchased from Sigma (A 4669). It was dissolved in sterile deionized water and further diluted in culture medium. MTT was purchased from Sigma. Virus infectivity was measured by a dilution method using a 96-well microtitre plate and expressed as 50% tissue culture infections dose ($TCID_{50}$). Cells grown in 96-well microtitre were inoculated with virus at input 1 PFU (plaque-forming unit)/cell for 2 h at 37°C. After virus adsorption, virus inoculum was replaced by a culture medium containing quinolone acyclonucleobases carboxylic acid and their correspondent esters at the concentration of 50 µM. Control cultures were incubated with media without compounds. After 3 days of incubation at 37°C in 5% CO_2 atmosphere, the culture medium was harvested and the virus titre of each sample was determined in terms of 50% tissue culture dose (TCID 50/mL) by endpoint dilution.

Cytotoxicity

The cytotoxicity of the compounds was tested in Vero cells using two methods, namely, MTT and trypan blue dye exclusion assay. Monolayers of uninfected cells were incubated with culture medium containing different concentrations of compounds for 72 h at 37°C. The medium was then removed, the cells trypsinized and viable cells counted by trypan blue dye exclusion test. The 50% cytotoxic concentration (CC_{50}) was calculated by linear regression analysis of the dose-response curves generated from these data. In the second method, monolayer of Vero cells in 96-multiwell plates were incubated with MTT (5 µg/mL) at 37°C for 4 h. After this period, SDS 10% and 0.01 N HCl were added to each well and incubated overnight. The plates were read using an automatic plate reader with a 540-nm test wavelength and a 690-nm reference wavelength. Plaque reduction assay was performed utilizing Vero cells at a density of 3×10^5 infected with various dilutions of the supernatant from a yield reduction assay for 1 h at 37°C and 5% CO_2. After adsorption, the plates were washed and the medium was replaced with DMEM containing methylcellulose 1% and fetal bovine serum 5%. After incubation for 72 h, the monolayers were fixed with 1% formaldehyde in PBS, methylcellulose removed, and cell stained with a 0.1% solution of crystal violet in 70% methanol. The virus yield assay was performed as follows. Confluent Vero cells were washed with PBS and infected with HSV-1 at moi of 1 PFU/cell for 1 h at 37°C. The infected cells were washed with PBS and covered with a culture medium containing either no compounds or a different concentration of compounds. 20 h after adsorption, cells were lysed by freezing and thawing (three times), and the supernatant consisting of culture medium and lysed cells was obtained by centrifugation at 400*g* for 10 min at 4°C. Virus titre was determined by the plaque assay in Vero cells as described above. Data were statistically analyzed by Student's t-test for a significance level of $p < 0.05$.

Abbreviations

DMEM: Dulbecco's modified Eagle's medium; DMF *N*: *N*-dimethylformamide; HCMV: human cytomegalovirus; HSV-1: herpes simplex virus type-1; MTT: (3-(4,5-dimethylthiazol-2-yl)-2,5-diphenyl tetrazolium bromide; PBS: phosphate buffered saline; PFU: plaque-forming unit; SDS: sodium dodecyl sulphate.

Acknowledgements

This study was supported by the following Brazilian agencies and governmental institutions: Fundação de Amparo à Pesquisa do Estado do Rio de Janeiro (FAPERJ), Coordenação de Aperfeiçoamento de Pessoal de Nível Superior (CAPES), Conselho Nacional de Desenvolvimento Científico e Tecnológico (CNPq).

Author details

[1]Departamento de Química Orgânica, Instituto de Química, Programa de Pós-Graduação em Química, Universidade Federal Fluminense, Campus do Valonguinho, 24020-150, Niterói, RJ, Brazil [2]Departamento de Biologia Celular e Molecular, Instituto de Biologia, Universidade Federal Fluminense, Campus do Valonguinho, 24020-150, Niterói, RJ, Brazil [3]Programa de Pós-Graduação em Biologia Celular e Molecular, Fundação Oswaldo Cruz, Instituto Oswaldo Cruz, 21040-900, Rio de Janeiro, RJ, Brazil [4]Departamento de Física e Química, Instituto de Ciências Exatas, Universidade Federal de Itajubá, 37500-903, Itajubá, MG, Brazil

Competing interests

The authors declare that they have no competing interests.

References

1. James SH, Kimberlin DW, Whitley RJ (2009) Antiviral therapy for herpesvirus central nervous system infections: neonatal herpes simplex virus infection, herpes simplex encephalitis, and congenital cytomegalovirus infection. Antiviral Res 83:207–213. doi:10.1016/j.antiviral.2009.04.010.
2. Knizewski Ł, Kinch L, Grishin NV, Rychlewski L, Ginalski K (2006) Human herpesvirus 1 UL24 gene encodes a potential PD-(D/E)XK endonuclease. J Virol 80:2575–2577. doi:10.1128/JVI.80.5.2575-2577.2006.
3. Kang IJ, Wang LW, Hsu TA, Yueh A, Lee CC, Lee YC, Lee CY, Chao YS, Shih SR, Chern JH (2011) Isatin-b-thiosemicarbazones as potent herpes simplex virus inhibitors. Bioorg Med Chem Lett 21:1948–1952. doi:10.1016/j.bmcl.2011.02.037.
4. Jerome KR (2005) The road to new antiviral therapies. Clin Appl Immunol Rev 5:65–76. doi:10.1016/j.cair.2004.10.002.
5. Morfin F, Thouvenot D (2003) Herpes simplex virus resistance to antiviral drugs. J Clin Virol 26:29–37. doi:10.1016/S1386-6532(02)00263-9.
6. Mohamed SF, Flefel EM, Amr AEE, El-Shafy DNA (2010) Anti-HSV-1 activity and mechanism of action of some new synthesized substituted pyrimidine, thiopyrimidine and thiazolopyrimidine derivatives. Eur J Med Chem 45:1494–1501. doi:10.1016/j.ejmech.2009.12.057.
7. Ju HQ, Xiang YF, Xin BJ, Pei Y, Lu JX, Wang QL, Xia M, Qian CW, Ren Z, Wang SY, Wang YF, Xing GW (2011) Synthesis and in vitro anti-HSV-1 activity of a novel Hsp 90 inhibitor BJ-B11. Bioorg Med Chem Lett 21:1675–1677. doi:10.1016/j.bmcl.2011.01.098.
8. Jordão AK, Ferreira VF, Souza TML, Faria GGS, Machado V, Abrantes JL, Souza MCBV, Cunha AC (2011) Synthesis and anti-HSV-1 activity of new 1,2,3-triazole derivatives. Bioorg Med Chem 19:1860–1865. doi:10.1016/j.bmc.2011.02.007.
9. Gudmundsson KS, Johns BA, Weatherhead J (2009) Pyrazolopyrimidines and pyrazolotriazines with potent activity against herpesviruses. Bioorg Med Chem Lett 19:5689–5692. doi:10.1016/j.bmcl.2009.08.009.
10. Lowden CT, Bastow KF (2003) Anti-Herpes simplex virus activity of substituted 1-hydroxyacridones. J Med Chem 46:5015–5020. doi:10.1021/jm030206l.
11. Hammond JL, Koontz DL, Bazmi HZ, Beadle JR, Hostetler SE, Kini GD, Aldern KA, Richman DD, Hostetler KY, Mellors JW (2001) Alkylglycerol prodrugs of phosphonoformate are potent in vitro inhibitors of nucleoside-resistant human immunodeficiency virus type 1 and select for resistance mutations that suppress zidovudine resistance. Antimicrob Agents Chemother 45:1621–1628. doi:10.1128/AAC.45.6.1621-1628.2001.
12. Ramkumar K, Serrao E, Odde S, Neamati N (2010) HIV-1 integrase inhibitors: 2007-2008 update. Med Res Rev 30:890–954. doi:10.1002/med.20194.
13. Johns BA, Weatherhead JG, Allen SH, Thompson JB, Garvey EP, Foster SA, Jeffrey JL, Miller WH (2009) 1,3,4-Oxadiazole substituted naphthyridines as HIV-1 integrase inhibitors. Part 2: SAR of the C5 position. Bioorg Med Chem Lett 19:1807–1810. doi:10.1016/j.bmcl.2009.01.089.
14. Melamed JY, Egbertson MS, Varga S, Vacca JP, Moyer G, Gabryelski L, Felock PJ, Stillmock KA, Witmer MV, Schleif W, Hazuda DJ, Leonard Y, Jin L, Ellis JD, Young SD (2008) Synthesis of 5-(1-H or 1-alkyl-5-oxopyrrolidin-3-yl)-8-hydroxy-[1,6]-naphthyridine-7-carboxamide inhibitors of HIV-1 integrase. Bioorg Med Chem Lett 18:5307–5310. doi:10.1016/j.bmcl.2008.08.038.
15. Egbertson MS, Moritz HM, Melamed JY, Han W, Perlow DS, Kuo MS, Embrey M, Vacca JP, Zrada MM, Cortes AR, Wallace A, Leonard Y, Hazuda DJ, Miller MD, Felock PJ, Stillmock KA, Witmer MV, Schleif W, Gabryelski LJ, Moyer G, Ellis JD, Jin L, Xu W, Braun MP, Kassahun K, Tsou NN, Young SD (2007) A potent and orally active HIV-1 integrase inhibitor. Bioorg Med Chem Lett 17:1392–1398. doi:10.1016/j.bmcl.2006.11.080.
16. Falardeau G, Lachance H, Pierre AS, Yannopoulos CG, Drouin M, Bédard J, Chan L (2005) Design and synthesis of a potent macrocyclic 1,6-napthyridine anti-human cytomegalovirus (HCMV) inhibitors. Bioorg Med Chem Lett 15:1693–1695. doi:10.1016/j.bmcl.2005.01.050.
17. Chan L, Jin H, Stefanac T, Lavallée JF, Falardeau G, Wang W, Bédard J, May S, Yuen L (1999) Discovery of 1,6-Naphthyridines as a novel class of potent and selective human cytomegalovirus inhibitors. J Med Chem 42:3023–3025. doi:10.1021/jm9902483.
18. Thompson AM, Connolly CJC, Hamby JM, Boushelle S, Hartl BG, Amar AM, Kraker AJ, Driscoll DL, Steinkampf RW, Patmore SJ, Vincent PW, Roberts BJ, Elliott WL, Klohs W, Leopold WR, Showalter HDH, Denny WA (2000) 3-(3,5-Dimethoxyphenyl)-1,6-naphthyridine-2,7-diamines and related 2-urea derivatives are potent and selective inhibitors of the FGF receptor-1 tyrosine kinase. J Med Chem 43:4200–4211. doi:10.1021/jm000161d.
19. Vanlaer S, Voet A, Gielens C, De Maeyer M, Compernolle F (2009) Bridged 5,6,7,8-tetrahydro-1,6-naphthyridines, analogues of huperzine a: synthesis, modeling studies and evaluation as inhibitors of acetylcholinesterase. Eur J Org Chem 2009:643–654
20. Brown DJ (ed) (2008) Chemistry of heterocyclic compounds: the naphthyridines. John Wiley & Sons, New Jersey
21. Jachak MN, Bagul SM, Kazi MA, Toche RB (2011) Novel synthetic protocol toward pyrazolo[3,4-*h*]-[1,6]naphthyridines *via* Friedlander condensation of new 4-aminopyrazolo[3,4-*b*]pyridine-5-carbaldehyde with reactive α-methylene ketones. J Het Chem 48:295–300. doi:10.1002/jhet.242.
22. Rote RV, Bagul SM, Shelar DP, Patil SR, Toche RB, Jachak MN (2011) Synthesis of benzo[3,4-*h*][1,6]naphthyridines *via* Friedlander condensation with active methylenes. J Het Chem 48:301–307. doi:10.1002/jhet.391.
23. Toche RB, Pagar BP, Zoman RR, Shinde GB, Jachak MN (2010) Synthesis of novel benzo[h][1,6]naphthyridine derivatives from 4-aminoquinoline and cyclic b-ketoester. Tetrahedron 66:5204–5211. doi:10.1016/j.tet.2010.04.085.
24. Chandra A, Singh B, Upadhyay S, Singh RM (2008) Copper-free Sonogashira coupling of 2-chloroquinolines with phenyl acetylene and quick annulation to benzo[b][1,6]naphthyridine derivatives in aqueous ammonia. Tetrahedron 64:11680–11685. doi:10.1016/j.tet.2008.10.010.
25. Bernardino AMR, Castro HC, Frugulhetti ICPP, Loureiro NIV, Azevedo AR, Pinheiro LCS, Souza TML, Giongo V, Passamani F, Magalhães UO, Albuquerque MG, Cabral LM, Rodrigues CR (2008) SAR of a series of anti-HSV-1 acridone derivatives, and a rational acridone-based design of a new anti-HSV-1 3H-benzo[b]pyrazolo[3,4-h]-1,6-naphthyridine series. Bioorg Med Chem 16:313–321. doi:10.1016/j.bmc.2007.09.032.
26. Leal B, Afonso IF, Rodrigues CR, Abreu PA, Garrett R, Pinheiro LCS, Azevedo AR, Borges JC, Vegi PF, Santos CCC, Silveira FCA, Cabral LM, Frugulhetti ICPP, Bernardino AMR, Santos DO, Castro HC (2008) Antibacterial profile against drug-resistant *Staphylococcus epidermidis* clinical strain and structure-activity relationship studies of 1H-pyrazolo[3,4-b]pyridine and thieno[2,3-b]pyridine derivatives. Bioorg Med Chem 16:8196–8204. doi:10.1016/j.bmc.2008.07.035.
27. Mello H, Echevarria A, Bernardino AM, Cavalheiro MC, Leon LL (2004) Antileishmanial pyrazolopyridine derivatives: synthesis and structure-activity relationship analysis. J Med Chem 47:5427–5432. doi:10.1021/jm0401006.

28. Bernardino AMR, Azevedo AR, Pinheiro LCS, Borges JC, Carvalho VL, Miranda MD, Meneses MDF, Nascimento M, Ferreira D, Rebello MA, Silva VAGG, Frugulhetti ICPP (2007) Synthesis and antiviral activity of new 4-(phenylamino)/4-[(methylpyridin-2-yl)amino]-1-phenyl-1*H*-pyrazolo[3,4-*b*] pyridine-4-carboxylic acids derivatives. Med Chem Res 16:352–369. doi:10.1007/s00044-007-9035-6.
29. Pinheiro LCS, Borges JC, Oliveira CD, Ferreira VF, Romeiro GA, Marques IP, Abreu PA, Frugulhetti ICPP, Rodrigues CR, Albuquerque MG, Castro HC, Bernardino AMR (2008) Synthesis of new 4-(phenylamino)thieno[2,3-b] pyridines and derivatives of the novel benzo[b]thieno[3,2-h]-1,6-naphthyridine tetracyclic system. Arkivoc 14:77–87
30. Bernardino AMR, Pinheiro LCS, Rodrigues CR, Loureiro NI, Castro HC, Rangel AL, Lopes JS, Borges JC, Carvalho JM, Romeiro GA, Ferreira VF, Frugulhetti ICPP, Santos MAV (2006) Design, synthesis, SAR, and biological evaluation of new 4-(phenylamino)thieno[2,3-b]pyridine derivatives. Bioorg Med Chem 14:5765–5770. doi:10.1016/j.bmc.2006.03.013.

2

Antimicrobial studies of unsymmetrical *bis*-1,2,3-triazoles

Abid H Banday[1*], Shameem A Shameem[1] and Bashir A Ganai[2]

Abstract

Aryl azides were treated with allenylmagnesium bromide to generate 1,5-disubstituted butynyl 1,2,3-triazoles in a domino fashion, which upon Cu(I) catalyzed 1,3-dipolar cycloaddition with aryl azides afforded novel *bis*-1,2,3-triazoles in quantitative yields. The final products were analyzed for their antimicrobial activities against a panel of bacterial and fungal strains which revealed the products to be potent antimicrobials.

Keywords: azides, *bis*-triazoles, antimicrobials, microbial strains

1. Introduction

Most of the nitrogen-containing molecules are pharmacologically very active which can be attributed to the fact that nitrogenous compounds are part and parcel of the biomolecular diversity [1-7]. Amongst the pharmacologically active nitrogenous compounds, a large number of 1,2,3-triazoles and their derivatives attracted considerable attention for the past few decades due to their chemotherapeutical value. Many 1,2,3-triazoles, including bis-triazoles, are found to be potent antimicrobial, analgesic, anti-inflammatory, local anesthetic, anti-convulsant, anti-neoplastic, anti-malarial, and antiviral agents [8-10]. Some of them exhibited anti-proliferative, anticancer activity, and several are used as DNA cleaving agents and potassium channel activators. Such type of diverse biological functions is also reported with a variety of *bis*-triazoles. The 'click chemistry' approach has been the most widely used method for the synthesis of libraries of a large number of biologically active molecular frameworks particularly for the regioselective synthesis of 1,2,3-triazoles, which involves the copper(I)-catalyzed cycloaddition reaction between azides and terminal alkynes (CuAAC). This reaction has been termed as the 'cream of the crop' of 'click reactions' and has found application in various facets of drug discovery as it enables a modular approach to generate novel pharmacophores utilizing a collection of reliable chemical reactions [11,12]. Thus, the development of the copper(I)-catalyzed 'triazole click chemistry' has led to many interesting applications including the synthesis, medicinal chemistry, molecular biology, and material science. The bioorthogonality of azide and alkynes [13] has allowed the use of their [3 + 2] cycloaddition in various biological applications including target guided synthesis [14] and activity-based protein profiling [15]. Of particular interest would be the dimeric heterocycle-based ligands which are designed for specific target interactions. Various approaches reported for the synthesis of biologically relevant *bis*-triazoles include Cu(I)-catalyzed 1,3-dipolar cycloaddition of monoazides with diacetylenes or that of monoacetylenes with diazides. For example, the synthesis of *bis*-triazoles is reported by the reactions of *bis*(azidomethyl)benzenes with several substituted acetylenes [16]. Recently, much attention has been paid toward the synthesis and pharmacological evaluation of triazoles and *bis*-triazoles as potent HIV-1 protease inhibitors [17,18] and size-specific ligands for mRNA Hairpin loops [19], respectively. Keeping into consideration the tremendous biological potence of triazoles and *bis*-triazoles in general and the antimicrobial activity in particular, we, in our continuous endeavor toward the synthesis of pharmacologically active molecules, designed the synthesis of novel unsymmetrical *bis*-1,2,3-triazoles and then evaluated them for antimicrobial activities. The biological results obtained were very interesting and revealed most of the synthesized molecules to be potent antimicrobials.

* Correspondence: abidrrl@gmail.com
[1]Department of Chemistry, Islamia College of Science and Commerce, Srinagar 190009, J&K, India
Full list of author information is available at the end of the article

2. Experimental

2.1. General methods

Melting points were recorded on Buchi Melting point apparatus D-545; IR spectra (KBr disks) were recorded on Bruker Vector 22 instrument. NMR spectra were recorded on Bruker DPX200 instrument in $CDCl_3$ with TMS as internal standard for protons and solvent signals as internal standard for carbon spectra. Chemical shift values are mentioned in δ (ppm) and coupling constants are given in Hz. Mass spectra were recorded on EIMS (Shimadzu) and ESI-esquire 3000 Bruker Daltonics instrument. The progress of all reactions was monitored by TLC on 2 × 5 cm pre-coated silica gel 60 F254 plates of thickness of 0.25 mm (Merck). The chromatograms were visualized under UV 254-366 nm and iodine.

2.2.1. Chemical synthesis

2.2.1.1. General procedure for the synthesis of bis-1,2,3-triazoles (5) To a suspension of Mg turnings (1.6 g, 0.66 mol, 10 equiv.) in specially dried THF with $HgCl_2$ (5 mg, 1% w/w of propargyl bromide) was added propargyl bromide (3.05 ml of an 80% wt. soln. in toluene, 4 mmol, 5 equiv.) in small portions while stirring the mixture at r.t. (*Note*: A small grain of $HgCl_2$ is generally required to promote formation of the reagent.) The mixture was stirred at r.t. for 2 h to give a cloudy light green solution. The allenylmagnesium bromide generated as above was cooled to 0°-5° and added dropwise to a solution of 3-methylphenyl azide (1 g, 0.007 mol) maintaining the temperature between 0 and 5°C. The mixture was allowed to attain r.t., and stirring was continued at ambient temperature for 30 min, followed by quenching with aq. NH_4Cl solution (10 mL) and diluting with AcOEt (50 mL). The org. layer was separated and the aq. layer extracted with AcOEt (2 × 20 mL). The combined org. layers were dried (anh. Na_2SO_4) and evaporated under reduced pressure to afford crude product, which was subjected to chromatography (silica gel, 60-120 mesh, elution; hexane/AcOEt gradient) to afford pure 5-(But-3-yn-1-yl)-1-(3-methylphenyl)-1H-1,2,3-triazoles 3 as a colorless liquid. 3-Methyl butynyl triazole (10 mmol) was stirred in 5 mL of *tert*-butanol and H_2O (1:1 mixture). $CuSO_4$ (12 mmol) and sodium ascorbate (50 mmol) were charged into the reaction mixture. After 15 min, 3-methylphenyl azide (10 mmol) was added to the above mixture, and stirred for 8 h. The mixture was diluted with AcOEt, the org. layer was separated, and the aq. layer extracted with AcOEt (2 × 20 mL). The combined org. layers were dried (anh. Na_2SO_4) and evaporated under reduced pressure to afford crude product 5 (Scheme 1), which was subjected to precipitation in hexane–AcOEt, affording pure *bis*-triazole 5 as an amorphous brown solid (only entries 2 and 13, see Table 1) (Scheme 2).

The analytical data of all the isolated *bis*-triazoles is given as under.

1-(4-methoxyphenyl)-5-(2-(1-*m*-tolyl-1H-1,2,3-triazol-4-yl)ethyl)-1H-1,2,3-triazole (5a)

Syrupy brownish liquid. IR (KBr) cm^{-1}: 3453, 2913, 2865, 1593, 1212, 1080, and 685; ^1H NMR ($CDCl_3$): δ 2.44 (s, 3H); 3.12 (m, 4H); 3.87 (s, 3H); 7.02 (d, 2H, *J* = 8.89 Hz); 7.35 (m, 6H); 7.50 (s, 1H), 7.60 (s, 1H); ^{13}C NMR (500 MHz, $CDCl_3$): δ 21.40, 23.44, 24.53, 55.63, 114.74, 117.53, 119.41, 121.14, 126.71, 128.00, 129.53, 138.11, 140.03, 148.22, 161.12.; ESI-MS: 383 (M^+ + Na); Anal. Calcd. for $C_{20}H_{20}N_6O$: C, 66.65; H, 5.59; N, 23.32; Found: C, 66.83; H, 5.38; N, 23.51.

4-(4-(2-(3-(4-methoxyphenyl)-3H-1,2,3-triazol-4-yl) ethyl)-1H-1,2,3-triazol-1-yl)benz-oic acid (5b)

Amorphous white solid. m. p. 195-197°C; IR (KBr) cm^{-1}: 3413, 2922, 2860, 1593, 1234, 1017, and 690; ^1H NMR (CDCl3): δ δ 3.10 (t, 2H, *J* = 5.97); 3.12 (t, 2H, *J* = 5.97); 3.84 (s, 3H); 7.08 (d, 2H, *J* = 8.90 Hz); 7.37 (d, 2H, *J* = 8.90 Hz); 7.72 (s,1H), 7.93 (d, 2H, *J* = 8.63 Hz), 8.21 (d, 2H, *J* = 8.90 Hz); 8.33 (s, 1H); ^{13}C NMR (500 MHz, CDCl3): δ 22.50, 23.59, 54.45, 114.15, 115.43, 119.17, 119.21, 120.13, 126.36, 127.43, 130.78, 131.06, 147.23, 200.12; ESI-MS: 391 (M^+ + H); Anal. Calcd. for $C_{20}H_{18}N_6O_3$: C, 61.53; H, 4.65; N, 21.53; Found: C, 61.71; H, 4.82; N, 21.79.

1-(4-methoxyphenyl)-5-(2-(1-(3-nitrophenyl)-1H-1,2,3-triazol-4-yl)ethyl)-1H-1,2,3-triazole (5c)

Syrupy grayish semisolid. IR (KBr) cm^{-1}: 3393, 2897, 2867, 1582, 1244, 1018, and 689; ^1H NMR (CDCl3): δ 3.10 (t, 2H, *J* = 5.78); 3.23 (t, 2H, *J* = 5.78); 3.85 (s, 3H); 7.05 (d, 2H, *J* = 8.94 Hz); 7.38 (d, 2H, *J* = 8.94 Hz); 7.73-7.88 (m, 2H); 8.22-8.32 (m, 2H); 8.42 (s, 1H); 8.68 (m, 1H); ^{13}C NMR (500 MHz, CDCl3): δ 22.20, 23.69, 55.45, 113.15, 116.43, 118.17, 119.41, 120.13, 127.36, 127.43, 130.78, 132.06, 142.33, 148.25; ESI-MS: 392 (M^+ + H); Anal. Calcd. for $C_{19}H_{17}N_7O_3$: C, 58.31; H, 4.38; N, 25.05; Found: C, 58.54; H, 4.5; N, 25.21.

1-(4-methoxyphenyl)-5-(2-(1-*p*-tolyl-1H-1,2,3-triazol-4-yl)ethyl)-1H-1,2,3-triazole (5d)

Syrupy grayish semisolid. IR (KBr) cm^{-1}: 3423, 2932, 2876, 1593, 1234, 10179, and 694; ^1H NMR ($CDCl_3$): δ 2.45 (s, 3H); 3.15 (m, 4H); 3.87 (s, 3H); 7.02 (d, 2H, *J* = 8.89 Hz); 7.18 (d, 2H, *J* = 8.89 Hz), 7.37 (d, 2H, *J* = 8.90 Hz); 7.47 (d, 2H, *J* = 8.90 Hz); 7.50 (s,1H), 7.80 (s, 1H); ^{13}C NMR (500 MHz, $CDCl_3$): δ 18.50, 22.23, 23.59, 54.45, 114.15, 115.43, 119.17, 119.51, 120.13, 126.36, 127.33, 130.78, 135.06, 147.23; ESI-MS: 383 (M^+ + Na); Anal. Calcd. for $C_{20}H_{20}N_6O$: C, 66.65; H, 5.59; N, 23.32; Found: C, 66.42; H, 5.68; N, 23.54.

Table 1 *Bis*-triazoles prepared by 'Domino-Click' reaction

Entry	Triazole	Azide	Bis-triazole[a]	Yield (%)
a	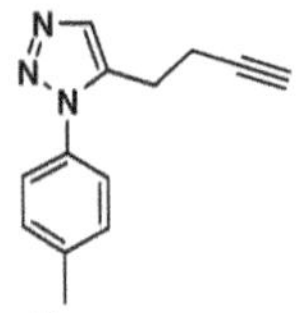	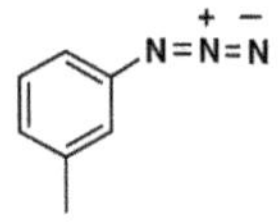	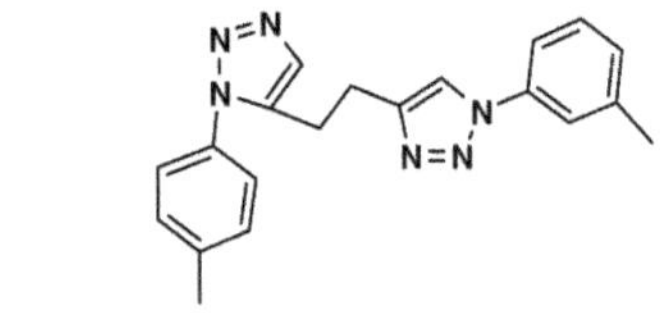	92
b	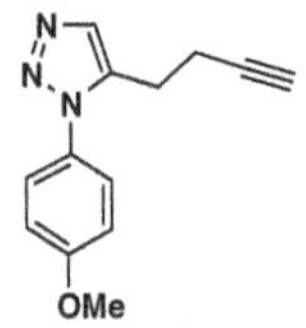	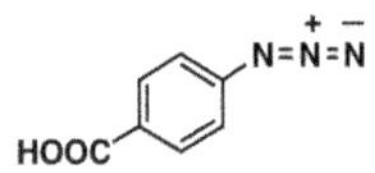	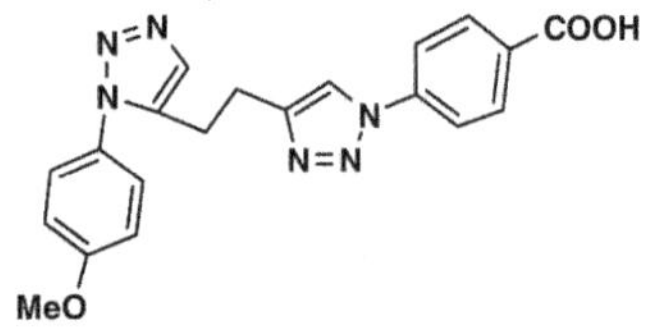	91[b]
c	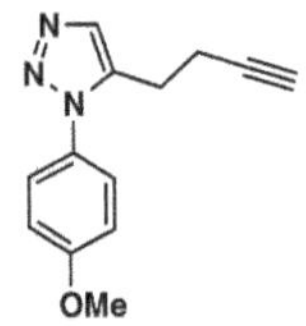	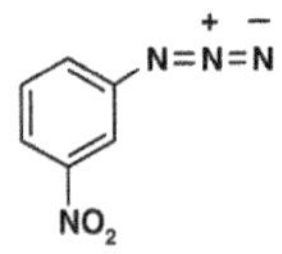	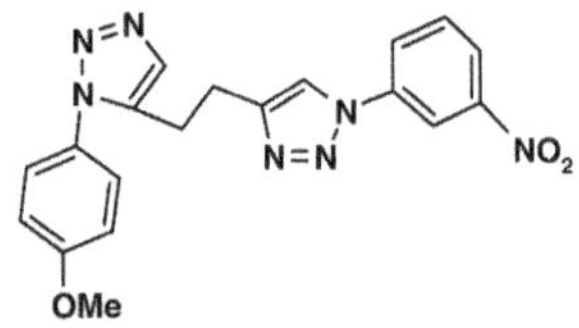	89
d	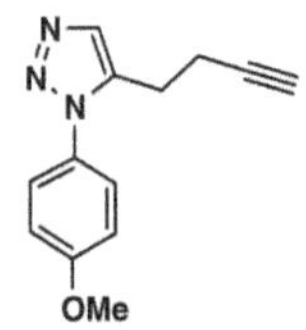	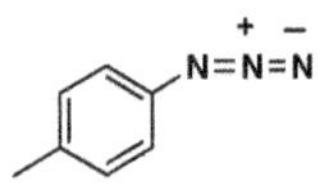	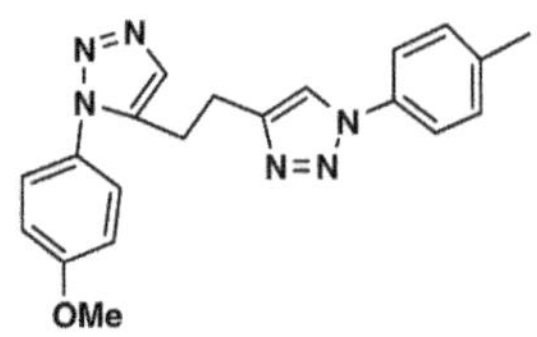	91
e	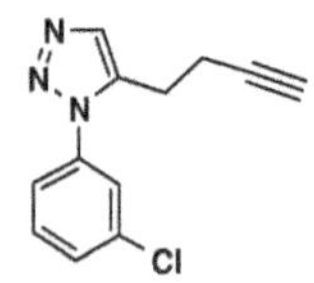	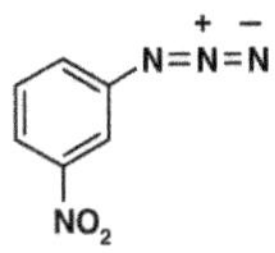	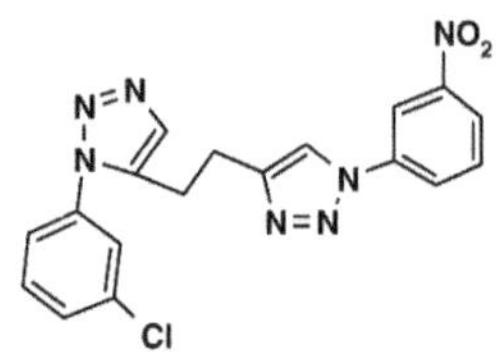	88
f	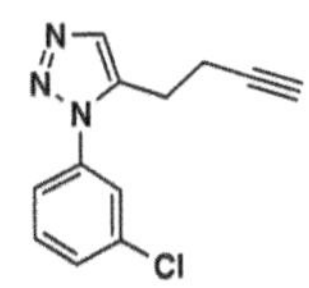	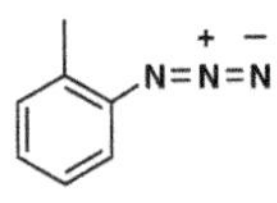	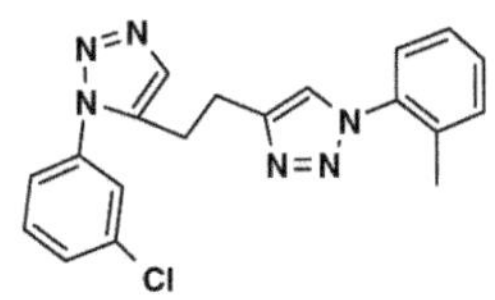	92
g	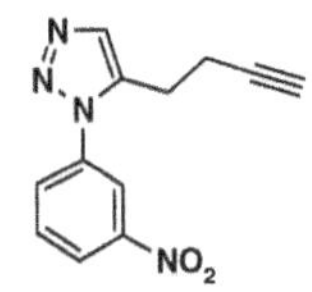	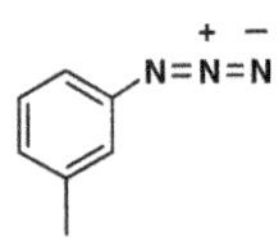	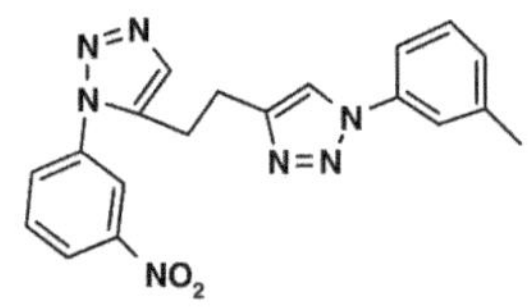	90
h	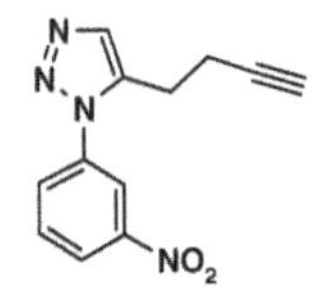	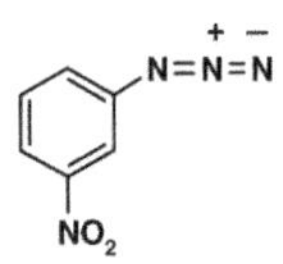	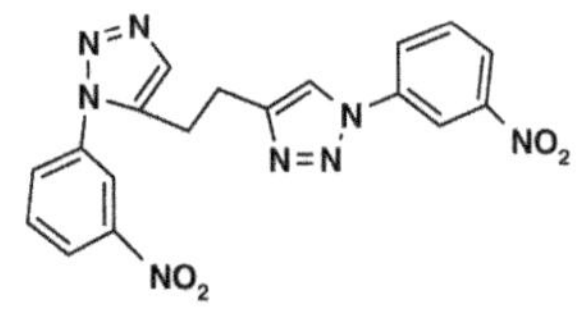	90

Table 1 ***Bis*****-triazoles prepared by ?'?Domino-Click?'? reaction** *(Continued)*

i	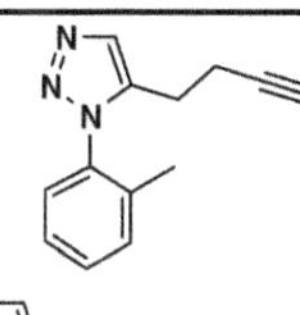	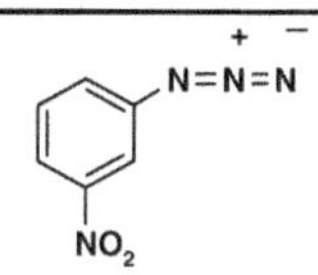	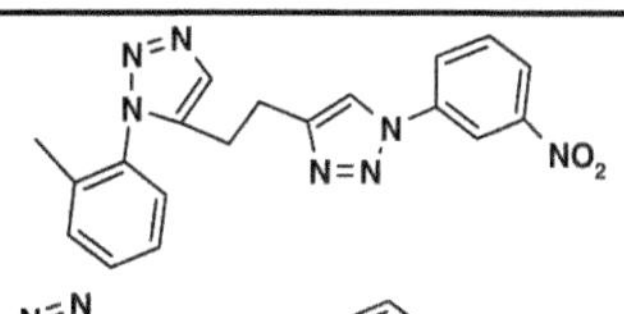	91
j	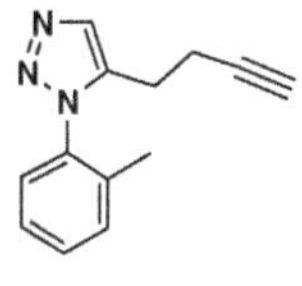	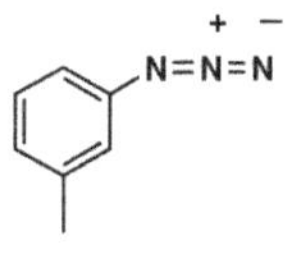	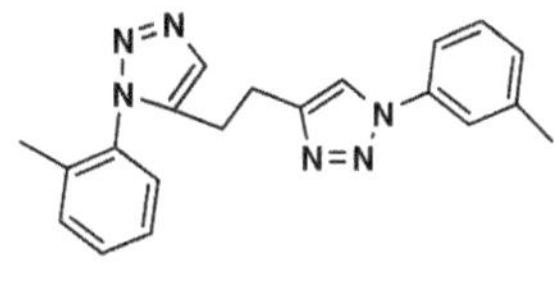	93
k	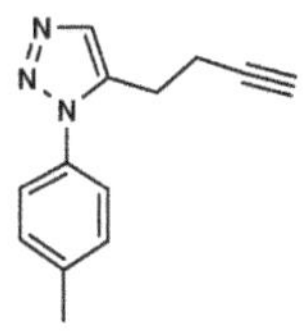	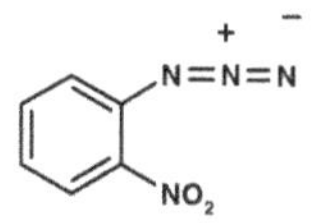	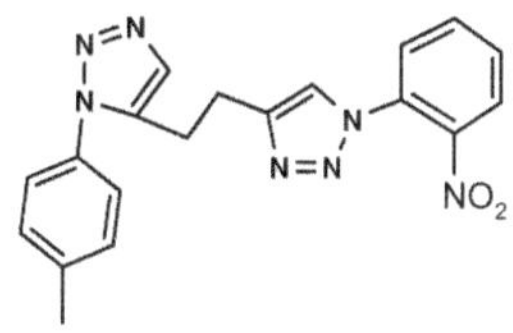	92
l	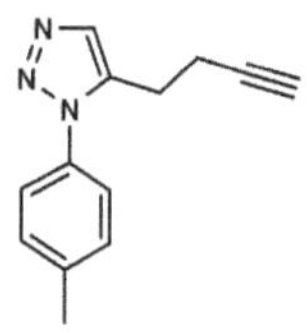	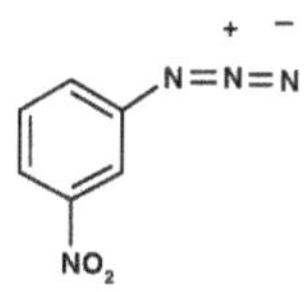	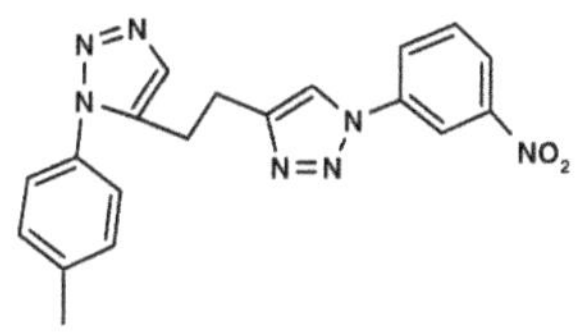	89
m	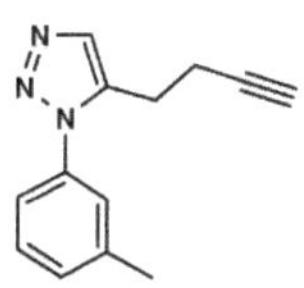	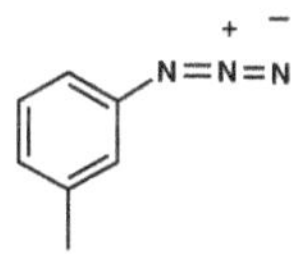	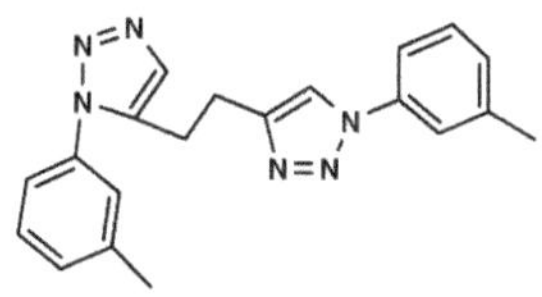	90[c]

1-(3-chlorophenyl)-5-(2-(1-*p*-nitrophenyl-1H-1,2,3-triazol-4-yl)ethyl)-1H-1,2,3-triazole (5e)

Syrupy grayish semisolid. IR (KBr) cm^{-1}: 3411, 2945, 2898, 1597, 1265, 1067, and 702; ^{1}H NMR ($CDCl_3$): δ 3.17-3.40 (m, 4H); 7.34-7.57 (m, 2H); 7.77 (m, 2H), 7.86 (s, 1H); 8.17 (d, 2H, *J* = 7.85 Hz); 8.30 (d, 2H, *J* = 7.85), 8.55 (s, 1H); ^{13}C NMR (500 MHz, $CDCl_3$): δ 19.25, 21.23, 23.56, 114.15, 115.43, 119.17, 119.51, 120.13, 126.36, 128.33, 130.87, 136.06, 146.23; ESI-MS: 418 (M$^+$ + Na); Anal. Calcd. for $C_{18}H_{14}ClN_7O$: C, 54.62; H, 3.57; N, 24.77; Found: C, 54.85; H, 3.38; N, 24.86.

1-(3-nitrophenyl)-5-(2-(1-*m*-tolyl-1H-1,2,3-triazol-4-yl)ethyl)-1H-1,2,3-triazole (5f)

Syrupy brownish semisolid. IR (KBr) cm^{-1}: 3417, 2954, 2856, 1587, 1235, 1079, and 698; ^{1}H NMR (CDCl3): δ 2.44 (s, 3H); 3.17-3.25 (m, 4H); 7.39 (d, 2H, *J* = 7.40 Hz); 7.50 (s, 2H), 7.70-7.82 (m, 4H); 8.36 (m, 2H); ^{13}C NMR (500 MHz, CDCl3): δ 19.54, 21.23, 23.59, 114.15, 116.41, 119.17, 119.51, 120.13, 128.32, 127.35, 130.88, 136.06, 146.23, 153.22.; ESI-MS: 398 (M$^+$ + Na); Anal. Calcd. for $C_{19}H_{17}N_7O_2$: C, 60.79; H, 4.56; N, 26.12; Found: C, 60.95; H, 4.72; N, 26.34.

1-(3-nitrophenyl)-5-(2-(1-(3-nitrophenyl)-1H-1,2,3-triazol-4-yl)ethyl)-1H-1,2,3-triazole (5g)

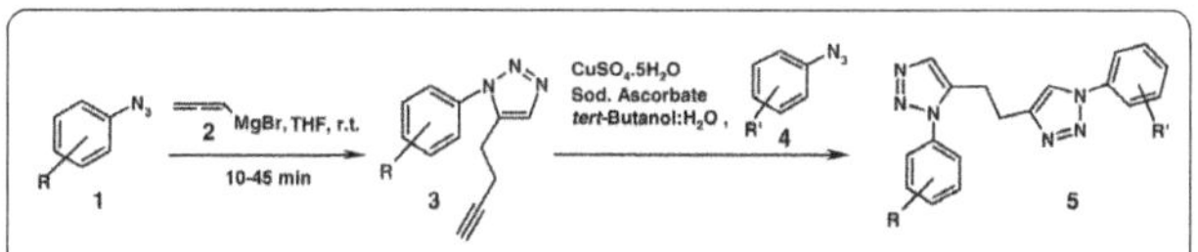

Scheme 1 Domino-click method for the synthesis of unsymmetrical bis 1,2,3-Triazoles.

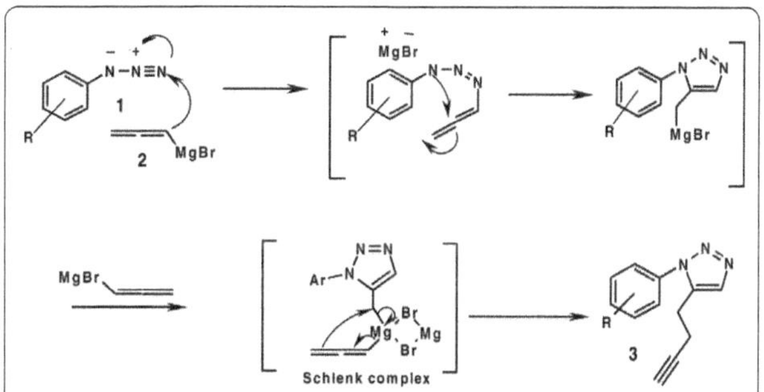

Scheme 2 Plausible mechanism for the formation of 5-butynyl triazoles 3.

Syrupy brownish semisolid. IR (KBr) cm^{-1}: 3419, 2965, 2857, 1580, 1265, 1099, and 714; ^1H NMR (CDCl3): δ 3.21 (t, 2H, J = 5.44); 3.30 (t, 2H, J = 5.44); 7.79 (m, 4H, J = 7.40 Hz); 7.87 (s, 1H), 8.15 (d, 2H, J = 7.82 Hz); 8.38 (m, 2H), 8.54 (s, 1H); ^{13}C NMR (500 MHz, CDCl3): δ 19.47, 21.34, 22.89, 114.15, 116.67, 119.77, 118.52, 120.13, 127.32, 128.35, 130.32, 136.18, 146.56, 154.31; ESI-MS: 407 (M^+ + H); Anal. Calcd. for $C_{18}H_{14}N_8O_4$: C, 53.20; H, 3.47; N, 27.57; Found: C, 53.11; H, 3.62; N, 27.34.

5-(2-(1-(3-nitrophenyl)-1H-1,2,3-triazol-4-yl)ethyl)-1-*o*-tolyl-1H-1,2,3-triazole (5h)

Syrupy brownish semisolid. IR (KBr) cm^{-1}: 3418, 2954, 2856, 1587, 1235, 1079, and 698; ^1H NMR (CDCl3): δ 2.36 (s, 3H); 3.09 (m, 4H); 7.22 (m, 2H); 7.43 (m, 4H), 7.68 (s, 1H); 7.71-7.84 (m, 2H), 8.17 (d, 1H, J = 7.66); ^{13}C NMR (500 MHz, CDCl3): δ 18.54, 21.23, 23.59, 114.15, 117.41, 119.17, 119.51, 120.13, 128.32, 127.35, 130.88, 136.06, 146.23, and 155.23; ESI-MS: 398 (M^+ + Na); Anal. Calcd. for $C_{19}H_{17}N_7O_2$: C, 60.79; H, 4.56; N, 26.12; Found: C, 60.95; H, 4.72; N, 26.34.

1-*o*-tolyl-5-(2-(1-*m*-tolyl-1H-1,2,3-triazol-4-yl)ethyl)-1H-1,2,3-triazole (5i)

Syrupy brownish semisolid. IR (KBr) cm^{-1}: 3417, 2944, 2856, 1587, 1235, 1079, and 695; ^1H NMR (CDCl3): δ 2.07 (s, 3H); 2.15 (s, 3H); 3.12 (m, 2H); 7.54 (m, 2H); 7.63 (s, 1H); 7.74 (m, 3H), 8.08-8.23 (m, 3H); 8.57 (s,1H); ^{13}C NMR (500 MHz, CDCl3): δ 19.68, 19.19, 21.58, 23.38, 116.10, 121.14, 122.22, 124.7, 129.82, 130.30, 131.31, 132.0, 135.80, 136.80, 137.83, 140.01, 148.20; ESI-MS: 367 (M^+ + Na); Anal. Calcd. for $C_{20}H_{20}N_6$: C, 69.75; H, 5.85; N, 24.40; Found: C, 69.90; H, 5.52; N, 24.61.

5-(2-(1-(2-nitrophenyl)-1H-1,2,3-triazol-4-yl)ethyl)-1-*p*-tolyl-1H-1,2,3-triazole (5j)

Syrupy greyish semisolid. IR (KBr) cm^{-1}: 3427, 2966, 2865, 1576, 1235, 1079, and 687; ^1H NMR ($CDCl_3$): δ 2.45 (s, 3H); 3.21-3.23 (m, 4H); 7.38-7.45 (d, 2H, J = 8.00 Hz); 7.70 (d, 2H, J = 8.00 Hz), 7.81 (m, 1H); 7.90 (m, 3H), 8.14 (m, 2H); ^{13}C NMR (500 MHz, $CDCl_3$): δ 19.85, 23.00, 23.54, 125.19, 125.27, 127.31, 129.71, 129.97, 130.89, 133.80, 134.97, 140.39, 144.60; ESI-MS: 367 (M^+ + Na); Anal. Calcd. for $C_{19}H_{17}N_7O_2$: C, 60.79; H, 4.56; N, 26.12; Found: C, 60.61; H, 4.72; N, 26.29.

5-(2-(1-(3-nitrophenyl)-1H-1,2,3-triazol-4-yl)ethyl)-1-*p*-tolyl-1H-1,2,3-triazole (5k)

Syrupy greyish semisolid. IR (KBr) cm^{-1}: 3417, 2986, 2865, 1576, 1233, 1089, and 677; ^1H NMR ($CDCl_3$): δ 2.45 (s, 3H); 3.08-3.22 (m, 4H); 7.33 (s, 4H); 7.50 (s, 1H), 7.52-7.72 (m, 4H), 7.89 (d, 1H, J = 7.89 Hz); ^{13}C NMR (500 MHz, $CDCl_3$): δ 15.82, 21.24, 23.33, 118.90, 122.73, 125.56, 130.23, 132.51, 133.69, 133.80, 135.61, 136.81, 139.97, 142.41, 144.43, 151.16; ESI-MS: 398 (M^+ + Na); Anal. Calcd. for $C_{19}H_{17}N_7O_2$: C, 60.79; H, 4.56; N, 26.12; Found: C, 60.92; H, 4.30; N, 26.26.

1-*m*-tolyl-5-(2-(1-*m*-tolyl-1H-1,2,3-triazol-4-yl)ethyl)-1H-1,2,3-triazol (5l)

Amorphous brown solid; m.p. 175°C. IR (KBr) cm^{-1}: 3429, 3138, 2922, 2860, 1612, 1593, 1549, 1494, 1383, 1234, 1165, 1089, 1047, 1017, 980, 873, 849, 786, 690, and 618; ^1H NMR (CDCl3): 2.33 (s, 3H); 2.43 (s, 3H); 3.05 (t, 2H, J = 6.2 Hz); 3.20 (t, 2H, J = 6.2 Hz); 7.25-7.59 (m, 8H); 7.73 (s, 1H); 8.36 (s, 1H). ^{13}C NMR (500 MHz, CDCl3): 19.8, 19.9, 22.8, 23.8, 117.0, 120.4, 122.2, 125.7, 129.1, 129.8, 130.3, 132.0, 135.8, 136.8, 137.8, 140.0, 146.2. ESI-MS: 367 (M^+ + Na). Anal. calc. for $C_{20}H_{20}N_6$: C, 69.75; H, 5.85; N, 24.40; Found: C, 69.80; H, 5.82; N 24.51.

2.2.2. Biology

The bacterial strains used for the analysis were *Bacillus subtilis* (MTCC 619), *Staphylococcus epidermidis* (MTCC 435), *Proteus vulgaris* (MTCC 426), and *Pseudomonas aeruginosa* (MTCC 424). The fungal strains used were *Aspergillus niger* (MTCC 1344) and *Penicillium chrysogenum* (MTCC 947). All the bacterial and fungal strains were obtained from The Microbial Type Culture Collection and Gene Bank (MTCC), Institute of Microbial Technology (IMTECH), Chandigarh, India. Kenamycin and flucanazole were used as standard antibacterial and antifungal substances, respectively, under similar conditions for comparison. Dimethyl sulfoxide (DMSO) was used as negative control.

The test organisms were cultured on agar slants, incubated 24 h at 37 ± 0.5°C and 24-48 h at 27 ± 0.2°C for bacteria and fungi, respectively, to get the freshly prepared cultures. The steroidal derivatives were evaluated for antimicrobial activity against these freshly prepared strains of test organisms by agar diffusion method [20,21]. Muller Hinton Agar (MHA) and Potato Dextrose Agar (PDA) were used as nutrient media for bacterial and fungal strains, respectively. The media (MHA &PDA) were prepared using distilled water and 20 mL of it was transferred into 50-mL test tubes, the test tubes were tightly plugged with cotton and sterilized in autoclave at 15 lb/in^2 for 15 min as directed by the manufacturer. After sterilization, the medium was inoculated with freshly cultured bacterial strains under sterile condition, i.e., under Laminar Flow. The inoculation was done when the temperature of the medium reached 50-40°C, so that test organism may not die at higher temperature. The medium inoculated with test microorganisms was transferred into the plates of 90-mm size under sterile conditions. The medium was allowed to solidify and the wells (4/plate) of 6-mm-diameter and 50 μL volume were bored on it using sterile cork borer. The solution of test compound 1000 μg/mL

Table 2 Antibacterial and antifungal screening data of compounds 5a-l

Compounds	Zone of inhibition (mm)					
	Antibacterial activities				Antifungal activities	
	B. subtilis (MTCC 619)	*S. epidermidis* (MTCC 435)	*P. Vulgaris* (MTCC 426)	*P. aeruginosa* (MTCC 424)	*A. niger* (MTCC1344)	*P. chrysogenum* (MTCC 947)
3a	08	09	10	12	-	10
3b	07	12	07	03	11	10
3c	-	11	10	12	10	10
3d	11	12	-	12	12	12
3e	12	10	13	10	10	16
3f	09	14	14	-	13	14
3g	12	-	08	11	12	09
3h	14	12	10	10	11	10
3i	10	12	-	09	13	12
3j	08	-	10	11	11	12
3k	07	16	11	11	12	13
3l	10	09	11	08	09	13
Control	-	-	-	-	-	-
Kenamycin	23	24	22	17	-	-
Flucanazole	-	-	-		18	14

P. vulgaris, Proteus vulgaris; B. subtilis, Bacillus subtilis; S. epidermidis, Staphylococcus epidermidis; P. aeruginosa, Pseudomonas aeruginosa; DMSO, negative control; well diameter/vol.- 6 mm/50 µl; Kenamycin, standard for antibacterial activity. Flucanazole, standard for anti fungal activity.

was prepared in DMSO and the wells bored on the medium were each filled (50 µg) with test compound using micropipette (20-200 µL). Four wells were bored on the plates and each filled with same compound and two plates for each test compound were taken and the experiment was repeated twice. The disks of Kenamycin and Flucanazole were also incorporated into the medium for comparison (10-30 µg). The plates containing test organism and test material in contact were incubated at 37 ± 0.5°C for 24 h. Same procedure was employed for antifungal activity; however, the culture strains of fungi were maintained on PDA and spores were transferred into the PDA medium and the plates were incubated at 27 ± 0.2°C for 24-48 h. Inhibition of growth of test organisms (bacterial & fungal) in presence of test material and standard was measured with the help of standard scale and the mean values of inhibition zones are reported in Table 2.

Table 2 gives the antimicrobial screening data obtained after treating different microbial strains with test doses of the different *bis*-triazolyl derivatives and the values are reported in terms of zone of inhibition in "mm".

It is clear from the above data that all the compounds **3a-l** showed significant antimicrobial activity against all microbial strains used for testing. It is evident from the data that even the position of substituent on the aromatic ring influences the relative activity which can be attributed to their differences in either the bioavailability or the protein-binding properties.

3. Results and discussions

The wide range of pharmacological activities especially the antimicrobial potential [14,22-27] of triazole and *bis*-triazole systems prompted us to design the synthesis of a library of unsymmetrical *bis*-1,2,3-triazoles based on a stepwise synthetic route involving domino addition of allenylmagnesium bromide to aryl azides resulting in a serendipitous formation of 5-butynylated triazoles in good yields (> 70%) instead of 4-butynylated triazoles. 5-Butynylated triazoles upon Cu(I) catalyzed 1,3-dipolar cycloaddition with aryl azides generated bis-1,2,3-triazoles in quantitative yields. The products together with the approach for their synthesis being novel, the intermediate 5-butynylated triazoles and the final product, the bistriazole, were characterized by IR, $^{1}H/^{13}C$ NMR, and mass spectral analysis. The intermediate 3 undergoes a high yielding regioselective Cu(I) catalyzed 1,3-dipolar cycloaddition with aryl azides (click reaction) to afford quantitative yields of the product, i.e., *bis*-1,2,3-triazoles, which were isolated in pure form after precipitation. The isolated products were evaluated for their antimicrobial activities against a panel of bacterial and fungal cell lines. The biological results were highly encouraging paving a way for the futuristic medicinal chemistry work based on these scaffolds.

4. Conclusion

In conclusion, we have developed an unprecedented, convenient strategy for the synthesis of novel, biologically important *bis*-1,2,3-triazoles employing a domino reaction followed by the copper catalyzed 'click' protocol. The products thus obtained were found to be potent antimicrobial agents.

Acknowledgements
The authors thank the Principal, ICSC, for his interest and encouragement.

Author details
[1]Department of Chemistry, Islamia College of Science and Commerce, Srinagar 190009, J&K, India [2]Department of Biochemistry, University of Kashmir, Srinagar 190009, J&K, India

Competing interests
The authors declare that they have no competing interests.

References

1. Wahe H, Asobo PF, Chekasov RA, Fomum ZT, Doepp D (2004) Heterocycles of biological importance: Part 8.1. Formation of pyrimido[1,2-*a*] benzimidazoles and oxazolo[3,2-*a*]benzimidazoles by conjugate addition of 2-aminobenzimidazoles to 4-hydroxy-2-alkynenitriles. ARKIVOC 2004(i):130–137
2. Chauhan PM, Srivastava SK (2001) Recent developments in the combinatorial synthesis of nitrogen heterocycles using solid phase technology. Comb Chem High Throughput Screen 4(1):35–51
3. Larock RC, Babu S (1987) Synthesis of nitrogen heterocycles via palladium-catalyzed intramolecular cyclization. Tetrahedron Lett 28:5291. doi:10.1016/S0040-4039(00)96710-8.
4. Banday AH, Bhupinder SA, Alam MS, kumar HMS (2007) A novel 'Domino-Click approach' to unsymmetrical bis-triazoles. Helv Chem Acta 90(12):2368–2374. doi:10.1002/hlca.200790242.
5. Butler MS (2004) The Role of Natural Product Chemistry in Drug Discovery? J Nat Prod 67:2141. doi:10.1021/np040106y.
6. Martin R, Rivero MR, Buchwald SL (2006) A general, highly flexible Cu-catalyzed domino C-N coupling/hydroamination reaction constitutes a straightforward alternative to existing methodology for the preparation of pyrroles and pyrazoles. Angew Chem Int Ed 45:7079–7082. doi:10.1002/anie.200602917.
7. Srinivasan M, Perummal S (2007) (l)-Proline-catalysed novel tandem reactions of 1-substituted piperidin-4-ones with (E)-4-arylbut-3-en-2-ones: N-substituent mediated product selectivity and synthesis of novel nitrogen heterocycles. Tetrahedron 63(13):2865–2874 and the references cited therein. doi:10.1016/j.tet.2007.01.038.
8. Modzelewska BB, Jagiello WE (2000) Synthesis and biological activity of BIS-1,2,4-triazole and BIS-1,3,4-thiadiazole derivatives. Acta Pol Pharm 57(3):199–204
9. Jin JY, Zhang LX, Chen XX, Zhang AJ, Zhang HL (2007) Syntheses and Biological Activities of 6-Aryl-3-(3-hydroxy- propyl)-7H-1,2,4-triazolo[3,4-b][1,3,4]thiadiazines. Molecules 12:297–303. doi:10.3390/12030297.
10. Sanghvi YS, Bhattacharya BK, Kini GD, Matsumoto SS, Larson SB, Jolley WB, Robins RK, Revankar GR (1990) Growth inhibition and induction of cellular differentiation of human myeloid leukemia cells in culture by carbamoyl congeners of ribavirin. J Med Chem 33:336. doi:10.1021/jm00163a054.
11. Rostovtsev W, Green LG, Fokin W, Sharpless KB (2002) A Stepwise Huisgen Cycloaddition Process: Copper(I)-Catalyzed Regioselective Ligation of Azides and Terminal Alkynes. Angew Chem Int Ed 41:2596. doi:10.1002/1521-3773(20020715)41:143.0.CO;2-4.
12. Wang Q, Chan RC, Hilgraf R, Fokin W, Sharpless KB, Finn MG (2003) Bioconjugation by Copper(I)-Catalyzed Azide-Alkyne [3 + 2] Cycloaddition. J Am Chem Soc 125:3192. doi:10.1021/ja021381e.
13. Kolb HC, Sharpless KB (2003) The growing impact of click chemistry on drug discovery. Drug Discov Today 8:1128. doi:10.1016/S1359-6446(03)02933-7.
14. Lewis WG, Green LG, Grynszpan F, Radic Z, Carlier PR, Taylor P, Finn MG, Sharpless KB (2002) Click Chemistry In Situ: Acetylcholinesterase as a Reaction Vessel for the Selective Assembly of a Femtomolar Inhibitor from an Array of Building Blocks. Angew Chem Int Ed 41:1053
15. Speers AE, Adam GC, Cravatt BF (2003) Activity-Based Protein Profiling in Vivo Using a Copper(I)-Catalyzed Azide-Alkyne [3 + 2] Cycloaddition. J Am Chem Soc 125:4686. doi:10.1021/ja034490h.
16. Abu-Orabi TS, Atfah MA, Jibril I, Marii F, Ali AS (1991) Dipolar Cycloaddition Reactions of Organic Bisazides with Some Acetylenic Compounds. Gazz Chim Ital 121:397
17. Whiting M, Tripp JC, Lin YC, Lindstorm W, Olson AJ, Elder JH, Sharpless KB, Fokin W (2006) Rapid Discovery and Structure?Activity Profiling of Novel Inhibitors of Human Immunodeficiency Virus Type 1 Protease Enabled by the Copper(I)-Catalyzed Synthesis of 1,2,3-Triazoles and Their Further Functionalization. J Med Chem 49:7697. doi:10.1021/jm060754+.
18. Whiting M, Muldoon J, Lin YC, Silverman SM, Lindstrom W, Olson AJ, Kolb HC, Finn MG, Sharples KB, Elder JH, Fokin W (2006) Inhibitors of HIV-1 Protease by Using In Situ Click Chemistry. Angew Chem Int Ed 45:1435. doi:10.1002/anie.200502161.
19. Thomas JR, Liu X, Hergenrother PJ (2005) Size-Specific Ligands for RNA Hairpin Loops. J Am Chem Soc 127:12434. doi:10.1021/ja051685b.
20. Dawane BS, Konda SG, Shaikh BM, Chobe SS, Khandare NT, Kamble VT, Bhosale RB (2010) Synthesis and in vitro antimicrobial activity of some new 1-thiazolyl-2-pyrazoline derivatives. Int J Pharm Sci Rev Res 1:2
21. Gurubasavaraja PMS, Agasimundin YS (2008) Synthesis and antimicrobial activity of some novel chalcones containing 3-hydroxy benzofuran. Acta Pharmaceutica Sciencia 50:197–202
22. Brik A, Alexandratos J, Lin YC, Elder JH, Olson AJ, Wlodawer A, Goodsell DS, Wong CH (2005) 1,2,3-Triazole as a Peptide Surrogate in the Rapid Synthesis of HIV-1 Protease Inhibitors. ChemBioChem 6:1167. doi:10.1002/cbic.200500101.
23. Shafi S, Banday AH, Ismail T, Kumar HMS (2007) Domino addition/N-C heterocyclization of Azides with allenyl magnesium bromide: Rapid synthesis of 5-butynyl- 1,2,3-triazoles. Synlett 7:1109–1111
24. Talekar RR, Wightman RH (1997) Synthesis of some pyrrolo[2,3-d]pyrimidine and 1,2,3-triazole isonucleosides. Tetrahedron 53:3831. doi:10.1016/S0040-4020(97)00102-6.
25. Bertelli L, Biagi G, Giorgi I, Manera C, Livi O, Scartoni V, Betti L, Giannaccini G, Trincavelli L, Barili PL (1998) 1,2,3-Triazolo[1,5-a]quinoxalines: synthesis and binding to benzodiazepine and adenosine receptors. Eur J Med Chem 33:113. doi:10.1016/S0223-5234(98)80036-6.
26. Contelles JM, Fernandez MR (2000) Novel synthesis of 2-thiazolines. Tetrahedron Lett 41:381. doi:10.1016/S0040-4039(99)01981-4.
27. Fox PG, Lewis G, Boden PJ (1979) Some chemical aspects of the corrosion inhibition of copper by benztriazole. Corros Sci 4:425

3

Microwave-assisted polystyrene sulfonate-catalyzed synthesis of novel pyrroles

Rosario Astrid Vargas Cárdenas, Blanca Olinda Quintanilla Leal, Ashwini Reddy, Debasish Bandyopadhyay and Bimal K Banik*

Abstract

Background: Pyrroles are widely distributed in nature and important biologically active molecules. The reaction of amines with 2,5-dimethoxytetrahydrofuran is a promising pathway for the synthesis of pharmacologically active pyrroles under microwave irradiation.

Results: Microwave-induced polystyrenesulfonate-catalyzed synthesis of pyrroles from amines and 2,5-diemthoxytetrahydrofuran has been accomplished with excellent yield. This method produces pyrroles with polyaromatic amines.

Conclusion: The present procedure for the synthesis of *N*-aromatic substituted pyrroles will find useful application in the area of pharmacologically active molecules.

Keywords: Pyrrole, Polystyrene sulfonate, Microwave, 2,5-dimethoxytetrahydrofuran

Background

Pyrrole is one of the most significant heterocyclic structural scaffold present in a large number of biologically active molecules [1,2] with a wide range of applications in medicinal chemistry [3]. Besides its pharmacological activity, pyrrole derivatives play a crucial role in material science [4]. The traditional methods rely on the cyclization of amines with ketones or diketones discovered by Knorr and Paal in 1880 s [5,6]. Since then, a number of publications have appeared on this reaction, but still, this method is under active investigation because of its simplicity. Recently, a number of methods and catalysts have been reported, e.g., supercritical carbon dioxide [7], silver-salts promoted three component reaction [8], manganese(III)-catalyzed [3 + 2] annulation [9], rhodium(III)-catalyzed bond functionalization [10], palladium-induced three component reaction [11], gold (I)-catalyzed amino-Claisen rearrangement [12] and zinc chloride [13]. In contrast, many of these reported methods involve the use of expensive reagents, hazardous solvents, longer reaction times and tedious workup procedure. Therefore, it is desirable to develop an efficient and practical method for the synthesis of pyrrole derivatives. We have also reported several procedures in this area [14-19]. We report herein a simple microwave-assisted method for the synthesis of *N*-arylpyrroles using an aqueous solution of polystyrene sulfonate. Synthesis of pyrroles in aqueous solution is promising and demanding because of eco-friendly nature of the procedure (Figure 1).

Although the mechanism of this reaction is not investigated, we believe compound 2 (Figure 1) produces a diketo compound in the media due to acid-induced cleavage reaction. The intermediate diketo compound then undergoes reaction with aromatic amines through nucleophilic and dehydration pathways (Figure 2). It is interesting to note that dehydration occurs in the presence of aqueous acid. Pyrroles are sensitive under strong acidic conditions, and isolation of these types of products from acidic solution may prove to be problematic. However, this problem can be overcome by simply basifying the reaction mixture prior to extraction. Higher temperature (60°C) and high power microwave radiation (300 W) accelerate the reaction significantly (Table 1). The reaction proceeds well in ethanol, THF and acetonitrile.

* Correspondence: banik@utpa.edu
Department of Chemistry, The University of Texas-Pan American, 1201 West University Drive, Edinburg, TX 78539, USA

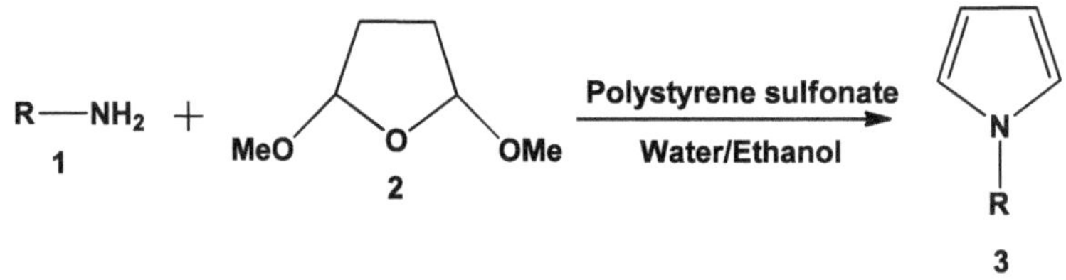

Figure 1 Polystyrene sulfonate-catalyzed simple synthesis of *N*-substituted pyrroles.

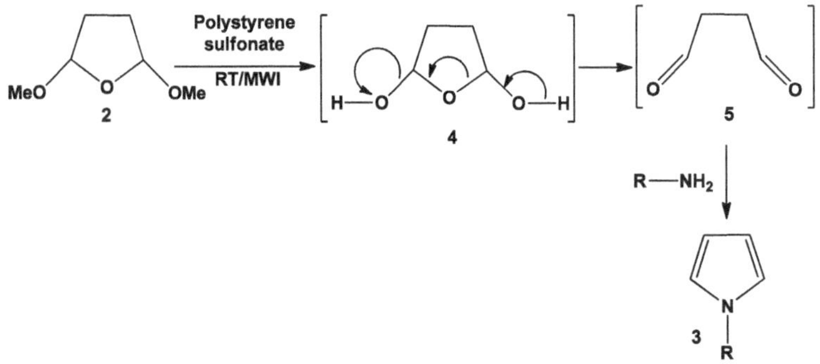

Figure 2 Polystyrene sulfonate- catalyzed synthesis of pyrroles: plausible mechanism of the reaction.

Table 1 Polystyrene sulfonate-catalyzed simple synthesis of *N*-substituted pyrroles under microwave irradiation (300 W, 60°C) following Figure 1

Entry	Amine	Product	Time (min)	Yield (%)[a]
1	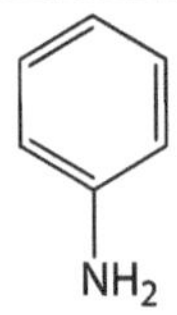	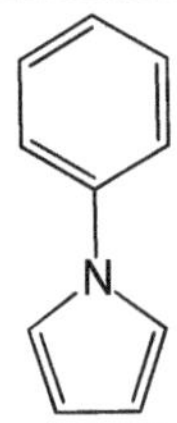	15	96
2	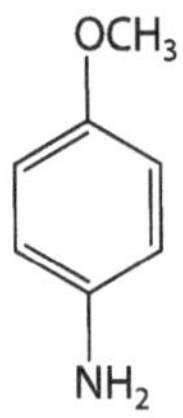	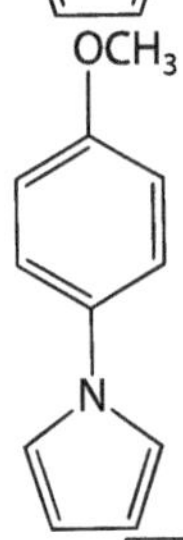	20	89
3	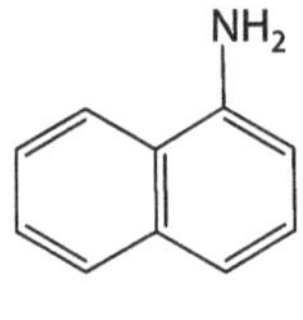	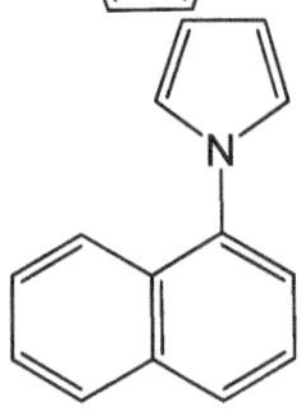	5	90

Table 1 Polystyrene sulfonate-catalyzed simple synthesis of *N*-substituted pyrroles under microwave irradiation (300 W, 60°C) following Figure 1 *(Continued)*

4	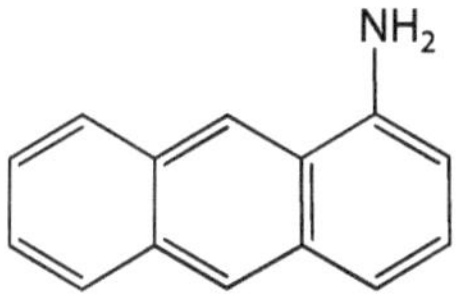	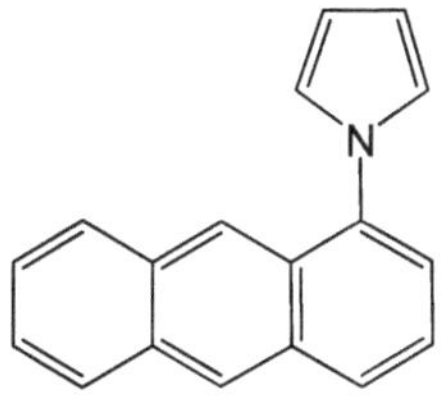	25	96
5	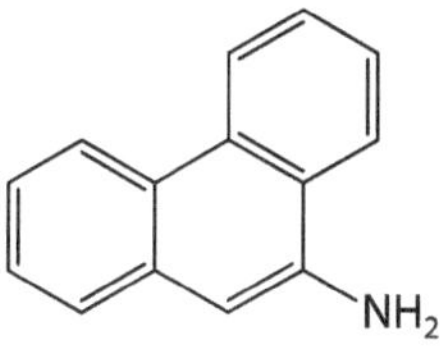	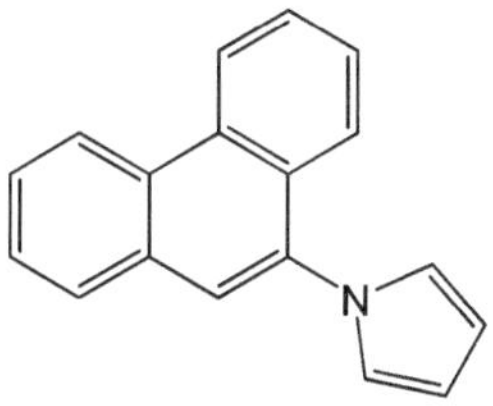	35	94
6	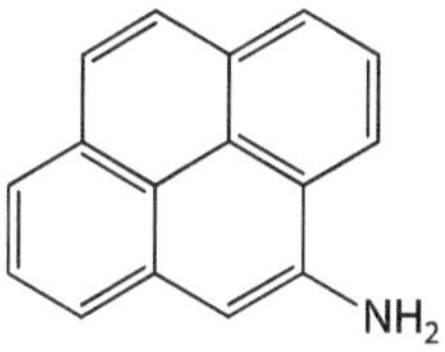	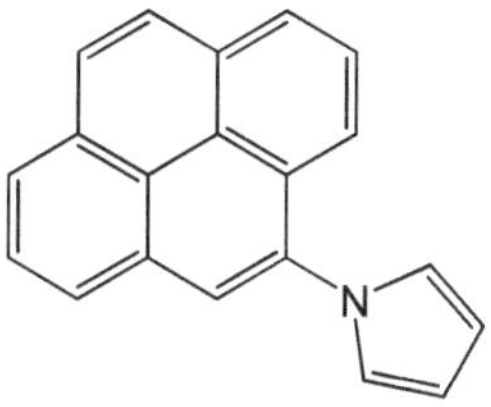	50	91
7	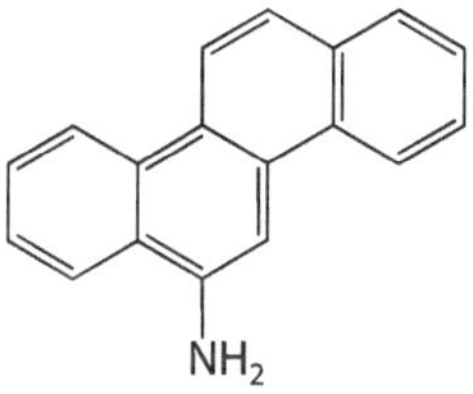	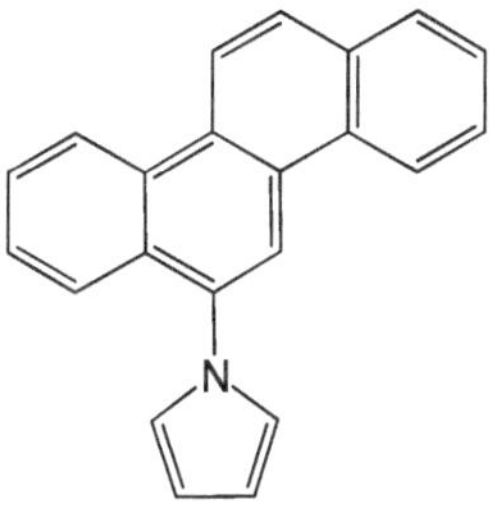	45	93

[a]Isolated yield.

Table 2 Polystyrene sulfonate-catalyzed simple synthesis of *N*-substituted pyrroles at room temperature following Figure 1

Entry	Amine	Product	Time (h)	Yield (%)[a]
1	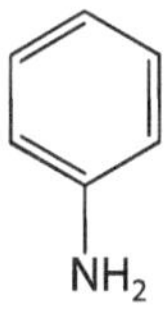	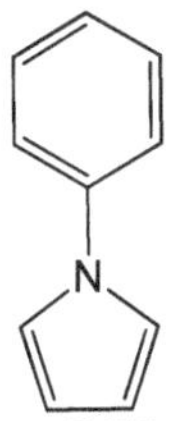	9	91
2	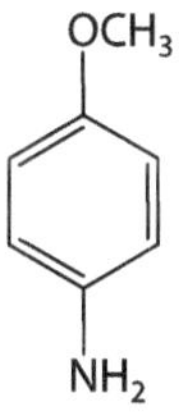	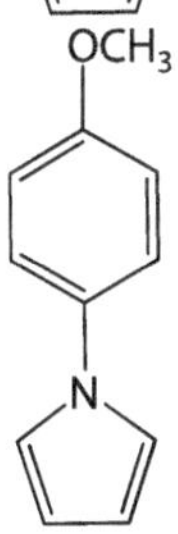	11	85

Table 2 Polystyrene sulfonate-catalyzed simple synthesis of *N*-substituted pyrroles at room temperature following Figure 1 *(Continued)*

3	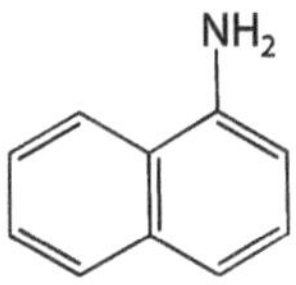	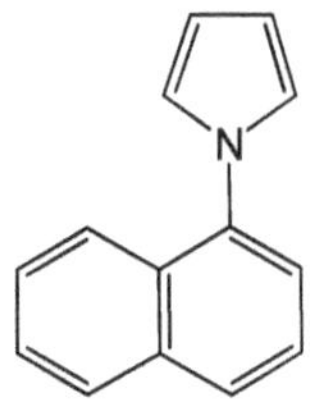	8	87
4	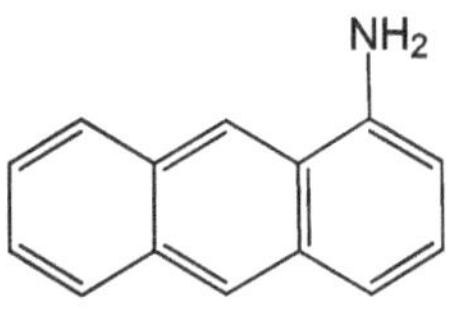	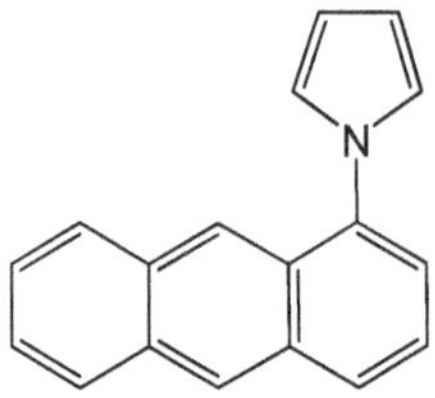	17	90
5	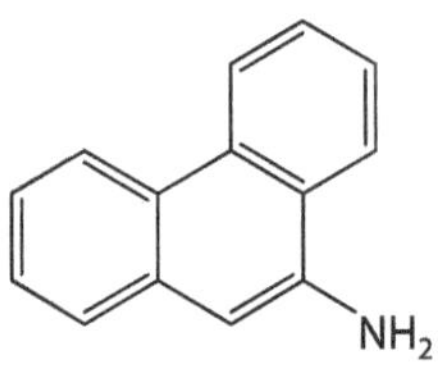	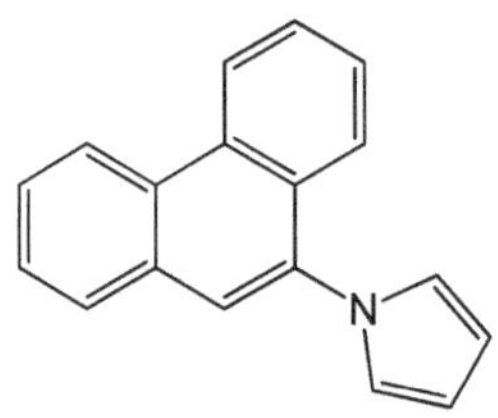	21	88
6	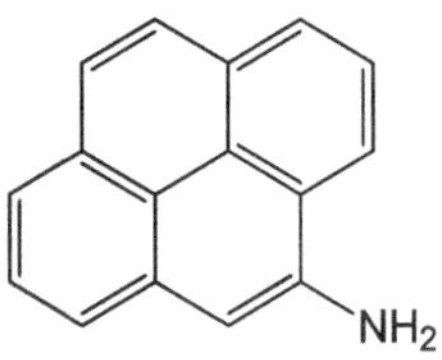	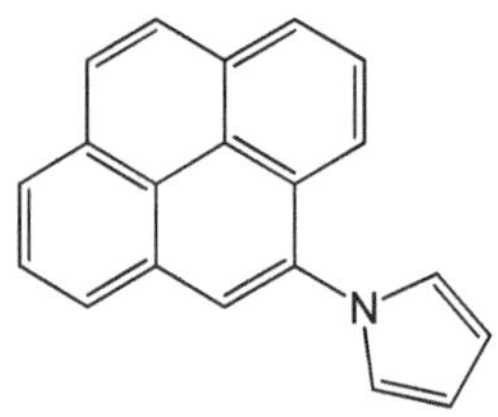	26	92
7	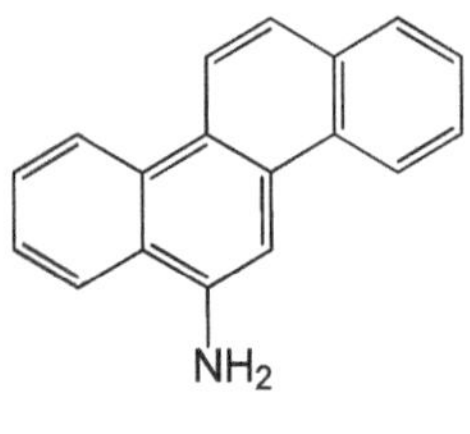	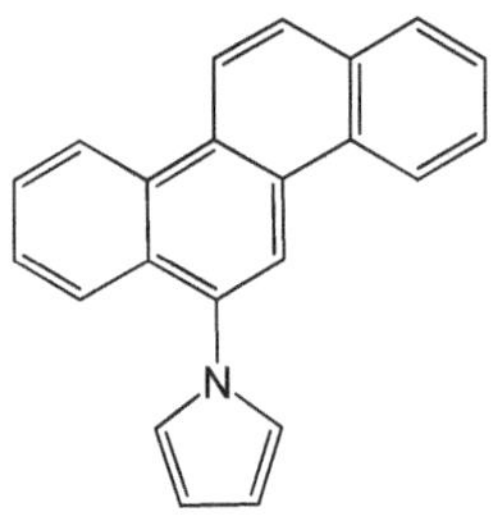	23	89

[a]Isolated yield.

Methods

FT-IR spectra were registered on a Bruker IFS 55 Equinox FTIR spectrophotometer (Bruker Corporation, Billerica, MA, USA) as KBr discs.^{1}H-NMR (600 MHz) and^{13}C-NMR (150 MHz) spectra were obtained at room temperature with Bruker-600 equipment (Bruker Corporation) using TMS as internal standard and $CDCl_3$ as solvent. Analytical grade chemicals (Sigma-Aldrich Corporation, St. Louis, MO, USA) were used throughout the project. Deionized water was used for the preparation of all aqueous solutions.

Results and discussion

In continuation of our research on environmentally benign reaction and biological evaluation of various polyaromatic compounds as novel anticancer agents [20-26], we have investigated reaction between aromatic amines (1) with 2,5-diemthoxytetrahydrofuran (2) using aqueous polystyrene sulfonate. After various experimentations, we have identified that this method works well under microwave-induced reaction conditions. Monocyclic, bicyclic, tricyclic and tetracyclic aromatic amines are used, and *N*-aryl pyrroles are produced in good yields (Figure 1).

At the beginning of the procedure, 2,5-diemthoxytetrahydrofuran (2), the amine (1) and aqueous solution of polystyrene sulfonate were mixed in ethanol. The mixture was then stirred at room temperature, and the progress of the reaction was monitored through TLC every after 30 min. After completion of the reaction, the reaction mixture was basified with aqueous-saturated sodium bicarbonate solution and extracted with dichloromethane. The organic part was then washed with brine, dried with sodium sulfate and evaporated. The yields of the products are shown in Table 2. The multi-cyclic aromatic amines needed longer reaction time compared to the amines which are more basic and superior nucleophilic reagents.

Experimental

General procedure for the synthesis of pyrroles (3)

Amine (1.0 mmol), 2, 5-dimethoxytetrahydrofuran (1.2 mmol) and polystyrene sulfonate (18 wt% solution in water) in ethanol/water (1:1) mixture was stirred at room temperature, and the progress of the reaction was monitored by TLC every 30 min. After completion of the reaction (Table 2), the reaction mixture was basified with saturated aqueous sodium bicarbonate solution and extracted with dichloromethane. The organic layer was then washed with brine, dried with sodium sulfate and evaporated to isolate the pure product.

Alternatively, amine (1.0 mmol), 2, 5-dimethoxytetrahydrofuran (1.2 mmol) and polystyrene sulfonate (18 wt% solution in water) in ethanol/water (1:1) were irradiated in an automated microwave oven (CEM Corporation, Matthews City, NC, USA). The reaction was monitored by TLC every 5 min. Depending upon the nature of the amines, the reaction was completed in different time. The result of the procedure was shown in Table 1. All the products have demonstrated satisfactory spectral and mp data with our reported compounds [16].

Conclusions

A new and simple method for the synthesis of *N*-substituted pyrroles in aqueous solution has been investigated with success. Based on our previous studies in this series, the compounds as reported herein may demonstrate anticancer activities.

Competing interests

The authors declare that they have no competing interests.

Authors' contributions

RAVC and BOQL performed the reactions with the help of AR and DB. BKB is the PI. All authors read and approved the final manuscript.

Acknowledgment

We gratefully acknowledge the funding support from the Kleberg Foundation, Texas.

References

1. Fan H, Peng J, Hamann MT, Hu J-F (2008) Lamellarins and related pyrrole-derived alkaloids from marine organisms. Chem Rev 108:264–287
2. Walsh CT, Garneau-Tsodikova S, Howard-Jones AR (2006) Biological formation of pyrroles: nature's logic and enzymic machinery. Nat Prod Rep 23:517–531
3. Aiello A, D'Esposito M, Fattorusso E, Menna M, Mueller WEG, Perovic-Ottstadt S, Schroeder HC (2006) Novel bioactive bromopyrrole alkaloids from the Mediterranean sponge *Axinella verrucosa*. Bioorg Med Chem 14:17–24
4. Domingo VM, Aleman C, Brillas E, Julia L (2001) Diradical dications of *m*- and *p*-phenylenebis[2,5-di(2-thienyl)-1-pyrrole]: weakly coupled diradicals. J Org Chem 66:4058–4061
5. Knorr L (1884) Synthesis of pyrroline-derivatives II. Chem Ber 17:1635–1642
6. Paal C (1885) Synthesis of thiophen and pyrolline derivatives. Chem Ber 18:367–371
7. Cardoso AL, Nunes RMD, Arnaut LG, Pinho M, Teresa MVD (2011) Synthesis of pyrroles in supercritical carbon dioxide: formal [3 + 2] cycloaddition of 2-benzoyl-aziridines and allenoates. Synthesis 21:3516–3522
8. Zeng J, Bai Y, Cai S, Ma J, Liu X-W (2011) Direct synthesis of pyrroles via a silver-promoted three-component reaction involving unusual imidazole ring opening. Chem Commun 47:12855–12857
9. Ng EPJ, Wang Y-F, Chiba S (2011) Manganese(III)-catalyzed formal [3 + 2] annulation of vinyl azides and β-keto acids for synthesis of pyrroles. Synlett 6:783–786
10. Stuart DR, Alsabeh P, Kuhn M, Fagnou K (2010) Rhodium(III)-catalyzed arene and alkene c-h bond functionalization leading to indoles and pyrroles. J Am Chem Soc 132:18326–18339
11. Lamande-Langle S, Abarbri M, Thibonnet J, Duchene A, Parrain J-L (2010) Domino allylic amination/Sonogashira/heterocyclisation reactions: palladium-catalysed three-component synthesis of pyrroles. Chem Commun 46:5157–5159
12. Saito A, Konishi T, Hanzawa Y (2010) Synthesis of pyrroles by gold(I)-catalyzed amino-Claisen rearrangement of *N*-propargyl enaminone derivatives. Org Lett 12:372–374
13. Wyrebek P, Sniady A, Bewick N, Li Y, Mikus A, Wheeler KA, Dembinski R (2009) Microwave-assisted zinc chloride-catalyzed synthesis of substituted pyrroles from homopropargyl azides. Tetrahedron 65:1268–1275
14. Banik BK, Samajdar S, Banik I (2004) Simple synthesis of substituted pyrroles. J Org Chem 69:213–216
15. Banik BK, Banik I, Renteria M, Dasgupta SK (2005) A straightforward highly efficient Paal–Knorr synthesis of pyrroles. Tetrahedron Lett 46:2643–2645
16. Bandyopadhyay D, Mukherjee S, Banik BK (2010) An expeditious synthesis of *N*-substituted pyrroles via microwave-induced iodine-catalyzed reaction under solventless conditions. Molecules 15:2520–2525
17. Andoh-Baidoo R, Danso R, Mukherjee S, Bandyopadhyay D, Banik BK (2011) Microwave-induced *N*-bromosuccinimide-mediated novel synthesis of pyrroles via Paal-Knorr reaction. Heterocycl Lett 1:107–109
18. Abrego D, Bandyopadhyay D, Banik BK (2011) Microwave-induced indium-catalyzed synthesis of pyrrole fused with indolinone in water. Heterocycl Lett 1:94–95
19. Rivera S, Bandyopadhyay D, Banik BK (2009) Facile synthesis of *N* via microwave-induced bismuth nitrate-catalyzed reaction under solventless conditions.-substituted pyrroles. Tetrahedron Lett 50:5445–5448
20. Banik I, Becker FF, Banik BK (2003) Stereoselective synthesis of β-lactams with polyaromatic imines: entry to new and novel anticancer agents. J Med Chem 46:12–15
21. Becker FF, Banik BK (1998) Polycyclic aromatic compounds as anticancer agents: synthesis and biological evaluation of some chrysene derivatives. Bioorg Med Chem Lett 8:2877–2880
22. Becker FF, Mukhopadhyay C, Hackfeld L, Banik I, Banik BK (2000) Polycyclic aromatic compounds as anticancer agents: synthesis and biological evaluation of dibenzofluorene derivatives. Bioorg Med Chem 8:2693–2699
23. Banik BK, Becker FF (2001) Polycyclic aromatic compounds as anticancer agents. 4. Structure-activity relationships of chrysene and pyrene derivatives. Bioorg Med Chem 9:593–605
24. Banik BK, Becker FF (2001) Synthesis, electrophilic substitution and structure-activity relationship studies of polycyclic aromatic compounds towards the development of anticancer agents. Curr Med Chem 8:1513–1533

25. Banik BK, Becker FF, Banik I (2004) Synthesis of anticancer β-lactams: mechanism of action. Bioorg Med Chem 12:2523–2528
26. Bandyopadhyay D, Granados JC, Short JD, Banik BK (2012) Polycyclic aromatic compounds as anticancer agents: evaluation of synthesis and *in vitro* cytotoxicity. Oncol Lett 3:45–49

4

Diversity oriented one-pot three-component sequential synthesis of annulated benzothiazoloquinazolines

Mahendra Kumar*, Kailash Sharma and Dinesh Kumar Sharma

Abstract

Annulated benzothiazoloquinazolines have been synthesized by a diversity oriented simple and convenient synthesis involving one-pot three-component reaction of substituted 2-aminobenzothiazoles with α-tetralone and aromatic/heteroaromatic aldehydes in ethanol in the presence of catalytic amount of triethylamine. The synthesized compounds have been characterized by their elemental analyses and spectral data.

Keywords: benzothiazoloquinazolines, one-pot, 2-aminobenzothiazoles, cyclic ketones, thiophene-2-carbaldehyde.

Background

The synthesis of fused heterocycles has attracted considerable interest in heterocyclic chemistry as the fusion of biodynamic heterosystems has proved to be a very attractive and useful for the design of new molecular framework of potential drugs with varying pharmacological activities. A major challenge of modern drug discovery is to design highly efficient chemical reaction sequences which provide molecules containing maximum complexity and structural diversity with interesting bioactivities in minimum number of synthetic steps. Recently, multicomponent reactions have attracted attention of chemical and pharmaceutical research and emerged as highly efficient and synthetically useful reactions for the preparation of structurally diverse drug-like heterocyclic compounds.

There has been an increasing interest in the chemistry of quinazolines [1-5] because of being present quinazoline heterocyclic system as a building block in many natural and synthetic products capable of exhibiting a wide variety of biological and pharmacological activities [6]. Quinazolines have been reported to exhibit anti-inflammatory [7], antihypertensive [8], anticancer [9], antitumor [10] and antibacterial [11] activities. Quinazoline and its derivatives have recently been evaluated as antagonist of various biological receptors such as 5-HT_{5A} [12] related disease calcitonin gene - related peptide [13] and vasopressin V3 receptors [14]. Benzothiazole has also been an interesting heterocyclic system in drug research on account of significant biological activities of its fused derivatives [15-17]. Thiazoloquinazolines, have shown significant activity against cancer [18]. Thiazoloquinazolines have also been identified as cyclin dependent kinase (CDK) and glycogen synthase kinase (GSK-3) inhibitors [19,20].

Result and discussion

The syntheses of heterocycles with fused heterosystems involve, in most of the cases, multistep synthetic methods which require a large number of synthetic operations including extraction and purification of each individual step. The multistep synthetic methodologies, therefore, led to the synthetic inefficiency with the generation of large amounts of waste. The methods reported in the literature [21,22] for the synthesis of thiazoloquinazolines irrespective of positions of attachment of both the heterocyclic systems involved multisteps in which the formation of thiazole ring before the quinazoline ring induced low subsequent reactivity. Thiazoloquinazolines prepared by reaction of 2-aminobenzylamine with aromatic amine and then with 2-mercaptopropionic acid also involved multistep reaction. However, after detailed literature survey it was observed that there were only limited publications devoted to the synthesis of especially benzothiazoloquinazolines which involved cyclocondensation of 2-aminobenzothiazoles

* Correspondence: mahendrakpathak@gmail.com
Department of Chemistry, University of Rajasthan, Jaipur 302 055, India

with Mannich bases obtained in the first step as a result of Mannich reaction [23]. The multistep synthesis of benzothiazoloquinazolines suffered from some flaws including low yields, side products and tedious workup. In continuation of our research programme on the synthesis of nitrogen and sulphur containing novel heterocycles [24-31] of pharmaceutical interest and in view of the operational simplicity and intrinsic convergence (atom economy) of multicomponent reactions [32-36] in addition to their potential to introduce considerable structural diversity, we have synthesized annulated benzothiazoloquinazolines incorporating three biodynamic privileged heterosystems by a simple and convenient method involving multicomponent reaction of substituted 2-aminobenzothiazoles with α-tetralone and aromatic/heteroaromatic aldehydes in ethanol in the presence of catalytic amount of triethylamine, wherein 2-aminobenzothiazoles with both endocyclic nitrogen and exocyclic amino group participate as 1,3-binucleophile synthones in the formation of annulated benzothiazoloquinazolines (Scheme 1).

The reaction is believed to proceed to involve Knoevenagal condensation between α-tetralone and aromatic/heteroaromatic aldehyde in the initial step to form α,β-unsaturated ketone which undergoes Michael type addition with the nucleophilic endocyclic nitrogen of 2-aminobenzothiazole under the reaction conditions. The adduct formed is then cyclised intramolecularly with the lose of water molecule to provide annulated benzothiazolo[2,3-*b*] quinazolines. These reactions have taken place in one-flask domino manner and the enone system generated in situ immediately undergoes Michael type addition with 2-aminobenzothiazoles and subsequent cyclization. The possibility of formation of isomeric product involving nucleophilic attack of exocyclic amino group has been completely discarded on the basis of spectral characteristics. Annulated benzothiazoloquinazolines have also been synthesized by a multistep synthesis involving the reaction of substituted 2-aminobenzothiazoles with chalcones obtained by the reaction of α-tetralone with thiophene-2-carbaldehyde/p-methoxybenzaldehyde in the presence of catalytic amount of triethylamine. It has been observed that with the use of chalcones the reaction occurs in two steps relatively in longer time (6-8 h) with the moderate yields (50-60%) of annulated benzothiazoloquinazolines. But

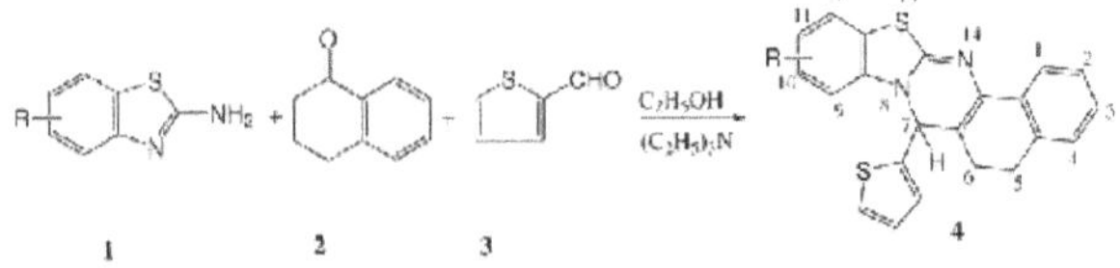

Scheme 1

when the chalcones are replaced by their synthetic precursors, α-tetralone and thiophene-2-carbaldehyde/p-methoxybenzaldehyde, annulated benzothiazoloquinazolines are obtained with excellent yields (75-85%). The synthesized annulated benzothiazoloquinazolines are presented in table 1.

The structures of the synthesized compounds were confirmed by their elemental analyses and spectral data. Infrared spectra of all the synthesized compounds exhibit an intense unsaturation absorption band in the region 1605-1610 cm^{-1} (C = C). The absorption band in the region 1620-1654 cm^{-1} in the IR spectra of all the compounds indicated the presence of C = N bond. Two absorption bands corresponding to asymmetric and symmetric stretching vibrations of $-NH_2$ group, which were present in the IR spectra of 2-aminobenzothiazoles, are absent in the IR spectra of the synthesized compounds. ^1H NMR spectra of the synthesized compounds showed a multiplet in the region δ 7.01-8.08 ppm due to aromatic protons. The singlet appeared in the region δ 5.90-6.80 was assigned to the aliphatic proton (C_7-H). The singlet observed in the region δ 3.69-3.84 ppm was attributed to the methoxy protons, whereas the methyl protons resonate as a singlet in the region δ 2.34-2.36 ppm in the ^1H NMR spectra of annulated benzothiazoloquinazolines containing $-OCH_3$ and $-CH_3$ groups respectively. The multiplets observed in the region δ 2.74-3.23 ppm were assigned to the methylene protons at C-5 and C-6. In the ^{13}C NMR spectra of the synthesized annulated benzothiazoloquinazolines, the δ values of most of the carbon atoms of CH_3, CH_2, CH, C = C, C = N, C-N, C-O, C-S, C-F and aromatic system could be determined by distinct resonance signals and were found to be in agreement with the proposed structures.

Conclusion

In conclusion, we have developed a simple and convenient diversity oriented one-pot three-component sequential synthesis for the synthesis of structurally diverse heterocycles, annulated benzothiazoloquinazolines, incorporating medicinally privileged heterosystems.

The present method with its mild reaction conditions and operational simplicity enables the sequential combination of three reactive components; α-tetralone, thiophene-2-carbaldehyde/p-methoxybenzaldehyde and 2-aminobenzothiazole in one-pot and efficiently incorporates structural diversity simply by varying the substituents or by slight structural modification in the components involved in the reaction. This new method has the advantages of higher yields, mild reaction conditions, shorter reaction time, and convenient procedure and can be extended to prepare a library of structurally diverse drug like small heterocyclic molecules.

Table 1 Reaction of 2-aminobenzothiazoles with α-tetralone and aromatic/heteroaromatic aldehydes.

2-aminobenzothiazole	α-tetralone	Aldehydes	product	m.p.°C	% yield
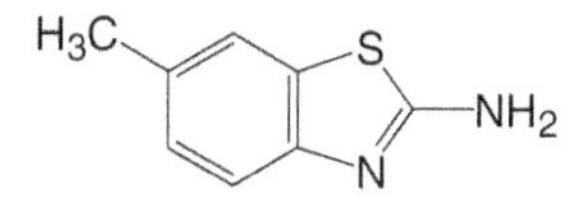	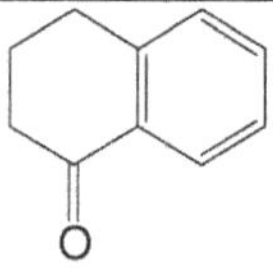	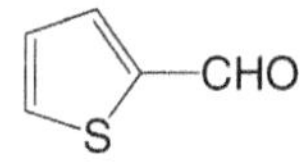	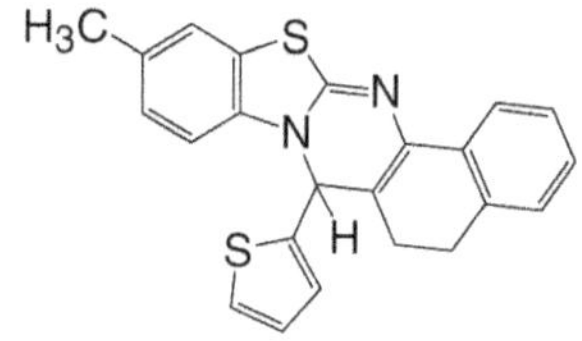 **4a**	210-212	76
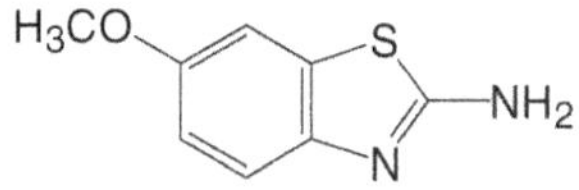	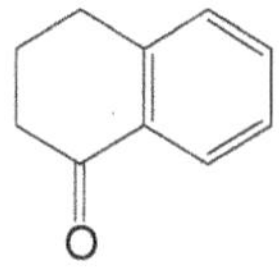	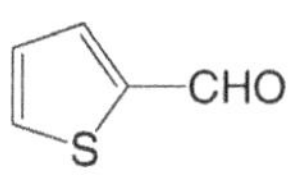	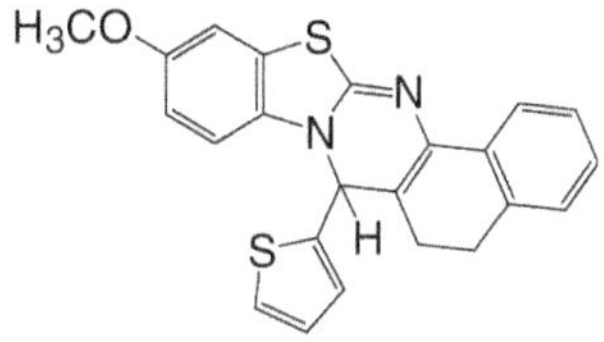 **4b**	220-222	80
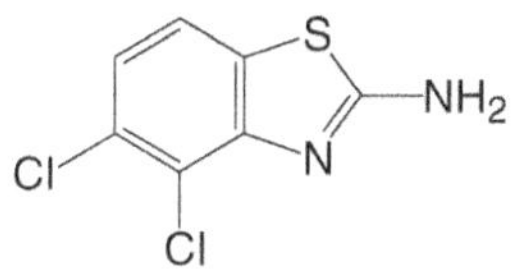	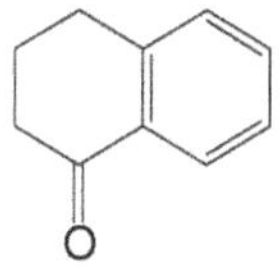	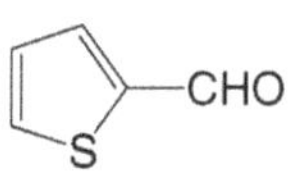	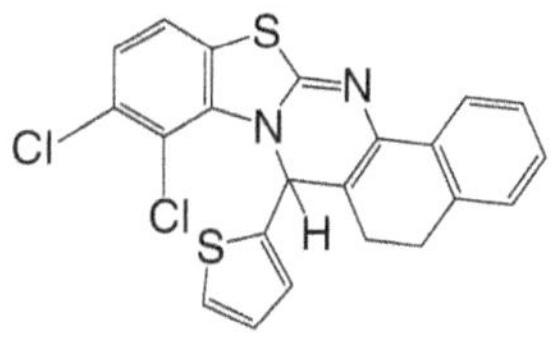 **4c**	205-207	77
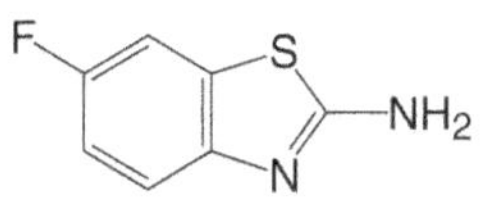	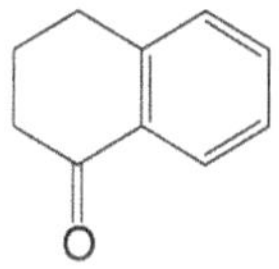	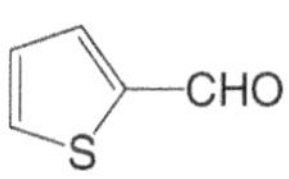	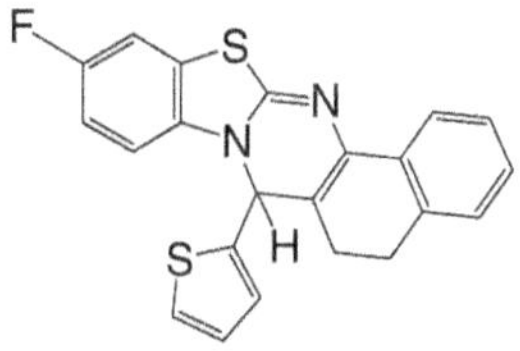 **4d**	190-192	75
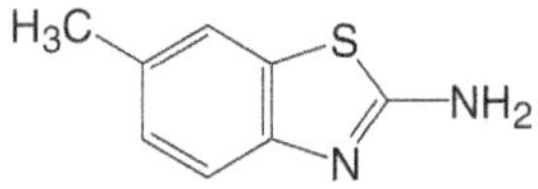	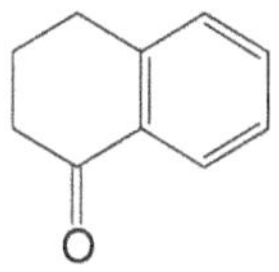	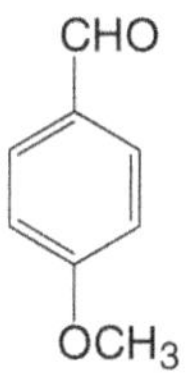	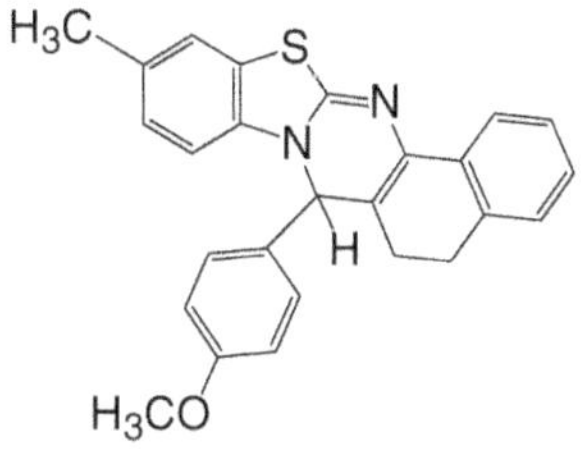 **4e**	215-217	80
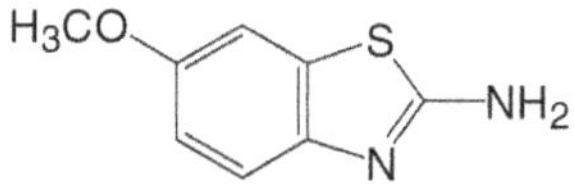	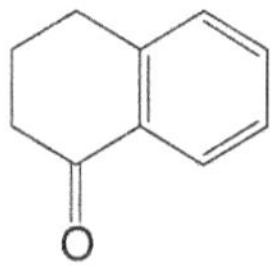	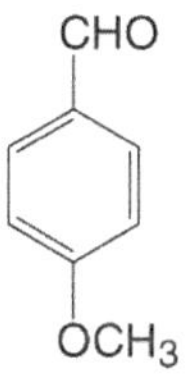	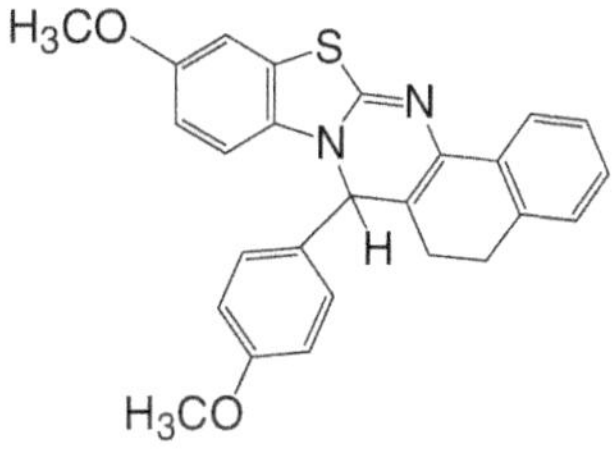 **4f**	227-229	80

Table 1 Reaction of 2-aminobenzothiazoles with α-tetralone and aromatic/heteroaromatic aldehydes. *(Continued)*

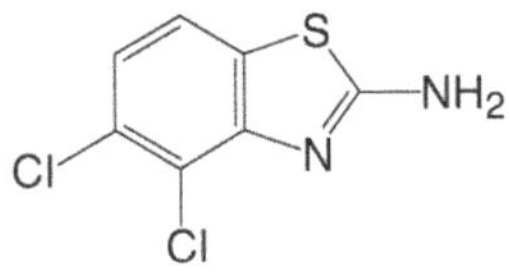	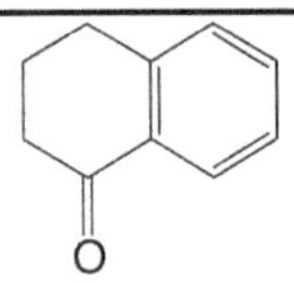	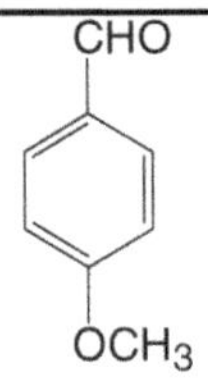	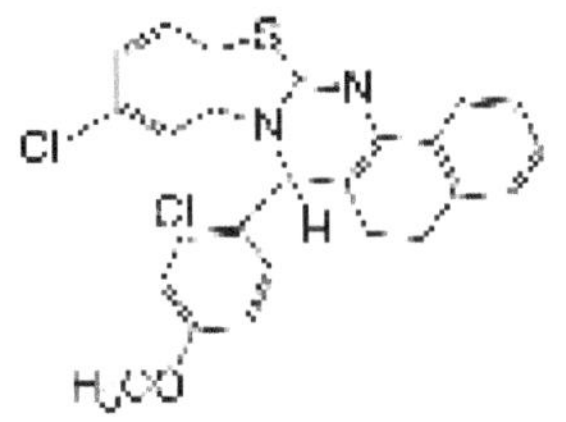 4g	192-194	74
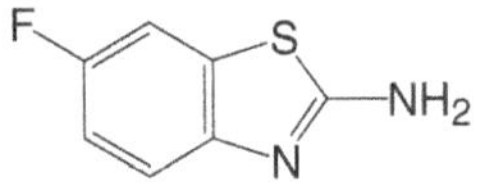	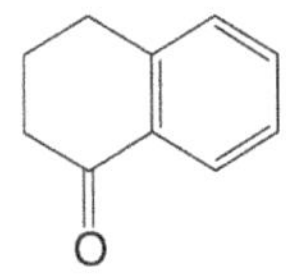	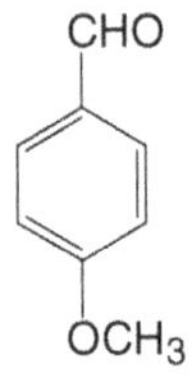	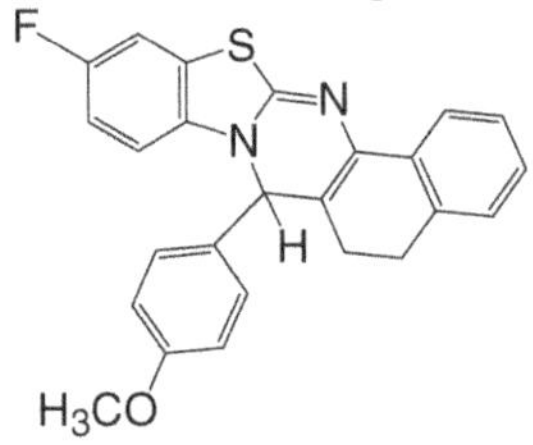 **4h**	189-191	75

Experimental

Melting points were determined on an electric melting point apparatus and are uncorrected. The purity of all the compounds was checked by thin layer chromatography using various non-aqueous solvents. IR spectra (KBr pellets) were recorded on Shimadzu-8400S FT-IR Spectrophotometer. The ^{1}H NMR and ^{13}C NMR spectra were scanned on Jeol AL 300 FT NMR in $CDCl_3$ using TMS as an internal standard. The chemical shifts are expressed as δ ppm.

Methods

Procedure for the preparation of 7-thien-2-yl/4′-methoxyphenyl-5, 6-dihydro-7H-benzo [h] benzothiazolo [2, 3-b] quinazolines

To a magnetically stirred solution of thiophene-2-carbaldehyde/p-methoxy benzaldehyde (0.01 mole) and α-tetralone (0.01 mole) in ethanol (20 ml), a catalytic amount of $(C_2H_5)_3N$ was added slowly and further stirred for 30 min. Then 2-aminobenzothiazole (0.01 mole) was added to the reaction mixture with stirring for 2 h and then refluxed for 60-90 min in a round bottom flask fitted with reflux condenser. The progress of the reaction was monitored by TLC. The precipitate formed after the completion of reaction was isolated by filtration. The solid separated out was washed well with ethanol, dried and finally crystallized from ethanol.

11-Methyl-7-(thien-2-yl)-5,6-dihydro-7H-benzo[h] benzothiazolo[2, 3-b]quinazoline (4a)

(4a). m.p. 210-212°C; yield: 76%; IR (KBr, cm^{-1}): 3100, 2980, 1620, 1605; ^{1}H NMR (300 MHz, $CDCl_3$) δppm: 7.10-7.68 (m, 10H, Ar-H), 5.86 (s, 1H, C_7), 3.18-3.23 (m, 2H, CH_2), 2.93-3.05 (m, 2H, CH_2), 2.36 (s, 3H, CH_3); ^{13}C NMR (75 MHz, $CDCl_3$) δppm: 18.38, 26.98, 28.10, 58.32, 119.43, 122.13, 125.34, 125.53, 126.23,126.56, 126.85, 127.80, 127.32, 127.54, 128.26, 130.20, 132.14, 133.65, 134.12, 137.34, 139.14,143.15, 167.35; Anal. Calcd. for $C_{23}H_{18}N_2S_2$: C, 71.47; H, 4.69; N, 7.25; Found: C, 73.65; H, 4.99; N, 7.19.

11-Methoxy-7-(thien-2-yl)-5,6-dihydro-7H-benzo[h] benzothiazolo [2, 3-b] quinazoline (4b)

(4b) m.p. 220-222°C; yield: 80%, IR (KBr, cm^{-1}): 3010-3080, 2975, 1620, 1615; ^{1}H NMR (300 MHz, $CDCl_3$) δppm: 7.09-7.84 (m, 10H, Ar-H), 5.98 (s, 1H,C_7-H), δ 3.84 (s, 3H, OCH_3), 2.96-3.22 (m, 4H, CH_2, C_5, and C_6); ^{13}C NMR (75 MHz, $CDCl_3$) δppm: 26.9, 28.06, 54.60, 57.20, 115.70, 122.52, 125.29, 125.62, 126.14, 126.45, 127.58, 127.69, 128.08, 129.44, 130.68, 133.12, 133.28, 134.60, 137.20, 139.04, 142.98, 155.61, 167.19 Anal. Calcd. for $C_{23}H_{18}N_2OS_2$: C, 68.63; H, 4.51; N, 6.96; Found: C, 70.65; H, 4.35; N, 6.99.

9,10-Dichloro-7-(thien-2-yl)-5,6-dihydro-7H-benzo[h] benzothiazolo-[2, 3-b]quinazoline (4c)

(4c) m.p. 205-207°C; yield: 77%, IR (KBr, cm^{-1}): 3060, 2972, 1622, 1615; ^{1}H NMR (300 MHz, $CDCl_3$) δppm: 7.08-7.45 (m, 9H, Ar-H), 5.96 (s, 1H,C_7-H), δ 3.12-3.24 (m, 2H,CH_2) 2.94-2.96 (m, 2H,CH_2); ^{13}C NMR (75 MHz, $CDCl_3$) δppm: 26.96, 28.16, 57.23, 119.92, 120.32, 123.46, 125.13, 125.24, 126.23, 126.52, 127.26, 127.46, 128.13, 130.32, 131.82, 133.65, 134.91, 138.03, 139.45, 143.98, 167.16; Anal. Calcd. for $C_{22}H_{14}Cl_2N_2S_2$: C, 59.86; H, 3.20; N, 6.35; Found: C, 62.09; H, 3.10; N, 6.45.

11-Fluoro-7-(thien-2-yl)-5,6-dihydro-7H-benzo[h] benzothiazolo-[2, 3-b]quinazoline (4d)

(4d) m.p. 190-192°C; yield: 75%, IR (KBr, cm^{-1}): 3075, 2978, 1620, 1610; ^{1}H NMR (300 MHz, $CDCl_3$) δ ppm:

6.92-7.40 (m, 10H, Ar-H), 5.95 (s, 1H, C_7-H), δ 3.18-3.23 (m, 2H,CH_2) 3.01-3.05 (m, 2H, CH_2); ^{13}C NMR (75 MHz, $CDCl_3$) δppm: 26.78, 28.13, 58.62, 119.23, 120.35, 122.16, 125.28, 125.69, 126.31, 126.65, 127.58, 127.67, 128.23, 131.98, 133.54, 134.46, 138.42, 139.68, 142.06, 153.72, 170.43; Anal. Calcd. for $C_{22}H_{15}FN_2S_2$: C, 67.67; H, 3.87; N, 7.17; Found: C, 67.65; H, 3.83; N, 7.13.

11-Methyl-7-(4-methoxyphenyl)-5,6-dihydro-7H-benzo[h] benzothiazolo[2, 3-b]quinazoline (4e)

(4e) m.p. 215-217°C; yield: 80%, IR (KBr, cm^{-1}): 3045, 2977, 1650, 1610,1275 ^{1}H NMR (300 MHz, $CDCl_3$) δppm: 7.20-7.54 (m, 11H, Ar-H), 5.90 (s, 1H, C_7-H), 3.76 (s, 3H, OCH_3), 2.94-3.01 (m, 2H, CH_2), 2.80-2.86 (m, 2H, CH_2), 2.26 (s, 3H, CH_3); ^{13}C NMR (75 MHz, $CDCl_3$) δppm: 18.26, 26.98, 28.68, 54.92, 57.23, 113.74, 114.96, 115.26, 123.64, 125.32, 125.76, 126.23, 126.64, 127.19, 127.84, 128.68, 128.96, 130.05, 132.92, 133.30, 134.52, 143.42, 156.39, 169.30; Anal. Calcd. for $C_{26}H_{22}N_2OS$: C, 76.07; H, 5.40; N, 6.82; Found: C, 76.01; H, 5.15; N, 6.92.

11-Methoxy-7-(4-methoxyphenyl)-5,6-dihydro-7H-benzo[h] benzothiazolo-[2, 3-b]quinazoline (4f)

(4f) m.p. 227-229°C; yield: 80%, IR (KBr, cm^{-1}): 3100, 3080-3050, 1648, 1612; ^{1}H NMR (300 MHz, $CDCl_3$) δppm: 7.15-7.52 (m, 11H, Ar-H), 5.90 (s, 1H, C_7-H), δ 3.73 (s, 3H, OCH_3), 3.69 (s, 3H, OCH_3), 2.94-3.00 (m, 2H, CH_2), 2.80-2.86 (m, 2H, CH_2); ^{13}C NMR (75 MHz, $CDCl_3$) δppm: 28.26, 28.95, 54.20, 55.09, 56.96, 115.52, 117.52, 119.32, 120.44, 125.18, 126.48, 127.32, 127.47, 127.80, 128.12, 128.76, 133.07, 133.40, 134.23, 136.35, 137.98, 153.62, 158.26, 169.39; Anal. Calcd. for $C_{26}H_{22}N_2O_2S$: C, 76.2; H, 5.2; N, 6.86; Found: C, 76.07; H, 5.40; N, 6.82.

9,10-Dichloro-7-(4-methoxyphenyl)-5,6-dihydro-7H-benzo [h]benzothiazolo[2, 3-b]quinazoline (4g)

(4g) m.p. 192-194°C; yield: 74%, IR (KBr, cm^{-1}): 3008-3050, 2972, 1645, 1612, 1270; ^{1}H NMR (300 MHz, $CDCl_3$) δppm: 7.12-7.54 (m, 10H, Ar-H), 5.92 (s, 1H, C_7-H), δ 3.73 (s, 3H,OCH_3), 2.74-2.99 (m, 4H, CH_2 at C_5 and C_6); ^{13}C NMR (75 MHz, $CDCl_3$) δppm: 26.98, 28.12, 55.08, 58.74, 115.26, 115.35, 119.62, 120.43, 125.63, 127.48, 127.32, 127.58, 128.11, 128.45, 128.69, 130.24, 131.67, 133.40, 133.86, 134.26, 144.53, 155.62, 167.38; Anal. Calcd. for $C_{25}H_{18}Cl_2N_2OS$: C, 64.49; H, 3.88; N, 6.06; Found: C, 64.52; H, 3.90; N, 6.02.

11-Fluoro-7-(4-methoxyphenyl)-5,6-dihydro-7H-benzo[h] benzothiazolo-[2, 3-b]quinazoline (4h)

(4h) m.p. 189-191°C; yield: 75%, IR(KBr, cm^{-1}): 3010-3072, 2974, 1648, 1612, 1242; ^{1}H NMR (300 MHz, $CDCl_3$) δppm: 7.12-7.54 (m, 11H, Ar-H), 5.95 (s, 1H, C_7-H), δ 3.69 (s, 3H, OCH_3), 2.82-2.96 (m, 4H, CH_2 at C_5 and C_6); ^{13}C NMR (75 MHz, $CDCl_3$) δppm: 26.98, 28.56, 55.63, 57.39, 115.47, 118.78, 119.12, 121.45, 125.73, 126.63, 127.32, 127.58, 128.16, 128.73, 128.97, 131.43, 133.26, 133.89, 134.38, 142.19, 153.76, 170.43; Anal. Calcd. for $C_{25}H_{19}FN_2OS$: C, 72.40; H, 4.60; N, 6.72; Found: C, 72.44; H, 4.62; N, 6.76.

Acknowledgements

The authors were thankful to the Head, Department of Chemistry, University of Rajasthan, Jaipur for providing laboratory and instrumentation facilities. RSIC, CDRI, Lucknow is also acknowledged for providing analytical and spectral data of the compounds. One of the authors (KS) thanks University of Rajasthan Jaipur (India) for the research fellowship.

Competing interests

The authors declare that they have no competing interests.

References

1. Witt A, Bergman J (2003) Recent Developments in the field of quinazoline chemistry. Curr Org Chem 7:659–677. doi:10.2174/1385272033486738.
2. Connolly DJ, Cusack D, O'Sullivan TP, Guiry PJ (2005) Synthesis of quinazolinones and quinazolines. Tetrahedron 61:10153–10202. doi:10.1016/j.tet.2005.07.010.
3. Michael JP (1999) Quinoline, quinazoline and acridone alkaloids. Nat Prod Rep 16:697–709. doi:10.1039/a809408j.
4. Michael JP (2002) Quinoline, quinazoline and acridone alkaloids. Nat Prod Rep 19:742–760. doi:10.1039/b104971m.
5. Michael JP (2003) Quinoline, quinazoline and acridone alkaloids. Nat Prod Rep 20:476–493. doi:10.1039/b208140g.
6. Maritinei-Viturro CM, Dominguez D (2001) Synthesis of the antitumoural agents batracylin and related isoindolo[1,2-b]quinazoline-12(10H)-ones. Tetrahedron Lett 48:1023–1026
7. Alagarsamy V, Raja SV, Dhanabal K (2007) Synthesis and pharmacological evaluation of some 3-phenyl-2-substituted-3H-quinazolin-4-one as analgesic, anti-inflammatory agents. Bioorg Med Chem 15:235–241. doi:10.1016/j.bmc.2006.09.065.
8. Alagarsamy V, Pathak US (2007) Synthesis and antihypertensive activity of novel 3-benzyl-2-substituted-3H-[1,2,4]triazolo[5,1-b]quinazolin-9-ones. Bioorg Med Chem 15:3457–3462. doi:10.1016/j.bmc.2007.03.007.
9. Murugan V, Kulkarni M, Anand RM, Kumar EP, Suresh B, Reddy VM (2006) Synthesis of 2-[bis-2(chloroethyl)amino}methyl]-6,8-dinitro-1-(4-substituted phenyl)-1H-quinazolin-4-one derivatives as possible antineoplastic agents. Asian J Chem 18:900–906
10. Godfrey AAA (2005) Preparation of Quinazolin-4-ones via Cyclization of N-(cyanophenyl) acetamide Derivatives. PCT Int Appl WO 2005012260 A2. Chem Abstr. 142, 198095, 10 Feb 2005
11. Selvam P, Girija K, Nagarajan G, De Clerco E (2005) Synthesis, antibacterial, and anti-HIV activities of 3-[5-amino-6-(2,3-dichloro-phenyl)-[1,2,4]triazin-3-yl]-6,8- dibromo-2-substi tuted-3H-quinazolin-4-one. Indian J Pharm Sci 67:484–487
12. Alanine A, Gobbi LC, Kolczewski S, Luebbers T, Peters JU, Steward L (2006) Preparation of 8-Alkoxy or Cycloalkoxy-4-methyl-3,4-dihydro-quinazolin-2-ylamines for Treating 5-HT5A Receptor Related Diseases. US Patent 2006293350 A1. Chem Abstr. 146,100721, 28 Dec 2006
13. Chaturvedula PV, Chen L, Civiello R, Degnan AP, Dubowchik GM, Han X, Jiang XJ, Macor JE, Poindexter GS, Tora GO, Luo G (2007) Preparation of Piperidine-1-carboxamideDerivatives and Spirocycles Thereof as Antagonists of Calcitonin Gene-relatedPeptide Receptors. US Patent 2007149503 A1. Chem Abstr. 147,118256. 28 Jun 2007
14. Letourneau J, Riviello C, Ho KK, Chan JH, Ohlmeyer M, Jokiel P, Neagu I, Morphy JR, Napier SE (2006) Preparation of 2-(4-Oxo-4H-quinazolin-3-yl) acetamides as Vasopressin V3 Receptor Antagonists. PCT Int Appl WO 2006095014 A1. Chem Abstr. 145,315012, 14 Sep 2006

15. Molinski TF (1993) Marine pyridoacridine alkaloid: Structure, synthesis and biological chemistry. Chem Rev 93:1825–1838. doi:10.1021/cr00021a009.
16. Robin M, Fature R, Perichaud A, Galy JP (2000) Synthesis of new thiazolo [5,4-a]acridine derivatives. Heterocycles 53:387–395. doi:10.3987/COM-99-8794.
17. Khan RH, Rastogi RC (1991) Condensed heterocycles: synthesis and antifungal activities of pi-deficient pyrimidines linked with pi-rich heterocycles. J Agricult Food Chem 39:2300–2303. doi:10.1021/jf00012a042.
18. Grasso S, Micale N, Anna-aria Monforte, Monforte P, Polimeni S, Zappala M (2000) Synthesis and in vitro antitumour activity evaluation of 1-aryl-1H,3Hthiazolo[4,3-b]quinazolines. Eur J Med Chem 35:115–1119
19. Testard A, Picot L, Lozach O, Blairvacq M, Meijer L, Murillo L, Piot JM, Thiery V, Besson T (2005) Synthesis and evaluation of the antiproliferative activity of novel thiazolquinazolinone kinase inhibitors. J Enzyme Inhib Med Chem 20:557–568. doi:10.1080/14756360500212399.
20. Testard A, Loge C, Leger B, Robert JM, Lozach O, Blairvacq M, Meijer L, Thiery V, Besson T (2006) Thiazolo[5,4-f]quinazolin-9-ones, inhibitors of glycogen synthase kinase-3. Bioorg Med Chem Lett 16:3419–3423. doi:10.1016/j.bmcl.2006.04.006.
21. Alexandre FR, berecibar A, Wrigglesworth R, Besson T (2003) Efficient synthesis of thiazoloquinazolinone derivatives. Tetrahedron Lett 44:4455–4458. doi:10.1016/S0040-4039(03)01026-8.
22. Besson T, Guillard J, Rees CW (2000) Multistep synthesis of thiazoloquinazolines under microwave irradiation in solution. Tetrahedron Lett 41:1027–1030. doi:10.1016/S0040-4039(99)02221-2.
23. Quiroga J, Hernández P, Insuasty B, Abonía R, Cobo J, Sánchez A, Nogueras M, Low NL (2002) Control of the reaction between 2-aminobenzothiazoles and Mannich bases. Synthesis of pyrido[2,1-b][1,3] benzothiazoles versus [1,3]benzothiazolo[2, 3-b]quinazolines. J Chem Soc Perkin Trans 1:555–559
24. Rathore BS, Kumar M (2006) Synthesis of 7-chloro-5-trifluoromethyl/7-fluoro/7-trifluoromethyl-4H-1,4-benzothiazines as antimicrobial agents. Bioorg Med Chem 14:5678–5682. doi:10.1016/j.bmc.2006.04.009.
25. Rathore BS, Gupta V, Gupta RR, Kumar M (2007) Synthesis of 7-chloro-5-trifluoromethyl/7-fluoro/7-trifluoromethyl-4H-1,4-phenothiazines. Heteroatom Chem 18:81–86. doi:10.1002/hc.20235.
26. Kumar M, Sharma K, Samarth RM, Kumar A (2010) Synthesis and antioxidant activity of quinolinobenzothaizinones. Eur J Med Chem 45:4467–4472. doi:10.1016/j.ejmech.2010.07.006.
27. Arya AK, Kumar M (2011) An efficient green chemical approach for the synthesis of structurally diverse spiroheterocycles with fused heterosystems. Green Chem 13:1332–1338. doi:10.1039/c1gc00008j.
28. Arya AK, Kumar M (2011) Base catalyzed multicomponent synthesis of spiroheterocycles with fused heterosystems. Mol Divers 15:781–789. doi:10.1007/s11030-011-9309-2.
29. Dandia A, Arya K, Khaturia S, Jain AK (2010) Microwave-induced preparation of biologically important benzothiazolo[2, 3-b]quinazolines, and comparison with ultrasonic and classical heating. Monatsh Chem 141:979–985. doi:10.1007/s00706-010-0361-x.
30. Sharma BK, Sharma PK, Kumar M (2010) One-Pot, Multicomponent Sequential Synthesis of Benzothiazoloquinazolinones. Synth Commun 40:2347–2352. doi:10.1080/00397910903243807.
31. Dandia A, Khaturia S, Jain AK, Arya K (2008) Statement of a methodology for the microwave-induced preparation of biologically important benzothiazolo [2, 3-b] quinazolines and its comparison with ultrasonic and classical heating. 12th International Electronic Conference on Synthetic Organic Chemistry ECSOC-12 http://www.usc.es/congresos/ecsoc/11/ECSOC11.htm. 1-30 November 2008
32. Nefzi A, Ostresh JM (1997) The Current status of heterocyclic combinatorial liberies. Chem Rev 97:449. doi:10.1021/cr960010b.
33. Roth HJ, Kleemann A (1988) In pharmaceutical chemistry. In Drug Synthesis, vol 1.New York: Wiley
34. Zhu J (2003) Recent developments in the isonitrile-based multicomponent synthesis of heterocycles. Eur J Org Chem 7:1133–1144
35. Orm RVA, de Greef M (2003) Recent advances in solution phase multicomponent methodology for the synthesis of heterocyclic compounds. Synthesis 10:1471–1499
36. Domling A, Ugi I (2000) Multicomponent reaction with isocyanides. Angew Chem Int Ed 39:3168–3210. doi:10.1002/1521-3773(20000915)39:183.0.CO;2-U.

5

Facile and efficient one-pot synthesis of benzimidazoles using lanthanum chloride

Yekkirala Venkateswarlu, Sudhagani Ramesh Kumar and Panuganti Leelavathi*

Abstract

Background: We report the synthesis of benzimidazoles using lanthanum chloride as an efficient catalyst. One-pot synthesis of 2-substituted benzimidazole derivatives from *o*-phenylenediamine and a variety of aldehydes were developed under mild reaction conditions.

Results: We have examined the effect of different solvents using the same reaction conditions. The yield of the product varied with the nature of the solvents, and better conversion and easy isolation of products were found with acetonitrile. In a similar manner, the reaction with *o*-phenylenediamine and 3,4,5-trimethoxybenzaldehyde was carried out without any solvents. The observation shows that the reaction was not brought into completion, even after starting for a period of 9 h, and the reaction mixture showed a number of spots in thin-layer chromatography.

Conclusions: In conclusion, lanthanum chloride has been employed as a novel and efficient catalyst for the synthesis of benzimidazoles in good yields from *o*-phenylenediamine and a wide variety of aldehydes. All of the reactions were carried out in the presence of lanthanum chloride (10 mol%) in acetonitrile at room temperature.

Keywords: Benzimidazoles; Aldehydes; *o*-Phenylenediamine; Lanthanum chloride

Background

Benzimidazole nucleus is found in a variety of naturally occurring compounds such as vitamin B12 and its derivatives; it is structurally similar to purine bases. Benzimidazoles and its derivatives represent one of the most biologically active classes of compounds, possessing a wide spectrum of activities, and these are well documented in the literature. They show selective nonpeptide luteinizing hormone-releasing hormone antagonist, lymphocyte-specific kinase inhibitor, *N*-methyl-D-aspartate antagonist, 5-liopoxygenase inhibitor, NS5B polymerase inhibitor (Figure 1), neuropeptide YY1 receptor antagonist, nonpeptide thrombin inhibitor, γ-aminobutyric acid receptor, factor Xa inhibitor, and poly (ADP-ribose) polymerase inhibitor. DNA-minor groove-binding agents possess antitumor activity, topoisomerase I inhibitors, angiotensin II inhibitors, and proliferation inhibitors. Several benzimidazole derivatives find applications that include antimicrobial, antihypertensive, anticancer antiulcer, antifungal, antihistamine activity, herbicides, and other veterinary applications as promising drugs in different therapeutic categories. The benzimidazole moieties express a significant activity against several viruses such as HIV, herpes (HSV-1), RNA influenza, human cytomegalovirus, selective angiotensin II inhibitors, and 5-HT3 antagonists. In addition, benzimidazoles are very impotent intermediates in synthetic routes and serve as ligands for asymmetric catalysts [1-8]. The high profile of biological applications of the benzimidazole compounds has prompted the emergence of extensive studies of their syntheses. In this context, numerous efforts have been made to synthesize benzimidazole derivatives. One of the most common methods for the preparation of benzimidazole derivatives involves the condensation of an *o*-phenylenediamine and carbonyl compounds such as aldehydes and acid derivatives. The condensation of *o*-phenylenediamine with carboxylic acid often requires strong acidic conditions and high temperatures [9,10]. The other method involves the oxidative cyclodehydrogenation of Schiff bases, which is generated from *o*-phenylenediamine and aldehydes in the presence of various catalysts.

This is the most popular approach in general for the synthesis of benzimidazole derivatives. The catalysts used are CAN, K_3PO_4, oxone, sulfamic acid, DDQ, $PhI(OAc)_2$, iodine, and $KHSO_4$ [11-17]. In addition, several

* Correspondence: ameshteja_2001@yahoo.co.in
Department of Chemistry, Osmania University College for Women, Koti, Hyderabad 500095, India

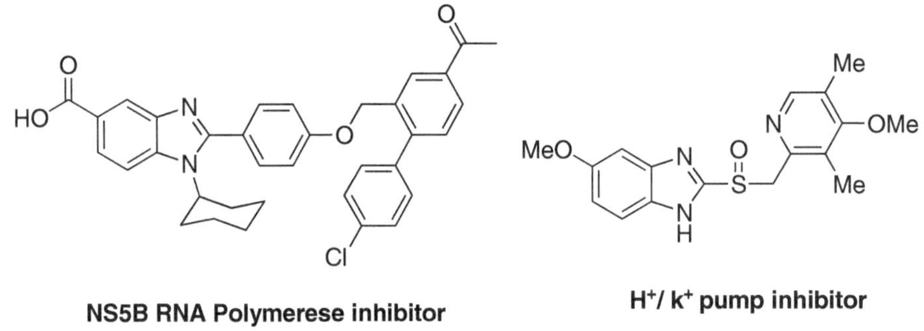

Figure 1 Scheme of NS5B polymerase and H^+/K^+ inhibitors.

catalysts such as metal halides and metal oxychlorides, [18-22] metal oxides, PTSA, metal triflates, air, [23-30] ionic liquid, heteropoly acid, BDSB [31-33], proline, solid-supported catalysts, polymer-supported catalysts [34,35], and microwave-promoted [36-39] and clayzic [40] reactions have been reported in the literature. Unfortunately, many of these methods suffer from drawbacks such as drastic reaction conditions, low yields, tedious workup procedures, and co-occurrence of several side reactions. As a consequence, the introduction of an efficient and mild method is still needed to overcome these limitations.

As part of our research program in developing various synthetic methodologies [41-46], we report the synthesis of benzimidazoles using lanthanum chloride ($LaCl_3$) as an efficient catalyst. The catalyst is known as an efficient catalyst in the literature for various organic transformations [47-52].

Methods

Melting points were recorded on a Buchi R-535 apparatus (BUCHI Labortechnik AG, Flawi, Switzerland) and were uncorrected. Infrared (IR) spectra were recorded on a PerkinElmer FT-IR 240-c spectrophotometer (PerkinElmer Instruments, Branford, CT, USA) using KBr discs. Hydrogen-1 nuclear magnetic resonance (^1H NMR) spectra were recorded on a Gemini-200 spectrometer (Varian Medical Systems, Palo Alto, CA, USA) in $CDCl_3$ using TMS as internal standard. Mass spectra were recorded on a Finnigan MAT 1020 (Thermo Fisher Scientific, Waltham, MA, USA) mass spectrometer operating at 70 eV.

Results and discussion

In a typical experiment, a reaction was made to occur between 1,2-phenylenediamine (OPD) (**1**) and 3,4,5-trimethoxybenzaldehyde (**2**) in the presence of $LaCl_3$ in acetonitrile at room temperature to afford the corresponding product, **2**-(3,4,5-trimethoxyphenyl)-1*H*-benzo [d]imidazole (**3**), in excellent yield. The reaction was completed within 2 h (Scheme 1).

We have examined the effect of different solvents using the same reaction conditions, as shown in Table 1. The yield of the product varied with the nature of the solvents; better conversion and easy isolation of products were found with acetonitrile. Acetonitrile dissolves a wide range of ionic and nonpolar compounds. In a similar manner, the reaction with *o*-phenylenediamine and 3,4,5-trimethoxybenzaldehyde was carried out without any solvents. The observation shows that the reaction was not brought into completion, even after starting for a period of 9 h, and the reaction mixture showed a number of spots in thin-layer chromatography (TLC).

In a similar manner, a comparative study on the role and requirement of the catalyst for condensation has been carried out, and the obtained results are clearly shown in Table 2. The reactants for this reaction are also *o*-phenylenediamine and 3,4,5-trimethoxybenzaldehyde in acetonitrile. From our observation, a catalytic amount

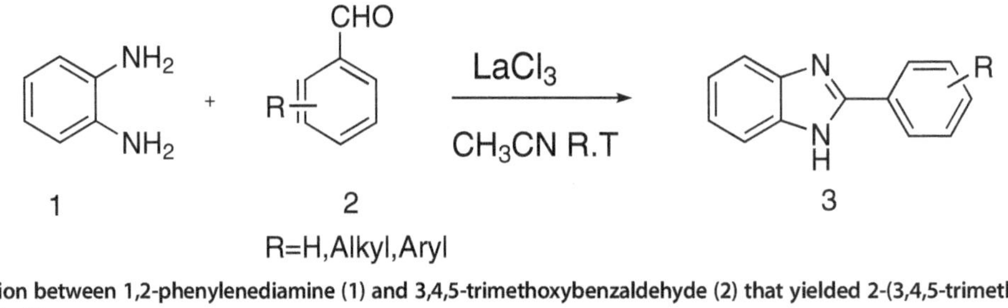

Scheme 1 Reaction between 1,2-phenylenediamine (1) and 3,4,5-trimethoxybenzaldehyde (2) that yielded 2-(3,4,5-trimethoxyphenyl)-1*H*-benzo[d]imidazole (3).

Table 1 Comparative study of the solvent system

Number	Solvent	Time (h)	Yield (%)
1	CH_3CN	2.0	95
2	CH_3OH	4.0	80
3	Dioxane	5.0	75
4	THF	6.0	70
5	Toluene	7.0	65
6	DMF	5.0	6
7	DCM	8.0	50
8	-	9.0	-

(10 mol%) of $LaCl_3$ was enough to complete the conversion of aldehyde and *o*-phenylenediamine into the required condensation product.

A blank experiment was carried out with *o*-phenylenediamine and 3,4,5-trimethoxybenzaldehyde in the absence of the catalyst $LaCl_3$, and the required 3,4,5-trimethoxybenzimidazole product was not found even after stirring for 15 h. Finally, it was decided that the suitable conditions for condensation is in a solvent and in the presence of an activator or promoter. As shown in Table 3, aromatic, heteroaromatic, α-unsaturated and β-unsaturated aldehydes, and aliphatic aldehydes were reacted very well to afford the corresponding products of benzimidazole derivatives in very good to excellent yields. In general, the aromatic aldehydes having electron-donating groups and heteroaromatic compounds are reacting a little faster when compared with other aldehydes. In a similar manner, the aliphatic aldehydes and aromatic aldehydes containing electron-withdrawing groups are reacting comparatively a little slower in terms of conversion as well as yields, benzaldehyde and OPD, in the presence of the catalyst $Lacl_3$. In general, all the reactions were completed within 2 to 4 h, and the obtained yields were 85% to 95%.

Experimental

General procedure

A mixture of *o*-phenylenediamine (1.0 mmol) and aldehyde (1.2 mmol) in the presence of lanthanum chloride (10 mol%) was stirred in acetonitrile (5 ml) at room temperature. The progress of the reaction was monitored by TLC. After completion of the reaction as indicated by TLC, the solvent was removed under reduced pressure. The residue was dissolved in ethyl acetate and washed with water and brine. The organic layer was dried over Na_2SO_4 and concentrated under reduced pressure. The crude products were purified by column chromatography. All the products were identified by their ^{1}H NMR, IR, and mass spectroscopy data.

Table 2 Comparative study of catalyst

Number	Amount of catalyst ($LaCl_3$) (eq)	Time (h)
1	0.1	2.0
2	0.2	2.0
3	0.4	3.5
4	0.6	3.5
5	0.8	3.0
6	1.0	3.0
7	No catalyst	15

Spectral data for selected compounds

2-(3,4,5-Trimethoxyphenyl)-1H-benzo[d]imidazole (3a)

For this compound, the white solid's melting point was 259°C. The IR (KBr) frequency (*υ*) values were as follows: 2,924, 2,851, 1,601, 1,495, 1,463, 1,416, 1,282, 1,096, 1,020, 899, 801, 749, and 693 cm$-^1$. The ^{1}H NMR (DMSO-d_6) chemical shift (*δ*) values were as follows: 3.90 (s, 3H), 4.00 (s, 6H), 7.43 to 7.60 (m, 2H), 7.65 (s, 2H), and 7.85 to 7.95 (m, 2H). The electron ionized mass spectrometry (EIMS) mass-to-ratio (*m/z*) values and corresponding percentage were as follows: 285 (m^{+1} 100%), 269 (10%), 255 (10%), and 224 (5%).

4-(1H-Benzo[d]imidazol-2-yl)-N,N-dimethyl benzenamine (3b)

For this compound, the white solid's melting range was 288°C to 290°C. The IR (KBr) *υ* values were as follows: 2,853, 2,800, 1,740, 1,611, 1,561, 15,276, 1,446, 1,389, 1,362, 1,324, 1,278, 1,230, 1,200, 1,167, 1,106, 1,064, 948, 819, 800, 744, 769, and 583 cm^{-1}. The ^{1}H NMR (DMSO-d_6) *δ* values were as follows: 2.90 (s, 6H), 6.70 (dd, 2H), 6.95 (d, 2H), 7.10 to 7.25 (m, 2H), and 7.60 (dd, 2H). The EIMS *m/z* values and percentage were as follows: 238 (m^{+1} 100%), 157 (30%), 134 (80%), and 109 (10%).

2-(4-(Allyoxy)-3-methoxyphenyl)-1H-benzo[d]imidazole (3c)

For this compound, the solid's IR (KBr) *υ* values were as follows: 3,063, 2,923, 2,853, 1,886, 1,747, 1,649, 1,607, 1,580, 1,449, 1,460, 1,422, 1,387, 1,316, 1,250, 1,215, 1,180, 1,138, 1,027, 991, 924, 866, 805, 763, 743, 628, and 594 cm^{-1}. The ^{1}H NMR (DMSO-d_6) *δ* values were as follows: 3.75 (s, 3H), 4.55 (d, 2H), 5.25 (d, 1H), 5.40 (t, 2H), 5.95 to 6.10 (m, 1H), 6.60 (d, 1H) 6.73 (t, 1H), 7.15 to 7.35 (m, 2H), 7.50 to 7.60 (m, 2H), and 7.80 (d, 2H). The EIMS *m/z* values and corresponding percentage were as follows: 280 (m^{+1} 100%) and 242 (80%).

2-(Furan-2-yl)-1H-benzo[d]imidazole (3d)

For this compound, the solid's melting point was 296°C. The IR (KBr) *υ* values were as follows: 2,927, 2,857, 1,741, 1,609, 1,545, 1,462, 1,379, 1,189, 1,069, 751, and

Table 3 Lanthanum chloride-catalyzed synthesis of benzimidazoles

Entry	Diamine	Aldehyde	Product (3a-3q)	Time (h)	Yields (%)
a	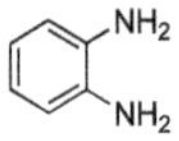	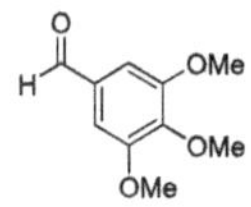	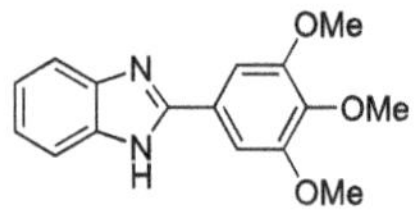	2.0	95
b	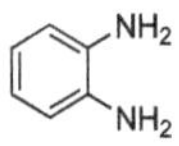	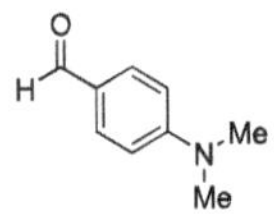	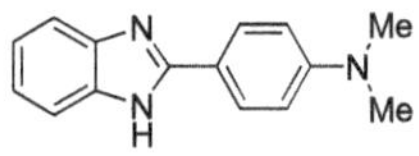	2.5	88
c	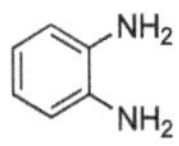	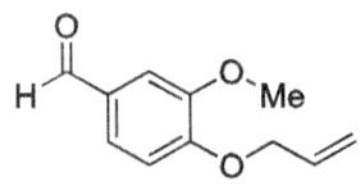	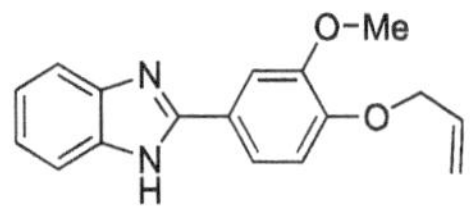	2.0	91
d	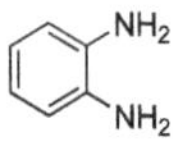	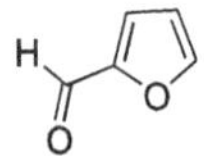	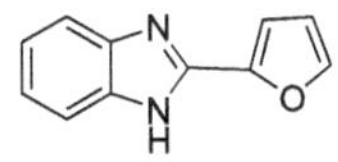	2.0	9.0
e	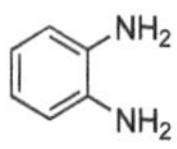	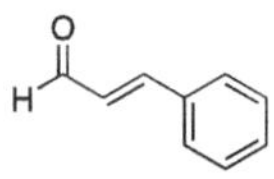	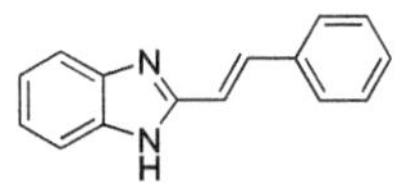	3.0	87
f	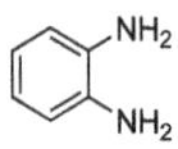	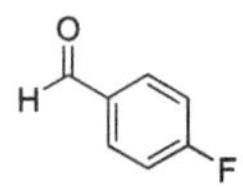	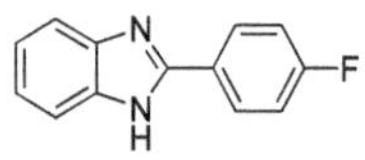	2.0	85
g	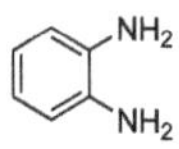	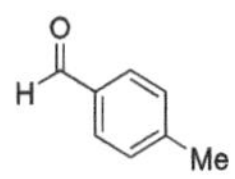	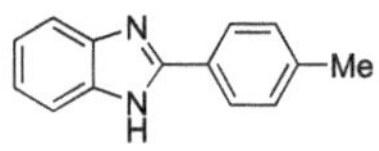	2.5	92
h	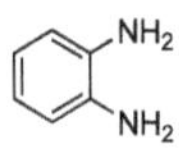	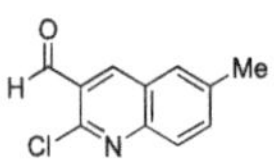	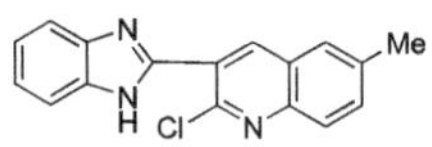	4.0	90
i	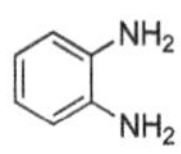	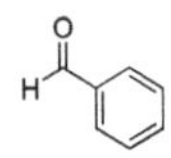	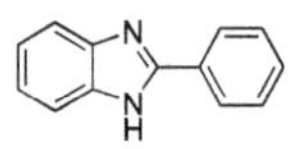	3.0	88
j	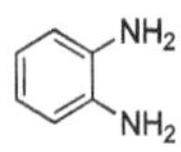	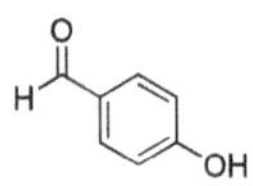	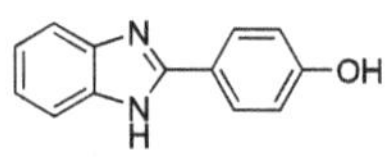	2.5	86
k	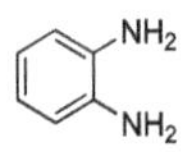	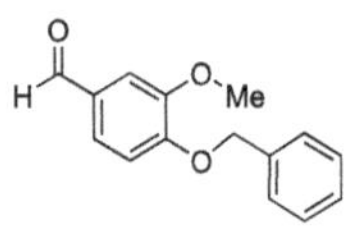	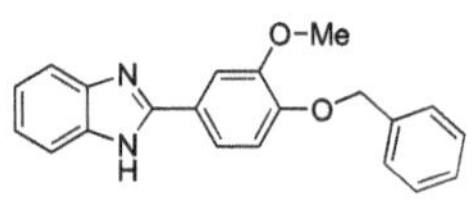	3.0	90
l	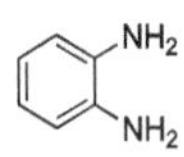	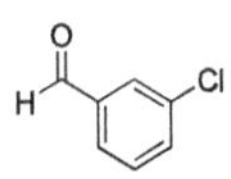	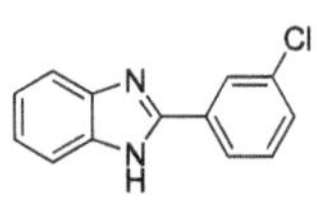	2.5	91
m	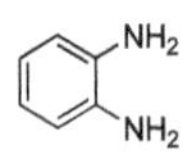	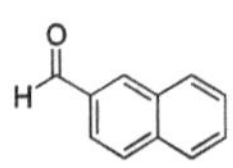	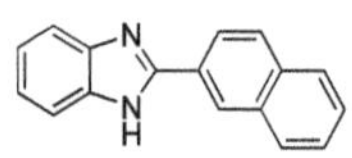	3.0	87

Table 3 Lanthanum chloride-catalyzed synthesis of benzimidazoles *(Continued)*

n	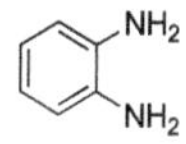	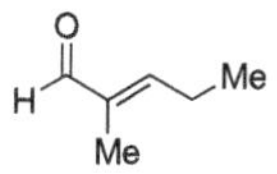	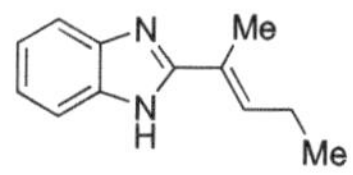	4.0	85
o	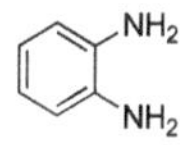	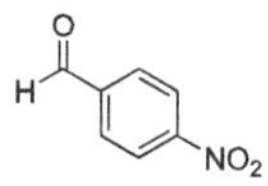	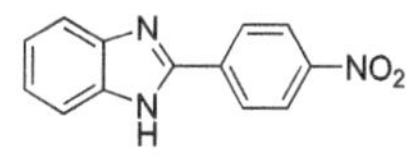	3.0	88
p	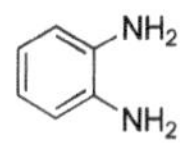	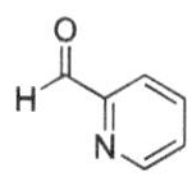	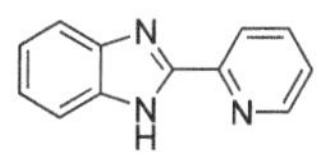	2.5	86
q	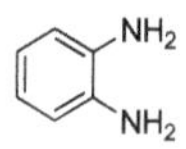	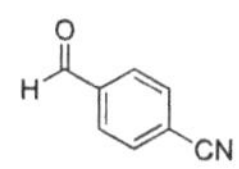	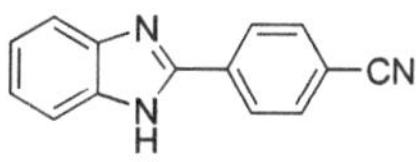	2.5	89

597 cm^{-1}. The ^{1}H NMR (DMSO-d$_6$) δ values were as follows: 6.30 (d, 2H), 7.15 to 7.35 (m, 2H), 7.40 (d, 1H), and 7.65 (d, 2H). The EIMS *m/z* values and corresponding percentage were as follows: 184 (m^{+1} 100%), 158 (20%), 137 (5%), and 133 (5%).

(E)-2-Styryl-1H-benzo[d]imidazole (3e)

For this compound, the solid's melting range was 201°C to 203°C. The IR (KBr) υ values were as follows: 3,377, 3,027, 2,924, 2,853, 1,948, 1,805, 1,633, 1,598, 1,495, 1,449, 1,402, 1,355, 1,326, 1,284, 1,194, 1,153, 1,070, 1,018, 963, 918, 841, 737, 691, and 558 cm^{-1}. The ^{1}H NMR (DMSO-d$_6$) δ values were as follows: 6.40 (dd, 1H), 6.55 (d, 1H), 7.15 to 7.55 (m, 7H), and 7.70 (d, 2H). The EIMS *m/z* values and corresponding percentage were as follows: 220 (m^{+1} 15%), 195 (5%), 174 (5%), 155 (5%), 144 (5%), and 134 (5%).

2-(4-Fluorophenyl)-1H-benzo[d]diazole (3f)

For this compound, the white solid's melting point was 248°C. The IR (KBr) υ values were as follows: 3,053, 2,930, 1,663, 1,624, 1,545, 1,486, 1,440, 1,315, 1,277, 1,229, 1,094, 1,034, 1,004, 972, 833, 795, 746, 690, 618, and 568 cm^{-1}. The ^{1}H NMR (DMSO-d$_6$) δ values were as follows: 7.15 to 7.20 (m, 2H), 7.20 to 7.40 (m, 2H), 7.45 to 7.52 (m, 2H), 7.60 to 7.70 (m, 2H), and 8.00 (brs, 1H). The EIMS *m/z* values and corresponding percentage were as follows: 212 (m$^+$ 100%), 193 (5%), 215 (15%), 168 (5%), 155 (5%), 136 (5%), 129 (5%), and 95 (5%).

2-p-Tolyl-1H-benzo[d]imidazole (3g)

For this compound, the white solid's melting point was 275°C. The IR (KBr) υ values were as follows: 3,397, 3,027, 2,922, 2,858, 1,813, 1,514, 1,481, 1,452, 1,412, 1,383, 1,348, 1,282, 1,250, 1,183, 1,157, 1,114, 1,021, 987, 823, 746, and 612.cm^{-1}. The ^{1}H NMR (DMSO-d$_6$) δ values were as follows: 2.35 (s, 3H), 4.42 (brs, 1 NH), 6.95 (d, 2H), 7.10 (d, 2H), 7.28 (d, 2H), and 7.55 (d, 2H). The EIMS *m/z* values and corresponding percentage were as follows: 208 (m$^+$ 100%), 195 (15%), 179 (20%), 161 (10%), 153 (10%), 149 (5%), 140 (20%), 136 (5%), 126 (10%), and 122 (5%).

3-(1H-Benzo[d]imidazol-2-yl)-2-chloro-6-methylquinoline (3h)

For this compound, the solid's IR (KBr) υ values were as follows: 3,073, 1,585, 1,493, 1,435, 1,392, 1,331, 1,280, 1,227, 1,147, 1,031, 929, 816, 748, 711, 646, 579, and 483 cm^{-1}. The ^{1}H NMR (DMSO-d$_6$) δ values were as follows: 2.60 (s, 3H), 7.25 (d, 2H), 7.70 (d, 1H), 7.80 (d, 2H), 7.90 (d, 2H), and 8.80 (s 1H). The EIMS *m/z* values and corresponding percentage were as follows: 294 (m$^+$ 70%), 290 (10%), 274 (40%), 258 (5%), 246 (5%), 230 (5%), 212 (5%), 191 (10%), and 169 (5%).

2-Phenyl-1H-benzo[d]imidazole (3i)

For this compound, the white powder's melting point was 295°C. The IR (KBr) υ values were as follows: 3,406, 3,047, 1,589, 1,540, 1,443, 1,409, 1,483, 1,275, 1,118, 736, and 704 cm^{-1}. The ^{1}H NMR (DMSO-d$_6$) δ values were 4.50 (brs, 1H), 7.20 to 7.40 (m, 2H), 7.50 to 7.75 (m, 5H), 7.70 (d, 2H), and 8.25 (d, 2H). EIMS *m/z* values and corresponding percentage were as follows: 195 (m$^+$ 10%), 175 (5%), and 160 (5%).

4-(1H-Benzo[d]imidazole-2yl) phenol (3j)

For this compound, the white powder's melting range was 229°C to 230°C. The IR (KBr) υ values were as follows: 3,376, 3,290, 3,027, 2,807, 1,697, 1,611, 1,591, 1,515, 1,443, 1,394, 1,268, 1,246, 839, and 745 cm^{-1}. The ^{1}H NMR (DMSO-d$_6$) δ values were as follows: 6.90 (d, 1H), 7.05 to 7.15 (m, 4H), and 7.75 (d, 2H). The EIMS *m*/*z* values and corresponding percentage were as follows: 210 (m^+ 100%), 193 (5%), 191 (20%), 183 (10%), 181 (5%), 169 (40%), 154 (5%), 137 (5%).

2-(4-(Benzyloxy)-3-methoxyphenyl)-1H-benzo[d]imidazole (3k)

For this compound, the IR (KBr) *υ* values were as follows: 3,036, 2,924, 2,853, 1,738, 1,604, 1,497, 1,458, 1,384, 1,321, 1,240, 1,209, 1,175, 1,132, 1,028, 992, 905, 802, 740, 697, 641, and 572, and 465 cm^{-1}. The ^1H NMR (DMSO-d_6) *δ* values were as follows: 3.73 (s, 3H), 5.15 (s, 2H), 6.55 (d, 1H), 6.55 (d, 1H), 6.75 (dd, 2H) 7.10 to 7.50 (m, 7H), and 7.80 (d, 2H). The EIMS *m*/*z* (first set) values and corresponding percentage were as follows: 330 (m^+ 60%), 313 (10%), 305 (20%), 289 (5%), 261 (30%), 245 (20%), 227 (100%), 210 (20%), 201 (50%), 195 (20%), 157 (20%), 100 (30%), 91 (10%), and 89 (5%). The EIMS *m*/*z* (second set) values and corresponding percentage were as follows: 245 (m^+ 100%), 243 (5%), and 141 (10%). The EIMS *m*/*z* (third set) values and corresponding percentage were as follows: 245 (m^+ 100%), 243 (5%), and 141 (10%).

2-(3-Chlorophenyl)-1H-benzo[d]imidazole (31)

For this compound, the white powder's melting range was 232°C to 234°C. The IR (KBr) *υ* values were as follows: 3,059, 1,619, 1,593, 1,440, 1,421, 1,269, 836, and 750 cm^{-1}. The ^1H NMR (DMSO-d6 MHz) *δ* values were as follows: 7.45 to 7.60 (m, 4H), 7.62 to 7.72 (m, 2H), and 8.30 to 8.45 (m, 2H). The EIMS *m*/*z* value with its corresponding percentage was 229 (m^+ 100%).

2-(Naphthalene-2yl)-1H-benzo[d]imidazole (3m)

For this compound, the white powder's melting range was 218°C to 219°C. The IR (KBr) *υ* values were as follows: 3,425, 3,047, 2,924, 2,853, 1,624, 1,605, 1,447, 1,385, and 748 cm^{-1}. The ^1H NMR (DMSO-d6) *δ* values were as follows: 6.70 to 6.90 (m, 2H), 7.20 to 7.35 (m, 2H), 7.55 to 7.80 (m 4H), and 7.90 to 8.10 (m, 2H). The EIMS *m*/*z* values and corresponding percentage were as follows: 245 (m^+ 100%), 243 (5%), and 141 (10%).

(E)-2-(Pent-en-2-yl)-1H-benzo[d]imidazole (3n)

For this compound, the IR (KBr) *υ* values were as follows: 3,064, 2,963, 2,923, and 1,648 cm^{-1}. The ^1H NMR (DMSO-d6) *δ* values were as follows: 1.10 (t, 3H), 1.80 (m, 2H), 1.95 to 2.10 (m, 2H), 5.90 (dd, 1H), 7.30 (d, 2H), and 7.75 (d, 2H). The EIMS *m*/*z* value was 187.

2-(4-Nitrophenyl)-1H-benzo[d]imidazole (3o)

For this compound, the yellow powder's melting point was 314°C. The IR (KBr) *υ* values were 3,042, 1,604, 1,515, 1,434, 1,353, 854, 745, and 710 cm^{-1}. The ^1H NMR (DMSO-d6) *δ* values were as follows: 7.10 to 7.15 (m, 2H), 7.30 (d, 1H), 7.35 (d, 1H), 7.40 (t, 1H), 7.45 (t, 1H), 8.0 (dd, 2H), and 13.0 (brs, 1H). The EIMS *m*/*z* values and corresponding percentage were as follows: 240 (m^+ 100%), 226 (5%), 211 (10%), 194 (20%), and 182 (5%).

2-(Pyridine-2-yl)-1H-benzo[d]imidazole (3p)

For this compound, the solid's melting range was 245°C to 248°C. The IR (KBr) *υ* values were as follows: 3,068, 1,449, 1,402, 1,280, and 746 cm^{-1}. The ^1H NMR (DMSO-d6) *δ* values were as follows: 6.85 (m, 2H), 7.00 to 7.10 (m, 1H), 7.45 to 7.55 (m, 1H), 7.80 to 7.90 (m, 2H), 8.10 (t, 1H), and 8.65 (d, 1H). EIMS *m*/*z* value with its corresponding percentage was 196 (m^+ 15%).

4-(1H-Benzo[d]imidazole-2yl) benzonitrile (3q)

For this compound, the white crystal solid's melting point was 262°C. The IR (KBr) *υ* values were as follows: 3,417, 3,047, 2,912, 2,222, 1,605, 1,454, 1,408, and 748 cm^{-1}. The ^1H NMR (DMSO-d6) *δ* values were as follows: 5.50 (brs, 1H), 7.45 to 7.60 (m, 2H), 7.82 to 7.90 (m, 2H), 8.05 (d, 2H), and 8.50 (d, 2H). The EIMS *m*/*z* values and corresponding percentage were as follows: 220 (m^+ 100%), 211 (10%), 196 (5%), and 186 (5%).

Conclusions

In conclusion, lanthanum chloride has been employed as a novel and efficient catalyst for the synthesis of benzimidazoles in good yields from *o*-phenylenediamine and a wide variety of aldehydes. All the reactions were carried out at room temperature while using the catalyst lanthanum chloride in 10 mol%. The reaction conditions were very mild, and the isolation of products was also very easy.

Competing interests

The authors declare that they have no competing interests.

Authors' information

YV and SRK are research scholars, and PL is a professor at the Department of Chemistry, University College for Women, Koti Osmania University, Hyderabad 500095, India.

Acknowledgments

The authors are thankful to the director of IICT for providing the working space and chemicals.

References

1. Nakano H, Inoue T, Kawasaki N, Miyataka H, Matsumoto H, Taguchi T, Inagaki N, Nagai H, Satoh T (2000) Synthesis of biologically activities of novel anti-allergic agents with 5-lipoxygenase inhibiting action. Bioorg Med Chem 8:373–380
2. Hauel HN, Nar H, Priepke H, Ries U, Stassen J, Wienen W (2002) Structure-based design of novel potent nonpeptide thrombin inhibitors. J Med Chem 45:1757–1766

3. He Y, Wu B, Yang J, Robinson D, Risen L, Ranken R, Blyn L, Sheng S, Swayze EE (2003) 2-Piperidin-4-yl-benzimidazoles with broad spectrum antibacterial activities. Bioorg Med Chem Lett 13:3253–3256
4. Porcari RA, Devivar RV, Kucera LS, Cdreach J, Townsend BL (1998) Design, synthesis and antiviral evaluations of 1-(substituted benzyl)-2-substituted-5, 6-dichlorobenzimidazoles as non nucleoside analogues of 2,5,6-trichloro-1-(β-D-ribofuranosyl) benzimidazole. J Med Chem 41:1252–1262
5. Roth T, Morningstar LM, Boyer LP, Hughes MS, Buckheitjr RW, Michejda JC (1997) Synthesis and biological activity of novel nonnucleoside inhibitors of HIV-1 reverse transcriptase. 2-Aryl-substituted benzimidazoles. J Med Chem 40:4199–4207
6. Migawa TM, Girardet LJ, Walker AJ, Koszalka WG, Chamberjain DS, Drach C, Townsend BL (1998) Design, synthesis, and antiviral activity of α-nucleosides: D-and L-isomers of lyxofuranosyl and (5-deoxylyxofuranosyl) benzimidazoles. J Med Chem 41:1242–1251
7. Mann J, Baron AY, Opoku-Boahen Y, Johansoon E, Parkmson G, Kelland RL, Neidle S (2001) A new class of symmetric bisbenzimidazole based DNA minor groove-binding agents showing antitumor activity. J Med Chem 44:138–144
8. Figge A, Altenbach JH, Brauer DJ, Tielmann P (2002) Synthesis and resolution of 2-(2-diphenylphosphinyl-naphthalen-1-yl)-1-isopropyl-1H-benzimidazole: a new atropisomeric P, N-chelating ligand for asymmetric catalysis. Tetrahedron-Asymmetry 13:137–144
9. Hisano T, Ichikawa M, Tsumoto K, Tasaki M (1982) Synthesis of benzoxazoles, benzothiazoles and benzimidazoles and evaluation of their antifungal, insecticidal and herbicidal activities. Chem Pharm Bull 30:2996–3004
10. Kumar BVS, Vaidya SD, Kumar RV, Bhirud SB, Mane RB (2006) Synthesis and anti-bacterial activity of some novel 2-(6-fluorochroman-2-yl)-1-alkyl/acyl/aroyl-1*H*-benzimidazoles. Eur J Med Chem 41:599–604
11. Bahrami K, Khodaei MM, Naali F (2008) Mild and highly efficient method for the synthesis of 2-arylbenzimidazoles and 2-arylbenzothiazoles. J Org Chem 73:6835–6837
12. Buchwald SL, Zheng N, Anderson KW, Huang X, Nguyen HN (2007) A palladium-catalyzed regiospecific synthesis of *N*-arylbenzimidazoles. Angew Chem 46:7509–7512
13. Beaulieu PL, Hache B, Moon VE (2003) A practical oxone-mediated, high-through, solution-phase synthesis of benzimidazoles from 1,2-phenylenediamines and aldehydes and its application to preparative-scale synthesis. Synthesis 11:1683–1692
14. Eynde JJV, Delfosse F, Lor P, Van YH (1995) 2,3-Dichloro-5, 6-dicyano-1,4-benzoquinone, a mild catalyst for the formation of C-N bonds. Tetrahedron 51:5813–5818
15. Du LH, Wang YG (2007) A rapid and efficient synthesis of benzimidazoles using hypervalent iodine as oxidant. Synthesis 5:675–678
16. Du HL, Luo AP (2010) Efficient and one-pot synthesis of and benzimidazoles under solvent free conditions. Synth Commun 40:2880–2886
17. Gogoi P, Konwar D (2006) An efficient and one-pot synthesis of imidazolines and benzimidazoles via anaerobic oxidation of C-N bonds in water. Tetrahedron Lett 47:79–82
18. Singh PM, Sasmal S, Lu W, Chatterjee NM (2000) Synthetic utility of catalytic Fe(III)/Fe(II) redox cycling towards fused heterocycles: a facile access to substituted benzimidazoles, bisbenzimidazoles and imidazopyridine derivatives. Synthesis 10:1380–1390
19. Wang XJ, Zhang L, Xu Y, Murthy DK, Senanayake CS (2004) A practical synthesis of 2-(*N*-substituted)-amino-benzimidazoles utilizing CuCl-promoted intramolecular cyclization of *N*-(2-aminoaryl)thioureas. Tetrahedron Lett 45:7167–7170
20. Alloum AB, Bougrin K, Soufiaoui M (2003) Synthese chimioselective des benzimidazoles sursilice traitee parlechlorure du thionyle. Tetrahedron Lett 44:5935–5937
21. Yang D, Fu H, Hu L, Jiang Y, Zhao Y (2008) Copper-catalyzed synthesis of benzimidazoles via cascade reactions of *o*-halo acetanilide derivatives with amidine hydrochlorides. J Org Chem 73:7841–7844
22. Subramanyam SC, Narayanan S (2010) Yttrium (III) chloride: a mild and efficient catalyst for the synthesis of benzimidazoles. Int J Apples Bio and Phar Tech 1:689–694
23. Tandon VK, Kumar M (2004) BF_3-Et_2O-promoted one-pot expeditious and convenient synthesis of 2-substituted benzimidazoles and 3,1, 5-benzoxadiazepines. Tetrahedron Lett 45:4185–4187
24. Shinde B, Nagawade RR (2006) BF_3-Et_2O promoted solvent free synthesis of benzimidazole derivatives. Chin Chem Lett 17:453–456
25. Yulu W, Huiqiang M, Xiangming H (2007) *p*-TsOH catalyzed synthesis of 2-arylsubstituted benzimidazoles. ARKIVOC 2007(13):150–154
26. Trivedi R, De SK, Gibbs RA (2006) A convenient one-pot synthesis of 2-substituted benzimidazoles. J Mol Catal A 245:8–11
27. Currini M, Epifano F, Motanari F, Rosati O, Taccone S (2004) Yttrium triflate promoted synthesis of benzimidazole derivatives. Synlett 10:1832–1834
28. Chari MA, Sadanandam P, Shobha D, Mukkanti K (2010) A Simple mild, and efficient procedure for benzimidazoles using copper triflate as catalyst. Heterocyclic Chem 47:153–155
29. Reddy AR, Narasaiah AV, Yadav JS (2011) Mild and efficient protocol for the synthesis of benzimidazoles using samarium triflate. Synth Commun 41:262–267
30. Lin S, Yang L (2005) A simple and efficient procedure for the synthesis of benzimidazoles using air as the oxidant. Tetrahedron Lett 46:4315–4319
31. Nadaf RN, Siddiqui SA, Daniel T, Lahoti RJ, Srinivasan KV (2004) Room-temperature ionic liquid-promoted region selective synthesis of 2-aryl benzimidazoles, benzoxazoles and benzthiazoles under ambient conditions. J Mol Catal A 214:155–160
32. Heravi MM, Sadjadi S, Oskooie HA, Shoar RH, Bamoharram FF (2008) Heteropoly acids as heterogeneous and recyclable catalysts for the synthesis of benzimidazoles. Catal Commun 8:504–507
33. Das B, Holla H, Srinivas Y (2007) Efficient (bromodimethysulfonium bromide mediated synthesis of benzimidazoles. Tetrahedron Lett 48:61–64
34. Zou B, Yuan Q, Ma D (2007) Synthesis of 1,2-disubstituted benzimidazoles by a Cu-catalyzed cascade aryl amination/condensation process. Angew Chem 46:2598–2601
35. Varala R, Nasreen A, Enugala R, Adapa SR (2007) L-Proline catalyzed selective synthesis of 2-aryl-1-arylmethyl-1*H*-benzimidazoles. Tetrahedron Lett 48:69–72
36. Wu CH, Sun CM (2006) Parallel synthesis of amino bis-benzimidazoles by multistep microwave irradiation. Tetrahedron Lett 47:2601–2604
37. Surpur MP, Singh PR, Patil SB, Samant SD (2007) One-pot synthesis of benzimidazoles from *o*-nitro anilines under microwaves via a reductive cyclization. Synth Commun 37:1375–1379
38. Wang Y, Sarris K, Sauer DR, Djuric SW (2006) A simple and efficient one step synthesis of benzoxazoles and benzimidazoles from carboxs. Tetrahedron Lett 47:4823–4826
39. Mao Z, Wang Z, Li J, Song X, Luo Y (2010) Rapid and cheap synthesis of benzimidazoles via intermittent microwave promotion: a simple and potential industrial application of air as oxidant. Synth Commun 40:1963–1977
40. Pitchumani K, Kanagaraj K, Dhakshinamoorthy A (2011) A Zn^{2+} K10-clay (clayzic) as an efficient water-tolerant, solid acid catalyst for the synthesis of benzimidazoles and quinoxalines at room temperature. Tetrahedron Lett 52:69–73
41. Kumar SR, Venkateswarlu Y, Leelavathi P (2011) Synthesis of 1, 5-benzodiazepines catalysed by $Zn(OTf)_2$ in solvent free medium. Asian J Chem 23:1611–1614
42. Venkateswarlu Y, Leelavathi P (2010) $NbCl_5$: an efficient catalyst for the synthesis of quinoxalines. Lett Org Chem 7:208–211
43. Venkateswarlu Y, Kumar SR, Leelavathi P (2012) $CdCl_2$: a simple and efficient catalyst for the synthesis of 1,4-dihydropyridine. (Hantzsch pyridines). Int J Ind Chem 3:18
44. Venkateswarlu Y, Kumar SR, Leelavathi P (2011) $Eu(OTf)_3$: an efficient catalyst for one-pot synthesis of 3,4-dihydropyrimidin-2(1*H*)-ones. Organic Synthesis and Medicinal Chemistry ASAP
45. Venkateswarlu Y, Kumar SR, Leelavathi P (2012) A simple and efficient protocol for the synthesis of quinolines catalyzed by chloramines-T. Org Commun 5(3):120
46. Kumar SR, Venkateswarlu Y, Leelavathi P (2012) $LaCl_3$: an efficient catalyst for the synthesis of substituted thiazoles. Organic synthesis and medicinal chemistry 1:11–14
47. Narsaiah AV (2007) Lanthanum trichloride ($LaCl_3$): accelerated conjugate addition of amines to electron-poor alkenes. Lett Org Chem 4(7):462–464
48. Luche JL, Gemal AL (1978) Efficient synthesis of acetals catalyzed by rare earth chlorides. Chem Commun 1978:976–977
49. Narsaiah AV, Nagaiah K (2003) $LaCl_3$: mediated regeneration of carbonyl compounds from oximes in water. Ind J Chem 42(9):2045–2047

50. Narsaiah AV, Nagaiah K (2003) An efficient Knoevenagel condensation catalyzed by $LaCl_3$ in heterogeneous medium. Synth Commun 33:3825–3832
51. Narsaiah AV (2007) $LaCl_3$: an efficient catalyst for the silylation of hydroxyl groups by activating HMDS. J Orgnomet Chem 692:3614
52. Lu J, Bai Y, Wang Z, Yang B, Ma H (2000) One-pot synthesis of 3, 4-dihydropyrimidin-2(1*H*)-ones using $LaCl_3$ as a catalyst. Tetrahedran Lett 41:9075–9078

Ultrasound-assisted synthesis of 2,4-thiazolidinedione and rhodanine derivatives catalyzed by task-specific ionic liquid: [TMG][Lac]

Suresh* and Jagir Singh Sandhu

Abstract

Background: Synthesized arylidene derivatives of rhodanine and 2,4-thiazolidiendione have potent pharmacological activities, and these are also key substrates for the preparation of clinically used antidiabetics.

Findings: Some 1,1,3,3-tetramethylguanidine-based task-specific ionic liquids (TSILs) **1a-1e** were prepared and employed to the catalyzed solvent-free Knoevenagel condensation of 2,4-thiazolidinedione **3a** and rhodanine **3b** with a variety of aldehydes.

Conclusions: Best results were obtained with 1,1,3,3-tetramethylguanidine lactate ([TMG][Lac]) **1c**. The TSIL used can be easily recovered and recycled, yielding products **4–5** in excellent yields under ultrasonic environment without the formation of any side products or toxic waste.

Keywords: 2,4-thiazolidinedione, Rhodanine, Knoevenagel condensation, Recyclability, Task-specific ionic liquid

Findings

Background

2,4-thiazolidenedione (TZD) is an attractive scaffold because of its prestigious position in medicinal chemistry as this unit is responsible for numerous pharmacological and biological activities, e.g., antidiabetic [1,2], antidiarrheal [3], anticonvulsant [4], antimicrobial [5], antihistaminic [6], anticancer [7], anti-HIV [8], 15-hydroxyprostaglandin dehydrogenase inhibitors [9], and anti-ischemic [10]. The position of these molecules seems to be most significant as they are a subset of commercially employed non-insulin-dependent diabetes mellitus and insulin-sensitizing agents (Figure 1) such as rosiglitazone, epalrestat, ciglitazone, AD-5061, pioglitazone, and so on.

Several methods have been developed for their condensation with aldehydes as this is a crucial step in the production of the above clinically used drugs (Figure 1), and thus, this condensation is of commercial value. To achieve this end, several production protocols are reported employing several catalysts used such as amines [11], amine derivatives [12], amines salts [13], baker's yeast [14], sodium acetate [15-17], glycine [18,19], KF-Al_2O_3 [20], and ionic liquids [21-25]. Several of these existing protocols for achieving this step have drawbacks like having long reaction times and low yields and leaving toxic residues on aqueous work-up; amine use is also now found to be carcinogenic. In addition, ionic liquids used earlier to accelerate this reaction are not environmentally benign because their preparation involves the harmful chemical intake, that is, volatile solvent and corrosive/toxic reagents [21-25]. Hence, a facile efficient process is still desirable. In search of greener chemical process development, ionic liquids are finding a prominent place [26-30]; herein, we report the first-ever sonically enhanced procedure using the environmentally benign ionic liquid 1,1,3,3-tetramethylguanidine lactate ([TMG][Lac]).

This ionic liquid based on TMGs is stable and easy to prepare in the laboratory, e.g., [TMG][Lac] **1c** is prepared by neutralizing TMG with lactic acid [31]. [TMG][Lac] has already been reported to accelerate important reactions such as Henry reactions, hydrogenation of olefins, hydrogenolysis of glycerol, aldol reaction, and so on [32-38]. Our own interest in ionic liquids (ILs) and in green synthetic transformations [29,30] prompted us to explore the catalytic activities of TMG-based ILs in the synthesis of 2-TZD and rhodanine derivatives. On top of

* Correspondence: jind_suresh7@rediffmail.com
Department of Chemistry, Punjabi University, Patiala, Punjab 147 002, India

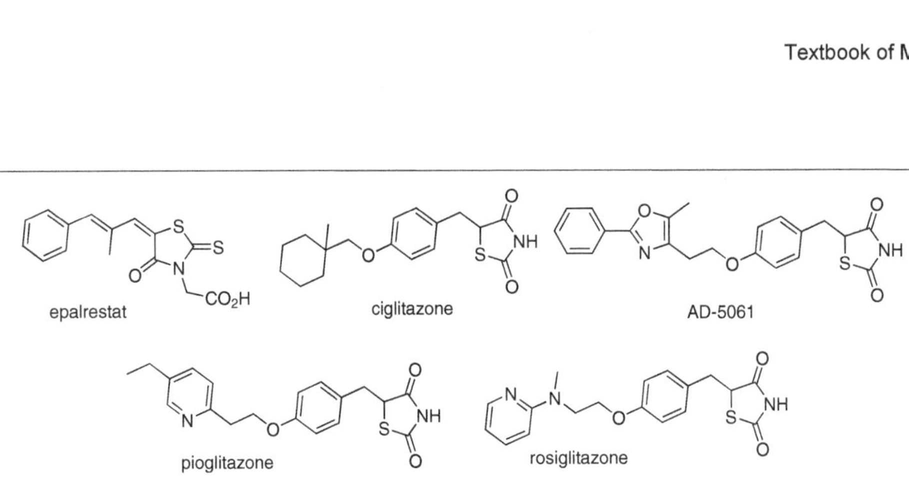

Figure 1 Clinically used molecules having 5-arylidene rhodanines and 2,4-thiazolidenediones.

all these factors, sonication is finding extensive use as it saves time and is environmentally friendly [39-41].

Results and discussion

In our initial pilot experiments, ionic liquids **1a-1e** based on TMGs were used to catalyze condensation of 4-methoxybenzaldehyde **2a** with 2,4-thiazolidinedione **3a** (Table 1). The best results were obtained when the reaction was catalyzed by task-specific ionic liquid (TSIL) [TMG][Lac] **1c** under ultrasound irradiations at 80°C for 20 min (Table 1, entry 3) among the ILs **1a-1e**. The amount of catalyst **1c** was also established as 20 mol% by carrying out reactions of **2a** with **3a** using different amounts of catalyst (5 to 50 mol%).

To check the effect of catalyst, temperature, and ultrasound irradiations, a set of reactions was performed using different reaction conditions such as heating alone (Table 2, entry 2), ultrasound alone (Table 2, entries 6 and 7), heating along with ultrasound irradiations (Table 2, entries 5 to 10), and in the absence of both (Table 2, entry 1). Conclusively, catalyst, temperature, and ultrasound irradiations are all equally important to accelerate the Knoevenagel condensation of arylaldehydes **2** and 2,4-thiazolidenedione/rhodanine **3** to afford 5-arylidene-2,4-thiazolidinediones and 5-arylidenerhodanines **4–5** with excellent yields (Table 2, entry 9).

Further, a variety of carbonyl compounds such as aromatic aldehydes **2a-2b**, heterocyclic aldehydes **2c-2e** (furan-2-carbaldehyde **2c**, thiophene-2-carbaldehyde **2d**, and 3-formylchromone **2e**) were condensed with 5-membered active hydrogen compounds 2,4-thiazolidinedione **3a** and rhodanine **3b** in the presence of 20 mol% **1c** under ultrasound irradiations at 80°C under solvent-free conditions to provide Knoevenagel products **4–5** in excellent yields (Scheme 1). Aromatic aldehydes **2a-2b** afforded excellent yields in a shorter reaction time, whereas heterocyclic **2c-2e** gave high yields in a slightly long reaction time (Table 3).

Active methylene compounds **3a-3b** afforded the Knoevenagel products selectively with exo-double bond without the formation of other side products/bis-products as shown in Scheme 2. Electron-withdrawing and electron-donating groups on aromatic aldehyde showed a slight diversion in the rate of reaction and yields, i.e.,

Table 1 Synthesis of (*Z*)-5-(4-methoxybenzylidene)thiazolidine-2,4-dione 4a via Knoevenagel condensation of 2a with 3a employing different ILs as catalyst

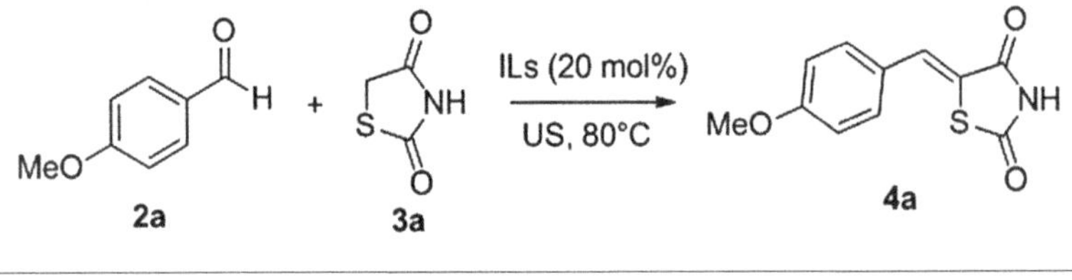

Entry	ILs (20 mol%)	Time (min)	Yield (%)[a]
1	[TMG][CH_3COO^-]: **1a**	50	92
2	[TMG][CF_3COO^-]: **1b**	120	85
3	[TMG][$CH_3CHOHCOO^-$]: **1c**	20	95
4	[TMG][$CH_3CH_2COO^-$]: **1d**	75	91
5	[TMG][$(CH_3)_2CH_2COO^-$]: **1e**	40	94

The reaction conditions for (*Z*)-5-(4-methoxybenzylidene)thiazolidine-2,4-dione **4a** are as follows: **2a** (1 mmol), **3a** (1 mmol), and catalysts (20 mol%) were irradiated under ultrasound irradiations at 80°C. The product was characterized by spectral techniques like IR, ^1H NMR, ^{13}C NMR, and mass spectra. [a]Isolated yields after recrystallization.

Table 2 Condensation of 2a and 3a in the presence of different reaction conditions

Entry	Catalyst	Time (min)	Yield[a]
1	No catalyst + No Heating + No US	180	-
2	No catalyst + Heating (50°C)	180	-
3	Catalyst (20 mol%) + Heating (50°C)	60	<55
4	Catalyst (20 mol%) + Heating (80°C)	60	68
5	No catalyst + Heating (50°C) + US	120	<10
6	Catalyst (20 mol%) + No Heating + US	50	74
7	Catalyst (50 mol%) + No Heating + US	50	72
8	Catalyst (20 mol%) + Heating (50°C) + US	40	80
9	Catalyst (20 mol%) + Heating (80°C) + US	20	95
10	Catalyst (20 mol%) + Heating (100°C) + US	30	92

The different reaction conditions are as follows: **1a** (1 mmol), **2a** (1 mmol), and catalysts were irradiated under ultrasound irradiations (US) at different temperatures. [a]Isolated yield.

the electron-withdrawing group containing aromatic aldehydes afforded arylidene compounds **4–6** with better yields in a shorter reaction time (Table 3).

Next, the recyclability of the catalyst **1c** was studied using **2a** and **3a** as the model substrate. We observed that **1c** could be recovered by extraction of the filtrate with a particular solvent, and pure IL (colorless oil) was obtained after drying the water-rich layer under vacuum. The recovered catalyst was successfully recycled and reused for five runs.

As plausible reaction mechanism is concerned, **1c** catalyzed synthesis of arylidene products **4–5** by facilitating the nucleophilic attack of **3a**-**3b** (lactate anion abstract the active hydrogen of **3**) on the electrophilic carbon of carbonyl compounds (activated by TGA cation) **2a**-**2e**, and subsequent dehydration leads to the product formation (Scheme 2).

Conclusion

In summary, we have disclosed a clean and efficient procedure for the synthesis of pharmacologically significant thiazolidine derivatives via Knoevenagel condensation of aldehydes with 2,4-thiazolidinedione/rhodanine. The task-specific ionic liquid [TMG][Lac] catalyst used is biodegradable, recyclable, and purely environmentally benign as it is easy to prepare, without the involvement of any harmful solvents/chemicals [31]; hence, it is better than already used imidazolium-based ionic liquids [21-25] as catalysts. The scope is fairly large as the range of aldehydes and active methylene compounds used afforded products in very good to excellent yields. Other prominent features are as follows: the reaction time is shorter, no polluting volatile solvents are used, reaction work-up is simple, no toxic by-products are formed during aqueous work-up, and all these green aspects place this method at an advantageous position compared to already reported methods for these molecules of commercial value.

Methods

General

All starting materials were commercial products and were used without further purification except liquid aldehydes, which were distilled before use. Yields refer to yield of the isolated products. Melting points were determined in open capillaries in a paraffin bath and are uncorrected. Nuclear magnetic resonance spectra were obtained on a 400 MHz Bruker AMX instrument (Bruker Corporation, Billerica, MA, USA) in DMSO-d_6 using TMS as a standard. HRMS analyses were carried out using a ESI-Q TOF instrument (Bruker Corporation). Infrared spectra were recorded using a Shimadzu FT-IR-8400 s spectrophotometer (Shimadzu Corporation, Kyoto, Japan) as KBr pellets. All the reactions were studied using a SIDILU Indian-made sonic bath (Sidilu Ultrasonic Technology, Bangalore India) working at 35 kHz (constant frequency, 120 W) maintained at 80°C without mechanical stirring.

General procedure for the synthesis of arylidene-thiazolidenes

A mixture of aldehyde (1 mmol), 2,4-thiazolidinedione/rhodanine (1 mmol), and [TMG][Lac] (20 mol%) was irradiated under ultrasonic irradiation at 80°C for a few

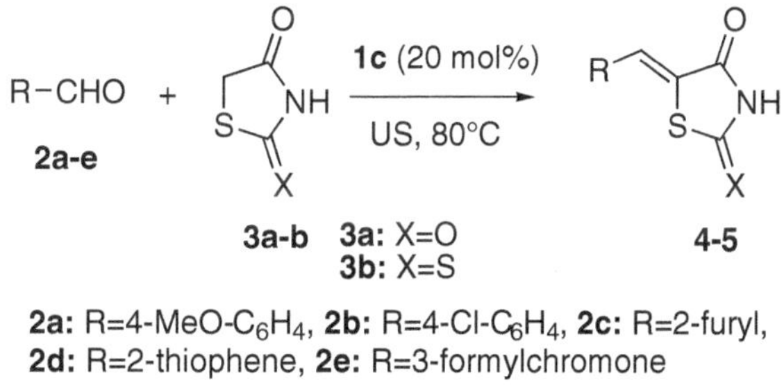

Scheme 1 Knoevenagel reaction of 2 and 3 catalyzed by 1c.

Table 3 [TMG][Lac]-catalyzed solvent-free reactions of thiazolidines 3 with aldehydes 2

Entry	Aldehydes	Thiazolidenes	Product[a]	Time (min)	Yield (%)[b]
1	2a	3a	**4a**	20	95
2	2b	3a	**4b**	15	98
3	2c	3a	**4c**	25	91
4	2d	3a	**4d**	30	92
5	2e	3a	**4e**	20	96
6	2a	3b	**5a**	15	97
7	2b	3b	**5b**	10	99
8	2c	3b	**5c**	20	92
9	2d	3b	**5d**	25	91
10	2e	3b	**5e**	15	98

[a]Reaction conditions: **2a-2e** (1 mmol), **3a-3b** (1 mmol), and **1c** (20 mol%) were irradiated under ultrasound irradiations at 80°C. The products were characterized by spectral techniques like IR, ^{1}H NMR, ^{13}C NMR, and mass spectra. [b]Isolated yields after recrystallization.

minutes (see Table 3). The progress of the reaction was monitored via thin layer chromatography. After the reaction completion, the reaction mass was cooled (15°C to 20°C) and stirred with water (10 mL) for 30 min. The solid product was filtered and dried. The obtained products were recrystallized in EtOH/DMF (3:2). The products **4–5** were confirmed by their spectral data after comparison with authentic samples, infrared (IR), proton nuclear magnetic resonance (1H NMR), mass spectra, and melting points.

General procedure for the recovery of [TMG][Lac]

Further, the obtained filtrate was extracted with diethyl ether (3 × 10 mL), and the aqueous layer was dried under pressure. IL as a colorless oil was obtained which was further reused to catalyze more reactions.

Spectral data of reprehensive compounds

The following are the spectral data for **4a**, **4e**, **5b**, and **5e**:

- (4a): Mp. 249°C to 250°C, IR (KBr, cm^{-1}): 3393, 1671, 1605, 1434, 1201; ^{1}H NMR (300 MHz, DMSO-d$_6$) δ 3.09 (s, 3H), 7.08 (d, 2H, J = 8.2 Hz), 7.52 (d, 2H, J = 8.2 Hz), 7.61 (s, 1H), 13.71 (s, 1H). Analysis calculated for $C_{11}H_9NO_2S_2$: C, 52.57%; H, 3.61%; N, 5.57%; S, 25.52%; found: C, 52.78%; H, 3.95%; N, 5.48%; S, 25.79%
- (4e) Mp.: 259°C to 260°C, IR (KBr, cm^{-1}): 1647 (γ pyrone CO); ^{1}H NMR δ 7.54 (ddd, 1H, 6-H), 7.62 (s, 1H, C = C-H), 7.71 (d, 1H, $J_{8,7}$ = 8.41 Hz, 8-H), 7.98 (ddd, 1H, 7-H), 8.17 (dd, 1H, $J_{5,6}$ = 8.41 Hz, $J_{5,7}$ = 1.68 Hz, 5-H), 8.83 (s, 1H, 2-H), 12.41 (s, 1H, NH). Analysis calculated for $C_{13}H_7NO_3S_2$: C, 53.98%; H, 2.42%; N, 4.84%; S, 22.15%; found: C, 53.84%; H, 2.74%; N, 4.95%; S, 21.96%
- (5b): Mp. 268°C to 269°C. IR (KBr, cm^{-1}): 3148, 1719, 1610; ^{1}H NMR (300 MHz, DMSO-d$_6$) δ_H: 7.53 (2H, m), 7.72 (2H, m), 7.76 (1H, s), 12.65 (1H, bs). Analysis calculated for $C_{10}H_6ClNO_2S$: C, 50.11%; H, 2.52%; N, 5.84%; S, 13.38%; found: C, 49.87%; H, 2.63%; N, 5.92%; S, 13.78%
- (5e) Mp.: 290°C, IR (KBr, cm^{-1}): 1637 (γ pyrone CO); ^{1}H NMR: δ 7.58 (ddd, 1H, 6-H), 7.61 (s, 1H, C = C-H), 7.74 (d, 1H, $J_{8,7}$ = 8.40 Hz, 8-H), 7.88 (ddd, 1H, 7-H), 8.13 (dd, 1H, $J_{5,6}$ = 8.40 Hz, $J_{5,7}$ = 1.60 Hz, 5-H), 8.85 (s, 1H, 2-H), 12.48 (s, 1H, NH). Analysis calculated for $C_{13}H_7NO_4S$: C 57.14%, H 2.58%, N 5.13%, S 11.73%; found: C 56.84%, H 2.74%, N 5.25%, S 11.46%

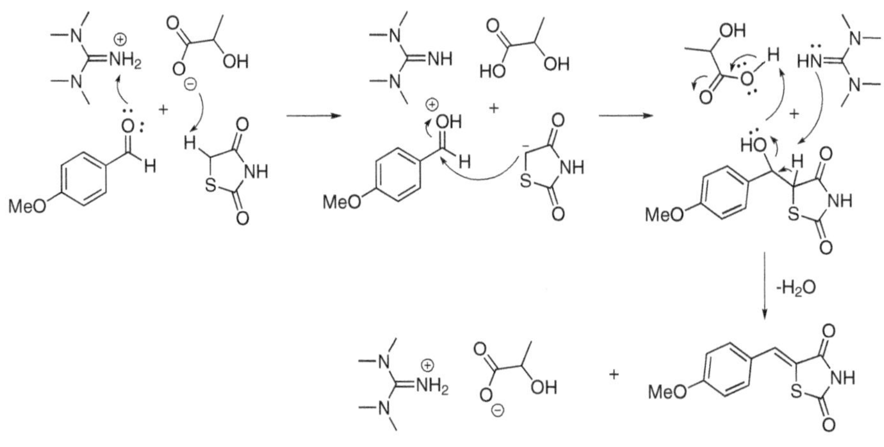

Scheme 2 The possible reaction mechanism for the Knoevenagel reaction catalyzed by TSIL.

Competing interests

The authors declare that they have no competing interests.

Acknowledgments

The authors are also thankful to the Sophisticated Analytical Instrument Facility Central Instrument Laboratory (SAIF-CIL), Panjab University, Chandigarh for the spectral analysis.

References

1. Carroll RT, Dluzen DE, Stinnet H, Awale PS, Funk MO, Geldenhuys WJ (2011) Structure-activity relationship and docking studies of thiazolidinedione-type compounds with monoamine oxidase B. Bioorg Med Chem Lett 21:4798–4803. doi:10.1016/j.bmcl.2011.06.060
2. Bruno G, Costantino L, Curinga C, Maccari R, Monforte F, Nicolò F, Ottanà R, Vigorita MG (2002) Synthesis and aldose reductase inhibitory activity of 5-arylidene-2,4-thiazolidinediones. Bioorg Med Chem 10:1077–1084. http://dx.doi.org/10.1016/S0968-0896(01)00366-2
3. Diurno MV, Mazzoni O, Correale G, Monterrey IG, Calignano A, Rana GL, Bolognese A (1999) Synthesis and structure-activity relationships of 2-(substituted phenyl)-3-3-(*N,N*-dimethylamino)propyl.-1,3-thiazolidin-4-ones acting as H1-histamine antagonists. IL Farmaco 54:579–583. http://dx.doi.org/10.1016/S0014-827X(99)00064-6
4. Ergenc N, Capan G (1994) Synthesis and anticonvulsant activity of new 4-thiazolidone and 4-thiazoline derivatives. IL Farmaco 49:133–135
5. Piscapo E, Diurno MV, Gagliardi R, Mazzoni O (1989) Studies on heterocyclic compounds: 1,3-thiazolidin-4-one derivatives. IV. Biological activity of variously substituted 2,3-diaryl-1,3-thiazolidin-4-ones. Boll Soc Ital Niol Sper 65:853–859
6. Previtera T, Vigorita MG, Bisila M, Orsini F, Benetolla F, Bombieri G () 3,3′-di1,3-thiazolidine-4-one.system. VI: Structural and conformational studies on configurational isomers with antihistaminic activity. Eur J Med Chem 29:317–324. http://dx.doi.org/10.1016/0223-5234(94)90102-3
7. Havrylyuka D, Zimenkovskya B, Lesyka R (2009) Synthesis and anticancer activity of novel nonfused bicyclic thiazolidinone derivatives. Phosphorus, sulfur, and silicon and the related elements. 184:638–650. doi:10.1080/10426500802247563
8. Rawal RK, Prabhakar YS, Katti SB, De Clercq E (2005) 2-(Aryl)-3-furan-2-ylmethyl-thiazolidin-4-ones as selective HIV-RT inhibitors. Bioorg Med Chem 13:6771–6776. http://dx.doi.org/10.1016/j.bmc.2005.07.063
9. Wu Y, Karna S, Choi CH, Tong M, Tai HH, Na DH, Jang CH, Cho H (2011) Synthesis and biological evaluation of novel thiazolidinedione analogues as 15-hydroxyprostaglandin dehydrogenase inhibitors. J Med Chem 54:5260–5264. doi:10.1021/jm200390u
10. Adachi Y, Suzuki Y, Homma N, Fukazawa M, Tamura K, Nishie I, Kuromaru O (1999) The anti-ischemic effects of CP-060S during pacing-induced ischemia in anesthetized dogs. Eur J Pharmacol 367:267–273. http://dx.doi.org/10.1016/S0014-2999(98)00938-8
11. Safonov IG, Heerding DA, Keenan RM, Price AT, Erickson-Muller CL, Hopson CB, Levin JL, Lord KA, Tapley PM (2006) New benzimidazoles as thrombopoietin receptor agonists. Biorg Med Chem Lett 16:1212–1216. http://dx.doi.org/10.1016/j.bmcl.2005.11.096
12. Lohray BB, Bhushan V, Rao PB, Madhavan GR, Murali N, Rao KN, Reddy KA, Rajesh BM, Reddy PG, Chakrabarti R, Rajagopalan R (1997) Novel indole containing thiazolidinedione derivatives as potent euglycemic and hypolipidaemic agents. Bioorg Med Chem Lett 7:785–788. http://dx.doi.org/10.1016/S0960-894X(97)00118-2
13. Zhou JF, Zhu FX, Song YZ, Zhu YL (2006) Synthesis of 5-arylalkylidenerhodanines catalyzed by tetrabutylammonium bromine in water under microwave irradiation. Arkivoc 14:175–180
14. Pratap UR, Jawale DV, Waghmare RA, Lingampalle DL, Mane RA (2011) Synthesis of 5-arylidene-2,4-thiazolidinediones by Knoevenagel condensation catalyzed by baker's yeast. New J Chem 35:49–51. doi:10.1039/C0NJ00691B
15. Powers JP, Piper DE, Li Y, Mayorga V, Anzola J, Chen JM, Jaen JC, Lee G, Liu J, Peterson MG, Tonn GR, Ye QY, Walker NPC, Wang Z (2006) SAR and mode of action of novel non-nucleoside inhibitors of hepatitis C NS5b RNA polymerase. J Med Chem 49:1034–1046. doi:10.1021/jm050859x
16. Wrobleski ML, Reichard GA, Paliwal S, Shah S, Tsui HC, Duffy RA, Lachowicz JE, Morgan CA, Varty GB, Shih NY (2006) Cyclobutane derivatives as potent NK1 selective antagonists. Bioorg Med Chem Lett 16:3859–3863. http://dx.doi.org/10.1016/j.bmcl.2006.04.031
17. Song Y, Connor DT, Doubleday R, Sorenson RJ, Sercel AD, Unangst PC, Roth BD, Gilbertsen RB, Chan K, Schrier DJ, Guglietta A, Bornemeier DA, Dyer RD (1999) Synthesis, structure-activity relationships, and in vivo evaluations of substituted di-tert-butylphenols as a novel class of potent, selective, and orally active cyclooxygenase-2 inhibitors. 1. Thiazolone and oxazolone series. J Med Chem 42:1151–1160. doi:10.1021/jm9805081
18. Chowdhy MM, Michael D, Mingas P, White AJP, William DJ (2000) Syntheses and characterization of 5-substituted hydantoins and thiazolines-implications for crystal engineering of hydrogen bonded assemblies. Crystal structures of 5-(2- pyridylmethylene)hydantoin, 5-(2-pyridylmethylene)-2-thiohydantoin, 5-(2-pyridylmethylene) thiazolidine-2,4-dione, 5-(2-pyridylmethylene) rhodanine and 5-(2-pyridylmethylene) pseudothiohydantoin. J Chem Soc Perkin Trans 1:3495–3504. doi:10.1039/B004312P
19. Yang BY, Yang DH (2011) Solvent-free synthesis of 5-benzylidene-2-thioxothiazolidin-4-ones and thiazolidine-2,4-diones catalysed by glycine under microwave irradiation. J Chem Res 4:238–239. doi:10.3184/174751911X13025104502362
20. Yang DH, Yang BY, Chen BC, Chen SYA (2006) Convenient synthesis of 5-arylidenethiazolidine-2,4-diones on potassium fluoride-aluminium oxide. Org Prep Pro Int 38:81–85. doi:10.1080/00304940609355982
21. Alizadeh A, Khodaei MM, Eshghi A (2010) A solvent-free protocol for the green synthesis of arylalkylidenerhodanines in a task-specific ionic liquid. Can J Chem 88:514–518
22. Jawale DV, Pratap UR, Lingampalle DL, Mane RA (2011) Dicationic ionic liquid mediated synthesis of 5-arylidine-2,4-thiazolidinediones. Chin J Chem 29:942–946. doi:10.1002/cjoc.201190192
23. Gong K, He ZW, Xu Y, Fang D, Liu Z-L (2008) Synthesis of 5-benzylidene rhodanine derivatives catalyzed by 1-butyl-3-methyl imidazolium hydroxide in water. Monatsh Chem 139:913–915. doi:10.1007/s00706-008-0871-y
24. Shelke KF, Sapkal SB, Madje BR, Shingate BB, Shingare MS (2009) Ionic liquid promoted an efficient synthesis of 5-arylidene-2,4-thiazolidinedione. Bull Catal Soc India 8:30–34
25. Yang D-H, Chen Z-C, Chen S-Y, Zheng Q-G (2003) Organic reactions in ionic liquids; ionic liquid-accelerated three-component reaction: a rapid one-pot synthesis of 3-alkyl-5-(Z)-arylmethylidene-1,3-thiazolidine-2,4-diones 1891–1894. Synthesis. doi:10.1055/s-2003-40980
26. Welton T (1999) Room-temperature ionic liquids: solvents for synthesis and catalysis. Chem Rev 99:2071–2084. doi:10.1021/cr980032t
27. Wasserscheid P, Keim W (2000) Ionic liquids—new "Solutions" for transition metal catalysis. Angew Chem Int Ed 39:3772–3789. doi:10.1002/1521-3773(20001103)39:21<3772::AID-ANIE3772>3.0.CO;2-5
28. Dupont J, de Souza RF, Suarez PAZ (2002) Ionic liquid (molten salt) phase organometallic catalysis. Chem Rev 102:3667–3691. doi:10.1021/cr010338r
29. Suresh SJS (2011) Recent advances in ionic liquids: green unconventional solvents of this century Part I. Green Chem Lett Rev 4:289–310. doi:10.1080/17518253.2011.572294
30. Suresh SJS (2011) Recent advances in ionic liquids: Green unconventional solvents of this century Part II. Green Chem Lett Rev 4:311–320. doi:10.1080/17518253.2011.572295
31. Gao H, Han B, Li J, Jiang T, Liu Z, Wu W, Chang Y, Zhang J (2004) Preparation of room-temperature ionic liquids by neutralization of 1,1,3, 3-tetramethylguanidine with acids and their use as media for Mannich reaction. Synth Commun 34:3083–3089. doi:10.1081/SCC-200028532
32. Jiang T, Gao H, Han B, Zhao G, Chang Y, Wu W, Gao L, Yang G (2004) Ionic liquid catalyzed Henry reactions. Tetrahedron Lett 45:2699–2701. doi:10.1016/j.tetlet.2004.01.129
33. Huang J, Jiang T, Gao H, Han B, Liu Z, Wu W, Chang Y, Zhao G (2004) Pd nanoparticles immobilized on molecular sieves by ionic liquids: heterogeneous catalysts for solvent-free hydrogenation. Angew Chem Int Ed 43:1397–1399. doi:10.1002/ange.200352682
34. Jiang T, Zhou Y, Liang S, Liu H, Han B (2009) Hydrogenolysis of glycerol catalyzed by Ru-Cu bimetallic catalysts supported on clay with the aid of ionic liquids. Green Chem 11:1000–1006. doi:10.1039/B901425J
35. Zhu A, Jiang T, Han B, Huang J, Zhang J, Ma X (2006) Study on guanidine-based task-specific ionic liquids as catalysts for direct aldol reactions without solvent. New J Chem 30:736–740. doi:10.1039/B600277C

36. Zhu A, Jiang T, Wang D, Han B, Liu L, Huang J, Zhang J, Sun D (2005) Direct aldol reactions catalyzed by 1,1,3,3-tetramethylguanidine lactate without solvent. Green Chem 7:514–517. doi:10.1039/B501925G
37. Chavan SS, Degani MS (2011) Ionic liquid catalyzed 4,6-disubstituted-3-cyano-2-pyridone synthesis under solvent-free conditions. Catal Lett 141:1693–1697. doi:10.1007/s10562-011-0700-5
38. Liang S, Liu H, Zhou Y, Jiang T, Han B (2010) The tetramethylguanidine-based ionic liquid-catalyzed synthesis of propylene glycol methyl ether. New J Chem 34:2534–2536. doi:10.1039/C0NJ00502A
39. Li JT, Wang SX, Chen GF, Li TS (2005) Some applications of ultrasound irradiation in organic synthesis. Curr Org Synth 2:415–436. doi:10.1002/chin.200541232
40. Cravotto G, Cintas P (2006) Power ultrasound in organic synthesis: moving cavitational chemistry from academia to innovative and large-scale applications. Chem Soc Rev 35:180–196. doi:10.1039/B503848K
41. Cella R, Stefani H (2009) Ultrasound in heterocycles chemistry. Tetrahedron 65:2619–2641. http://dx.doi.org/10.1016/j.tet.2008.12.027

Synthesis and evaluation of antitumor activities of novel chiral 1,2,4-triazole Schiff bases bearing γ-butenolide moiety

Xiang Li[1,3], Xue-Qiang Li[1*], He-Mei Liu[1], Xue-Zhang Zhou[2] and Zhi-Hui Shao[3*]

Abstract

Background: 1,2,4-Triazole derivatives have received much attention due to their versatile biological properties including antibacterial, antifungal, anticonvulsant, antiinflammatory, anticancer, and antiproliferative properties. 1,2,4-Triazole nucleus has been incorporated into a wide variety of therapeutically interesting molecules to transform them into better drugs. Schiff bases of 1,2,4-triazoles have also been found to possess extensive biological activities. On the other hand, γ-substituted butenolide moiety represents a biological important entity that is present in numerous biologically active natural products.

Results: We have described herein the synthesis of 12 hybrid 1,2,4-triazole Schiff bases bearing γ-substituted butenolide moiety. These compounds were synthesized by utilizing the tandem asymmetric Michael addition/elimination reaction as the key step. All the new compounds were evaluated for their *in vitro* anticancer activity.

Conclusions: Tandem asymmetric Michael addition/elimination approach has offered an easy access to new chiral 1,2,4-triazole compounds **7a-7l**. All these chiral 1,2,4-triazole derivatives exhibited good anticancer activities towards Hela. Of all the tested compounds, the chiral compound **7l** with an IC_{50} of 1.8 μM was found to be the most active.

Keywords: 1,2,4-triazole, Schiff base, γ-butenolide, A activity, HeLa cells

Background

Cancer, a diverse group of diseases characterized by the proliferation and spread of abnormal cells, is a major worldwide problem. Therefore, the discovery and development of new potent and selective anticancer drugs are of high importance in modern cancer research.

1,2,4-Triazole derivatives have received much attention due to their versatile biological properties including antibacterial, antifungal, anticonvulsant, antiinflammatory, anticancer, and antiproliferative properties [1-10]. 1,2,4-Triazole nucleus has been incorporated into a wide variety of therapeutically interesting molecules to transform them into better drugs [11-13]. Schiff bases of 1,2,4-triazoles have also been found to possess extensive biological activities [14-18]. On the other hand, γ-substituted butenolide moiety represents a biological important entity that is present in numerous biologically active natural products [19-24].

Recently, we reported on the synthesis of a series of hybrid 1,3,4-thiadiazoles derivatives possessing γ-substituted butenolide moiety, which exhibited good anticancer activities against cervical cancer cells [25]. In continuation of our studies on the identification of potential active antitumor compounds, herein we report the synthesis and evaluation of a new series of hybrid 1,2,4-triazole Schiff bases bearing γ-substituted butenolide moiety as potential anticancer agents (Figure 1). To the best of authors' knowledge, the synthesis and anticancer activities of this types of compounds have not been reported so far.

* Correspondence: lixq@nxu.edu.cn; zhihui_shao@hotmail.com
[1]Key Laboratory of Energy Sources & Chemical Engineering, Development Center of Natural Products and Medication and School of Chemistry and Chemical Engineering, Ningxia University, Yinchuan 750021, China
[3]Key Laboratory of Medicinal Chemistry for Natural Resource (Yunnan University), Ministry of Education, Yunnan University, Kunming 650091, China
Full list of author information is available at the end of the article

Results and discussion

The enantiomerically pure γ-substituted butenolides **1** were synthesized via acetalization of mucobromic acid by employing (−)-menthol and (+)-borneol as a chiral

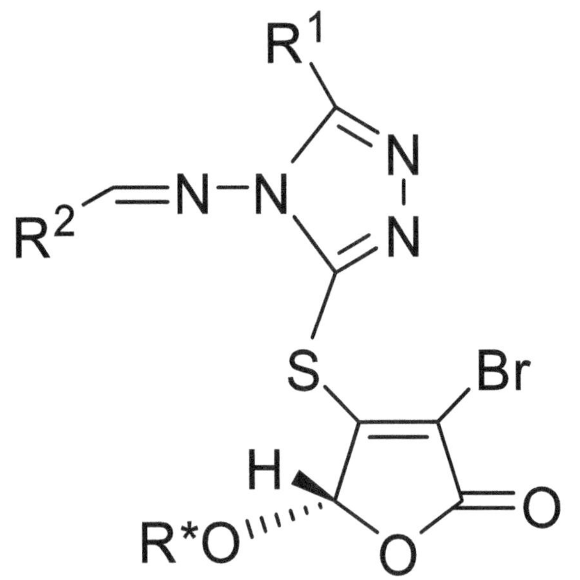

Figure 1 The general structure of target compounds.

auxiliary, respectively, and followed by resolution of the resulting diastereomers [25-27].

The 1,2,4-triazole Schiff bases **6** were synthesized by condensation 4-amino-5-substituted-4*H*-1,2,4-triazol-3-thiols **5** with aromatic aldehydes in glacial acetic acid (Scheme 1) [14]. The 4-amino-5-substituted-4*H*-1,2,4-triazol-3-thiols **5** were prepared according to the previous procedure [28,29]. When R^1 is methyl, the compound **5a** was prepared by heating a mixture of thiocarbohydrazide with acetic acid [28]. When R^1 are aryl, a different procedure was employed as aromatic carboxylic acids are generally solid, have high melting points, and are difficult to react with thiocarbohydrazide fully [29]. Thus, staring from aromatic carboxylic acid esters **2**, the aroyl hydrazides **3** were obtained by reaction with hydrazine in EtOH. Treatment of the aroyl hydrazides **3** with CS_2 under a basic condition (KOH/EtOH) gave the corresponding potassium aroyl dithiocarbazates **4**. Then, the resulting compounds **4** were cyclized with hydrazine to provide the compounds **5b–d** in good yields.

The target compounds **7a–l** were prepared via tandem Michael addition–elimination reaction of γ-substituted butenolides **1** with 5-substituted 1,2,4-triazole Schiff bases **6** under phase-transfer catalysis conditions (Scheme 2).

The structures of these new compounds **7a–l** were characterized with IR, ^{1}H, ^{13}C NMR, and LC-MS spectra. In addition, the molecular structure of **7a** was unambiguously confirmed through X-ray crystallography (Figure 2).[a]

All newly synthesized compounds **7a–l** were initially evaluated for their *in vitro* anticancer activities against cervical cancer cell lines (HeLa) using the MTT assay, and the results were summarized in Table 1. All the compounds **7a–l** displayed good inhibition activities on HeLa cell lines. Of all the studied compounds, the compound **7l** exhibited the best inhibitory activity with an IC_{50} of 1.8 μM.

Then, the growth inhibition rates of HeLa cell lines with compounds **7a–l** at different concentrations (0.1–20 μM) were evaluated (Table 2). After being treated with 20 μg/mL compound **7l** for 24 h, the growth inhibition rate was the highest (90.0%).

Experimental

All the chemicals were used as-received without further purification unless otherwise stated. IR spectra were

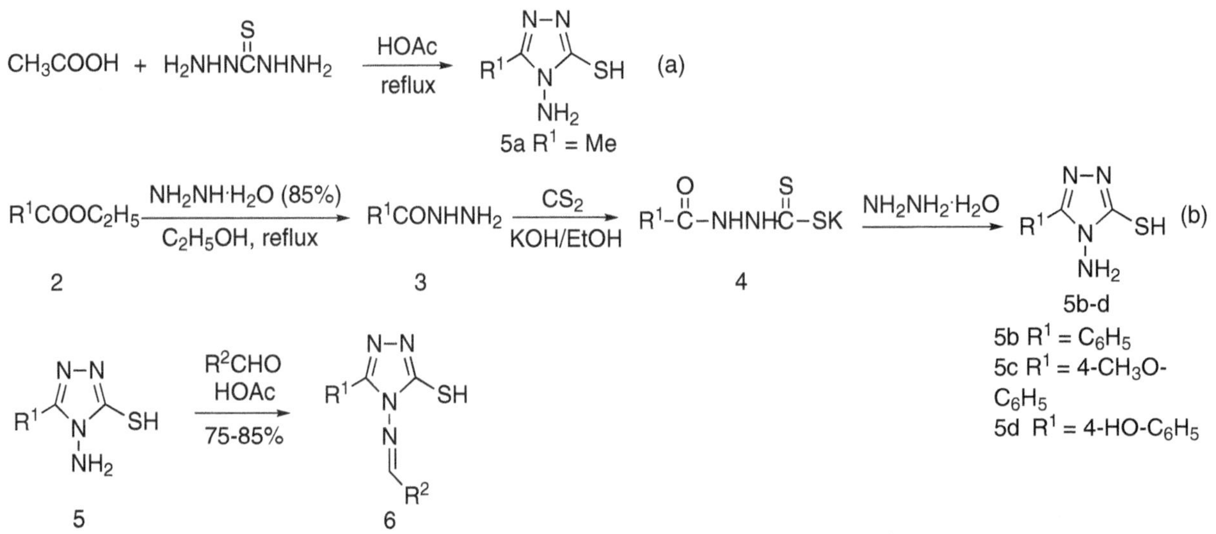

Scheme 1 Synthesis of 1,2,4-triazole Schiff bases 6.

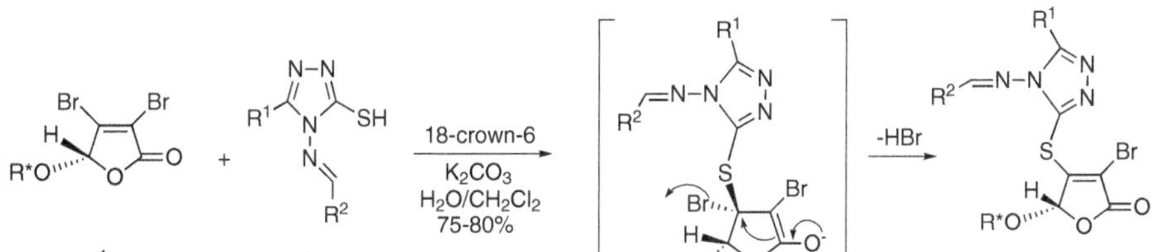

1 6 7

7a	7b	7c	7d
R* = 1-menthyl	R* = 1-menthyl	R* = 1-menthyl	R* = 1-menthyl
$R^1 = C_6H_5$	$R^1 = 4\text{-}CH_3O\text{-}C_6H_5$	$R^1 = C_6H_5$	$R^1 = 4\text{-}CH_3O\text{-}C_6H_5$
$R^2 = 4\text{-Cl-}C_6H_5$	$R^2 = 4\text{-Cl-}C_6H_5$	$R^2 = 4\text{-}O_2N\text{-}C_6H_5$	$R^2 = 4\text{-}O_2N\text{-}C_6H_5$
7e	7f	7g	7h
R* = 1-menthyl	R* = 1-menthyl	R* = 1-menthyl	R* =1-menthyl
$R^1 = C_6H_5$	$R^1 = 4\text{-}CH_3O\text{-}C_6H_5$	$R^1 = CH_3$	$R^1 = 4\text{-HO-}C_6H_5$
R^2 = 2-furanl	R^2 = 2-furanl	$R^2 = 4\text{-Cl-}C_6H_5$	$R^2 = 4\text{-}CH_3O\text{-}C_6H_5$
7i	7j	7k	7l
R* = 1-menthyl	R* = bornyl	R* = bornyl	R* = bornyl
$R^1 = C_6H_5$	$R^1 = C_6H_5$	$R^1 = 4\text{-HO-}C_6H_5$	$R^1 = CH_3$
$R^2 = 4\text{-HO-}C_6H_5$	$R^2 = 4\text{-Cl-}C_6H_5$	$R^2 = 4\text{-}CH_3O\text{-}C_6H_5$	$R^2 = 2\text{-HO-}C_6H_5$

Scheme 2 Synthesis of target compounds 7a–l.

recorded on a FTIR-8400S spectrometer as KBr disks. ^{1}H NMR and ^{13}C NMR spectra were obtained with a Bruker Avance III 400 MHz spectrometer in chloroform-d ($CDCl_3$) and tetramethylsilane was used as an internal standard. Diffraction measurement was made on a Bruker AXS SMART 1000 CCD diffractometer with graphite-monochromatized Mo Kα radiation (λ = 0.71073 Å). All the melting points were determined on a WRS-1B digital melting point apparatus and are uncorrected. Thin-layer chromatography (TLC) was carried out on silica GF254 plates (Qingdao Haiyang Chemical Co., Ltd., China).

General procedure for the synthesis of compounds 7

To an aqueous solution of dichloromethane was sequentially added the compounds **1** (1.0 mmol), potassium carbonate (1.0 mmol), 18-crown-6 (0.1 mmol), and the compounds **6** (1.1 mmol). The resulting mixture was stirred at room temperature, and the reaction was monitored by TLC. On completion of the reaction (10–20 h), the mixture was exacted and the organic layer was washed with saturated brine. Then the organic layer was dried over anhydrous $MgSO_4$, filtered, and concentrated *in vacuo* The purification of the residue by silica gel column chromatography or crystallizations yielded the desired compounds **7a-l** in 65-89% yields (For the characterization of compound **7a-7l**, please see the Additional file 1: Supporting Information). Compound **7 l**: white solid, 76% yield, $[\alpha]_D^{20} = -37.2$ ($c = 0.5$ M, $CHCl_3$). mp 131–132°C. IR (KBr) 3210, 1780, 1603, 1523, 1440, 1421, 1319, 1212, 1134, 993 cm^{-1}. ^{1}H NMR (400 MHz, $CDCl_3$) 10.04 (s, 1H), 8.73 (s, 1H), 7.59-7.04 (m, 2H), 7.14-7.06 (m, 2H), 6.20 (s, 1H), 3.81 (m, 1H), 2.59 (s, 3H), 2.25-2.22 (m, 1H), 1.69-1.09 (m, 6H), 0.78-0.74 (m, 6H), 0.53 (s, 3H). ^{13}C NMR (100 MHz, $CDCl_3$) 170.4, 164.0, 160.3, 152.9, 151.0, 138.2, 136.3, 133.7, 120.6, 118.1, 115.4, 112.8, 103.1, 88.8, 49.3, 47.6, 44.7, 36.7, 27.9, 26.5, 19.5, 18.7, 13.3, 11.2. HRMS calcd. for $C_{24}H_{27}Br N_4O_4S$ $[M]^+$: 546.0936, found 546.0933.

Pharmacology

Cells (1 × 10^4 in 100 μL) were seeded on 96-well plates in triplicate. Following a 24-h culture at 37°C, the medium was replaced with fresh medium at various concentrations (1.25, 2.5, 5, 10, 20 μg/mL) of compounds **7a–l** in a final volume of 110 μL. At the same time, set drug-free medium negative control well, and solvent control well of the same volume of dimethyl sulfoxide (DMSO). Cells were incubated at 37°C for 24 h. Then, 20 μL of 3-(4,5-dimethylthiazol-2-yl)-2,5-diphenyltetrazolium bromide (MTT) (2 mg/mL in a phosphate buffer solution) was added to each well, incubated for an additional 4 h, the plates were centrifuged at 1000 r/min for 10 min, then the medium was removed. MTT formazan precipitates were dissolved in 100 μL of DMSO, shaken mechanically for 10 min and then read immediately at 492 nm in a plate reader (Opsys MR,

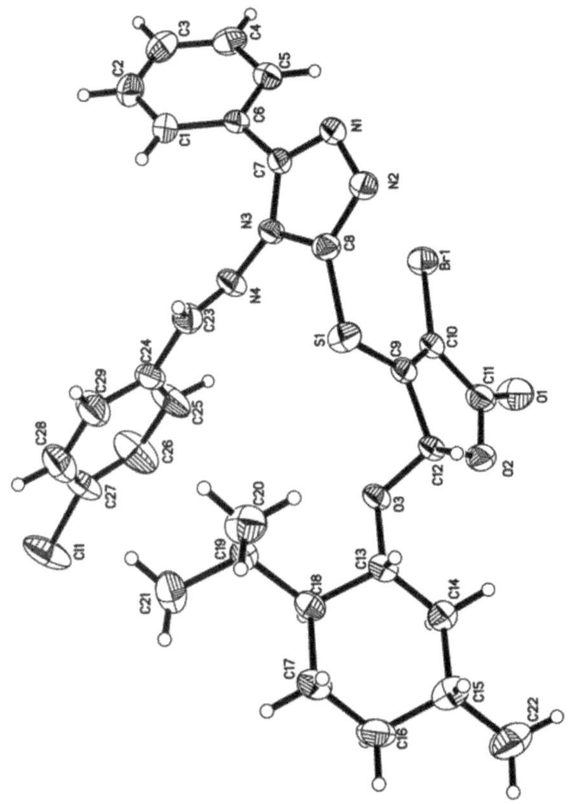

Figure 2 ORTEP view of the crystal structure of compound 7a.

Denex Technology, USA).

$$\text{Cell inhibition rate} = [A_{492}(\text{negative control well}) - A_{492}(\text{dosing well})]/A_{492}(\text{negative control well})\ 100\%.$$

Conclusions

In summary, a new type of chiral 1,2,4-triazole Schiff bases bearing γ-substituted butenolide moiety have been synthesized and their *in vitro* anticancer activities against have been evaluated. These chiral 1,2,4-triazole derivatives exhibited good anticancer activities towards HeLa. The compound **7l** with an IC_{50} of 1.8 μM was found to be the most active. Further studies of anticancer activities of these compounds are in progress in our group.

Table 1 *In vitro* anticancer activities against HeLa cell lines with compounds 7a–l (*n* = 3)

Compound	IC_{50} (μM)	Compound	IC_{50} (μM)
7a	19.7	**7h**	7.1
7b	4.4	**7i**	3.7
7c	11.6	**7j**	4.5
7d	11.2	**7k**	6.2
7e	6.8	**7l**	**1.8**
7f	5.1	DDP (Cisplatin)	2.6
7g	8.2		

The IC_{50} values represent the compound concentration (μM) required to inhibit tumor cell proliferation by 50%.

Table 2 Growth inhibition rates of HeLa cell lines with compounds 7a–l at different concentrations

Compounds	Inhibition rates (%)				
	1.25 μM	**2.5 μM**	**5 μM**	**10 μM**	**20 μM**
7a	1.2	8.7	16.1	30.2	41.9
7b	26.2	30.2	53.8	65.2	85.7
7c	9.4	35.3	21.3	52.3	60.2
7d	17.9	11.0	34.8	47.7	65.5
7e	10.9	11.4	24.3	76.0	85.2
7f	10.3	27.4	56.9	73.4	85.1
7g	18.0	30.9	43.4	49.7	67.1
7h	8.3	14.3	40.7	77.5	71.7
7i	14.3	35.6	67.8	85.4	87.7
7j	24.0	32.5	54.1	67.6	81.2
7k	14.8	36.2	60.0	56.7	67.3
7l	47.5	45.4	74.1	88.6	90.0

Endnote

[a]The molecular structure of the product **7a** was determined by means of X-ray crystallographic studies. CCDC 829447 (**7a**) contains the supplementary crystallographic data for this article. These data can be obtained free of charge from The Cambridge Crystallographic Data Centre via www.ccdc.cam.ac.uk/data_request/cif.

Additional file

Additional file 1: Supporting Information Available. Experimental procedures, spectral data of new compounds.

Competing interests

The authors declare that they have no competing interests.

Authors' contributions

ZS and XL carried out the design of the project, and drafted the manuscript. XL and HL synthesized target compounds. XZ evaluated in vitro anticancer activities against cervical cancer cell lines (HeLa). All authors read and approved the final manuscript.

Supporting information available

Experimental procedures, spectral data of new compounds.

Acknowledgments

We gratefully acknowledge the financial support from the National Natural Science Foundation of China (20962023, 21062014, 21162034), the Major State Basic Research Development Program of China (2007CB21602), the Program for New Century Excellent Talents in University (NCET-10-0907), the Key Project of Chinese Ministry of Education (210237), and the Natural Science Foundation of Ningxia Province of China (NZ0606).

Author details
[1]Key Laboratory of Energy Sources & Chemical Engineering, Development Center of Natural Products and Medication and School of Chemistry and Chemical Engineering, Ningxia University, Yinchuan 750021, China. [2]Key Lab of Ministry of Education for Protection and Utilization of Special Biological Resources in Western China, School of Life Science, Ningxia University, Yinchuan 750021, China. [3]Key Laboratory of Medicinal Chemistry for Natural Resource (Yunnan University), Ministry of Education, Yunnan University, Kunming 650091, China.

References

1. Sztanke K, Tuzimski T, Rzymowska J, Pasternak K, Kandefer-Szerszen M (2008) Synthesis, determination of the lipophilicity, anticancer and antimicrobial properties of some fused 1,2,4-triazolederivatives. Eur J Med Chem 43:404–419
2. Sadana AK, Mirza Y, Aneja KR, Prakash O (2003) Hypervalent iodine mediated synthesis of 1-aryl/hetryl-1,2,4-triazolo[4,3-a]pyridines and 1-aryl/hetryl5-methyl-1,2,4-triazolo[4,3-a]quinolines as antibacterial agents. Eur J Med Chem 38:533–536
3. Amir M, Kumar H, Javed SA (2008) Condensed bridge head nitrogen heterocyclic system: synthesis and pharmacological activities of 1,2,4-triazolo-[3,4-b]-1,3,4-thiadiazole derivatives of ibuprofen and biphenyl-4-yloxyaceticacid. Eur Med Chem 43:2056–2066
4. Turan-Zitouni G, Kaplancıklı ZA, Yıldız MT, Chevallet P, Kaya D (2005) Synthesis and antimicrobial activity of 4-phenyl/cyclohexyl-5-(1-phenoxyethyl)-3-[*N*-(2-thiazolyl)acetamido]thio-4H-1,2,4-triazole derivatives. Eur J Med Chem 40:607–613
5. Mavrova AT, Wesselinova D, Tsenov YA, Denkova P (2009) Synthesis, cytotoxicity and effects of some1,2,4-triazole and 1,3,4-thiadiazole derivatives on immunocompetent cells. Eur J Med Chem 44:63–69
6. Al-Soud YA, Al-Masoudi NA, Ferwanah AE-RS (2003) Synthesis and properties of new substituted 1,2,4-triazoles: potential antitumor agents. Bioorg Med Chem 11:1701–1708
7. Almasirad A, Tabatabai SA, Faizi M, Kebriaeezadeh A, Mehrabi N, Dalvandi A, Shafiee A (2004) Synthesis and anticonvulsant activity of new 2-substituted-5-[2-(2-fluorophenoxy)phenyl]-1,3,4-oxadiazoles and 1,2,4-triazoles. Bioorg Med Chem Lett 14:6057–6059
8. Padmavathi V, Thriveni P, Reddy GS, Deepti D (2008) Synthesis and antimicrobial activity of novel sulfone-linked bis heterocycles. Eur J Med Chem 43:917–924
9. Bhat KS, Poojary B, Prasad DJ, Naik P, Holla BS (2009) Synthesis and antitumor activity studies of some new fused 1,2,4-triazole derivatives carrying 2,4-dichloro-5-fluorophenylmoiety. Eur J Med Chem 44:5066–5070
10. Romagnoli R, Baraldi PG, Cruz-Lopez O, Cara CL, Carrion MD, Brancale A, Hamel E, Chen L, Bortolozzi R, Basso G, Viola G (2010) Synthesis and antitumor activity of 1,5-disubstituted 1,2,4-triazoles as cis-restricted combretastatin analogues. J Med Chem 53:4248–4258
11. Sun S, Lou H, Gao Y, Fan P, Ma B, Ge W, Wang X (2004) Liquid chromatography-tandem mass spectrometric method for the analysis of fluconazole and evaluation of the impact of phenolic compounds on the concentration of fluconazole in *Candida albicans*. J Pharm Biomed Anal 34:1117–1124
12. Clemons M, Coleman RE, Verma S (2004) Aromatase inhibitors in the adjuvant setting: bringing the gold to a standard. Cancer Treat Rev 30:325–332
13. Johnston GAR (2002) Medicinal chemistry and molecular pharmacology of GABAC receptors. Curr Top Med Chem 2:903–913
14. Li Z, Gu Z, Yin K, Zhang R, Deng Q, Xiang J (2009) Synthesis of substituted-phenyl-1,2,4-triazol-3-thione analogues with modified D-glucopyranosyl residues and their antiproliferative activities. Eur J Med Chem 44:4716–4720
15. Holla BS, Veerendra B, Shivananda MK, Poojary B (2003) Synthesis characterization and anticancer activity studies on some Mannich bases derived from 1,2,4-triazoles. Eur J Med Chem 38:759–767
16. Bayrak H, Demirbas A, Karaoglu SA, Demirbas N (2009) Synthesis of some new 1,2,4-triazoles, their Mannich and Schiff bases and evaluation of their antimicrobial activities. Eur J Med Chem 44:1057–1066
17. Bagihalli GB, Avaji PG, Patil SA, Badami PS (2008) Synthesis, spectra characterization, in vitro anti bacterial, antifungal and cytotoxic activities of Co(II), Ni(II) and Cu(II) complexes with 1,2,4-triazole Schiff bases. Eur J Med Chem 43:2639–2649
18. Bekircan O, Bektas H (2006) Synthesis of new bis-1,2,4-triazole derivatives. Molecules 11:469–477
19. Gunasekera SP, McCarthy PJ, Kelly-Borges M, Lobkovsky E, Clardy J (1996) Dysidiolide: a novel protein phosphatase inhibitor from the Caribbean sponge dysidea etheria de laubenfels. J Am Chem Soc 118:8759–8760
20. Avcibasi H, Anil H (1987) Four terpenoids from Cedrus libanotica. Phytochemistry 26:2852–2854
21. Miles DH, Chittawong V, Lho D-S, Payne AM, de La Cruz AA, Gomez ED, Weeks JA, Atwood JL (1991) Novel sesquiterpene lactones from the mangrove plant *Heritiera littoralis*. J Nat Prod 54:286–289
22. Marcos IS, Escola MA, Moro RF, Basabe P, Diez D, Sanz F, Mollinedo F, de la Iglesia-Vicente J, Sierrac BG, Urones JG (2007) Synthesis of novel antitumour alanalogues of dysidiolide from ent-halimicacid. Bioorg Med Chem 15:5719–5737
23. Takahashi M, Dodo K, Sugimoto Y, Aoyagi Y, Yamada Y, Hashimoto Y, Shirai R (2000) Synthesis of the novel analogues of dysidiolide and their structure–activity relationship. Bioorg Med Chem Lett 10:2571–2574
24. Brohm D, Philippe N, Metzger S, Bhargava A, Muller O, Lieb F, Waldmann H (2002) Solid-phase synthesis of dysidiolide-derived protein phosphatase inhibitors. J Am Chem Soc 124:13171–13178
25. Wei M, Feng L, Li X, Zhou X, Shao Z (2009) Synthesis of new chiral 2,5-disubstituted 1,3,4-thiadiazoles possessing gamma-butenolide moiety and preliminary evaluation of *in vitro* anticancer activity. Eur J Med Chem 44:3340–3344
26. van Oeveren A, Jansen JFGA, Feringa BL (1994) Enantioselective synthesis of natural dibenzylbutyrolactone lignans (–)-Enterolactone, (–)-Hinokinin, (–)-Pluviatolide, (–)-Enterodiol, and Furofuran Lignan (–)-Eudesmin via tandem conjugate addition to gamma-alkoxybutenolides. J Org Chem 59:5999–6007
27. Chen Q, Geng Z, Huang B (1995) Synthesis of enantiomerically pure 5-(*l*-menthyloxy)-3,4-dibromo-2(5 H)-furanone and its tandem asymmetric Michael addition–elimination reaction. Tetrahedron Asymmetry 6:401–404
28. Smicius R, Burbuliene MM, Jakubkiene V, Udrwėnaitė E, Vainilavičius P (2007) Convenient way to 5-substituted 4-amino-2,3-dihydro-4H-1,2,4-triazole-3-thiones. J Heterocyclic Chem 44:279–284
29. Reid JR, Heindel ND (1976) Improved synthesis of 5-substituted –4-amino-3-mercapto-4H-1,2,4-triazoles. J Heterocyclic Chem 13:925–926

8

Pharmacophore generation and atom-based 3D-QSAR of *N*-iso-propyl pyrrole-based derivatives as HMG-CoA reductase inhibitors

Mahesh Kumar Teli and Rajanikant G K*

Abstract

Background: Coronary heart disease continues to be the leading cause of mortality and a significant cause of morbidity and account for nearly 30% of all deaths each year worldwide. High levels of cholesterol are an important risk factor for coronary heart disease. The blockage of 3-hydroxy-3-methylglutaryl-coenzyme A (HMG-CoA) reductase activity by small molecule inhibitors has been shown to inhibit hypercholesterolemia. Herein, we describe the development of effective and robust pharmacophore model and the structure–activity relationship studies of 43N-iso-propyl pyrrole-based derivatives previously reported for HMG-CoA reductase inhibition.

Results: A 5-point pharmacophore model was developed and the generated pharmacophore model was used to derive a predictive atom-based 3D quantitative structure–activity relationship analysis (3D-QSAR) model for the studied dataset. The obtained 3D-QSAR model has an excellent correlation coefficient value ($r^2 = 0.96$) along with good statistical significance as shown by high Fisher ratio ($F = 143.2$). The model also exhibited good predictive power confirmed by the high value of cross validated correlation coefficient ($q^2 = 0.672$). Further, pharmacophoric model was employed for virtual screening to identify four potential HMG-CoA reductase inhibitors.

Conclusions: The QSAR model suggests that electron-withdrawing character is crucial for the HMG-CoA reductase inhibitory activity. In addition to the electron-withdrawing character, hydrogen bond--donating groups, hydrophobic and negative ionic groups positively contribute to the HMG-CoA reductase inhibition. These findings provide a set of guidelines for designing compounds with better HMG-CoA reductase inhibitory potential.

Keywords: HMG-CoA reductase, Hypercholesterolemia, *N*-iso-propyl pyrrole-based derivatives, Pharmacophore, 3D-QSAR

Background

High levels of cholesterol are linked to atherosclerosis, which is the accumulation of cholesterol-rich fatty deposits in arteries. This can cause arteries to narrow or become blocked, slowing or stopping the flow of blood to vital organs, especially the heart, brain and kidney [1-5]. When atherosclerosis blocks arteries that supply blood to the brain, it can cause an ischemic stroke. Atherosclerotic heart disease is the leading cause of death, accounting for one-third of all deaths and atherosclerotic interference with blood supply to the brain (ischemic stroke) is the third most common cause of death after cancer [6-9]. The biosynthetic pathway for cholesterol involves more than 25 different enzymes and the major rate-limiting step in this pathway is regulated by the 3-hydroxy- 3-methylglutaryl Coenzyme A (HMG-CoA) reductase. Inhibition of HMG-CoA reductase leads to a decrease in intrahepatic cholesterol concentration [10-14].

In recent years, several successful strategies for the inhibition of cholesterol biosynthesis have effectively been demonstrated in preclinical and clinical settings. For examples, ezetimibe and statins have been approved for the treatment of hypercholesterolemia [15-17]. Up to now, there are still a lot of researches focusing on the development of novel inhibitors of HMG-CoA reductase [16,17]. Recently, a novel series of HMG-CoA reductase inhibitors, which can selectively inhibit HMG-CoA reductase with high inhibitory activities, has been reported by Pfefferkorn et al. [18].

* Correspondence: rajanikant@nitc.ac.in
School of Biotechnology, National Institute of Technology Calicut, Calicut, 673601 Kerala, India

Keeping the therapeutic significance of this class of inhibitors in mind and our continuing interest in the development of HMG-CoA reductase inhibitors, a 3D quantitative structure–activity relationship analysis (3D-QSAR) was proposed on the series of N-iso-propyl pyrrole-based derivatives reported for HMG-CoA reductase inhibitory activity [18]. The compounds reported were used for the purpose of 3D-QSAR modeling since they have a common scaffold and the biological assays have been carried out in the same lab.

3D-QSAR is widely used in the lead optimization stage and provides valuable insights about ligand–protein interactions [19,20]. In order to establish relationship between the spatial 3D pharmacophoric features and HMG-CoA reductase inhibitors activity of a group of N-iso-propyl pyrrole-based derivatives, a 3D-QSAR analysis was carried out on the combined dataset employing PHASE module of Schrodinger molecular modeling software [21].

In this study, we have developed a quantitative pharmacophore model based on HMG-CoA reductase inhibitors collected from the same laboratory [18]. The best quantitative model was used as a 3D search query for screening the ZINC database to identify new inhibitors of HMG-CoA reductase. Once identified, the candidate compounds were subsequently subjected to filtration by molecular docking.

Methods

Dataset

A set of 43N-iso-propyl pyrrole-based derivatives with well-defined HMG-CoA reductase inhibitory activity was used for the QSAR analysis [18]. In vitro inhibitory concentrations (IC_{50}) of the molecules against HMG-CoA reductase were converted into corresponding pIC_{50} [$-\log(IC_{50})$] and were used as dependent variables in the QSAR calculations (Additional file 1).

Molecular modeling

PHASE 3.0 module of Schrodinger molecular modeling software was used to generate pharmacophore models [21]. In QSAR studies, appropriate conformation (lowest energy) of the compound is required for accurate calculation of 3D descriptors. All the 43 compounds were sketched by Maestro. Further, geometry optimization was carried out using the semi-empirical OPLS_2005 force field. All the molecules were divided into a training set and test set to maintain the structure and activity diversity in both the sets for QSAR model and pharmacophore generation and validation.

PHASE incorporates a structure cleaning step utilizing LigPrep, which attaches hydrogens, converts 2D structures to 3D, generates stereoisomers and neutralizes charged structures or determines the most probable ionization state at a user-defined pH. It also allows for the importation of 3D structures prepared outside its own workflow. Because one does not generally know the structure that a given molecule will adopt if and when it binds to a target protein, it is customary to represent each molecule as a series of 3D structures that sample the thermally accessible conformational states. For the purposes of pharmacophore model development, PHASE provides two built-in approaches, both of which employ the MacroModel conformational search engine. Since most of the studied ligands were flexible, all possible conformations for a ligand were generated to consider a range of conformations in order to increase the chances of finding the most active conformer close to the bound structure. Accordingly, the prepared ligands were subjected to conformational analysis using Monte-Carlo Multiple Minimum method implemented in the Schrodinger software.

The ligands were assigned as active and inactive by giving an appropriate activity threshold value. The threshold value was 6 for active legend and 5 for inactive ligand. The activity threshold value was selected on the basis of dataset activity distribution (4.427–6.699) and the active ligands were chosen to derive a set of suitable pharmacophores. The so-prepared ligands were used for generating common pharmacophore and QSAR model building.

Creation of pharmacophore sites

The chemical features of all ligands were defined by six pharmacophorics features: H-bond acceptor (A), H-bond donor (D), hydrophobic group (H), negatively charged group (N), positively charged group (P), and aromatic ring (R). An active analog approach was used to identify common pharmacophore hypotheses (CPHs), in which common pharmacophores were culled from the conformations of the set of active ligands using a tree-based partitioning technique that groups together similar pharmacophores according to their intersite distances [21].

Scoring pharmacophores with respect to active and inactive ligands

The resulting pharmacophores were then scored and ranked. The scoring was done to identify the best candidate hypothesis, which provided an overall ranking of all the hypotheses. The scoring algorithm included the contributions from the alignment of site points and vectors, volume overlap, selectivity, number of ligands matched, relative conformational energy, and activity [22].

Perceiving common pharmacophores

After the careful analysis of the scores and alignment of the active ligands to the generated hypothesis, a best pharmacophore hypothesis AANRR (Figure 1a) was selected for further studies (Table 1). The selected 3D pharmacophore hypothesis (Figure 1b) encompassed the

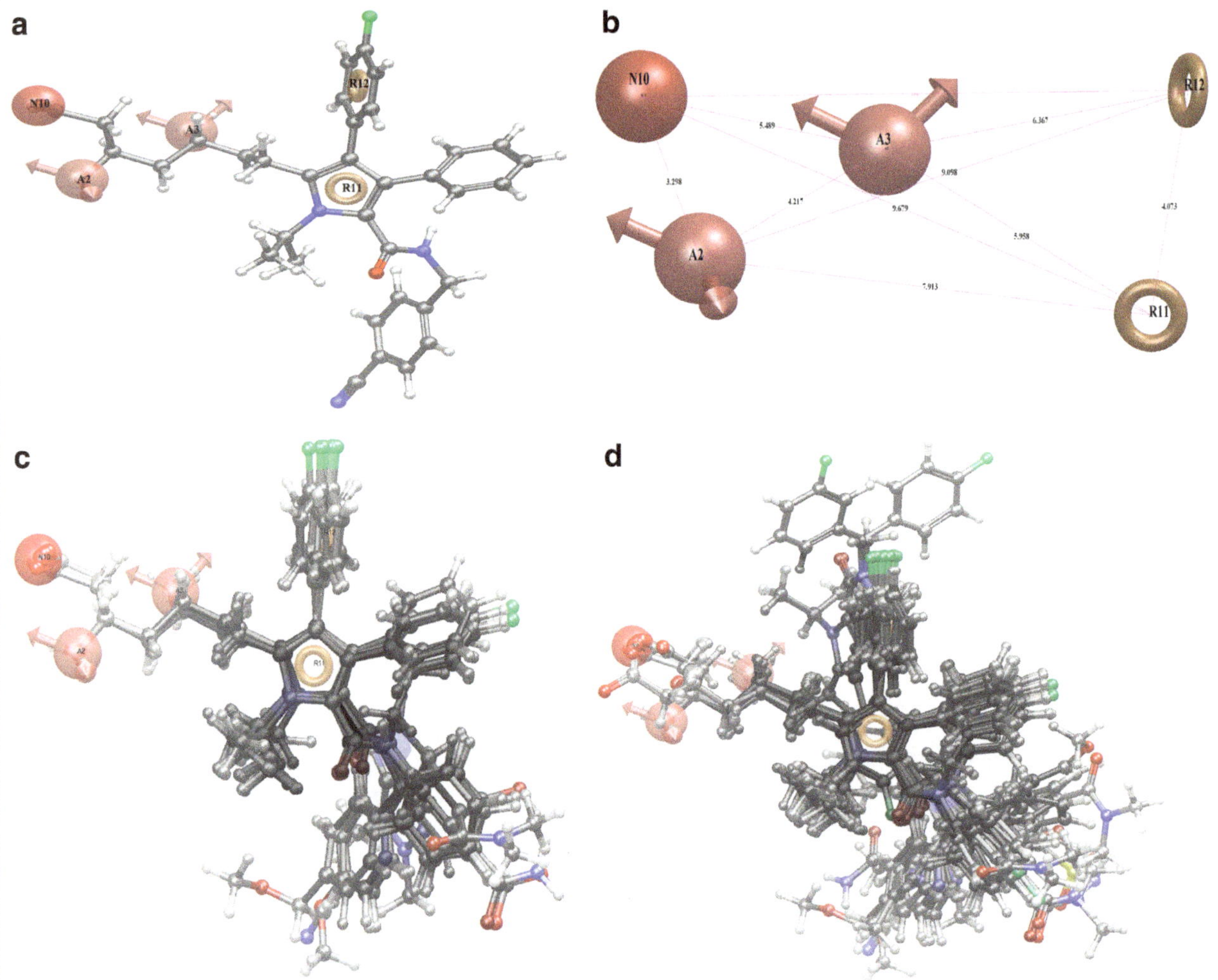

Figure 1 Common pharmacophore generation and validation: (a) Common pharmacophore aligned with most active ligand [two aromatic rings (dark yellow circle)], two acceptor [pink sphere with two arrows], and one negative ionic [pink sphere]; **(b)** common pharmacophoric sites of active ligand with distance. All distances are in Å unit; **(c)** alignment of all active ligands to the pharmacophore; and **(d)** alignment of all ligands (active and inactive) to the pharmacophore.

following features: Two hydrogen bond acceptor (A) (pink sphere with two arrows), one negatively charged group (N) (pink sphere), two aromatic rings (R) (grey circle). The 2D representation (Figure 1a) of the pharmacophore AANRR shows the two hydroxyl groups (pink sphere with two arrows) hydrogen bond acceptor (A), carboxyl group (pink sphere) negatively charged group (N), pyrrole and benzene side chain rings viz. R11 and R12 are as the key pharmacophoric elements present in the selected pharmacophore.

Building 3D-QSAR models

QSAR modeling was carried out using the selected hypothesis by dividing the dataset in to training set (70%) and test set (30%) in a random manner. PHASE presents two options for alignment of 3D structure of molecules: the pharmacophore based alignment and the atom-based alignment [21,23]. In this study, we have used an atom-based QSAR model, which is more useful in explaining the structure–activity relationship. In atom-based QSAR, a molecule is treated as a set of overlapping van der Waal's spheres. Each atom (and hence each sphere) is placed into one of six categories according to a simple set of rules: hydrogens attached to polar atoms are classified as hydrogen bond donors (D); carbons, halogens, and C–H hydrogens are classified as hydrophobic/non-polar (H); atoms with an explicit negative ionic charge are classified as negative ionic (N); atoms with an explicit positive ionic charge are classified as positive ionic (P); non-ionic nitrogen and oxygen are classified as electron-withdrawing (W); and all other types of atoms are classified as miscellaneous (X).

For the purpose of QSAR development, van der Waal's models of the aligned training set molecules were placed

Table 1 Score of different parameters of the AANRR hypothesis

ID	Survival	Survival-inactive	Site	Vector	Volume	Selectivity	Matches	Energy	Activity	Inactive
AANRR	3.603	1.593	0.9	0.967	0.732	2.077	12	4.741	6.097	2.011

in a regular grid of cubes, with each cube allotted zero or more 'bits' to account for different types of atoms in the training set that occupy the cube. This representation gives rise to binary-valued occupation patterns that can be used as independent variables to create partial least-squares (PLS) QSAR models. Atom-based QSAR models were generated for the selected hypothesis using the 31-member training set using a grid spacing of 1.0 Å. The best QSAR model was validated by predicting activities of the 12 test set compounds. A four-component (PLS factor) model with good statistics was obtained for the dataset whereas the maximum number of PLS factors in each model can be 1/5 of the total number of training set molecules. Further increase in the number of PLS factors did not improve the model statistics or predictive ability [19].

Protein preparation

The HMG-CoA reductase (PDB ID: 2R4F) was prepared using the Protein Preparation Wizard of the Schrödinger suite. H-atoms were added to the protein, including the protons necessary to define the correct ionization and tautomeric states of amino acid residues such as Asp, Ser, Glu, Arg, and His. The missing side chains of residues were corrected using Build interface incorporated in Maestro. For each structure, minimization was carried out with the Impact Refinement module, using the OPLS-2005 force field to alleviate steric clashes that may exist in the structures. The minimization was terminated when the energy converged or the Root Mean Square Deviation (RMSD) reached a maximum cutoff of 0.30 Å [24]. After protein preparation, receptor grid was set up, which was generated by employing the Receptor Grid Generation panel. Since this protein was associated with ligand, the ligand was selected to define the position and size of the active site.

Virtual screening

AANRR hypothesis was used to search a 3D database for structures that match the pharmacophoric features of the model. Virtual screening was carried out using ZincPharmer that uses the pharmacophore to efficiently search the ZINC database of fixed conformers for pharmacophore matches [25,26]. To accomplish the best 3D similarity search, we used constraints that included maximum of 0.7 RMSD, obeying 10 rotatable bond cut-off and molecular weight range of 180–500 Dalton. A molecule which fits well with the pharmacophoric features of the AANRR hypothesis was retrieved as a hit.

Docking methodology

All the hits with good RMSD value were enlisted and were incorporated to Maestro. Hits were subjected to hydrogen additions, removal of salt, ionization and generation of low-energy ring conformations using LigPrep. The chiralities of the original compounds were preserved. Finally, the low-energy 3D structures of all compounds were produced. The virtual screening workflow (VSW) in Maestro was used to dock and to score the lead-like compounds. In the first step, Glide was run in high-throughput virtual screen mode. 10% of the top-scoring ligands were kept to go onto the next, Glide Single Precision (SP), stage. The top-scoring 10% leads from GlideSP were retained and docked with Glide XP. All the Glide protocols were run using default parameters. An extensive search was carried out for generating all possible conformations. Minimization cycle for conjugate gradient and steepest descent minimizations were used with default value of 0.05 Å for initial step size and 1.0 Å for maximum step size. In convergence criteria for the minimization, both the energy change criteria and gradient criteria were used with default values of 10^{-7} and 0.001 kcal/mol, respectively. Then, all conformations were considered for docking. During the docking process, the Glide-score was used to select the best conformation for each ligand.

Results and discussion

The aim of this study was to elucidate the 3D structural features of N-iso-propyl pyrrole-based derivatives (Table 2) crucial for binding, by generating 3D pharmacophore and to quantify the structural features of HMG-CoA reductase inhibitors essential for biological activity by generating atom-based 3D QSAR model. For the pharmacophore modeling and QSAR studies, we have used Phase module of Schrodinger suite. This hypothesis generated by Phase will also convey the relative binding of the ligands inside the active site of the receptor. Hence, we have used conformation suggested by the hypothesis for generating 3D-QSAR model to identify overall aspects of molecular structure that govern the activity.

For the generation of pharmacophore model, we have considered 12 compounds having activity > 6 against HMG-CoA reductase as active as they contain important structural features crucial for binding to the receptors binding site. We used four minimum sites and five maximum sites to have optimum combination of sites or features common to the most active compounds. One hundred and two common pharmacophore models were

Table 2 PLS statistical parameters of the selected 3D-QSAR model

ID	PLS factors	SD	R^2	F	P	RMSE	Q^2	Pearson-R
AANRR	1	0.4323	0.5171	31	5.181e-006	0.4018	0.3971	0.6346
	2	0.3191	0.7459	41.1	4.687e-009	0.4157	0.3549	0.676
	3	0.2369	0.865	57.7	7.249e-012	0.3565	0.5255	0.7782
	4	0.1369	0.9566	143.2	2.609e-017	0.2965	0.6719	0.8371

SD, standard deviation of the regression; *R*, squared value of R^2 for the regression; *F*, variance ratio. Large values of *F* indicate a more statistically significant regression, *P*, significance level of variance ratio. Smaller values indicate a greater degree of confidence; RMSE,root-mean-square error, *Q*, squared value of Q^2 for the predicted activities, Pearson-*R*, Pearson *R* value for the correlation between the predicted and observed activity for the test set.

generated with different combination of variants in which all models were considered for further QSAR generation; the results were illustrated in (Additional file 2). Among these pharmacophores, the models which are showing the superior alignment with active compounds were identified by mapping to them and calculating the survival score. The survival scoring function identifies the best candidate hypothesis from the generated models and provides an overall ranking of all the hypotheses. The scoring algorithm includes contributions from the alignment of site points and vectors, volume overlap, selectivity, number of ligands matched, relative conformational energy, and activity. However, these pharmacophore models should also discriminate between the active (most active) and inactive (less active) molecules (Table 1). It is true that the hypothesis is incomplete if it lacks either a critical site that explains the binding or information on what prevents inactive ligands from binding. To identify the pharmacophore models with more active and less inactive features among these models, they were mapped to inactive compounds and scored. If inactive ligands score well, the hypothesis could be invalid because it does not discriminate between active and inactive ligands. Therefore, adjusted survival score was calculated by subtracting the inactive score from survival score of these pharmacophores (Additional file 2). Finally the models with maximum adjusted survival score and lowest relative conformational energy ware selected for generating pharmacophore (atom)-based alignment of HMG-CoA reductase inhibitors and model AANRR has been chosen because it produced good predictive power above other models. The special arrangement of features along with their distance present in five-featured pharmacophore, AANRR, was shown in Figure 1a. As depicted in the figure, among the two ring aromatic features, one feature is mapped to the pyrrole ring of all 12 active inhibitors and another on benzene side chain attached to pyrrole ring. The both hydrogen bond acceptor and negative ionic features are mapped to (the hydroxyl groups and carboxyl group) on N-iso-propyl side chain substituted on pyrrole ring.

For generating an atom-based 3D QSAR hypothesis, we have used a dataset of 31 (training set) compounds having inhibitory activity against HMG-CoA reductase. The model was validated using 12 (test set) compounds, which cover wide range of HMG-CoA reductase inhibitory activity. The alignment generated by the best pharmacophore model AANRR was used for QSAR model generation (Figure 1). Figure 1c presents good alignment of the active ligands and scattered alignment of inactive ligands to the developed pharmacophore model. Alignments of actives and of all inhibitors (active and inactive) are shown in Figure 1c,d, respectively. From Figure 1 we can easily identify that active ligand is having good alignment than inactive one. A four-PLS factor model with good statistics and predictive ability was generated for the dataset (Table 2). The number of PLS factor included in model development is four as incremental increase in the statistical significance and predictivity was observed for each incremental increase in the incorporated PLS factors up to four. The model express 95% variance exhibited by N-iso-propyl pyrrole-based derivatives, which is near to one and signifying a close agreement of fitting points on the regression line for the observed and PHASE-predicted activity that can be visualized from Figure 2 and is summarized in Table 3.

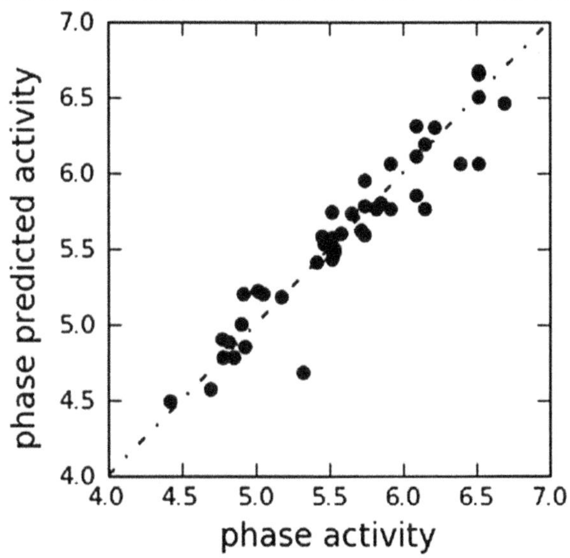

Figure 2 Fitness graph between observed activity versus phase-predicted activity for training and test set compounds.

Table 3 Fitness and predicted activity data for test and training set of compounds

Serial numbers	Ligand name	QSAR set	Activity	PLS factors	Predicted activity	Pharm set	Fitness
1	228583	Training	4.427	4	4.49	Inactive	1.61
2	228954	Training	4.932	4	4.85	Inactive	1.6
3	228955	Training	6.523	4	6.67	Active	2.33
4	249273	Training	5.469	4	5.53		2.85
5	249724	Training	6.097	4	6.31	Active	2.85
6	249884	Training	4.921	4	5.2	Inactive	2.85
7	250088	Training	5.18	4	5.18		1.58
8	250090	Training	4.699	4	4.57	Inactive	1.57
9	250317	Training	6.523	4	6.5	Active	2.32
10	250500	Training	4.824	4	4.88	Inactive	2.36
11	250707	Training	5.42	4	5.41		2.79
12	250749	Training	6.155	4	6.19	Active	2.79
13	250953	Training	5.538	4	5.5		2.29
14	251499	Training	5.921	4	5.76		2.67
15	389216	Training	5.538	4	5.47		2.53
16	389217	Training	4.785	4	4.78	Inactive	2.2
17	389442	Training	5.523	4	5.57		2.55
18	391002	Training	5.523	4	5.43		2.62
19	394937	Training	5.745	4	5.78		2.8
20	398239	Training	5.824	4	5.76		2.87
21	398551	Training	6.222	4	6.3	Active	2.37
22	399313	Training	6.097	4	6.11	Active	2.98
23	399315	Training	5.745	4	5.59		2.19
24	399360	Training	4.907	4	5	Inactive	1.51
25	399771	Training	5.056	4	5.2		2.86
26	400560	Training	5.585	4	5.6		2.89
27	400874	Training	6.699	4	6.46	Active	2.89
28	400973	Training	6.398	4	6.06	Active	2.75
29	401293	Training	5.658	4	5.73		1.5
30	403127	Training	5.854	4	5.8		2.3
31	437774	Training	6.523	4	6.65	Active	2.3
32	228528	Test	5.721	4	5.62		2.53
33	228667	Test	5.018	4	5.22		1.64
34	249906	Test	5.921	4	6.06		2.9
35	387514	Test	5.456	4	5.58		2.4
36	389002	Test	5.745	4	5.95		2.34
37	389441	Test	4.857	4	4.78	Inactive	2.19
38	389443	Test	5.328	4	4.68		1.62
39	398240	Test	6.097	4	5.85	Active	3
40	399773	Test	6.523	4	6.06	Active	2.29
41	400747	Test	6.155	4	5.76	Active	2.78
42	438662	Test	4.777	4	4.9	Inactive	2.22
43	438694	Test	5.523	4	5.74		2.39

A 3D-QSAR analysis was performed on the series of N-iso-propyl pyrrole-based derivatives to understand the effect of spatial arrangement of structural features on their HMG-CoA reductase inhibition. The large value of F (143.2) indicates a statistically significant regression model, which is also supported by the small value of the variance ratio (P), an indication of a high degree of confidence. Further, small values of standard deviation (0.137) of the regression and RMSE (RMSE = 0.296) makes an obvious implication that the data used for model generation are best for the QSAR analysis. Validity of the model can be expressed by cross-validated correlation coefficient ($q^2 = 0.672$) that was obtained by leave one out or leave N out method. The q^2 is more reliable and robust statistical parameter than r^2 because it is obtained by external validation method by dividing the dataset into training and test set.

The atoms visualize 3D characteristics of the ligands (atoms or pharmacophores) as that contribute positively or negatively to activity. The QSAR model displays 3D characteristics (Figure 3) as cubes that represent the model and color according to the sign of their coefficient values, which by default is blue for positive coefficients and red for negative coefficients. Positive coefficients indicate an increase in activity, negative coefficients a decrease. The visualization of the coefficients is useful to identify characteristics of ligand structures that tend to increase or to decrease the activity. This might give a clue to what functional groups are desirable or undesirable at certain positions in a molecule. The blue cubes in 3D plots of the 3D pharmacophore regions refer to ligand regions in which the specific feature is important for better activity, whereas the red cubes demonstrates that particular structural feature or functional group, which is not essential for the activity or likely the reason for decreased binding potency.

Visual analysis of Figure 3a demonstrates that the presence of the blue cubes at the A2, A3, N10 (N-iso-propyl side chain), cyano group, and amide group (carbamoyl side chain) attached to pyrrole ring is pointing out the positive potential of electron withdrawing characteristic of the molecules and is requisite for the activity at this particular place. It can be suggested that addition of appropriate electron withdrawing groups at the A2, A3, cyano, and amide (carbamoyl side chain) sites will append the HMG-CoA reductase inhibition, whereas the addition of electron-withdrawing groups near carboxy group attached to pyrrole ring position will contribute to decreased receptor binding, which in turn will result in lower potency of compounds because red color cubes are for negative effect of electron-withdrawing group to that particular place. Figure 3b illustrates that H-bond donor characteristic is necessary at A2 and A3 (N-iso-propyl side chain) present on the pyrrole ring. The red cubes at the benzene ring attached to the amide side chain of pyrrole ring demonstrate a negative potential of H-bond donor at that position on the compounds. Figure 3c demonstrates the effect of hydrophobic groups on HMG-CoA reductase inhibition. It can be deduced from the figure that hydrophobic groups are well tolerated near cyano benzene ring on carbamoyl side chain (blue cubes), while the substitution of hydrophobic groups in between amide (carbamoyl side chain) and cyano benzene ring site are unacceptable (red cubes) or may hinder the binding of the molecules to the receptor active site and will result in decreased HMG-CoA reductase inhibition. Further, Figure 3d showed combined effect of all the features. The presence of hydroxyl groups (N-iso-propyl side chain), cyano group, and amide group (carbamoyl side chain) will have the positive effect (blue cubes).

Virtual screening

One efficient approach to drug discovery is the virtual screening of the molecular libraries. Pharmacophore-based database searching is considered as a type of ligand-based virtual screening, which can efficiently be used to find novel and potential leads for further development. A potent pharmacophore model possesses the chemical functionalities responsible for bioactivities of potential drugs; therefore, it can be used to perform a database search by serving as a 3D query. The pharmacophore AANRR was used as a 3D structural query for retrieving potent molecules from the ZINC chemical database through ZincPharmer. To avoid possible incorrect predictions, the molecular weight cutoff of 180–500 Dalton range, RMSD of 0.7, and cutoff limit of 10 rotatable bonds filters were applied. Altogether, 3D structural query retrieved 17,283 compounds from the ZINC database.

Drug likeness analysis

The ZINC database was evaluated for drug-likeness of the lead molecules by assessing their physicochemical properties and by applying Lipinski's rule of five. Their molecular weights were <500 Daltons with <5H-bond donors, <10H-bond acceptors and a log p of <5; these properties were well within the acceptable range of the Lipinski rule for drug-like molecules.

These compounds were further evaluated for their drug-like behavior through the analysis of pharmacokinetic parameters required for absorption, distribution, metabolism, and excretion (ADME). For the four lead compounds, the partition coefficient (QPlogPo/w) and water solubility (QPlogS), critical for estimation of absorption and distribution of drugs within the body, ranged between −2 to 6.5 and −6 to −0.5, respectively. Further, the blood brain barrier permeability, which is prerequisite for the entry of drugs to the brain, was

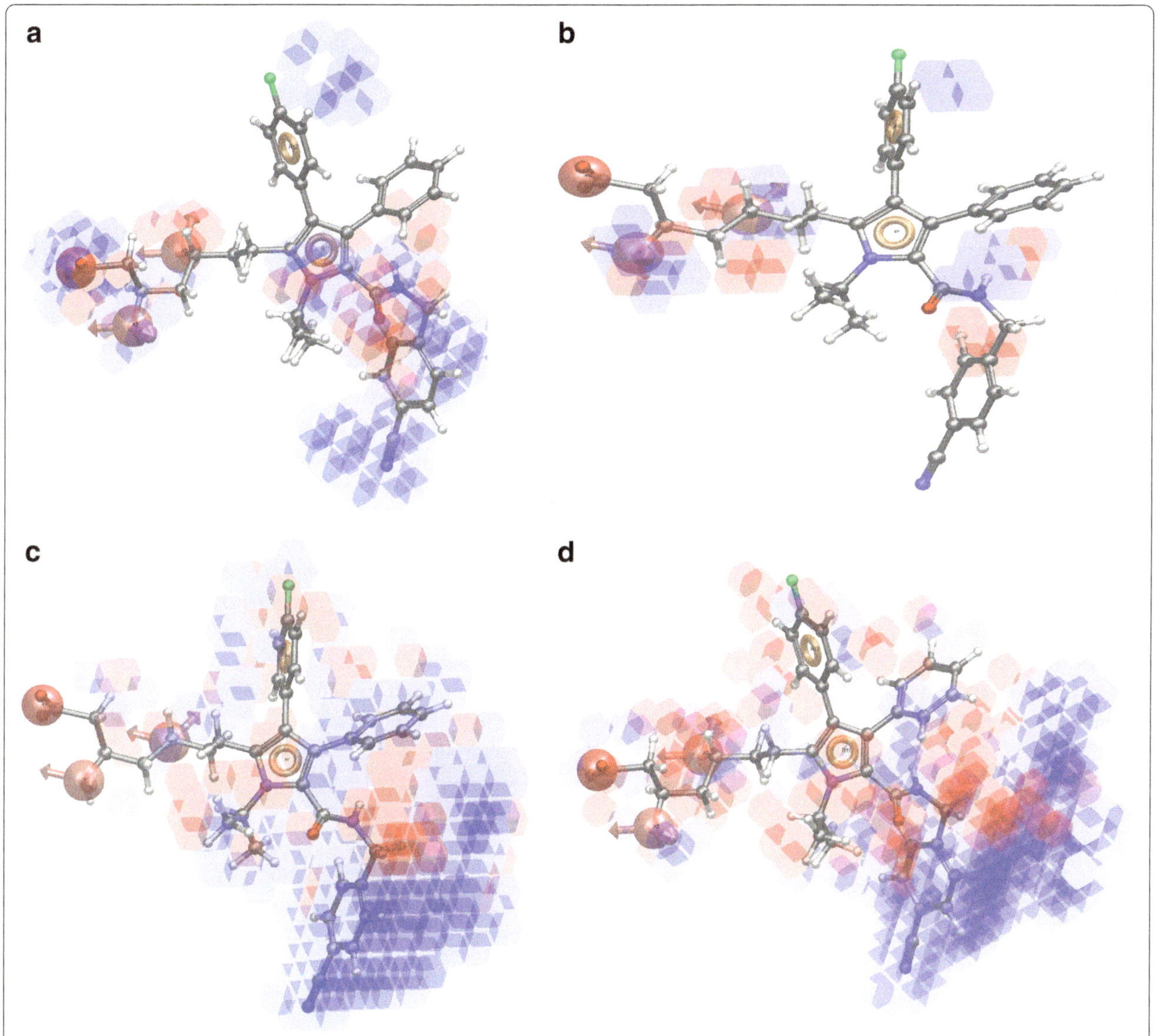

Figure 3 QSAR visualization of various substituents effect: (a) electron withdrawing feature; **(b)** hydrogen-bond donor; **(c)** hydrophobic features; and **(d)** combined effect (blue cubes showing positive potential while red cubes showing negative potential of particular substitution).

found to be in the acceptable range (−3 to 1.2). Overall, the percentage human oral absorption of all four compounds ranged from 30 to 79%. All these pharmacokinetic parameters were within the acceptable range defined for human use, thereby indicating their potential as drug-like molecules (Table 4).

Molecular docking

Docking was carried out to increase the power of the pharmacophore-based screening to discriminate between the active and inactive ligands (that could adopt poses to accomplish the pharmacophore features). The docking was especially useful during the second step of the VS workflow for the identification of molecules having at least one conformer that irrespective of its initial spatial orientation, can fit into the pharmacophore (because docking can be used to exclude those inactive molecules from the VS having at least one conformer, which matches the sites in the pharmacophore but is sterically hindered by other residues in the active site).

To further refine the retrieved candidates, the 17,283 candidates were docked (VSW) into the active site of HMG-CoA reductase and screened through developed QSAR model in order to predict the activities. The binding modes for these compounds identified by docking were ranked according to the information obtained by different scoring constraints. Based on the knowledge of existing HMG-CoA reductase inhibitors, ADME properties, docking score, and the active site requirements, we selected four compounds from highest

Table 4 ADME properties of selected hits with the docking score

ZINC ID	log*Po/w*[a]	log*S*[b]	logHERG[c]	logBB[d]	% Oral absorption[e]	Predicted activity	Docking score
14010678	3.61	−5.58	−3.61	−1.97	57.81	5.7	−9.22
35655503	2.05	−4.10	−2.87	−1.04	70.66	5.52	−9.34
26508465	−0.97	−2.25	−3.06	−2.22	32.50	5.98	−9.16
02554357	3.45	−6.05	−3.93	−0.92	79.57	5.23	−8.95

[a]Predicted octanol/water partition co-efficient log *p* (acceptable range: −2.0 to 6.5).
[b]Predicted aqueous solubility; *S* in mol/L (acceptable range: −6.5 to 0.5).
[c]Predicted IC_{50} value for blockage of HERG K+ channels (acceptable range: below −6.0).
[d]Predicted blood brain barrier permeability(acceptable range: −3 to 1.2).
[e]Percentage of human oral absorption (.25% is poor and .80% is high).

scoring structure. The four candidates were shown to exhibit highest binding affinities and the predicted activity (Table 4). The diversity of the candidates demonstrated that the pharmacophore model was able to retrieve candidates with similar features to the existing HMG-CoA reductase inhibitors as well as novel scaffolds (Figure 4).

Conclusion

A ligand-based pharmacophore model was generated for the series of N-iso-propyl pyrrole-based derivatives with HMG-CoA reductase inhibitory activity to reveal the structural features responsible for biological activity. With the help of pharmacophore-based alignment of HMG-CoA reductase inhibitors, a meaningful 3D-QSAR was derived to identify and how three-dimensional arrangements of various substituents will affect the HMG-CoA reductase inhibition. The selected model as shown by the correlation statistics and predictive statistics is very much significant to draw unambiguous inferences. Further, the generated 3D-QSAR model also explains how and at what extent electron withdrawing, hydrophobic and H-Donor moieties in the molecular structure influences HMG-CoA reductase inhibition showed by the title compounds. The model shows that HMG-CoA reductase inhibition can be increased, if the electron-withdrawing character near N-iso-propyl side chains is supplemented by appropriate functional groups and by the incorporation of H-donor, hydrophobic, and positive ionic groups at specific positions in the molecules. Finally, four potential hits with good fitness value and

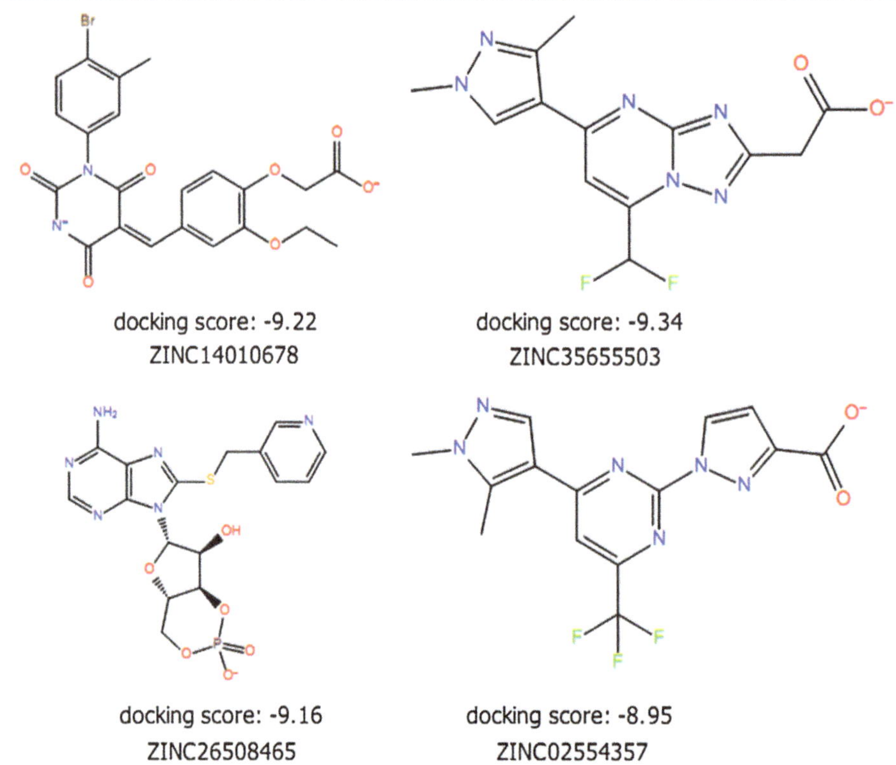

Figure 4 The chemical structures of final hits represented in 2D with docking scores.

predicted activity were identified by virtual screening and docking, whose activity can be further improved with the help of this QSAR model. This study provides a set of guidelines which will greatly help in designing the newer and more potent HMG-CoA reductase inhibitors of the N-iso-propyl pyrrole-based scaffold.

Additional files

Additional file 1: Inhibition data of N-iso-propyl pyrrole-based derivatives.

Additional file 2: Selected pharmacophore models with good survival score.

Competing interests

Both authors declare that they have no competing interests.

Authors' contributions

MKT designed methods and experiments, carried out the *in silico* experiments, analyzed the data, interpreted the results and wrote the paper. RGK was involved in the conception of the idea, drafting the manuscript or revising it critically and has given final approval of the version to be published. All authors have contributed to, seen and approved the manuscript.

References

1. Ballantyne CM, Houri J, Notarbartolo A, Melani L, Lipka LJ, Suresh R, Sun S, LeBeaut AP, Sager PT, Veltri EP (2003) Effect of ezetimibe coadministered with atorvastatin in 628 patients with primary hypercholesterolemia: a prospective, randomized, double-blind trial. Circulation 107:2409–2415
2. Bays HE, Moore PB, Drehobl MA, Rosenblatt S, Toth PD, Dujovne CA, Knopp RH, Lipka LJ, Lebeaut AP, Yang B, Mellars LE, Cuffie-Jackson C, Veltri EP (2001) Effectiveness and tolerability of ezetimibe in patients with primary hypercholesterolemia: pooled analysis of two phase II studies. Clin Ther 23:1209–1230
3. Bergström H, Andersson P (2008) Statins and polyneuropathy. Lakartidningen 105:826–827
4. Clader JW (2004) The discovery of ezetimibe: a view from outside the receptor. J Med Chem 47:1–9
5. Davidson MH, McGarry T, Bettis R, Melani L, Lipka LJ, LeBeaut AP, Suresh R, Sun S, Veltri EP (2002) Ezetimibe coadministered with simvastatin in patients with primary hypercholesterolemia. J Am Coll Cardiol 40:2125–2134
6. Davis HR Jr, Zhu LJ, Hoos LM, Tetzloff G, Maguire M, Liu J, Yao X, Iyer SP, Lam MH, Lund EG, Detmers PA, Graziano MP, Altmann SW (2004) Niemann-Pick C1 Like 1 (NPC1L1) is the intestinal phytosterol and cholesterol transporter and a key modulator of whole-body cholesterol homeostasis. J Biol Chem 279:33586–33592
7. Soliemani A, Nikoueinejad H, Tabatabaizade M, Mianehsaz E, Tamadon M (2011) Effect of hydroxymethylglutaryl-coa reductase inhibitors on low-density lipoprotein cholesterol, interleukin-6, and high-sensitivity C-reactive protein in end-stage renal disease. Iran J Kidney Dis 5:29–33
8. Notarnicola M, Messa C, Refolo MG, Tutino V, Miccolis A, Caruso MG (2010) Synergic effect of eicosapentaenoic acid and lovastatin on gene expression of HMGCoA reductase and LDL receptor in cultured HepG2 cells. Lipids Health Dis 9:135
9. Armitage J, Bowman L, Wallendszus K, Bulbulia R, Rahimi K, Haynes R, Parish S, Peto R, Collins R (2010) Intensive lowering of LDL cholesterol with 80 mg versus 20 mg simvastatin daily in 12,064 survivors of myocardial infarction: a double-blind randomised trial. Study of the effectiveness of additional reductions in cholesterol and homocysteine. Lancet 376:1658–1669
10. Lardizabal JA, Deedwania PC (2010) Benefits of statin therapy and compliance in high risk cardiovascular patients. Vasc Health Risk Manag 6:843–853
11. Gomes ME, Tack CJ, Verheugt FW, Smits P, Lenders JW (2010) Sympathoinhibition by atorvastatin in hypertensive patients. Circ J 74:2622–2626
12. Inadera H, Hamazaki T (2010) Cholesterol controversy: cutoff point of low-density lipoprotein cholesterol level in Guidelines by Japan Atherosclerosis Society. Nippon Eiseigaku Zasshi 65:506–515
13. Koniari IC, Tsamis K, Apostolakis E (2010) Simvastatin inhibits aortic valve calcification in hypercholesterolemic rabbits. Interact Cardiovasc Thorac Surg 11:301–302
14. Ghirlanda G, Oradei A, Manto A, Lippa S, Uccioli L, Caputo S, Greco A, Littarru G (1993) Evidence of plasma CoQ10-lowering effect by HMG-CoA reductase inhibitors: a double-blind, placebo-controlled study. J Clin Pharmacol 33:226–229
15. Grundy SM (1983) Absorption and metabolism of dietary cholesterol. Annu Rev Nutr 3:71–96
16. Knopp RH, Gitter H, Truitt T, Bays H, Manion CV, Lipka LJ, LeBeaut AP, Suresh R, Yang B, Veltri EP (2003) Effects of ezetimibe, a new cholesterol absorption inhibitor, on plasma lipids in patients with primary hypercholesterolemia. Eur Heart J 24:729–741
17. Rajanikant GK, Zemke D, Kassab M, Majid A (2007) The therapeutic potential of statins in neurological disorders. Cur Med Chem 14:103–112
18. Pfefferkorn JA, Song Y, Sun KL, Miller SR, Trivedi BK, Choi C, Sorenson RJ, Bratton LD, Unangst PC, Larsen SD, Poel TJ, Cheng XM, Lee C, Erasga N, Auerbach B, Askew V, Dillon L, Hanselman JC, Lin Z, Lu G, Robertson A, Olsen K, Mertz T, Sekerke C, Pavlovsky A, Harris MS, Bainbridge G, Caspers N, Chen H, Eberstadt M (2007) Design and synthesis of hepatoselective, pyrrole-based HMG-CoA reductase inhibitors. Bioorg Med Chem Lett 17:4538–4544
19. Mahipal TOP, Karthikeyan C, Moorthy NS, Trivedi P (2010) 3D QSAR of aminophenyl benzamide derivatives as histone deacetylase inhibitors. Med Chem 6:277–285
20. Leone S, Mutti C, Kazantsev A, Sturlese M, Moro S, Cattaneo E, Rigamonti D, Contini A (2008) SAR and QSAR study on 2-aminothiazole derivatives, modulators of transcriptional repression in Huntington's disease. Bioorg Med Chem 16:5695–5703
21. Dixon SL, Smondyrev AM, Rao S (2006) PHASE: A Novel Approach to Pharmacophore Modeling and 3D Database Searching. Chem Biol Drug Des 67:370–372
22. Dixon SL, Smondyrev AM, Knoll EH, Rao SN, Shaw DE, Friesner RA (2006) PHASE: a new engine for pharmacophore perception, 3D QSAR model development, and 3D database screening: 1. Methodology and preliminary results. J Comput Aided Mol Des 20:647–671
23. Teli MK, Rajanikant GK (2011) Pharmacophore generation and atom-based 3D-QSAR of novel quinoline-3-carbonitrile derivatives as Tpl2 kinase inhibitors. J Enzyme Inhib Med Chem 26.1–13
24. Teli MK, Rajanikant GK (2012) Identification of novel potential HIF-prolyl hydroxylase inhibitors by in silico screening. Mol Divers 16:193–202
25. Koes DR, Camacho CJ (2011) Pharmer: efficient and exact pharmacophore search. J Chem Inf Model 51:1307–1314
26. Irwin JJ, Shoichet BK (2005) ZINC—a free database of commercially available compounds for virtual screening. J Chem Inf Model 45:177–182

Design and synthesis of tetrahydrophthalimide derivatives as inhibitors of HIV-1 reverse transcriptase

Ashok Penta[1], Swastika Ganguly[2] and Sankaran Murugesan[1*]

Abstract

Background: Non-nucleoside reverse transcriptase inhibitors (NNRTIs) are one of the key components in highly active anti-retroviral therapy because of their high specificity and less toxicity. NNRTIs inhibit reverse transcriptase enzyme by binding to the allosteric site, which is 10Å away from the active site. Rapid emergence of resistance is the major problem with all anti-HIV agents. Hence, there is continuous need to develop novel anti-HIV agents active against both drug sensitive and resistance strains.

Results: All the 16 synthesized 2-(1,3-dioxo-3a,4-dihydro-1*H*-isoindol-2(3*H*,7*H*,7a*H*)-yl)-*N*-(substitutedphenyl) acetamide **4(a-p)** analogs were characterized by Fourier transform infrared spectroscopy, proton nuclear magnetic resonance spectroscopy, mass spectroscopy, and elemental analysis. Lipinski rule of five parameters and molecular parameters like solubility, drug likeness, and drug score were derived for designed analogs using online servers like Molinspiration and Osiris property explorer. Synthesized compounds were evaluated for their HIV-1 reverse transcriptase inhibitor activity by HIV-1 RNA-dependent DNA polymerase activity assay at 2 and 20 μM concentrations.

Conclusions: Among the 16 synthesized compounds, **4a**, **4b**, **4f**, **4g**, **4k**, and **4l** showed weak reverse transcriptase inhibitor activity at 20 μM concentration. For the designed compounds, there was no correlation observed between molecular modeling and *in vitro* studies.

Keywords: NNRTIs; HAART; HIV-1 reverse transcriptase; Docking; Molecular properties; Autodock; Tetrahydrophthalimide

Background

Acquired immune deficiency syndrome (AIDS) is the advance stage of infection caused by the human immunodeficiency virus (HIV-1). AIDS and AIDS-ailed infections are major leading causes of death. According to *UNAIDS*-2012 report, 33 million people are living with AIDS and 1.7 million people died in the year 2011 [1]. Highly active antiretroviral therapy (HAART), a combination of two nucleotide or nucleoside reverse transcriptase inhibitor (NRTIs) and one protease inhibitor (PI), is generally used for AIDS. Alternative combinations like two NRTIs and one non-nucleoside reverse transcriptase inhibitor (NNRTI) or two NRTIs and one integrase inhibitor are used. NNRTIs are the key components in HAART because of their high potency, selectivity, and less toxicity when compared to NRTIs and PIs [2,3]. Currently five NNRTIs are approved by United States Food and Drug Administration. Among them, nevirapine, delavirdine, and efavirenz are first generation, which already got resistance. Etravirine and rilpivirine are potent and currently using second generation NNRTIs. However, the occurrence of the high mutation rate of the virus and the resulting emergence of resistance make the researchers run a never-ending marathon to keep developing new drugs active against both drug-sensitive and drug-resistance strain with better therapeutic profile [4,5].

Many NNRTIs, including tetrahydroimidazo [4,5,1-jkj] [1,4] benzodiazepin-2(1*H*)-one and α-anilinophenyl acetamide derivatives, adapt typical butterfly-like conformations in non-nucleoside inhibitory binding pocket (NNIBP), with

* Correspondence: murugesaa789@gmail.com
[1]Department of Pharmacy, Birla Institute of Technology & Science, Pilani Rajasthan 333031, India
Full list of author information is available at the end of the article

one hydrophilic body and two hydrophobic wings (wing-1 and wing-2). Hydrophilic body contains mainly functional groups like -NH, -C=O, and -OH which are able to form hydrogen bonding interactions with active site amino acids like K101, K103, and P236. Hydrophobic wings are π-electron containing aromatic ring system, which can form hydrophobic interactions and pi-cationic interactions with amino acids Y181, Y188, W229, F227, V106, P236, L100, L234, and Y318 [6,7].

Compounds having phthalimide scaffold exhibit anti-inflammatory [8], anticancer [9], antibacterial [10], HIV-1 RT [11,12], and HIV-1 integrase inhibitory [13] activities. An extensive perusal of literature revealed that little work has been done on phthalimides and tetrahydrophthalimide as NNRTIs. In view of these facts and our interest on the development of novel NNRTIs, we have chosen tetrahydrophthalimide scaffold as one of the hydrophobic wings in butterfly-shape pharmacophore. All the newly synthesized compounds were designed based on the derived pharmacophoric model with acetamide moiety as hydrophilic body, and tetrahydrophthalimide and substituted aromatic amines as hydrophobic wings (general structure shown in Figure 1).

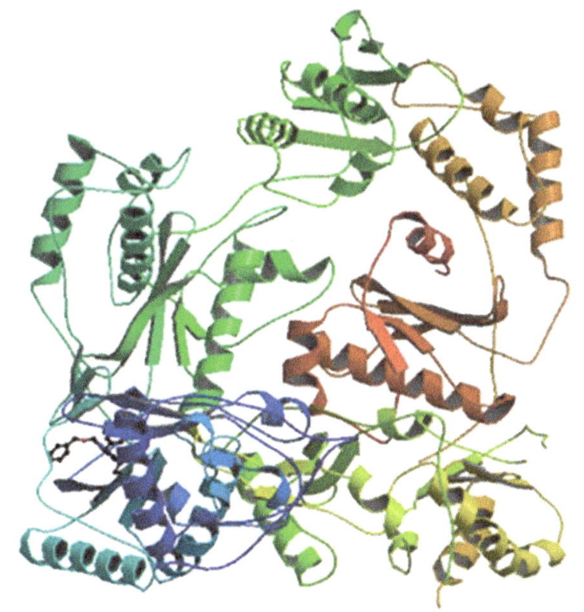

Figure 2 Structure of HIV-1 reverse transcriptase co-crystallized with TNK-651 [14].

Methods

Molecular docking study

The docking studies of all the derivatives **4(a-p)** were performed using molecular modeling software Autodock 4.2 (The Scripps Research Institute, CA, USA) [14] installed on a single machine running on a 3.4-GHz Pentium processor with Windows XP SP2 as the operating system. HIV-1 RT enzyme (pdb code 1rt2 (shown in Figure 2)) was taken from the RCSB, used as target protein [7]. Target protein pdb was further refined by removal of water molecules and by adding polar hydrogens and Kollmancharges. For the docking, a grid spacing of 0.375 Å and 63 × 63 × 63 number of points were used. The grid was centered on the active site. The auto grid program generated separate grid maps for all atom types of the ligand structures and one for electrostatic interactions. PRODRG online server was used to generate the energy minimized conformations of the ligands in pdb format [15]. Energy minimized conformation of ligands was subjected to calculation of Gasteiger-Huckel charges and saved in default format of Autodock. Autodock generated 50 possible binding conformations, i.e., 50 runs for each docking by using LGA search. Default protocol was applied, with initial population of 150 randomly placed individuals, a maximum number of 2.5×10^5 energy evaluations and 2.7×10^4 generations. A mutation rate of 0.02 and a crossover rate of 0.8 were used.

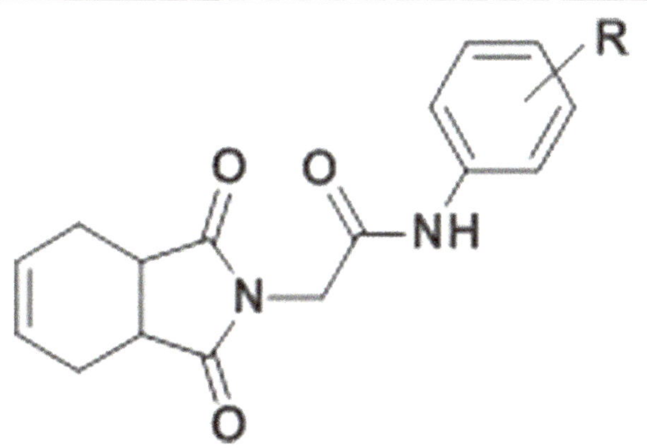

Figure 1 General structure of synthesized compounds.

Validation of docking

Initially, the receptor was docked with extracted ligand TNK 651 in order to validate the docking calculations, reliability, and reproducibility of the docking parameters for the study. It was evident that the docked pose of the re-docked ligand was almost superimposed with that of the co-crystallized ligand (Figure 3) with RMSD value of 0.5. Then, docking was performed with the standard drug efavirenz with 1tr2 for validation, and the mode of interaction was shown in Figure 4.

The binding free energies (docking score) and predicted inhibitory constant (Ki) values of the designed analogs were compared with binding free energies and inhibitory constants of the co-crystallized ligand TNK-651 and standard drug efavirenz. Binding free energies and predicted inhibitory constant values of TNK-651, efavirenz, and designed analogs were given in Table 1. Docking studies of

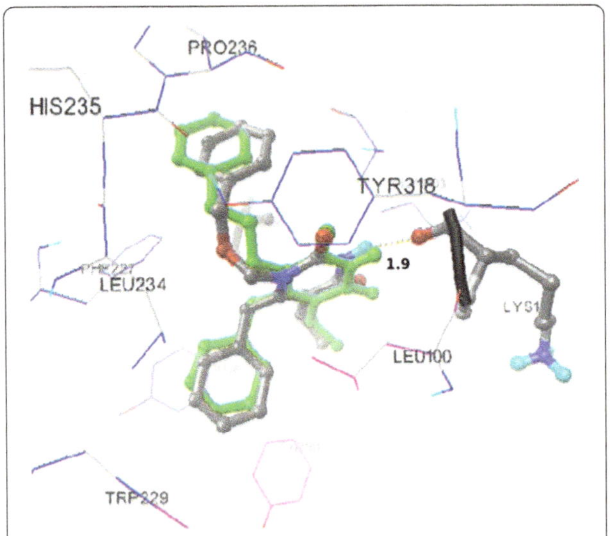

Figure 3 Redocked mode of TNK 651 (3) (green) superimposed with the co-crystallized ligand (gray). Ligand is shown as stick model, and the amino acid residues interacting with the ligands are shown as line model. Hydrogen bond interaction (1.9 Å) with LYS 103 amino acid residue of reverse transcriptase is shown as dotted spheres. The rest of the protein is suppressed for clarification purposes.

designed compounds have shown satisfactory results. Hydrophilic body of designed analogs showed hydrogen bonding interactions with amino acids of receptor protein 1rt2. Hydrogen bonding interactions of compound 4l with LYS 101 and LYS 103 are shown in Figure 5. All the

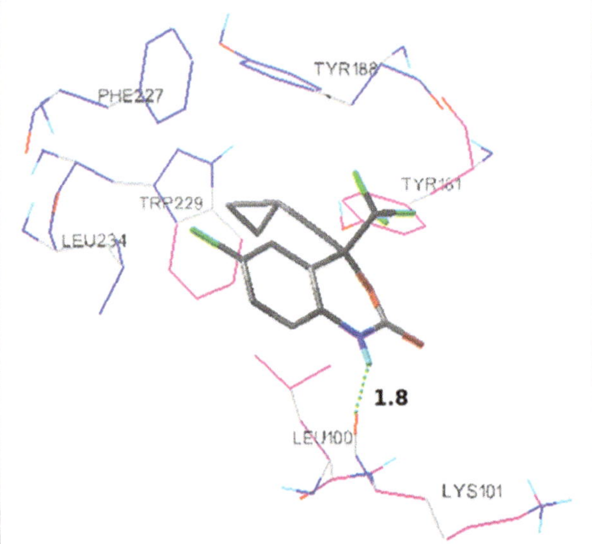

Figure 4 Binding mode of standard drug efavirenz in the NNIBP of HIV-1 RT (1rt2). Ligand is shown as stick model, and the amino acid residues interacting with the ligands are shown as line model. Hydrogen bond interactions (1.8 Å) with LYS 101 amino acid residues of reverse transcriptase respectively are shown as dotted spheres. The rest of the protein is suppressed for clarification purposes.

Table 1 Binding free energy and predicted inhibitory constant values of the synthesized compounds

Serial number	Compound code	*R*	Binding free energy (Kcal/mole)	Inhibitory constant (nM)
1	Efavirenz (standard)	-	−12.02	1.56
2	TNK-651	-	−11.88	1.95
3	4a	H	−8.13	1,100.0
4	4b	4-OCH_3	−7.65	2,460.0
5	4c	4-CH_3	−8.5	588.3
6	4d	4-Cl	−7.79	1,930.0
7	4e	3-OCH_3	−8.62	479.1
8	4f	3-CH_3	−8.61	484.7
9	4g	3-Cl	−8.87	315.7
10	4h	2-OCH_3	−7.94	1,510.0
11	4i	2-CH_3	−8.2	975.83
12	4j	2-Cl	−8.2	975.83
13	*4k*	*4-NO_2*	*−10.53*	*19.11*
14	*4l*	*3-NO_2*	*−10.89*	*10.38*
15	*4m*	*2-NO_2*	*10.46*	*22.86*
16	4n	2,4-diCH_3	−8.87	313.63
17	*4o*	*3,4-diCH_3*	*10.49*	*20.37*
18	*4p*	*2-Cl, 3-CH_3*	*−10.71*	*14.2*

4k, *4l*, *4m*, *4o*, and *4p* showed satisfactory and comparable docking results as that of standard drug efavirenz and TNK-651 (the same thing has been discussed under the subsection "*In vitro* HIV-1 RT inhibitory activity" of the "Results and discussion" section).

designed analogs showed similar orientation in NNIBP of receptor protein. The orientation of some designed compounds (having low binding free energy) in NNIBP of receptor is shown in Figure 6.

Molecular parameters

Lipinski rule of five parameters like ClogP, molecular weight, number of hydrogen bond acceptors (HBA), number of hydrogen bond donors (HBD), solubility, drug likeness, and drug score were derived through online servers Molinspiration (Molinspiration Cheminformatics, Nova Ulica, Slovak Republic) and OSIRIS (Organic Chemistry, Switzerland) property calculator [16,17]. All the calculated values were given in Table 2.

Results and discussion

Chemistry

Designed analogs were synthesized using a synthetic protocol shown in Scheme 1. In the first step, 2-chloro-*N*-(substituted phenyl) acetamide (**2a-p**) analogs were synthesized by treating substituted anilines with 2-chloroacetyl chloride in dichloromethane and triethylamine as base. 2-chloro-*N*-(substituted phenyl) acetamide (**2a-p**) intermediates were then treated with tetrahydrophthalimide (**3**)

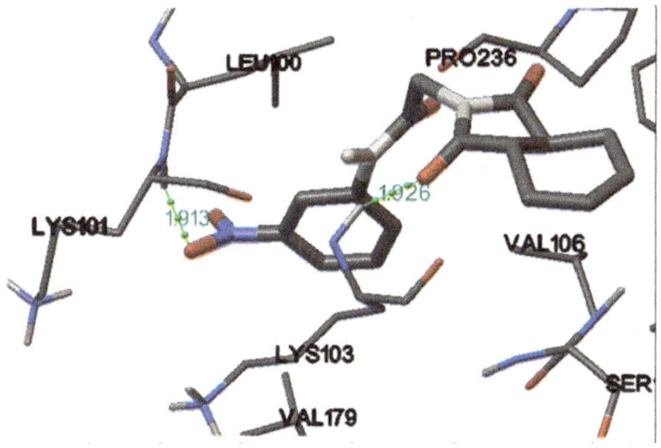

Figure 5 Binding mode of compound 4l in the NNIBP of HIV-1 RT (1rt2). Ligand and the amino acid residues interacting with the ligands are shown as ball-and-sticks model. Hydrogen bond interactions (1.913 Å) with LYS 101 and (1.926 Å) with LYS 103 amino acid residues of reverse transcriptase are shown as dotted spheres. The rest of the protein is suppressed for clarification purposes.

in presence of base potassium carbonate and acetonitrile as solvent to yield titled compounds as final products **4(a-p)** [18,19].

Synthesized compounds were isolated as pure and characterized by IR, ^{1}H NMR, mass, and elemental analysis data. In general, the IR spectra of the synthesized compounds showed N-H stretching at around 3,408 to 3,259 cm^{-1}, C = O (amide) absorption band at around 1,703 to 1,682 cm^{-1}, C = O (phthalimide) absorption band at around 1,786 to 1,768 and 1,712 to 1,702 cm^{-1}, C-O-C absorption (methoxy) band at around 1,249 to 1,234 cm^{-1}, and C-Cl absorption band at around 697 to 678 cm^{-1}. The ^{1}H NMR spectrum of the product **4c** (see 'Experimental' section) showed two characteristic singlets at δ 4.27 and δ 2.30 because of $COCH_2$-N and CH_3, respectively. One broad singlet at δ 7.36 indicates the presence of NH, two doublets at δ 7.32, and δ 7.10 confirms the presence of para-substituted benzene ring. Besides these, the aliphatic region also showed the characteristic multiplet peaks due to CH = CH, CH-CH, and =CH-CH_2 at δ 5.96 to 5.97, δ 3.21 to 3.23,δ 2.63 to 2.69, and δ 2.26 to 2.28, respectively. Mass spectral analysis of the compounds**4a** and **4c** showing the molecular ion peak at 285.6 and 299.6 (M + 1), respectively, confirms the molecular weight of the desired compounds.

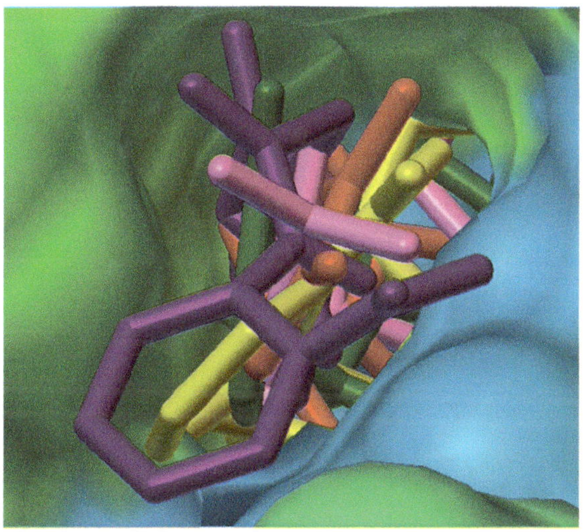

Figure 6 Overlay stereoview. 4k (pink), 4l (yellow), 4m (violet), 4o (red), and 4p (green)in the NNIBP of HIV-1 RT.

In vitro HIV-1 RT inhibitory activity

All the synthesized compounds **4(a-p)** were evaluated for HIV-1 RT inhibitory activity at concentrations 2 and 20 μM by using HIV-1 RT RNA-dependent DNA polymerase activity assay [20]. HIV-1 RT inhibitory activity results are shown in Table 3. Rilpivirine was used as standard drug in the assay.

Among the designed analogs, **4k**, **4l**, **4m**, **4o**, and **4p** showed satisfactory and comparable docking results such as free binding energy and predicted inhibitory constant (Ki) as that of standard drug efavirenz and TNK-651. Docking results encourage us towards their synthesis and *in vitro* RT inhibition evaluation. *In vitro* evaluation of these compounds (**4a**, **4b**, **4f**, **4g**, **4k**, and **4l**) showed weak HIV-1 RT inhibitory activity at 20 μM concentration. In this series of compounds **4a** (2-(1,3-dioxo-3a,4-dihydro-*1H*-isoindol-2(3*H*,7*H*,7aH)-yl)-*N*-phenylacetamide) having un-substituted phenyl ring (mentioned as wing 2 in pharmacophore) showed 25% inhibition of HIV-1 RT at tested concentration of 20 μM. Compound **4f** (2-(1,3-dioxo-3a,4-dihydro-1H-isoindol-2(3*H*,7*H*,7a*H*)-yl)-*N*-m-tolylacetamide), having m-tolyl (3-methylphenyl) group as wing 2, inhibited 20% of HIV-1 RT at 20 μM concentration. However, none of these compounds showed HIV-1 RT inhibition at 2 μM concentration.

Experimental

All solvents and reagents purchased from Sigma (Bangalore, India) or Merck (NJ, USA) companies are used as received without further purification. Solvent system used throughout experimental work for running thin layer chromatography was ethyl acetate and hexane mixture (30:70) in order to monitor the reaction.

Melting points are uncorrected and were determined in open capillary tubes on a Precision Buchi B530 (Flawil, Switzerland) melting point apparatus containing silicon oil. IR spectra were recorded using a Jasco FTIR spectrophotometer (JASCO, Inc., USA). ^{1}H NMR spectra were recorded on a Bruker DPX-400 spectrometer (Bruker India Scientific Pvt. Ltd., Mumbai) using TMS as an internal standard (chemical shifts

Table 2 Predicted molecular parameters of the synthesized compounds

Compound code	CLogP	Molecular weight	Number of HBA	Number of HBD	Solubility	Drug likeness	Drug score
4a	1.10	284	5	1	−2.45	2.29	0.7
4b	1.00	314	6	1	−2.47	2.67	0.34
4c	1.42	298	5	1	−2.79	2.54	0.42
4d	1.72	318	5	1	−3.19	4.71	0.69
4e	1.00	314	6	1	−2.47	3.65	0.43
4f	1.42	298	5	1	−2.79	3.56	0.71
4g	1.72	318	5	1	−3.19	3.93	0.69
4h	1.00	314	6	1	−2.47	4.05	0.72
4i	1.42	298	5	1	−2.79	4.07	0.71
4j	1.72	318	5	1	−3.19	4.17	0.55
4k	0.97	329	8	1	−2.91	−11.4	0.28
4l	0.97	329	8	1	−2.91	−1.34	0.27
4m	0.97	329	8	1	−2.91	−3.08	0.22
4n	1.74	312	5	1	−3.14	0.76	0.47
4o	1.74	312	5	1	−3.14	−0.22	0.32
4p	2.03	332	5	1	−3.53	3.93	0.66

in δ). The ESMS were recorded on MICROMASS Quattro-II LCMS system (Waters Corporation, Milford, USA). Elemental analysis was performed on Vario EL III M/s Elementar C, H, N, and S analyzer (Elementar Analysensysteme GmbH, Germany).

General procedure for synthesis of the compounds *3-(1,3-dioxo-3a,4-dihydro-1H-isoindol-2(3H,7H,7aH)-yl)-N-(substituted phenyl) acetamides 4*

To a solution of 3a,4,7,7a-tetrahydro-1*H*-isoindole-1,3 (2*H*)-dione (**3**) (2 mmol) in acetonitrile, potassium carbonate (6 mmol) and corresponding 2-chloro-*N*-(substituted phenyl) acetamides **2(a-p)** (2 mmol) were added and refluxed for 8 h. On completion of the reaction as monitored by TLC, the contents were poured on crushed ice. Resulted precipitate was filtered, dried, and recrystallized from ethanol to obtain pure product **4**.

2-(1,3-dioxo-3a,4-dihydro-1H-isoindol-2(3H,7H,7aH)-yl)-N-phenylacetamide (4a)

White solid (yield 84%, MP = 96°C to 98°C). IR (KBr, cm^{-1}): 3,271 (N-H), 1,776, and 1,712 (C = O, isoindole), 1,693 (C = O, amide). MS (ES^+): m/z = 285.6 [M + 1]. Analytically calculated for $C_{16}H_{16}N_2O_3$ (%) C, 67.80; H, 5.25; N, 9.60. Found: C, 67.75; H, 5.30; N, 9.55.

2-(1,3-dioxo-3a,4-dihydro-1H-isoindol-2(3H,7H,7aH)-yl)-N-(4-methoxyphenyl)acetamide (4b)

White solid (yield 92%, MP = 102°C to 104°C). IR (KBr, cm^{-1}): 3,305 (N-H), 1,778, and 1,710 (C = O, isoindole),

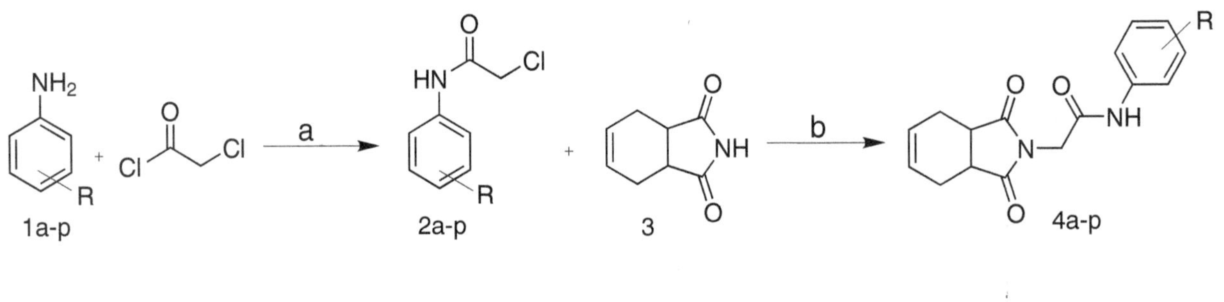

Scheme 1 Designed analogs synthesized using a synthetic protocol. (a) Triethylamine, dichloromethane, room temperature, 30 min; **(b)** K_2CO_3, acetonitrile, reflux, 7 to 8 h.

Table 3 HIV-1 RT inhibitory activity of synthesized compounds

Serial number	Compound code	%RT inhibition	
		2 μM	20 μM
1	4a	NA	25
2	4b	NA	10
3	4c	NA	NA
4	4d	NA	NA
5	4e	NA	NA
6	4f	NA	20
7	4g	NA	15
8	4h	NA	NA
9	4i	NA	NA
10	4j	NA	NA
11	4k	NA	15
12	4l	NA	10
13	4m	NA	NA
14	4n	NA	NA
15	4o	NA	NA
16	4p	NA	NA

NA indicates not active.

1,697 (C = O, amide), 1,249 (C-O-C). Analytically calculated for $C_{17}H_{18}N_2O_4$ (%) C, 64.70; H, 5.55; N, 8.70. Found: C, 64.75; H, 5.50; N, 8.65.

2-(1,3-dioxo-3a,4-dihydro-1H-isoindol-2(3H,7H,7aH)-yl)-N-p-tolylacetamide (4c)

White solid (yield 82%, MP = 100°C to 102°C). IR (KBr, cm^{-1}): 3,408 (N-H), 1,772, and 1,712 (C = O, isoindole), 1,698 (C = O, amide). ^1H NMR(400 MHz, $CDCl_3$) 7.36 (brs, 1H, N*H*), 7.32 (d, *J*= 7.3 Hz, 2H, Ar*H*), 7.10 (d, *J*= 7.1 Hz, 2H, Ar*H*), 5.96 to 5.97 (m, 2H, *CH* = *CH*), 4.27 (s, 2H, *CH*$_2$), 3.21 to 3.23 (m, 2H, *CH-CH*), 2.63 to 2.69 (m, 2H, C*H*H, C*H*H), 2.30 (s, 3H, *CH*$_3$), 2.26 to 2.28 (m, 2H, CH*H*, CH*H*). MS (ES$^+$): m/z = 299.6 [M + 1]. Analytically calculated for $C_{17}H_{18}N_2O_3$ (%) C, 68.60; H, 6.25; N, 9.70. Found: C, 68.65; H, 6.20; N, 9.65.

N-(4-chlorophenyl)-2-(1,3-dioxo-3a,4-dihydro-1H-isoindol-2 (3H,7H,7aH)-yl)acetamide (4d)

White solid (yield 84%, MP = 110°C to 112°C). IR (KBr, cm^{-1}): 3,363 (N-H), 1,768, and 1,706 (C = O, isoindole), 1,698 (C = O, amide), 689 (C-Cl). Analytically calculated for $C_{16}H_{15}ClN_2O_3$ (%) C, 60.35; H, 4.60; N, 8.85. Found: C, 60.40; H, 4.55; N, 8.90.

2-(1,3-dioxo-3a,4-dihydro-1H-isoindol-2(3H,7H,7aH)-yl)-N-(3-methoxyphenyl)acetamide (4e)

White solid (yield 78%, MP = 82°C to 84°C). IR (KBr, cm^{-1}): 3,259 (N-H), 1,774, and 1,712 (C = O, isoindole), 1,703 (C = O, amide), 1,234 (C-O-C). Analytically calculated for $C_{17}H_{18}N_2O_4$ (%) C, 64.80; H, 5.50; N, 8.65. Found: C, 64.75; H, 5.55; N, 8.70.

2-(1,3-dioxo-3a,4-dihydro-1H-isoindol-2(3H,7H,7aH)-yl)-N-m-tolylacetamide (4f)

White solid (yield 76%, MP = 86°C to 88°C). IR (KBr, cm^{-1}): 3,342 (N-H), 1,776, and 1,712 (C = O, isoindole), 1,682 (C = O, amide). Analytically calculated for $C_{17}H_{18}N_2O_3$ (%) C, 68.20; H, 6.35; N, 9.30. Found: C, 68.25; H, 6.30; N, 9.25.

N-(3-chlorophenyl)-2-(1,3-dioxo-3a,4-dihydro-1H-isoindol-2 (3H,7H,7aH)-yl)acetamide (4g)

White solid (yield 78%, MP = 92°C to 94°C). IR (KBr, cm^{-1}): 3,290 (N-H), 1,768, and 1,712 (C = O, isoindole), 1,697 (C = O, amide), 678 (C-Cl). Analytically calculated for $C_{16}H_{15}ClN_2O_3$ (%) C, 60.50; H, 4.20; N, 8.90. Found: C, 60.45; H, 4.15; N, 8.95.

2-(1,3-dioxo-3a,4-dihydro-1H-isoindol-2(3H,7H,7aH)-yl)-N-(2-methoxyphenyl)acetamide (4h)

White solid (yield 76%, MP = 78°C to80°C). IR (KBr, cm^{-1}): 3,345 (N-H), 1,774, and 1,712 (C = O, isoindole), 1,703 (C = O, amide), 1,242(C-O-C). Analytically calculated for $C_{17}H_{18}N_2O_4$ (%) C, 64.75; H, 5.80; N, 8.55. Found: C, 64.80; H, 5.75; N, 8.60.

2-(1,3-dioxo-3a,4-dihydro-1H-isoindol-2(3H,7H,7aH)-yl)-N-o-tolylacetamide (4i)

White solid (yield 74%, MP = 92°C to 94°C). IR (KBr, cm^{-1}). 3,265 (N-H), 1,772, and 1,705 (C = O, isoindole), 1,694 (C = O, amide). Analytically calculated for $C_{17}H_{18}N_2O_3$ (%) C, 68.55; H, 6.25; N, 9.40. Found: C, 68.50; H, 6.30; N, 9.45.

N-(2-chlorophenyl)-2-(1,3-dioxo-3a,4-dihydro-1H-isoindol-2 (3H,7H,7aH)-yl)acetamide (4j)

White solid (yield 76%, MP = 88°C to 90°C). IR (KBr, cm^{-1}): 3,302 (N-H), 1,784, and 1,702 (C = O, isoindole), 1,676 (C = O, amide), 697 (C-Cl). Analytically calculated for $C_{16}H_{15}ClN_2O_3$ (%) C, 60.10; H, 4.50; N, 8.95. Found: C, 60.15; H, 4.45; N, 8.90.

2-(1,3-dioxo-3a,4-dihydro-1H-isoindol-2(3H,7H,7aH)-yl)-N-(4-nitrophenyl)acetamide (4k)

Yellow solid (yield 86%, MP = 125°C to 127°C). IR (KBr, cm^{-1}): 3,325 (N-H), 1,779, and 1,710 (C = O, isoindole), 1,686 (C = O, amide), 1,542, 1,322 (C-NO_2). Analytically calculated for $C_{16}H_{15}N_3O_5$ (%) C, 58.60; H, 4.70; N, 12.55. Found: C, 58.55; H, 4.65; N, 12.60.

2-(1,3-dioxo-3a,4-dihydro-1H-isoindol-2(3H,7H,7aH)-yl)-N-(3-nitrophenyl)acetamide (4l)

Yellow solid (yield 70%, MP = 112°C to 114°C). IR (KBr, cm^{-1}): 3,338 (N-H), 1,774, and 1,712 (C = O, isoindole),

1,693 (C = O, amide), 1,537, 1,327 (C-NO_2). Analytically calculated for $C_{16}H_{15}N_3O_5$ (%) C, 58.45; H, 5.05; N, 12.45. Found: C, 58.50; H, 5.10; N, 12.50.

2-(1,3-dioxo-3a,4-dihydro-1H-isoindol-2(3H,7H,7aH)-yl)-N-(2-nitrophenyl)acetamide (4m)

Yellow solid (yield 64%, MP = 102°C to 104°C). IR (KBr, cm^{-1}): 3,331 (N-H), 1,774, and 1,714 (C = O, isoindole), 1,698 (C = O, amide), 1,531, 1,336 (C-NO_2). Analytically calculated for $C_{16}H_{15}N_3O_5$ (%) C, 58.65; H, 4.80; N, 12.50. Found: C, 58.70; H, 4.85; N, 12.55.

N-(2,4-dimethylphenyl)-2-(1,3-dioxo-3a,4-dihydro-1H-isoindol-2(3H,7H,7aH)-yl)acetamide (4n)

White solid (yield 86%, MP = 106°C to 108°C). IR (KBr, cm^{-1}): 3,284 (N-H), 1,782, and 1,712 (C = O, isoindole), 1,672 (C = O, amide). Analytically calculated for $C_{18}H_{20}N_2O_3$ (%) C, 69.45; H, 6.60; N, 8.75. Found: C, 69.40; H, 6.65; N, 8.70.

N-(3,4-dimethylphenyl)-2-(1,3-dioxo-3a,4-dihydro-1H-isoindol-2(3H,7H,7aH)-yl)acetamide (4o)

White solid (yield 80%, MP = 110°C to 112°C). IR (KBr, cm^{-1}): 3,286 (N-H), 1,778, and 1,708 (C = O, isoindole), 1,697 (C = O, amide). Analytically calculated for $C_{18}H_{20}N_2O_3$ (%) C, 69.65; H, 6.80; N, 8.60. Found: C, 69.60; H, 6.85; N, 8.65.

N-(2-chloro-3-methylphenyl)-2-(1,3-dioxo-3a,4-dihydro-1H-isoindol-2(3H,7H,7aH)-yl)acetamide (4p)

White solid (yield 84%, MP = 118°C to 120°C). IR (KBr, cm^{-1}): 3,356 (N-H), 1,786, and 1,714 (C = O, isoindole), 1,695 (C = O, amide), 694 (C-Cl). Analytically calculated for $C_{17}H_{17}ClN_2O_3$ (%) C, 61.50; H, 5.35; N, 8.65. Found: C, 61.55; H, 5.40; N, 8.70.

HIV-1 RNA-dependent DNA polymerase activity assay

Poly(rA)/oligo(dT) was used as a template for the RNA-dependent DNA polymerase reaction by HIV-1 RT, either wild type or carrying the mutations. For the activity assay, 25 μl final reaction volume contained TDB buffer (50 mM Tris-HCl (pH 8.0), 1 mM dithiothreitol, 0.2 mg/ml bovine serum albumin, 2% glycerol), 10 mM $MgCl_2$, 0.5 mg of poly(rA)/oligo(dT)10:1 (0.3 mM 3′-OH ends), and 10 mM ^{3}[H]-dTTP (1 Ci/mmol), and was introduced into tubes containing aliquots of different enzyme concentrations (5 to 10 nM RT). After incubation at 37°C for indicated time, 20 μL from each reaction tube were spiked on glass fiber filters GF/C and immediately immersed in 5% ice-cold trichloroacetic acid (TCA) (AppliChem GmbH, Darmstadt). Filters were washed three times with 5% TCA and once with ethanol for 5 min, then dried, and finally added with EcoLume scintillation cocktail (ICN, Research Products Division, Costa Mesa, CA, USA) to detect the acid precipitable radioactivity by PerkinElmer Trilux MicroBeta 1450 Counter (Waltham, MA, USA).

Conclusion

All the synthesized 3-(1,3-dioxo-3a,4-dihydro-1*H*-isoindol-2(3*H*,7*H*,7a*H*)-yl)-*N*-(substituted phenyl) acetamide **4(a-p)** analogs were evaluated for HIV-1 reverse transcriptase inhibitor activity.

Among these synthesized compounds, **4a**, **4b**, **4f**, **4g**, **4k**, and **4l** showed weak HIV-1 RT inhibitor activity at 20 μM concentration. There was no correlation observed between molecular modeling and *in vitro* studies for these synthesized compounds.

Abbreviations

AIDS: Acquired immune deficiency syndrome; HIV: Human immunodeficiency virus; RT: Reverse transcriptase; HAART: Highly active anti-retroviral therapy; NRTI: Nucleoside reverse transcriptase inhibitor; NNRTI: Non-nucleoside reverse transcriptase inhibitor; PI: Protease inhibitor; NNIBP: Non-nucleoside inhibitory binding pocket.

Competing interests

The authors declare that they have no competing interests.

Acknowledgements

We thank SAIF, Punjab University for providing NMR spectra and SAIF-CDRI for mass spectra. We greatly acknowledge Nicolas Cremor, Pittsburgh University, USA for HIV-1 RT screening of our compounds. One of the authors, AP, acknowledges the financial support from UGC-BSR, New Delhi in the form of Junior Research Fellowship.

Author details

[1]Department of Pharmacy, Birla Institute of Technology & Science, Pilani Rajasthan 333031, India. [2]Department of Pharmaceutical Sciences, Birla Institute of Technology, Mesra-Jharkhand 835215, India.

References

1. UNAIDS (2012) Report on the global AIDS epidemic 2012. http://www.unaids.org/. Accessed 21 Feb 2013
2. Sun LQ, Zhu L, Qian K, Qin B, Huang L, Chen CH, Lee KH, Xie L (2012) Design, Synthesis and preclinical evaluations of novel 4-substituted 1,5-diarylanilines as potent HIV-1 non-nucleoside reverse transcriptase inhibitor (NNRTI) drug candidates. J Med Chem 55:7219–7229
3. Chong P, Sebahar P, Youngman M, Garrido D, Zhang H, Eugene L, Robert ST, Wang NL, Ferris RG, Edelstein M, Weaver K, Mathis A, Peat A (2012) Rational design of potent non-nucleoside inhibitors of HIV-1 reverse transcriptase. J Med Chem 55:10601–10609
4. Bethune MP (2010) Non-nucleoside reverse transcriptase inhibitors (NNRTIs), their discovery, development and use in the treatment of HIV-1 infection: a review of the last 20 years (1989–2009). Antiviral Res 85:75–90
5. Li D, Zhan P, Clercq ED, Liu X (2012) Strategies for the design of HIV-1 non-nucleoside reverse transcriptase inhibitors: lessons from the development of seven representative paradigms. J Med Chem 55:3595–3613
6. Paul AJ, Janssen PAJ, Lewi PJ, Arnold E, Daeyaert F, Jonge M, Heeres J, Koymans L, Vinkers M, Guillemont J, Pasquier E, Kukla M, Ludovici D, Andries K, Béthune MPD, Pauwels R, Das K, Clark AD, Frenkel YV, Hughes SH, Medaer B, Knaep FD, Bohets H, Clerck FD, Lampo A, Williams P, Stoffels P (2005) In search of a novel anti-HIV drug: multidisciplinary coordination in the discovery of 4-[[4-[[4-[(1E)-2-cyanoethenyl]-2,6-dimethylphenyl]amino]-2-pyrimidinyl]amino] benzonitrile (R278474, rilpivirine). J Med Chem 48:1901–1909
7. Hopkins AL, Ren J, Esnouf RM, Willcox BE, Jones EY, Ross C, Miyasaka T, Walker RT, Tanaka H, Stammers DK, Stuart DI (1996) Complexes of HIV-1 reverse transcriptase with inhibitors of the HEPT series reveal

conformational changes relevant to the design of potent non-nucleoside inhibitors. J Med Chem 39:1589–1600

8. Lima LM, Castro P, Machado AL, Fraga CAM, Lugnier C, Moraesc VLGD, Barreiro EJ (2002) Synthesis and anti-inflammatory activity of phthalimide derivatives, designed as new thalidomide analogues. Bioorg Med Chem 10:3067–3073
9. Dos Santos JL, Lanaro C, Chelucci RC, Gambero S, Bosquesi PL, Reis JS, Lima LM, Cerecetto H, Gonzalez M, Costa FF, Chung MC (2012) Design, synthesis and pharmacological evaluation of novel hybrid compounds to treat sickle cell disease symptoms. Part II: furoxan derivatives. J Med Chem 55:7583–7592
10. Bhambi D, Salvi VK, Bapna A, Pemawat G, Talesara GL (2009) Synthesis and antimicrobial evaluation of some alkoxyphthalimide derivatives of naphthyridine. Indian J Chem 48B:697–704
11. Ranise A, Spallarossa A, Schenone S, Bruno O, Bondavalli F, Vargiu L, Marceddu T, Mura M, Colla PL, Pani A (2003) Design, synthesis, structure-activity relationship and molecular modeling studies of acylthiocarbamates: a novel series of potent non-nucleoside HIV-1 reverse transcriptase inhibitors structurally related to phenethylthiazolylthiourea derivatives. J Med Chem 46:768–781
12. Ranise A, Spallarossa A, Cesarini S, Bondavalli F, Schenone S, Bruno O, Menozzi G, Fossa P, Mosti L, Colla ML, Sanna G, Murreddu M, Collu G, Busonera B, Marongiu ME, Pani A, Colla PL, Loddo R (2005) Structure-based design, parallel synthesis, structure-activity relationship and molecular modeling studies of thiocarbamates, new potent non-nucleoside HIV-1 reverse transcriptase inhibitor isosteres of phenethylthiazolylthiourea derivatives. J Med Chem 48:3858–3873
13. Verschueren WG, Dierynck I, Amssoms KIE, Hu L, Boonants PMJG, Pille GME, Daeyaert FFD, Hertogs K, Surleraux DLNG, Wigerinck PBTP (2005) Design and optimization of tricyclic phthalimide analogues as novel inhibitors of HIV-1 integrase. J Med Chem 48:1930–1940
14. Lindstrom W, Morris GM, Weber C, Huey R (2008) AutoDock 4.2. The Scripps Research Institute, Molecular Graphics Laboratory, California, USA. http://autodock.scripps.edu. Accessed 21 Feb 2013
15. Schuettelkopf AW, Aalten DMFV (2004) PRODRG: a tool for high-throughput crystallography of protein-ligand complexes. Acta Crystallogrphica D60:1355–1363
16. Molinspiration Cheminformatics (1986) Molinspiration. http://www.molinspiration.com/cgi-bin/properties. Accessed 22 Feb 2013
17. Organic Chemistry Portal ( ) Molecular property explorer, OSIRIS. http://www.organic-chemistry.org/prog/peo. Accessed 23 Feb 2013
18. Ganguly S, Murugesan S, Maga G (2009) Synthesis, evaluation and molecular modeling studies of some novel tetrahydroisoquinoline derivatives targeted at the HIV-1 reverse transcriptase. Indian J Heterocycl Chem 18:357–360
19. Murugesan S, Ganguly S, Maga G (2010) Synthesis, evaluation and molecular modeling studies of some novel 3-(3,4-dihydroisoquinolin-2(*1H*)-yl)-*N*-(substituted phenyl) propanamides as HIV-1 non-nucleoside reverse transcriptase inhibitors. J Chem Sci 122:169–176
20. Cremer NS, Hamamouch N, Felix AS, Velazquez S, Balzarini J, Camarasa MJ (2006) Structure activity relationship of [2′,5′-bis-O-(tert-butyl dimethyl silyl)-β-D-ribofuranosyl]-3′-spiro-5-(4-amino-1,2-oxathiole-2,2-dioxide) thymine derivatives as inhibitors of HIV-1 reverse transcriptase dimerization. J Med Chem 49:4834–4841

Novel indole-bearing combretastatin analogues as tubulin polymerization inhibitors

Sunil Kumar[1*], Samir Mehndiratta[1], Kunal Nepali[1], Manish K Gupta[1], Surrinder Koul[2], Parduman R Sharma[2], Ajit K Saxena[2] and Kanaya L Dhar[1]

Abstract

Background: The combretastatins are a class of natural stilbenoids. These molecules generally share three common structural features: a trimethoxy "A"-ring, a "B"-ring containing substituent often at C3′ and C4′, and an ethene bridge between the two rings, which provides necessary structural rigidity. Members of the combretastatin family possess varying ability to cause vascular disruption in tumors. Combretastatin binds to the colchicine binding site of β-subunit of tubulin. Despite having a similar name, combretastatin is unrelated to statins, a family of cholesterol-lowering drugs.

Results: New combretastatin 2-(1-acetyl-1*H*-indole-3-yl)-3-(phenyl) propenoic analogues (**2a** to **2y**), bearing indole moiety at the place of ring A of combretastatin (CA4), were synthesized and evaluated for anticancer activity against various cancer cell lines such as THP-1 (leukemia), A-549 (lung), IGROV-1 (ovary), HEP-2 (liver), MCF-7 (breast), and DU-145 (prostate). Compound **2d** showed anti-cancer activity against THP-1 and MCF-7 with IC_{50} 0.80 and 0.37 μM, respectively, and **2y** showed against MCF-7 with IC_{50} 3.60 μM comparable to paclitaxel.

Conclusions: The target compounds bind to the colchicine binding site which is situated at α and β interface of tubulin and prevent polymerization as it was confirmed by immunofluorescence technique. The molecular docking further confirmed the binding of the potent compound **2d** to the colchicine binding site at α and β interface of tubulin.

Keywords: Colchicine binding site, Indole-based combretastatin, Molecular docking, Tubulin inhibitors

Background

Tubulin is a useful biochemical target for various clinically used anticancer drugs like paclitaxel, vincristine, and vinblastine (Figure 1) [1]. It plays an important role in the formation of the mitotic spindle which provides the structural framework for the physical segregation of the chromosomes during the mitosis [2]. Microtubules, made from tubulin are highly dynamic cytoskeleton elements in eukaryotic cells and play a critical role in various processes like mitosis, cell shape, intracellular organelle, transport and cell-cell interactions, and signal transduction [3,4]. They have highly polar structure and favor growth at the plus (+) end and shrinkage at the minus (−) end. This dynamic equilibrium can be affected by treatment with some agents like phenstatin, chalcone, lignan, colchicine, and podophyllotoxin ultimately prevent mitosis, thus used for cancer treatment [5,6]. Drugs which target tubulin interact with mitotic spindle and act by binding to the following binding sites: (1) colchicine binding site, (2) vinca alkaloid binding site, (3) rhizoxin/maytansine binding site, (4) tubulin sulfhydryl binding site, and (5) unknown binding sites [1]. Taxol binds to the β-tubulin of colchicine binding site and stabilizes microtubule against depolymerization. Colchicine binds to the α-tubulin of colchicine binding site and blocks the polymerization of microtubule [7]. Combretastatins binds to β-tubulin of colchicine binding site, strongly inhibits tubulin polymerization [8-10], and disrupts the normal mitotic spindle function [11]. It was first isolated from the bark of African willow tree *Combretum caffrum* [12]. Various analogues have been synthesized and showed very good anticancer activity by inhibiting tubulin polymerization [13]. Earlier synthesized

* Correspondence: suniliftm1982@gmail.com
[1]Laboratory for Drug Design and Synthesis, Department of Pharmaceutical Chemistry, Indo-Soviet Friendship (ISF) College of Pharmacy, Moga, Punjab 142 001, India
Full list of author information is available at the end of the article

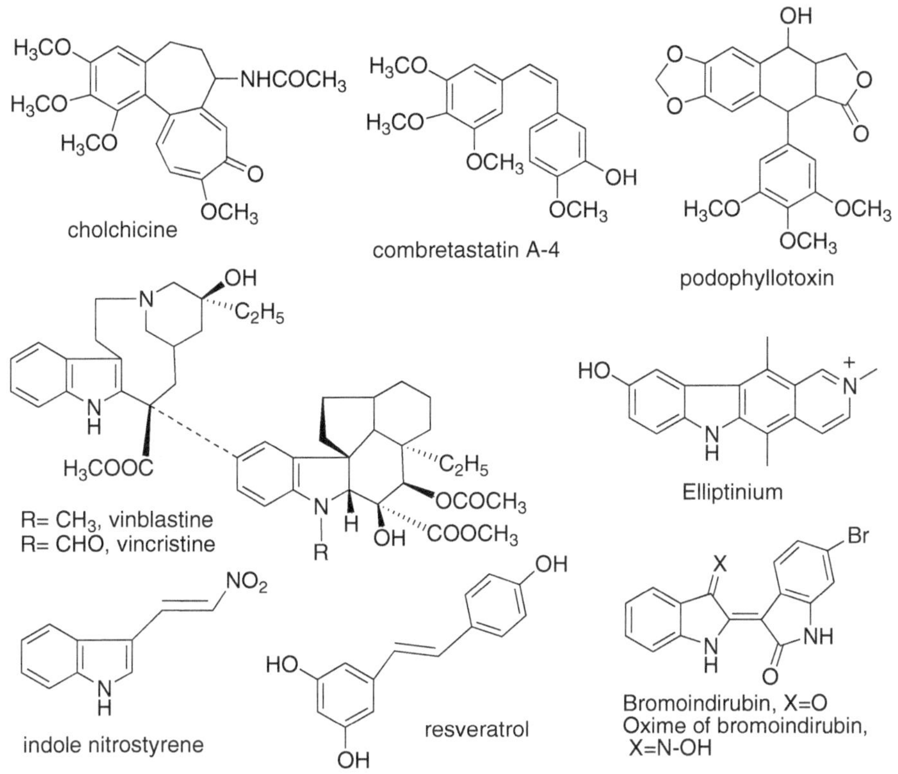

Figure 1 Some reported tubulin inhibitors.

compounds were having two rings in *cis*-configuration, but Pettit et al. have synthesized resveratrol type of compounds, β-nitrostyrenes, in which two rings are in *trans*-configuration and have marked antitumor activity. They also have synthesized E-indole nitrostyrene which showed marked anticancer activity [14]. Anticancer agents vincristine and vinblastine derived from *Catheranthus roseus* have been useful in cancer treatment, and this effect is due to the interaction of these drugs with tubulin [8,15]. It was thought worthwhile to incorporate another ring system having indole nucleus to rationally design combretastatin-like compounds replacing one ring with indole moiety because vincristine, vinblastine, elliptinium [16], and bromoindirubin contain indole moiety and have good tubulin polymerization inhibitory property [17]. Resistance remains a significant problem in the treatment of cancer with taxol like many chemotherapeutic agents, and it is caused by alterations in microtubule dynamics [18]. Our aim was to synthesize tubulin inhibitors having indole ring as basic moiety.

Methods

Combretastatin 2-(1-acetyl-1*H*-indole-3-yl)-3-(phenyl) propenoic analogues (**2a** to **2y**) were synthesized by condensation of indole-3-acetic acid with different substituted aldehydes using triethyl amine and acetic anhydride (shown in Scheme 1). For anticancer activity, seven cancer cell lines like lung (A-549), ovary (IGROV-1), prostate (DU-145), liver (HEP-2), leukemia (THP-1), and breast (MCF-7) were used.

Materials and methods of immunofluorescence confocal microscopy

THP1 cells (8 × 10 [4] cells/well) were seeded onto 18-mm square coverslips in six well plates. Cells were allowed to adhere for 24 h before dosing with required concentrations of **2d**. Paclitaxel 1 μM was used as a positive control. After the treatment period, cells were fixed in 4% paraformaldehyde for 10 min at room temperature and permeabilized using 0.5% Triton-X (Sigma-Aldrich, MO, USA) in PBS for 5 min. The cells were blocked with 10% goat serum for 20 min at room temperature. Microtubules were detected with a monoclonal α-tubulin antibody (Sigma Corporation, Cream Ridge, USA) diluted 1:100 in 0.1% Triton X-100 in PBS for 1 hr 37°C and Alexa Fluor 488 conjugated secondary antibody (Invitrogen, Carlsbad, USA) diluted 1:1,000 in PBS for 1 hr at room temperature. Cells were then washed three times in PBS and stained with DAPI diluted 1:1,000 in PBS [5]. The coverslips were mounted over glass slides, and the cells were imaged by confocal microscopy using

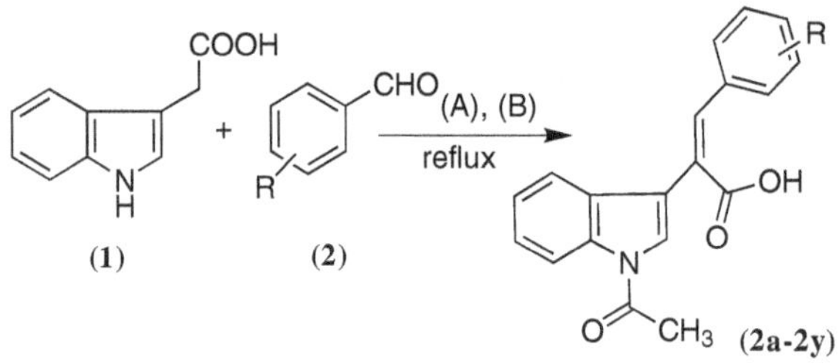

Scheme 1 Reagents and conditions. (**A**) Triethylamine; (**B**) acetic anhydride, refluxed for 6 to 10 h.

an Olympus Fluoview FV1000 laser scanning microscope (Olympus Inc., Center Valley, USA).

Material and methods for molecular docking

The coordinates of tubulin were obtained from protein data bank [PDB:1SA0] [19,20]. The structure of **2d** was drawn in ChemDraw [21] and subjected to energy minimization in the MOPAC module, using the AM1 procedure and implemented in the CS Chem3D Ultra (Cambridge Soft Corporation, Cambridge, USA). The **2d** was docked in to the colchicine binding site of tubulin using the GOLD 5.0.1 software [22]. GOLD performs genetic algorithm-based ligand docking to optimize the conformation of the ligand at the receptor binding site. It utilizes Gold score fitness function to evaluate the various conformations of the ligand at the binding site and comprises four components: protein-ligand hydrogen bond energy, protein-ligand van der Waals (vdw) energy, ligand internal vdw energy, and ligand torsional strain energy. The compound was docked ten times, and each pose was ranked according to its Gold score fitness function. The conformation with the highest score was selected for discussion.

Results and discussion

Chemistry

Twenty-five combretastatin analogues (**2a** to **2y**) were synthesized by condensation of indole-3-acetic acid (1) with different substituted aldehydes (2) using triethyl amine and acetic anhydride as reported previously (shown in Scheme 1) [23]. The reaction was monitored by TLC. The compounds were purified (yield 48% to 63%) by column chromatography using silica gel mesh size of 60 to 120. All the synthesized compounds (Figure 2) were characterized by spectroscopic techniques like infrared spectrometry (IR), mass spectrometry (MS), and nuclear magnetic resonance spectroscopy (NMR) (1H NMR, 13C NMR, heteronuclear multiple bond correlation (HMBC) NMR (Figure 3 and Table 1), and heteronuclear single quantum coherence (HSQC). 1H NMR indicates that H-7′ is highly deshielded as it appears to lie in the deshielding cone of N-acetyl group. H-3 is deshielded because of its nearby carbonyl of N-acetyl. H-3 is also deshielded because of its β position to carbonyl, but it is less deshielded than H-7′ because it does not come under the influence of magnetic anisotropy of carbonyl. No change in the integration of the H-3 was observed when H-2′ was doubly irradiated. These results indicated that H-2′ and H-3 are not in the close proximity. This is possible only when two rings are *trans* to each other. If two rings would have been in *cis* configuration, double irradiation of H-2′ would have resulted in signal enhancement of H-3 due to nuclear Overhauser effect (nOe). It was further confirmed that when a compound with hydroxyl located at 2″ was synthesized, the free OH (at 2″) is used in the formation of lactone because the geometry is such where OH and C = O are close in space and prefer to form lactone. H-3 gets more deshielded than H-7′ because it comes in the deshielding cone in the plane of benzene ring as well as the deshielding cone of carbonyl. IR value of carbonyl shifted to 1,763 from 1,710 because of lactone formation. Further Pschorr reaction [24] is fully supported in the condensation of phenyl acetic acid with aldehyde, resulting into combretastatin with *cis* configuration. When 2-hdroxybenzaldehyde is used for the condensation with phenyl acetic acid, no lactone formation occurred (Figure 4). From the above observations, it was thus concluded that synthesized compounds are having two rings in *trans*-configuration.

Anticancer activity

All the synthesized compounds were evaluated for anticancer activity (Table 2) against lung (A-549), ovary (IGROV-1), prostate (DU-145), liver (HEP-2), leukemia (THP-1), and breast (MCF-7) cancer cell lines. Compounds **2j**, **2 k**, and **2r** showed good anticancer activity against THP-1, DU-145, and MCF-7 cell lines. However, compounds **2d** (IC_{50} = 0.80 and 0.37 μM) and **2y** (IC_{50} = 3.6 μM) showed marked anticancer activity.

The italicized values indicate significant activity.

Synthesized compounds, in spite of having basic indole moiety, bind to colchicine binding site instead of

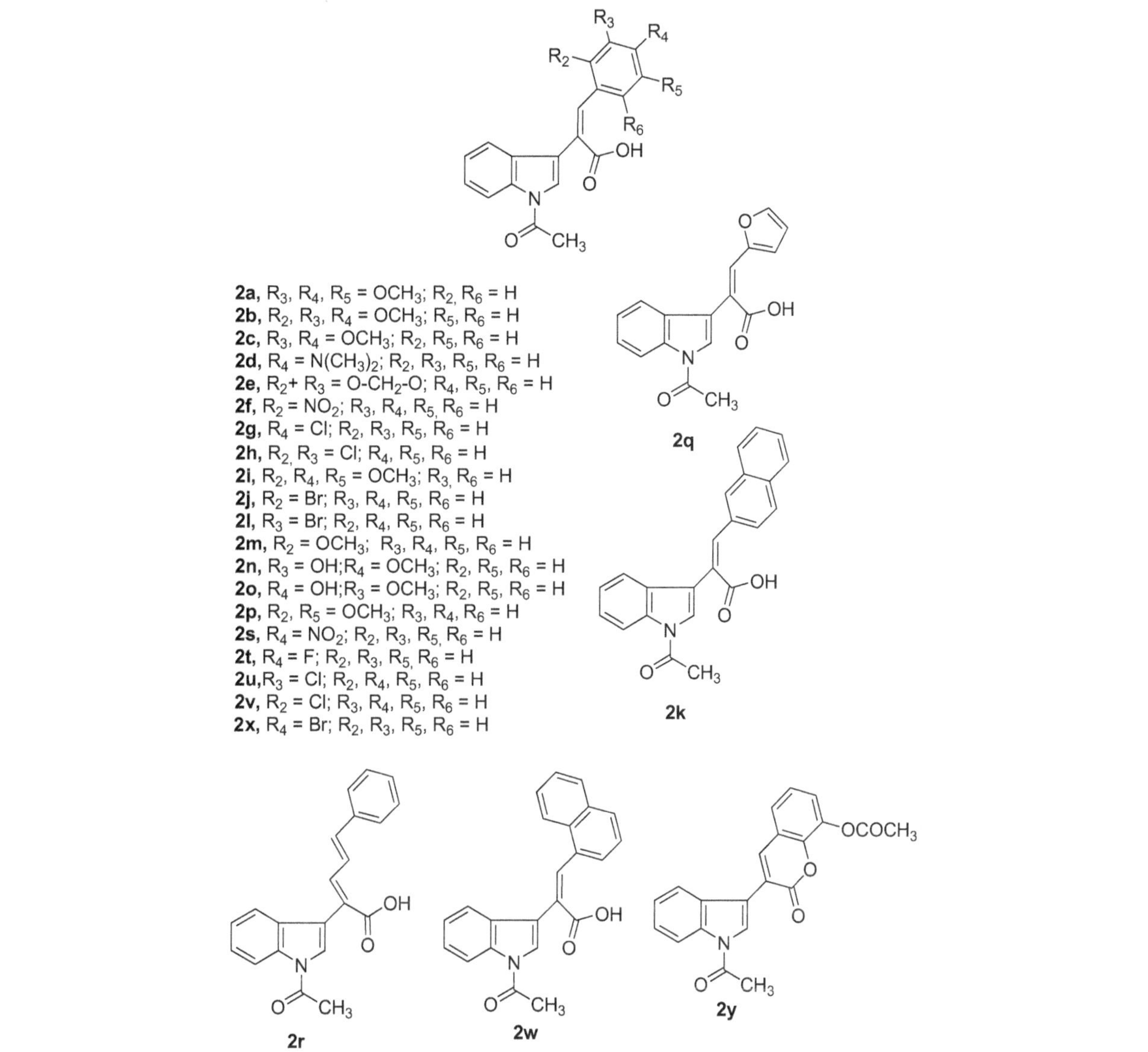

Figure 2 Chemical structures of the synthesized compounds.

vinblastine binding site because vincristine and vinblastine molecules are very large molecules, and thus, their binding sites have enlarged cavity as the binding site, while the present synthesized compounds, being much smaller in overall dimensions, appear to roll around in the vinblastine site. Further, this was confirmed by immunofluorescence confocal microscopy.

Immunofluorescence confocal microscopy

The immunofluorescence technique was used to evaluate the effect of **2d** on microtubules. The effect on microtubule structure was determined using confocal microscopy. Figure 5 shows representative images of microtubule structures and nuclei at 24 h of treatment. Minor changes in the microtubule structure were observed for 10 μM of **2d** at 24 h of treatment. At 30 μM, **2d** treatment at 24 h induced complete loss of microtubules. At the 48 h time point, cells treated with 10 and 20 μM **2d** showed a dose-dependent disruption and loss of microtubules compared to the control. Paclitaxel 1 μM was used as positive control. These results indicate that apoptosis induced by **2d** involves a severe loss of microtubule structure.

Molecular docking of 2d

In order to investigate the recognition process of these inhibitors at the colchicine-binding site of tubulin, a flexible docking study was performed on the most potent compound **2d** with the help of GOLD software [22]. The colchicine binding site encompasses the residues of both α and β subunits of tubulin (Figure 6). To validate the docking procedure for the prediction of the correct

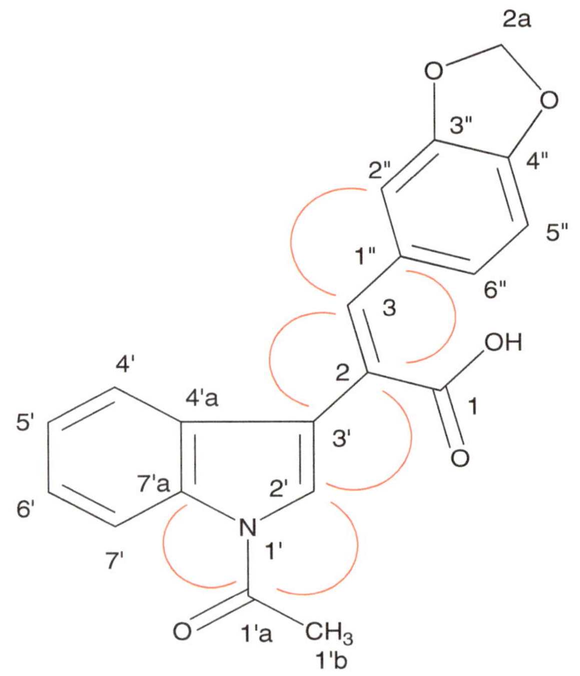

Figure 3 Selected HMBCs of 2e. Red ring indicates the correlation of two carbons or hydrogens which are near to each other.

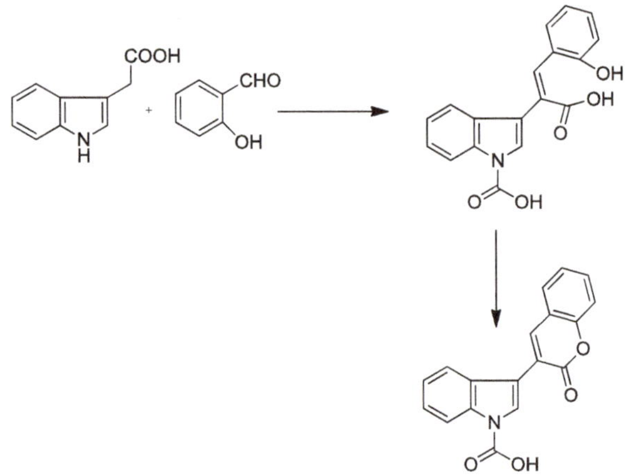

Figure 4 Lactonization of combretastatin analogue.

binding mode of inhibitor at the colchicine-binding site, the colchicine was extracted from the original X-ray structure [PDB:1SA0] [19,20] and re-docked using GOLD.21. The highest scoring conformation was selected and compared with X-ray structure conformation. The docked conformation of colchicine using GOLD was found to be similar with the original X-ray structure (Figure 7A). The root mean square deviation between the best scored conformers from docking and X-ray structure was found to be 0.72 Å. The compound **2d** was docked at the colchicine binding site of tubulin, and the best fit conformation was selected on the basis of Gold score and visual inspection. The Figure 7B shows the binding conformation of **2d** at the colchicine binding site. The compound **2d** gets stabilized at the colchicine-binding site of tubulin by hydrophobic and hydrogen bond interactions. The aromatic part of indole ring gets positioned in a hydrophobic cavity formed by Leu255*β*, Ala250*β*, Ala316*β*, Val318*β*, and Ala354*β*. The carbonyl oxygen (carbonyl group at indole) forms a hydrogen bond with sulfhydryl group of Cys241*β*. This is similar to the interaction of colchicines with the tubulin [25]. Another hydrogen bond was formed between the hydroxyl group of the carboxylic acid part of **2d** and nitrogen of Leu255*β*. These two hydrogen bonds play crucial role in stabilizing the conformation of **2d** at the colchicine-binding site. The unsaturated intermediate chain between rings A and B of **2d** is placed in close vicinity of the side-chain of Leu248*β* (Figure 7B). The ring B of **2d** is extended towards the *α*-chain of the tubulin. The docking study was helpful to find the binding conformation of **2d** at the colchicine binding site of tubulin.

Table 1 Three-bond [1] H- ^{13}C coupling (HMBC) in 2e

Serial number	H	C
1	H-3	C-3′, C-2″
2	H-2′	C-1′a, C-2
3	H-4′	C-3′
4	H-7′	C-1′a
5	H-2″	C-3
6	H-6″	C-3, C-1

Experimental

The reagents were purchased from Sigma-Aldrich (MO, USA), LobaChemie (Mumbia, India), and Central Drug House (New Delhi, India) and used without further purification. All yields refer to isolated products after purification. Products were characterized by spectroscopic data (IR, [1] H NMR, and [13] C NMR spectra). The spectra were measured in DMSO-d_6 relative to TMS (0.00 ppm). IR (KBr pallets) spectra were recorded on a Fourier transform infrared Thermo spectrophotometer (ThermoFisher Scientific Inc., Waltham, USA). Melting points were determined in open capillaries and were found to be uncorrected.

Typical experimental procedure for the synthesis combretastatin 2-(1-acetyl-1H-indole-3-yl)-3-(phenyl) propenoic analogues (2a to 2y)

A mixture of IAA (0.0057 mmol), substituted benzaldehyde (0.0057 mmol) and triethylamine (2 ml) in Ac_2O (4 ml), was heated until the reaction was complete. After cooling, the reaction mixture was acidified with 35% aqueous HCl (6 ml) and kept at room temperature overnight when precipitates appeared as such or on dilution with

Table 2 Anticancer activity of synthesized compounds

Compound code	IC$_{50}$ of cell line types (tissue/cell)					
	THP-1	A-549	MCF-7	IGROV-1	HEP-2	DU-145
	(WBC)	(lung)	(breast)	(ovary)	(liver)	(prostrate)
2a	>100	>100	86.9	>100	>100	>100
2b	>100	>100	>100	>100	-	-
2c	89.2	71.0	>100	>100	-	-
2d	*0.80*	>100	*0.37*	38.0	63.4	40.4
2e	73.0	>100	>100	>100	-	-
2f	81.3	>100	>100	>100	>100	>100
2 g	70.6	>100	>100	-	89	>100
2 h	>100	>100	>100	-	>100	-
2i	-	-	>100	-	-	-
2j	>100	>100	76.1	-	-	16.4
2 k	>100	>100	50.0	-	-	43.9
2 l	86.0	>100	76.4	>100	>100	>100
2 m	67.0	75.7	>100	>100	>100	>100
2n	>100	>100	>100	>100	-	-
2o	>100	>100	>100	>100	-	-
2p	>100	>100	>100	>100	-	-
2q	68.0	>100	79.0	>100	>100	>100
2r	40.8	38.7	51.9	>100	>100	>100
2 s	>100	90.3	>100	>100	>100	>100
2 t	-	>100	>100	-	>100	>100
2u	>100	>100	>100	>100	>100	>100
2v	>100	>100	95.2	>100	-	-
2w	>100	>100	51.8	>100	-	-
2x	92.0	>100	>100	>100	>100	>100
2y	81.8	49.8	*3.6*	>100	85.3	-
Adriamycin	*0.12*	*0.11*	*0.16*	*0.19*	-	-
Mitomycin	*0.23*	*0.19*	*0.27*	*0.25*	*0.31*	
Paclitaxel	*0.15*	-	-	*0.15*	*0.14*	-
5-fluorouracil	*9.7*	*8.6*	*9.9*	*8.3*	*9.7*	*9.1*

water. The products were purified by column chromatography using silica gel of mesh size 60 to120.

Characterization data

2a. (Z)-2-(1-acetyl-1H-indol-3-yl)-3-(3,4,5-trimethoxyphenyl) propenoic acid

Mp: 177°C to 178°C; I.R. (KBr, cm^{-1}): 1722 (C = O), 1681 (C = O, N-acetyl) 1636 (C = C), 1542 (C = C, phenyl ring), [1] H NMR (500 MHz, DMSO-d$_6$, δ, TMS = 0, J = Hz): 8.44 (d, 1H, J = 8.25, H-7′), 8.03 (s, 1H, H-3), 7.90 (s, 1H, H-2′), 7.42 (1H, dd, J = 7.9 and 7.8, H-5′), 7.31 (dd, 1H, J = 7.7 and J = 7.8, H-6′), 7.25 (d, 1H, J = 8.0, H-4′), 6.64 (s, 1H, H-2″), 6.57 (s, 1H, H-6″), 3.63 (s, 3H, OMe) 3.34 (s, 6H, 2× OMe) 2.71 (s, 3H, N-acetyl); [13] C NMR (125 MHz, DMSO-d$_6$, δ, TMS = 0, J = Hz): 169.40, 168.30, 152.20, 141.51, 138.38, 134.86, 129.35, 129.22, 125.95, 124.92, 123.46, 122.61, 119.84, 116.64, 115.97, 107.87, 59.96, 55.02, 23.70; MS: 418 (M + Na)$^+$; Anal. calcd. For $C_{22}H_{21}NO_6$: C, 66.83; H, 5.35; N, 3.54 found C: 66.73; H, 5.34; N, 3.34.

2b. (Z)-2-(1-acetyl-1H-indol-3-yl)-3-(2,3,4-trimethoxyphenyl) propenoic acid

Mp: 210°C to 212°C; I.R. (KBr, cm^{-1}): 1718 (C = O), 1668 (C = O, N-acetyl) 1637 (C = C), 1545 (C = C, phenyl ring); [1] H NMR (500 MHz, DMSO-d$_6$, δ, TMS = 0, J = Hz): 8.36 (d, 1H, J = 8.3, H-7′), 8.16 (s, 1H, H-3) 7.84 (s, 1H, H-2′), 7.31 (dd, 1H, J = 7.3 and 8.0, H-6′), 7.14 (m, 2H, H-5′, 4′), 6.66 (d, 1H, J = 8.9, H-6″), 6.47 (d, 1H, J = 8.9, H-5″), 3.89 (s, 3H, OMe), 3.71 (s, 3H, OMe) 3.65 (s, 3H, OMe) 2.64 (s, 3H, N-acetyl); [13] C NMR (125 MHz, DMSO-d$_6$, δ, TMS = 0, J = Hz): 169.40, 168.41, 154.55,

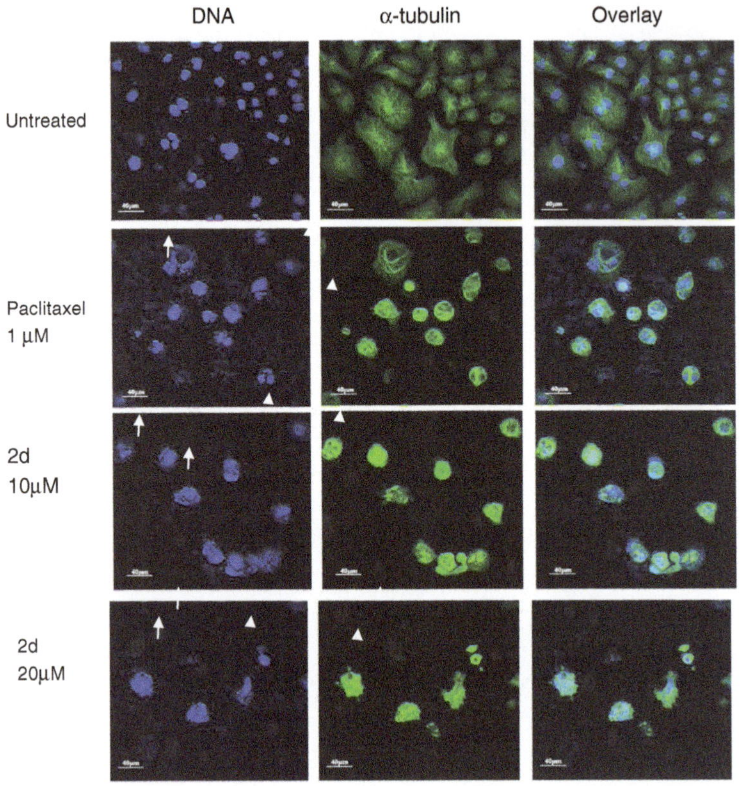

Figure 5 Effects of paclitaxel and 2d on microtubules in THP-1 cells. Cells were plated on coverslips and treated with 1 µM paclitaxel and 10 and 20 µM **2d** for 48 h. After treatment, cells were fixed and processed for immunofluorescence/confocal microscopy using monoclonal *α*-tubulin antibody and secondary antibody conjugated with Alexa-488 (Invitrogen, Carlsbad, USA). 4′,6-diamidino-2-phenylindole (DAPI) was used for nuclear staining. The untreated cells show normal nuclear morphology and microtubules. Paclitaxel treatment causes the condensation and fragmentation of nuclei due to apoptosis (arrow) and also causes loss of microtubules (arrowhead). **2d** treatment induces concentration-dependent increase in condensation and fragmentation of nuclei (arrow) due to apoptosis and also concentration-dependent loss of microtubules (arrowhead). Similar results were obtained in two separate experiments.

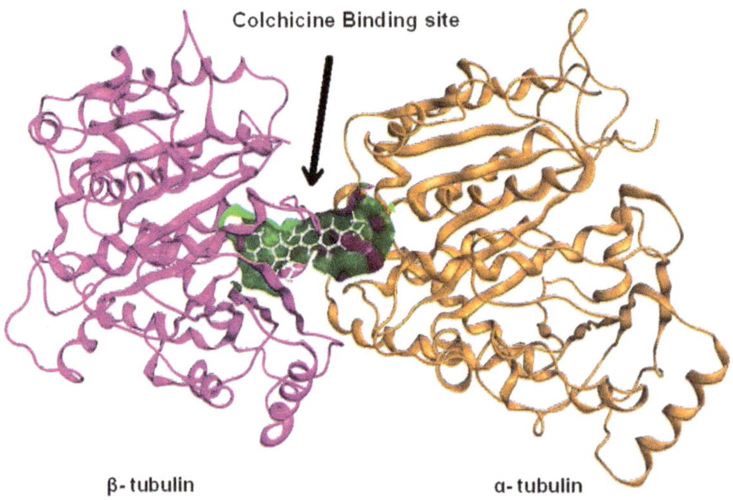

Figure 6 Colchicine binding site at the interface between *α* and *β* subunits of tubulin. The inhibitor **2d** is shown in silver color.

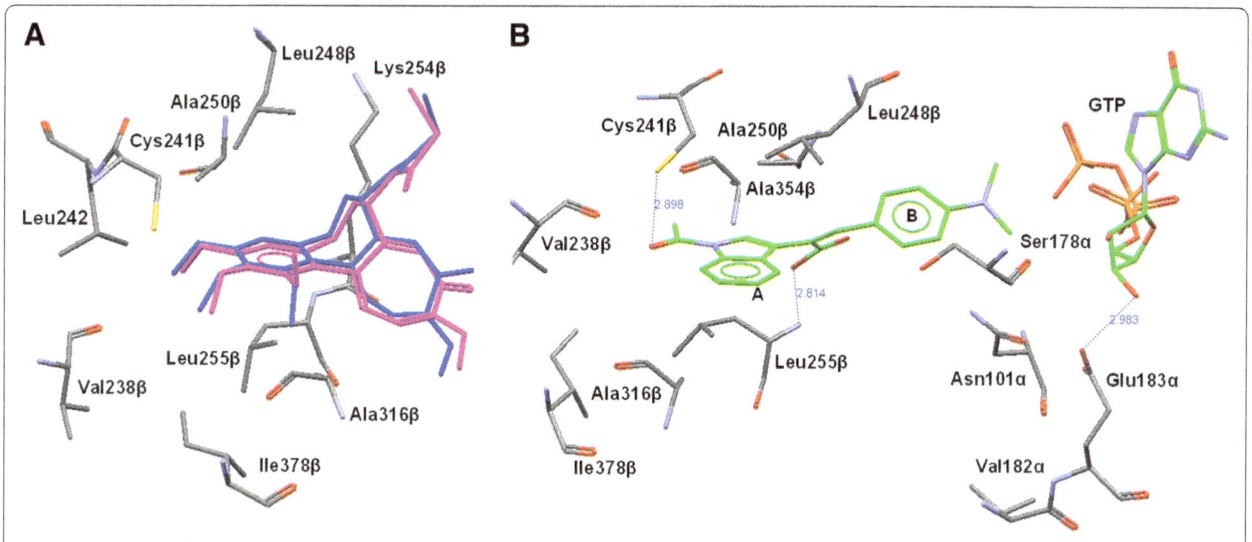

Figure 7 Overlay of crystal structure and binding conformation. (**A**) Overlay of crystal structure (blue) and docked (purple) conformation of colchicines, (**B**) binding conformation of **2d** (green) at the colchicine-binding site of tubulin.

152.73, 141.32, 135.58, 134.94, 129.29, 126.02, 124.74, 123.99, 123.40, 122.00, 120.78, 119.52, 116.75, 116.03, 107.71, 61.52, 60.39, 55.74, 24.30; MS: 418 $(M + Na)^+$; Anal. calcd. For $C_{22}H_{21}NO_6$: C, 66.83; H, 5.35; N, 3.54 found C: 66.73; H, 5.34; N, 3.34.

2c. (Z)-2-(1-acetyl-1H-indol-3-yl)-3-(3,4-dimethoxyphenyl) propenoic acid

Mp: 245°C to 247°C; I.R. (KBr, cm^{-1}): 1712 (C = O), 1681 (C = O, N-acetyl) 1638 (C = C), 1554 (C = C, phenyl ring); [1] H NMR (500 MHz, DMSO-d_6, δ, TMS = 0, *J* = Hz): 8.38 (d, 1H *J* = 8.3, H-7′), 7.96 (1H, s, H-3), 7.87 (1H, s, H-2′), 7.32 (dd, 1H, *J* = 7.3 and 7.2, H-6′), 7.16 (dd, 1H, *J* = 7.1, H-5) 7.12 (d, 1H, *J* = 7.6, H-4′) 6.97 (dd, 1H, *J* = 8.4 and 8.5, H-6″), 6.83 (d, 1H, *J* = 8.5, H-5″) 6.68 (d, 1H, *J* = 1.7, H-5″) 3.68 (s, 3H, OMe) 3.09 (s, 3H, OMe) 2.64 (s, 3H, N-acetyl); [13] C NMR (125 MHz, DMSO-d_6, δ, TMS = 0, *J* = Hz): 168.36, 167.30, 148.80, 146.75, 140.50, 133.85, 128.20, 125.64, 124.80, 123.76, 123.63, 122.34, 119.73, 118.71, 115.79, 114.91, 111.40, 110.12, 54.27, 53.12, 22.70; MS: 388 $(M + Na)^+$; Anal. calcd. For $C_{21}H_{19}NO_5$: C, 69.03; H, 5.24; N, 3.83 found C: 69.0; H, 5.30; N, 3.74.

2d. (Z)-2-(1-acetyl-1H-indol-3-yl)-3-(4-(dimethylamino) phenyl) propenoic acid

Mp: 246°C to 248°C; I.R. (KBr, cm^{-1}), 3423 (NH), 1702 (C = O), 1682 (C = O, N-acetyl), 1659 (C = C), 1583 (C = C, phenyl ring); [1] H NMR (200 MHz, DMSO-d_6, δ, TMS = 0, *J* = Hz): 8.43 (d, 1H *J* = 8.2, H-7′), 7.99 (s, 1H, H-3), 7.68 (s, 1H, H-2′), 7.14 to 7.30 (m, 5H, 5′, 6′, 4′, 2″, 6″), 6.20 (d, 2H, *J* = 8.9), 2.91 (s, 6H, 2× Me) 2.59 (s, 3H, N-acetyl); [13] C NMR (125 MHz, DMSO-d_6, δ, TMS = 0, *J* = Hz); 169.62, 168.66, 150.83, 143.06, 135.55, 132.59, 132.11, 129.69, 124.88, 124.59, 123.43, 121.89, 120.30, 118.39, 117.08, 116.37, 111.24, 23.96; MS: 371 $(M + Na)^+$; Anal. calcd. For $C_{21}H_{20}N_2O_3$: C, 72.4; H, 5.79; N, 8.04 found C: 72.1; H, 5.80; N, 8.14.

2e. (Z)-2-(1-acetyl-1H-indol-3-yl)-3-(benzo[d][1,3]dixol-6-yl) propenoic acid

Mp: 243°C to 245°C; I.R. (KBr, cm^{-1}): 1710 (C = O), 1683 (C = O, N-acetyl) 1637 (C = C), 1555 (C = C, phenyl ring); [1] H NMR (500 MHz, DMSO-d_6, δ, TMS = 0, *J* = Hz): 8.38 (d, 1H *J* = 8.3, H-7′), 7.94 (s, 1H, H-3), 7.86 (s, 1H, H-2′), 7.33 (dd, 1H, *J* = 7.2 and 8.2, H-5′), 7.17 (dd, 1H, *J* = 7.7 and 7.3, H-6′) 7.11 (d, 1H, *J* = 7.8, H-4′) 6.93 (dd, 1H, *J* = 7.1 and 1.2, H-6″), 6.80 (d, 1H, *J* = 8.1, H-5″) 6.67 (s, 1H, H-2″) 5.90 (s, 2H, O-CH_2-O) 2.65 (s, 3H, N-acetyl); [13] C NMR (125 MHz, DMSO-d_6, δ, TMS = 0, *J* = Hz):169.50, 168.36, 148.26, 147.15, 141.30, 134.94, 129.12, 128.42, 126.17, 126.04, 124.85, 123.46, 121.42, 119.64, 116.51, 116.06, 108.76, 108.32, 101.35, 23.84; MS: 372 $(M + Na)^+$; Anal. calcd. For $C_{20}H_{15}NO_5$: C, 68.76; H, 4.33; N, 4.01 found C: 68.75; H, 4.41; N, 4.11. For further information, please refer to Additional file 1: Figures S1, Additional file 2: Figure S2, Additional file 3: Figure S3, Additional file 4: Figure S4, Additional file 5: Figure S5 and Additional file 6: Figure S6.

2 f. (Z)-2-(1-acetyl-1H-indol-3-yl)-3-(2-nitrophenyl) propenoic acid

Mp: 209°C to 210°C; I.R. (KBr, cm^{-1}): 1701 (C = O), 1683 (C = O, N-acetyl), 1655 (C = C), 1560 (C = C, phenyl ring); [1] H NMR (200 MHz, DMSO-d_6, δ, TMS = 0, *J* = Hz): 8.39 (d, 1H *J* = 8.3, H-7′) 7.94 (s, 1H, H-3) 7.88 (s, 1H, H-2′) 7.6 to 7.70 (m, 4H, 3″, 4″, 5″, 6″) 7.39 (m, 3H, H-5′, 6′, 4′) 2.7 (s, 3H, N-acetyl); [13] C NMR

(125 MHz, DMSO-d_6, δ, TMS = 0, J = Hz): 168.58, 167.00 148.13, 138.99, 133.58, 133, 42, 130.76, 130.31, 129.04, 128.08, 125.31, 124.76, 124.57, 124.31, 123.36, 119.85, 119.57, 116.46, 23.90; MS: 373 $(M + Na)^+$; Anal. calcd. For $C_{19}H_{14}N_2O_5$: C, 65.14; H, 4.03; N, 8.0 found C: 65.12; H, 4.03; N, 8.12.

2 g. (Z)-2-(1-acetyl-1H-indol-3-yl)-3-(4-chlorophenyl) propenoic acid

Mp: 208°C to 209°C; I.R. (KBr, cm^{-1}): 1713 (C = O), 1673 (C = O, N-acetyl), 1633 (C = C), 1580 (C = C, phenyl ring); [1] H NMR (200 MHz, DMSO-d_6, δ, TMS = 0, J = Hz): 8.38 (d, 1H J = 8.9, H-7′), 7.99 (s, 1H, H-3) 7.58 to 7.61 (m, 4H, H-2′, 2″, 3″, 5″) 7.38 to 7.47 (m, 3H, H-5′, 6′, 6″), 7.26 (d, 1H, J = 7.9, 4′) 6.46 (s, 1H, NH, D_2O exchangeable) 2.63 (s, 3H, N-acetyl); [13] C NMR (125 MHz, DMSO-d_6, δ, TMS = 0, J = Hz): 168.67, 167.20, 142.78, 140.25, 135.51, 134.58, 133.49, 131.50, 129.53, 129.13, 128.55, 125.76, 125.15, 124.63, 123.59, 120.20, 119.98, 116.67, 23.71; MS: 362 $(M + Na)^+$; Anal. calcd. For $C_{19}H_{14}NO_3Cl$: C, 67.16; H, 4.15; N, 4.12 found C: 67.12; H, 4.23; N, 4.10.

2 h. (Z)-2-(1-acetyl-1H-indol-3-yl)-3-(2,3-dichlorophenyl) propenoic acid

Mp: 225°C to 227°C; I.R. (KBr, cm^{-1}): 1688 (C = O), 1624 (C = C), 1673 (C = O, N-acetyl), 1559 (C = C, phenyl ring); [1] H NMR (200 MHz, DMSO-d_6, δ, TMS = 0, J = Hz): 8.43 (d, 1H J = 8.1, H-7′), 8.09 (s, 1H, H-3) 8.01 (s, 1H, H-2′), 7.51 to 7.6 (m, 4H, H-6′, 4″, 5″, 6″), 7.26 (d, 2H, J = 7.9, H-5′, 4′) 6.5 (s, 1H, NH, D_2O exchangeable), 2.63 (s, 3H, N-acetyl); [13] C NMR (125 MHz, DMSO-d_6, δ, TMS = 0 J = Hz): 167.67, 140.04, 135.17, 133.70, 132.63, 131.30, 127.49, 125.87, 122.99, 23.90; MS: 397 $(M + Na)^+$; Anal. calcd. For $C_{19}H_{13}NO_3Cl_2$: C, 60.98; H, 3.50; N, 3.74 found C: 60.95; H, 3.50; N, 3.76.

2i. (Z)-2-(1-acetyl-1H-indol-3-yl)-3-(2,4,5-trimethoxyphenyl) propenoic acid

Mp: 229°C to 230°C; I.R. (KBr, cm^{-1}): 1701 (C = O), 1673 (C = O, N-acetyl), 1603 (C = C), 1514 (C = C, phenyl ring); [1] H NMR (200 MHz, DMSO-d_6, δ, TMS = 0, J = Hz): 8.40 (d, 2H, J = 7.2, H-3, 7′), 7.96 (s, 1H, 2′), 7.31 to 7.43 (m, 3H, H-5′, 6′, 4′), 6.47 (s, 1H, D_2O exchangeable), 6.40 (d, 2H, J = 7.6, H-5″, 6″), 3.89 (d, 6H, J = 11.3, 2× OMe), 2.9 (d, 3H, OMe) 2.73 (s, 3H, N-acetyl); [13] C NMR (100 MHz, DMSO-d_6, δ, TMS = 0, J = Hz): 169.54, 168.59, 153.80, 151.37, 142.03, 136.41, 135.47, 129.52, 125.09, 124.92, 123.61, 120.56, 119.91, 118.16, 116.40, 114.80, 112.69, 96.29, 56.42, 55.82, 55.01, 23.94; MS: 418 $(M + Na)^+$; Anal. calcd. For $C_{22}H_{21}NO_6$: C, 66.83; H, 5.35; N, 3.54 found C: 66.85; H, 5.35; N, 3.30.

2j. (Z)-2-(1-acetyl-1H-indol-3-yl)-3-(2-bromophenyl) propenoic acid

Mp: 199°C to 201°C; I.R. (KBr, cm^{-1}): 1708 (C = O), 1666 (C = O, N-acetyl), 1622 (C = C), 1556 (C = C, phenyl ring); [1] H NMR (200 MHz, DMSO-d_6, δ, TMS = 0,J = Hz): 8.43 (d, 1H, J = 8.7, H-7′), 7.98 (s, 1H, H-3), 7.48 (d, 1H, J = 9.0, H-2′), 7.32 to 7.20 (m, 3H, 6′, 3″, 6″), 7.01 (m, 4H, 5′, 4′, 4″, 6″), 2.64 (s, 3H, N-acetyl); [13] C NMR (125 MHz, DMSO-d_6, δ, TMS = 0, J = Hz): 168.81, 168.68, 140.01, 136.90, 135.53, 133.01, 131.82, 129.75, 128.10, 125.32, 125.28, 125.20, 123.57, 122.11, 120.24, 116.65, 116.51, 24.00; MS: 407 $(M + Na)^+$; Anal. calcd. For $C_{19}H_{14}BrNO_3$: C, 59.39; H, 3.67; N, 3.65 found C, 59.24; H, 3.56; N, 3.45.

2 k. (Z)-2-(1-acetyl-1H-indol-3-yl)-3-(naphthalene-2-yl) propenoic acid

Mp: 235°C to 237°C; I.R. (KBr, cm^{-1}): 1708 (C = O), 1676 (C = O, N-acetyl), 1637 (C = C), 1560 (C = C, phenyl ring); [1] H NMR (200 MHz, DMSO-d_6, δ, TMS = 0, J = Hz): 8.44 (d, 1H, J = 8.2, H-7′), 8.25 (s, 1H, H-3), 7.81 (s, 1H, H-2′), 7.68 (dd, 2H, J = 6.1 and 2.1, H-3″, 4″), 7.52 (1H, s, 1″) 7.44 to 7.30 (m, 4H, 8″, 7″, 6″, 4″), 7.11 (m, 3H, 5′, 6′, 4′) 2.6 (s, 3H, N-acetyl); [13] C NMR (125 MHz, DMSO-d_6, δ, TMS = 0, J = Hz); 169.26, 168.73, 142.17, 135.56, 133.27, 132.87, 132.40, 131.33, 129.38, 128.37, 127.64, 127.48, 127.03, 126.32, 126.10, 125.18, 125.13, 123.68, 123.57, 120.38, 117.43, 116.49, 24; MS: 378 $(M + Na)^+$; Anal. calcd. For $C_{23}H_{17}NO_3$: C, 77.73; H, 4.82; N, 3.94 found C, 77.54; H, 4.64; N, 3.73.

2 l. (Z)-2-(1-acetyl-1H-indol-3-yl)-3-(3-bromophenyl) propenoic acid

Mp: 226°C to 228°C; I.R. (KBr, cm^{-1}): 1708 (C = O), 1676 (C = O, N-acetyl), 1622 (C = C), 1555 (C = C, phenyl ring); [1] H NMR (200 MHz, DMSO-d_6, δ, TMS = 0, J = Hz): 8.41 (d, 1H, J = 7.6, H-7′), 7.95 (s, 1H, H-3) 7.75 (s, 1H, H-2′) 7.30 (dd, 2H, J = 7.1 and 3.3, H-6′), 7.21 to 7.00 (m, 4H, H-6′, 4″, 5″, 6″), 6.98 to 6.8 (m, 2H, H-5′, 4′), 2.65 (s, 3H, N-acetyl); [13] C NMR (100 MHz, DMSO-d_6, δ, TMS = 0, J = Hz): 168.80, 168.63, 139.53, 137.02, 135.45, 132.82, 131.66, 129.76, 128.80, 128.09, 125.76, 125.41, 125.06, 123.47, 122.00, 120.19, 116.69, 116.40, 23.95; MS: 407 $(M + Na)^+$; Anal. calcd. For $C_{19}H_{14}BrNO_3$: C, 59.39; H, 3.67; Br, 20.80; N, 3.65 found C, 59.56; H, 3.54; N, 3.44.

2 m. (Z)-2-(1-acetyl-1H-indol-3-yl)-3-(2-methoxyphenyl) propenoic acid

Mp: 229°C to 231°C; I.R. (KBr, cm^{-1}): 1707 (C = O),), 1677 (C = O, N-acetyl), 1603 (C = C), 1603 and 1450 (C = C, phenyl ring); [1] H NMR (200 MHz, DMSO-d_6, δ, TMS = 0, J = Hz): 8.44 (d, 1H, J = 8.3, H-7′), 7.96 (s, 1H, H-3) 7.81 (s, 1H, H-2′), 7.27 (dd, 1H, J = 8.1 and 8.0, H-6′), 7.23 (d, 2H, J = 7.3, H-4″, 6″), 7.13 (dd, 2H, J = 7.6 and 2.9,

5′, 4′) 6.82 (dd, 2H, J = 7.4 and 7.6, H-3″, 5″) 2.64 (s, 3H, N-acetyl); [13] C NMR (125 MHz, DMSO-d$_6$, δ, TMS = 0, J = Hz): 168.45, 160.00, 138.53, 136.19, 134.45, 130.87, 130.17, 129.53, 128.50, 127.89, 126.76, 125.51, 124.96, 123.45, 122.40, 121.09, 116. 23, 115.79, 24.10; MS: 378 (M + Na)$^+$; Anal. calcd. For $C_{20}H_{17}NO_4$: C, 71.63; H, 5.11; N, 4.18 found C, 71.63; H, 5.16; N, 4.26.

2n. (Z)-2-(1-acetyl-1H-indol-3-yl)-3-(3-hydroxy-4-methoxyphenyl) propenoic acid

Mp: 235°C to 237°C; I.R. (KBr, cm^{-1}): 2926 (O-H), 1702 (C = O), 1668 (C = O, N-acetyl), 1638 (C = C), 1504 (C = C, phenyl ring); [1] H NMR (200 MHz, DMSO-d$_6$, δ, TMS = 0, J = Hz): 8.45 (d, 1H, J = 8.2, H-7′), 7.89 (s, 1H, H-3), 7.63 (s, 1H, H-2′), 7.29 (dd, 1H, J = 7.0 and 7.1, H-6′), 7.15 (dd, 2H, J = 7.2 and 7.2, H-5′, 4′), 6.79 to 7.0 (m, 3H, H-2″, 5″, 6″), 3.75 (s, 3H, CH_3), 2.64 (s, 3H, N-acetyl); [13] C NMR (100 MHz, DMSO-d$_6$, δ, TMS = 0, J = Hz); 168.5, 168.46, 148.63, 145.65, 141.58, 135.03, 129.17, 127.01, 124.98, 124.31, 122.88, 122.82, 120.41, 119.64, 116.91, 116.15, 115.84, 110.86, 55.12, 23.70; MS: 374 (M + Na)$^+$; Anal. calcd. For $C_{20}H_{17}NO_5$: C, 68.37; H, 4.88; N, 3.99 found C, 68.21; H, 4.62; N, 4.13.

2o. (Z)-2-(1-acetyl-1H-indol-3-yl)-3-(4-hydroxy-3-methoxyphenyl) propenoic acid

Mp: 212°C to 213°C; I.R. (KBr, cm^{-1}): 2930 (OH), 1701 (C = O), 1681 (C = O, N-acetyl), 1599 (C = C), 1451 (C = C, phenyl ring); [1] H NMR (200 MHz, DMSO-d$_6$, δ, TMS = 0, J = Hz): 9.22 (s, 1H, OH, D_2O exchangeable), 8.43 (d, 1H, J = 8.2, H-7′), 8.03 (s, 1H, H-3), 7.83 (s, 1H, H-2′) 7.30 (dd, 2H, J = 7.2 and 7.3, H-5′, 6′) 6.90 (s, 1H, H-6″), 6.82 to 6.70 (m, 3H, 4′, 2″, 3″), 3.15 (s, 3H, OMe) 2.59 (s, 3H, N-acetyl); [13] C NMR (125 MHz, DMSO-d$_6$, δ, TMS = 0, J = Hz): 167.88, 167.50, 147.05, 145.72, 141.15, 134.05, 128.11, 124.56, 124.25, 123.93, 123.70, 122.20, 119.07, 118.36, 116.37, 113.91, 111.62, 53.37, 22.70; MS: 374 (M + Na)$^+$; Anal. calcd. For $C_{20}H_{17}NO_5$: C, 68.37; H, 4.88; N, 3.99 found C, 68.22; H, 4.71; N, 4.03.

2p. (Z)-2-(1-acetyl-1H-indol-3-yl)-3-(2,5-dimethoxyphenyl) propenoic acid

Mp: 246°C to 248°C; I.R. (KBr, cm^{-1}) 1710 (C = O), 1671 (C = O, N-acetyl), 1611 (C = C), 1452 (C = C, phenyl ring); [1] H NMR(200 MHz, DMSO-d$_6$, δ, TMS = 0, J = Hz): 8.79 (d, 1H, J = 7.2, H-7′), 8.37 (s, 1H, H-3), 8.02 (s, 1H, H-2′), 7.44 (dd, 1H, J = 8.1 and 8.0, H-6′), 7.17 to 7.20 (m, 2H, H-5′, 4′), 6.90 (d, 1H, J = 2.5, H-2″), 6.88 (d, 1H, J = 7.4, H-5″), 6.77 (d, 1H, J = 7.4, H-6″) 3.50 (s, 3H, OMe), 3.11 (s, 3H, OMe) 2.71 (s, 3H, N-acetyl); [13] C NMR (125 MHz, DMSO-d$_6$, δ, TMS = 0, J = Hz): 167.19, 167.00, 155.04, 150.65, 150.61, 134.72, 133.53, 128.73, 127.69, 124.00, 123.18, 122.07, 121.75, 118.45, 115.47, 115.31, 114.53, 112.28, 112.11, 110.27, 22.20; MS: 388 (M + Na)$^+$; Anal. calcd. For $C_{21}H_{19}NO_5$: C, 69.03; H, 5.24; N, 3.83 found C: 69.03; H, 5.37; N, 3.64.

2q. (Z)-2-(1-acetyl-1H-indol-3-yl)-3-(furan-2-yl) propenoic acid

Mp: 231°C to 232°C; I.R. (KBr, cm^{-1}): 1711 (C = O), 1671 (C = O, N-acetyl), 1640 (C = C), 1564 (C = C, phenyl ring); [1] H NMR (200 MHz, DMSO-d$_6$, δ, TMS = 0, J = Hz): 8.49 (d, 1H, J = 8.8, H-7′), 8.00 (s, 1H, H-3) 7.49 (s, 1H, H-2′) 7.35 (d, 1H, J = 5.3, H-2″), 7.27 to 7.10 (m, 3H, H-5′, 6′, 4′), 6.20 (dd, 2H, J = 3.4 and 3.5, H-3″, 4″) [13] C NMR (100 MHz, DMSO-d$_6$, δ, TMS = 0, J = Hz): 168.50, 167.42, 149.78, 142.94, 141.40, 136.61, 134.49, 130.82, 126.00, 125.20, 124.86, 123.28, 122.77, 121.00, 120.42, 111.60, 24.30; MS: 318 (M + Na)$^+$; Anal. calcd. For $C_{17}H_{13}NO_4$: C: 69.15; H, 4.44; N, 4.74 found C: 69.11; H, 4.53; N, 4.54.

2r. (2Z,4E)-2-(1-acetyl-1H-indol-3-yl)-5-phenylpenta-2, 4-dienoic acid

Mp: 232°C to 234°C; I.R. (KBr, cm^{-1}): 1725 (C = O), 1671 (C = O, N-acetyl), 1610 (C = C), 1449 (C = C, phenyl ring); [1] H NMR (200 MHz, DMSO-d$_6$, δ, TMS = 0, J = Hz): 8.52 (d, 1H, J = 8.4, H-7′), 7.91 (s, 1H, H-3), 7.52 (s, 1H, H-2′), 7.41 to 7.37 (m, 3H, 5′, 6′, 4′), 7.29 to 7.0 (m, 5H, 2″, 3″, 4″, 5″, 6″), 7.03 (dd, 1H, J = 15.5 and 15, H-4), 6.82 (d, 1H, J = 14, H-5), 2.68 (s, 3H, N-acetyl); [13] C NMR (100 MHz, DMSO-d$_6$, δ, TMS = 0, J = Hz): 170.89, 168.63, 144.60, 142.27, 135.93, 135.51, 130.14, 129.42, 128.82, 127.46, 125.67, 125.52, 124.86, 123.94, 122.09, 120.23, 116.69, 116.08, 24.00; MS: 318 (M + Na)$^+$; Anal. calcd. For $C_{17}H_{13}NO_4$: C: 76.12; H, 5.17; N, 4.23 found C: 76.23; H, 5.06; N, 4.33.

2 s. (Z)-2-(1-acetyl-1H-indol-3-yl)-3-(4-nitrophenyl) propenoic acid

Mp: 222°C to 223°C; I.R. (KBr, cm^{-1}): 1684 (C = O), 1671 (C = O, N-acetyl), 1629 (C = C), 1601 and 1450 (C = C, phenyl ring); [1] H NMR (200 MHz, DMSO-d$_6$, δ, TMS = 0, J = Hz): 8.41 (d, 1H, J = 8.2, H-7′), 8.32 (s, 1H, H-3), 8.26 (d, 1H, J = 4.7, H-2″), 7.58 to 7.63 (m, 2H, H-2′, 4″), 7.39 (d, 2H, H-4″, 5″), 7.31 to 7.11 (m, 3H, H-5′, 6′, 4′), 2.48 (s, 3H, N-acetyl); [13] C NMR (100 MHz, DMSO-d$_6$, δ, TMS = 0, J = Hz): 168.00, 167.62, 148.78, 141.94, 136.61, 134.49, 130.82, 124.86, 123.28, 122.77, 24.00; MS: 373 (M + Na)$^+$; Anal. calcd. For $C_{19}H_{14}N_2O_5$: C, 65.14; H, 4.03; N, 8.0 found C: 65.17; H, 4.12; N, 8.05.

2 t. (Z)-2-(1-acetyl-1H-indol-3-yl)-3-(4-fluorophenyl) propenoic acid

Mp: 228°C to 229°C; I.R. (KBr, cm^{-1}): 1711 (C = O), 1679 (C = O, N-acetyl), 1629 (C = C), 1599 and 1450 (C = C, phenyl ring); [1] H NMR (200 MHz, DMSO-d$_6$, δ,

TMS = 0, J = Hz): 8.37 (d, 1H, J = 8.2, H-7′), 8.00 (s, 1H, H-3), 7.87 (s, 1H, H-2′) 7.33 (m, 3H, 5′, 6′, 4′), 7.07 to 6.9 (m, 4H, 2″, 3″, 5″, 6″), 2.48 (s, 3H, N-acetyl); [13] C NMR (100 MHz, DMSO-d_6, δ, TMS = 0, J = Hz): 169.90, 168.63, 151.00, 140.53, 137.02, 135.45, 132.62, 132.66, 129.36, 126.60, 125.76, 123.47, 122.00, 120.19, 116.69, 116.40, 119.90, 115.70, 24.20: 346 $(M + Na)^+$; Anal. calcd. For $C_{19}H_{14}FNO_3$: C, 70.58; H, 4.36; N, 4.33 found C, 70.52; H, 4.31; N, 4.23.

2u. (Z)-2-(1-acetyl-1H-indol-3-yl)-3-(3-chlorophenyl) propenoic acid

Mp: 228°C to 229°C; I.R. (KBr, cm^{-1}): 1708 (C = O), 1665 (C = O, N-acetyl), 1623 (C = C), 1449 (C = C, phenyl ring); [1] H NMR (200 MHz, DMSO-d_6, δ, TMS = 0, J = Hz): 8.38 (d, 1H, J = 8.2, H-7′), 7.99 (s, 1H, H-3), 7.89 (s, 1H, H-2′), 7.31 to 7.50 (m, 6H, 5′, 6′, 4′, 3″, 4″, 5″), 2.48 (s, 3H, N-acetyl); [13] C NMR (125 MHz, DMSO-d $_6$, δ, TMS = 0, J = Hz): 169.90, 168.63, 151.00, 140.53, 137.02, 135.45, 132.62, 132.66, 129.36, 126.60, 125.76, 123.47, 122.00, 120.19, 116.69, 116.40, 119.90, 115.70, 19.30; MS: 362 $(M + Na)^+$; Anal. calcd. For $C_{19}H_{14}NO_3Cl$: C, 67.16; H, 4.15; N, 4.12 found C: 67.23; H, 4.11; N, 4.02.

2v. (Z)-2-(1-acetyl-1H-indol-3-yl)-3-(2-chlorophenyl) propenoic acid

Mp: 189°C to 190°C; I.R. (KBr, cm^{-1}): 1720 (C = O), 1685 (C = O, N-acetyl), 1621 (C = C), 1450 (C = C, phenyl ring); [1] H NMR (200 MHz, DMSO-d_6, δ, TMS = 0, J = Hz): 8.38 (d, 1H, J = 7.32, H-7′), 8.10 (s, 1H, H-3), 7.91 (d, 1H, J = 6.8, H-2′), 7.71 (d, 1H, H-3″), 7.43 to 7.30 (m, 3H, 5′, 6′, 4′), 6.80 to 6.9 (m, 3H, 4″, 5″, 6″), 2.62 (s, 3H, N-acetyl); [13] C NMR (100 MHz, DMSO-d_6, δ, TMS = 0, J = Hz): 169.80, 168.20, 139.53, 137.02, 135.45, 132.62, 132.66, 129.80, 126.60, 125.76, 123.47, 122.00, 119.00, 116.69, 116.40, 115.7, 24.20; MS: 362 $(M + Na)^+$; Anal. calcd. For $C_{19}H_{14}NO_3Cl$: C, 67.16; H, 4.15; N, 4.12 found C: 66.27; H, 4.11; N, 4.32.

2w. (Z)-2-(1-acetyl-1H-indol-3-yl)-3-(naphthalene-1-yl) propenoic acid

Mp: 190°C to 192°C; I.R. (KBr, cm¯1): 1703 (C = O), 1680 (C = O, N-acetyl), 1615 (C = C), 1449 (C = C, phenyl ring); [1] H NMR (200 MHz, DMSO-d_6, δ, TMS = 0, J = Hz): 8.23 (d, 1H, J = 7.9, H-7′), 8.16 (s, 1H, H-3), 8.00 (d, 1H, J = 6.2, H-2′), 7.64 to 7.3 (m, 7H, 2″, 3″, 4″, 5″, 6″, 7″, 8″) 6.93 to 6.80 (m, 3H, 5′, 6′, 4′), 2.60 (s, 3H, N-acetyl); [13] C NMR (100 MHz, DMSO-d_6, δ, TMS = 0, J = Hz); 168.50, 167.88, 140.66, 139.18, 135.56, 133.27, 132.87, 132.40, 131.20, 129.18, 127.64, 126.32, 126.10, 125.18, 123.68, 123.57, 120.38, 117.43, 116.49, 24.20; 378 $(M + Na)^+$; Anal. calcd. For $C_{23}H_{17}NO_3$: C, 77.73; H, 4.22; N, 3.94 found C, 77.45; H, 4.32; N, 3.83.

2x. (Z)-2-(1-acetyl-1H-indol-3-yl)-3-(4-bromophenyl) propenoic acid

Mp: 220°C to 222°C; I.R. (KBr, cm^{-1}): 1711 (C = O), 1676 (C = O, N-acetyl), 1632 (C = C), 1565 (C = C, phenyl ring); [1] H NMR (200 MHz, DMSO-d_6, δ, TMS = 0, J = Hz): 8.41 (d, 1H, J = 7.6, H-7′), 7.95 (s, 1H, H-3) 7.75 (s, 1H, H-2′) 7.30 (dd, 2H, J = 7.1 and 3.3, H-6′), 7.21 to 7.10 (m, 4H, H-6′, 3″, 5″, 6″), 6.98 to 6.80 (m, 2H, H-5′, 4′), 2.68 (s, 3H, N-acetyl); [13] C NMR (125 MHz, DMSO-d_6, δ, TMS = 0, J = Hz): 168.00, 168.53, 139.53, 137.02, 135.45, 132.82, 131.66, 129.76, 128.80, 128.09, 125.76, 125.41, 125.06, 123.47, 122.00, 120.19, 116.69, 116.40, 23.00: 407 $(M + Na)^+$;Anal. calcd. For $C_{19}H_{14}BrNO_3$: C, 59.39; H, 3.67; N, 3.65; found C, 59.22; H, 3.4; N, 3.45.

2y. 3-(N-acetyl-1H-indol-3-yl)-8-acetoxy-2H-chromen-2-one

Mp: 110°C to 112°C; I.R. (KBr, cm^{-1}): 1763 (C = O, lactone) 1710 (C = O, O-acetyl), 1703 (C = O, N-acetyl), 1684 (C = O), 1543 and 1453 (C = C, phenyl ring); [1] H NMR (200 MHz, DMSO-d_6, δ, TMS = 0, J = Hz): 8.51 (s, 1H, H-4), 8.45 (d, 1H, J = 7.0, H-7′), 8.35 (s, 1H, H-2′), 7.95 (dd, 1H, J = 5.2 and 7.2, H-6′) 7.95 (dd, 1H, J = 5.2 and 7.2, H-5′), 7.48 to 7.38 (m, 4H, H-4′, 5′, 6′, 7′), 2.67 (s, 3H, N-acetyl), 2.67 (s, 3H, O-acetyl); [13] C NMR (125 MHz, DMSO-d_6, δ, TMS = 0, J = Hz): 170.00, 168.93, 158.82, 148.78, 144.48, 139.62, 137.20, 135.50, 128.3, 128.27, 126.55, 125.70, 125.40, 125.00, 124.29, 12.05, 121.00, 120.90, 116.49, 114.98, 24.30, 20.81; MS: 386 $(M + Na)^+$; Anal. calcd. For $C_{20}H_{13}NO_6$: C, 66.12; H, 3.61; N, 3.86; found C, 66.24; H, 3.42; N, 3.88

Biological evaluation

In vitro cytotoxicity against five human cancer cell lines was determined using 96-well tissue culture plate [26]. The cells were allowed to grow in carbon dioxide incubator (37°C) for 24 h. Test materials in complete growth medium (100 μl) were added after 24 h of incubation to the wells containing cell suspension. The plates were further incubated for 48 h in a carbon dioxide incubator. The cell growth was stopped by gentle layering trichloroacetic acid (50%, 50 μl) on top of the medium in all the wells. The plates were incubated at 4°C for 1 h to fix the cells attached to the bottom of the wells. The liquid of all the wells was gently pipetted out and discarded. The plates were washed five times with distilled water to remove trichloroacetic acid, growth medium low-molecular weight metabolites, serum proteins, etc. and air-dried. The plates were stained with sulforhodamine B dye (0.4% in 1% acetic acid, 100 μl) for 30 min. The plates were washed five times with 1% acetic acid and then air-dried [27]. The adsorbed dye was dissolved in Tris–HCl buffer (100 μL, 0.01 M, pH 10.4), and the plates were gently stirred for 10 min on a mechanical stirrer. The optical density (OD) was recorded on ELISA reader at 540 nm. The cell growth was determined by subtracting the mean OD value of respective blank from the mean OD value of the experimental set. Percent growth in presence of test material was calculated considering the growth in the absence of any test material as 100%, and in turn, percent growth inhibition in presence of test material was calculated.

Conclusions

A series of novel combretastatin analogues have been synthesized by condensation of indole-3-acetic acid with different substituted aldehydes, and structures were established by various spectral techniques like IR, MS, and NMR ([1] H, [13] C, HMBC, and HSQC). Configuration was established by lactone formation when hydroxyl group was present on second position of aldehyde. Further, it was confirmed by nOe (H-4′ intensity increased on double irradiation of H-3). Compounds were evaluated for anticancer activity. The effect on microtubule structure was determined using confocal microscopy dose-dependent disruption, and loss of microtubules indicates apoptosis by **2d**. Binding of compound at colchicine binding site was established by molecular docking study. It was helpful to rationalize the inhibitory activity of these inhibitors. The carbonyl oxygen (carbonyl group at indole) forms a hydrogen bond with sulfhydryl group of Cys241*β*. This is similar to the interaction of colchicines with the tubulin. Another hydrogen bond was formed between the hydroxyl group of the carboxylic acid part of **2d** and nitrogen of Leu255*β*. These two hydrogen bonds play a crucial role in stabilizing the conformation of **2d** at the colchicine binding site. The activity of the synthesized compounds indicates that these can be promising anticancer drugs. To confirm their potency, further *in vivo* experiment will be required to address the anticancer property in cancer chemotherapy.

Additional files

Additional file 1: Compound 2e. C13 spectrum.
Additional file 2: Compound 2e. DEPT spectrum.
Additional file 3: Compound 2e. H1 NMR spectrum.
Additional file 4: Compound 2e. HMBC spectrum.
Additional file 5: Compound 2e. Expanded HMBC spectrum.
Additional file 6: Compound 2e. Expanded HSQC spectrum.

Competing interests

The authors declare that they have no competing interests.

Acknowledgments

The authors are grateful to the chairman of the ISF College of Pharmacy, Moga, and the director of the Indian Institute of Integrative Medicine, Jammu Tawi for providing facilities.

Author details

[1]Laboratory for Drug Design and Synthesis, Department of Pharmaceutical Chemistry, Indo-Soviet Friendship (ISF) College of Pharmacy, Moga, Punjab 142 001, India. [2]Division of Bio-Organic Chemistry and Pharmacology, Indian Institute of Integrative Medicine (IIIM), CSIR, Jammu Tawi 180 001, India.

References

1. Jordan A, Hadfield JA, Lawrence NJ, McGown AT (1997) Tubulin as a target for anticancer drugs: agent which interact with mitotic spindle. Inc Med Res Rev 18:259–296
2. Hadfield JA, Ducki S, Hirst N, McGown AT (2003) Tubulin and microtubules as target for anticancer drugs. Progress in Cell Cycle Res 5:309–325
3. Meng F, Cai X, Duan J, Matteuccki MG, Hart CP (2008) A novel class of tubulin inhibitors that exhibit potent antiproliferation and in vitro vessel-disrupting activity. Canc Chemoth Pharmacol 61:953–963
4. Toso RJ, Jordan MA, Farrel KW, Matsumoto B, Wilson L (1993) Kinetic stabilization of microtubule dynamic instability in vitro by vinblastine. Biochem 32:1285–1293
5. Wu R, Ding W, Liu T, Zhu H, Hu Y, Yang B, He Q (2009) XNO_5, a novel synthesized microtubule inhibitor, exhibits potent activity against human carcinoma cells in vitro. Canc Lett 285:13–22
6. Mitchison T, Kirschner M (1984) Dynamic instability of microtubule growth. Nature 312:237–242
7. Downing KH, Nogales E (1998) New insights into microtubule structure and function from the atomic model of tubulin. Eur Biophys J 27:431–436
8. Ouyang X, Piatnitski EL, Pattaropong V, Chen X, He HY, Kiselyov AS, Valankar A, Kwakami J, Labelle M, Smith L, Lohman J, Lee SP, Malikzay A, Fleming J, Gerlak J, Wang Y, Rosler RL, Zhou K, Mitelman S, Camara M, Surguladze D, Boody JF, Tuma MC (2006) Oxadiazole derivatives as novel class of antimitotic agents: synthesis, inhibition of tubulin polymerization and activity in tumor cell lines. Bioorg Med Chem Lett 16:1191–1196
9. Tron GC, Pirali T, Sorba G, Pagliai F, Busacca S, Genazzani AA (2006) Medicinal chemistry of combretastatin A4: present and future directions. J Med Chem 49:3033–3044
10. Woods JA, Hadfield JA, Pettit GR, Fox BW, McGown AT (1995) The interaction with tubulin of a series of stilbenes based on combretastatin A-4. Br J Canc 71:705–711
11. McGown AT, Fox BW (1989) Structural and biochemical comparison of the antimitotic agents colchicine, combretastatin A4 and amphethinile. Anticancer Drug Des 3:249–254
12. Petit GR, Rhodes MR, Herald DL, Hamel E, Schmidt JM, Petit RK (2005) Antineoplastic agents, 445, synthesis and evaluation of structural modifications of (Z), and (E)-combretastatin A-4. J Med Chem 48:4087–4099
13. Kaffy J, Pontikis R, Carrz D, Croisy A, Monneret C, Florent JC (2006) Isoxazole-type derivatives related to combretastatin A-4, synthesis and biological evaluation. Bioorg Med Chem 14:4067–4077
14. Pettit RK, Pettit GR, Hamel E, Hogan F, Moser BR, Wolf S, Pon S, Chapuis JC, Schmidt JM (2009) E-combretastatin and E-resveratrol structural modifications: antimicrobial and cancer cell growth inhibitory β-E -nitrostyrenes. Bioorg Med Chem 17:6606–6612
15. Gupta S, Bhattacharyya B (2003) Antimicrotubular drugs binding to vinca domain of tubulin. Mol Cell Biochem 253:41–47
16. Cragg GM, Newman DJ (2006) Ethnopharmacology. EOLSS, Oxford
17. Cragg GM, Newman DJ (2011) Anticancer agents from natural products. CRCnetBASE 2:699–728
18. Pinard PV, Wang F, Burd B, Angeletti RH, Horwitz SB, Orr GA (2003) Direct analysis of tubulin expression in cancer cell lines by electrospray ionization mass spectrometry. Biochem 42:12019–12027
19. Enroth C, Eger BT, Okamoto K, Nishino T, Nishino T, Pai EF (2000) Crystal structure of bovine milk xanthene dehydrogenase: structure based mechanism of conversion. Proc Natl Acad Sci USA 97:10723
20. Ravelli RB, Gigant B, Curmi PA, Jourdain I, Lachkar S, Sobel A, Knossow M (2004) Insight into tubulin regulation from a complex with colchicine and a stathmin-like domain. Nature 428:198–202
21. PerkinElmer, Inc (2000) ChemDraw Ultra 6.0 and Chem3D Ultra. Cambridge Soft Corporation, Cambridge, USA
22. CCDC (2011) GOLD 5.0.1. Cambridge Crystallographic Data Centre, Cambridge, UK

23. Cushman MS, Layfayette W, Hamel E (1995) Stilbene derivatives as anticancer agents.. US Patent 5,430,062, Bethesda, 4 July 1995
24. Leake PH (1956) Synthesis of phenanthrene. Chem Rev 56:27
25. Sylvie D, Grant M, Ben G, Simon A, Jérémie FDC, Elizabeth B, Jim N, James P, Nicholas JL (2009) Combretastatin-like chalcones as inhibitors of microtubule polymerisation. Part 2: Structure-based discovery of alpha-aryl chalcones. Bioor Med Chem 17:7711–7722
26. Monks A, Scudiero D, Skehan P, Shoemaker R, Paull K, Vistica D, Hose C, Langley J, Cronise P, Vaigro-Wolff A (1991) Feasibility of a high-flux anticancer drug screen using a diverse panel of cultured human tumor cell lines. J Natl Canc Inst 83:757–766
27. Skehan P, Storeng R, Scudiero D, Monks A, McMahon J, Vistica D, Warren JT, Bokesch H, Kenney S, Boyd MR (1990) New colorometric cytotoxicity assay for anticancer-drug screening. J Natl Canc Inst 82:1107–1112

Monastrol mimic Biginelli dihydropyrimidinone derivatives: synthesis, cytotoxicity screening against HepG2 and HeLa cell lines and molecular modeling study

Uttara Soumyanarayanan[1*], Varadaraj G Bhat[1], Sidhartha S Kar[1] and Jesil A Mathew[2]

Abstract

Biginelli dihydropyrimidinone derivatives as structural analogs of monastrol, a known human kinesin Eg5 inhibitor, were synthesized. IC_{50} values of the synthesized compounds against the proliferation of human hepatocellular carcinoma and human epithelial carcinoma cell lines were determined through MTT assay. Molecular docking study gave a clear insight into the structural activity relationship of the compounds in comparison with monastrol.

Keywords: Privileged structures, Amide coupling, Mitotic kinesin, Biginelli reaction

Background

1,4-Dihydropyrimidinones (DHPMs) comprise of a pyrimidine scaffold having a resemblance with the structures of the nucleic acid bases found in DNA and RNA. Their involvement as bases in nucleic acids has a great significance in drug design. Recent progress in the DHPM class of the anticancer agent monastrol, an inhibitor of human kinesin Eg5 [1,2], has led to the attention for efficient pharmacophore variation of Biginelli DHPMs. Human kinesin Eg5 plays a crucial role in bipolar spindle generation during mitosis, inhibition of which leads to mitotic arrest and subsequent apoptotic cell death [3]. It is therefore considered as one of the promising targets in cancer chemotherapy. Racemic dihydropyrimidinone is reported to be an allosteric inhibitor of Eg5 [4], and unlike taxanes, it is nontoxic to neuron cells [5,6].

Considerable work has also been devoted to gain insights into the structure-activity relationship in the monastrol derivative series [7]. Recently, Dennis Russowsky and coworkers described the differential effects of monastrol, oxo-monastrol and oxygenated analogs on seven human cancer cell lines [8]. However, anticancer activity profile of amide derivatives of dihydropyrimidinones with functional variations at aromatic ring has not been explored so far. This paper describes the synthesis and evaluation of monastrol-related racemic dihydropyrimidinones substituted with privileged structures [9] like pyrrolidine, piperidine and morpholine through an amide linkage. It was speculated that the introduction of cyclic amines through amide linkage at the side chain of the DHPM scaffold could mimic the interactions of the ester group of monastrol and might also provide improved metabolic stability to the moiety. In order to probe the effect of substitutions at the aromatic ring of Biginelli DHPMs on cytotoxicity, halogens were introduced at ortho and para positions. Physicochemical properties and biological activity of thiourea is closely related with urea, which possesses bioisosteric pharmacophore groups. Hence, thiourea motif of the DHPMs has been replaced by urea that may function as a bioisoster. In addition, the molecular docking and virtual physicochemical properties were studied to understand the structural activity relationship of the scaffold.

Methods

Chemistry

General remarks

Melting points were taken in capillary tubes, measured in the melting point apparatus and were uncorrected.

* Correspondence: uttarasn@gmail.com
[1]Department of Pharmaceutical Chemistry, Manipal College of Pharmaceutical Sciences, Manipal University, Manipal, Karnataka 576104, India
Full list of author information is available at the end of the article

Infrared spectra were recorded on a Shimadzu FTIR 8310 spectrometer. Nuclear magnetic resonance (NMR) spectra were recorded on Bruker 400/500 MHz spectrometer in $CDCl_3$/DMSO-d_6/CD_3OD. Chemical shifts are reported in parts per million (ppm) from tetramethylsilane with tetramethylsilane as the internal standard. Data reported are as follows: chemical shift, multiplicity as singlet (s), doublet (d), triplet (t), quartet (q), broad singlet (br s) and multiplet (m), and coupling constants (Hz). Mass spectra were obtained on a Shimadzu GCMS-QP5050A. Combustion analyses were performed on a Perkin-Elmer 2400-II analyzer. The progress of the reactions was monitored by thin layer chromatography using F254 silica gel pre-coated sheets (Merck, India). Column chromatography was performed on silica gel (100 to 200 mesh). Solvents for extraction and chromatography were AR/HPLC grade (Scheme 1).

General method for the preparation of compounds 1a to 1d

A solution of arylaldehyde (0.28 mmol), ethyl acetoacetate (0.28 mmol), urea (0.42 mmol) and boric acid (0.056 mmol) in glacial acetic acid (15 mL) was heated at 100°C, stirring for 9 h. Progress of the reaction was monitored by thin layer chromatography (TLC) using hexane: ethyl acetate (4:6) as mobile phase. Then, the reaction mixture was cooled to room temperature, poured into ice-cold water (150 to 200 mL) and stirred for 15 min. The solid precipitate obtained was filtered, washed with ice-cold water and recrystallized with absolute alcohol to afford white solid crystals with a quantitative yield [10].

Ethyl 4-methyl-2-oxo-6-phenylhexahydropyrimidine-5-carboxylate (1a): Colorless crystals, Yield 80%. Melting point (Mp.) 200°C to 202°C (Literature (Lit.) [11] Mp. 202°C to 204°C). R_f 0.56 (Hexane:ethyl acetate (4:6)). Infra

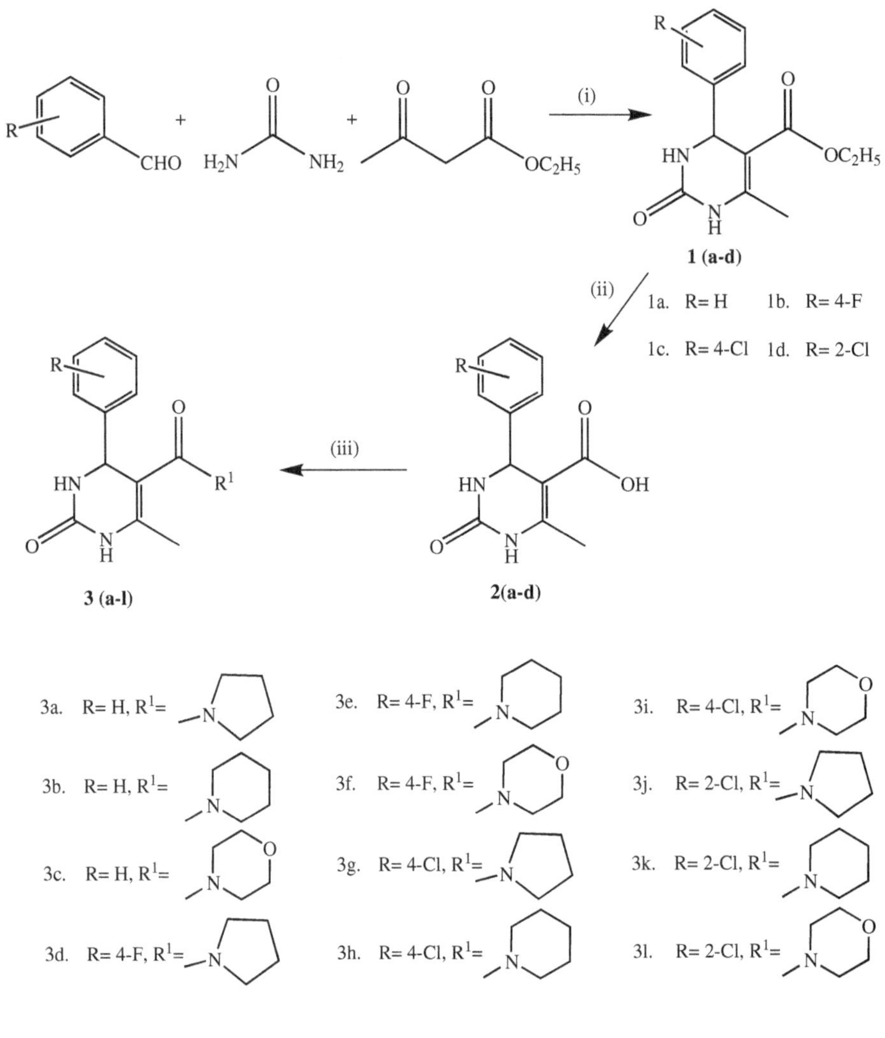

Scheme 1 Synthetic scheme for the preparation of compounds 3a to 3 l.

Red Spectra (IR) (KBr) cm^{-1}: 3,242 (N-H stretching (str.)), 1,645 (C = O str.). ^{1}H NMR (500 MHz, DMSO-d_6): δ 9.21 (s, 1 H), 7.46 (br s, 1 H), 7.35 to 7.14 (m, 5 H), 5.62 (s, 1 H), 3.95 (q, 2 H), 2.26 (s, 3 H), 0.997 (s, 3 H).

Ethyl 4-(4-fluorophenyl)-6-methyl-2-oxohexahydropyrimidine-5-carboxylate (1b): Colorless crystals, Yield 80%. Mp. 178°C to 180°C (Lit. [12] Mp. 175°C to 177°C). R_f 0.51 (Hexane:ethyl acetate (4:6)). IR (KBr) cm^{-1}: 3,242 (N-H str.), 1,718 (C = O str.), 1,645 (C = O str.). ^{1}H NMR (500 MHz, DMSO-d_6): δ 9.38 (s, 1 H), 7.86 (br s, 1 H), 7.46 to 7.36 (m, 2 H), 7.33 to 7.24 (m, 2 H), 5.56 (s, 1 H), 3.96 (q, 2 H), 2.27 (s, 3 H), 1.03 (s, 3 H).

Ethyl 4-(4-chlorophenyl)-6-methyl-2-oxohexahydropyrimidine-5-carboxylate (1c): Colorless crystals, Yield 81%. Mp. 214°C to 216°C. (Lit. [13] Mp. 214°C to 217°C). R_f 0.54 (Hexane:ethyl acetate (4:6)). IR (KBr) cm^{-1}: 3,350 (N-H str.), 1,637 (C = O str.). ^{1}H NMR (500 MHz, DMSO-d_6): δ 9.57 (s, 1 H), 7.76 (br s, 1 H), 7.43 to 7.38 (m, 2 H), 7.34 to 7.21 (m, 2 H), 5.68 (s, 1 H), 3.87 (q, 2 H), 2.33 (s, 3 H), 0.995 (s, 3 H).

Ethyl 4-(2-chlorophenyl)-6-methyl-2-oxohexahydropyrimidine-5-carboxylate (1d): Colorless crystals, Yield 78%. Mp. 213°C to 215°C. (Lit. [14] Mp. 212.5°C to 214.5°C). R_f 0.55 (Hexane:ethyl acetate (4:6)). IR (KBr) cm^{-1}: 3,350 (N-H str.), 1,637 (C = O str.). ^{1}H NMR (500 MHz, DMSO-d_6): δ 9.27 (s, 1 H), 7.71 (br s, 1 H), 7.40 (d, 1 H), 7.34 to 7.29 (m, 2 H), 7.28 to 7.25 (m, 1 H), 5.63 (s, 1 H), 3.91 (q, 2 H), 2.3 (s, 3 H), 0.998 (s, 3 H). MS (EI): 295 $[M]^+$.

General method for the preparation of compounds 2a to 2d

A solution of compounds 1a to 1d (2 mmol) in 10 mL methanol and NaOH (4 mmol) dissolved in 1 mL water was heated at 60°C to 62°C, stirring for 8 h. Progress of the reaction was monitored by TLC using chloroform: methanol (9:1) as mobile phase. The reaction mixture was cooled and concentrated under vacuum to remove methanol. The residue obtained was then added to 25 mL ice-cold water and was extracted with chloroform (3 × 10 mL) to remove the unreacted ester. The aqueous layer was acidified to pH 2 using 10% *v*/*v* HCl and then extracted with ethyl acetate (3 × 15 mL). The ethyl acetate layer was separated, pooled over anhydrous sodium sulfate and evaporated under vacuum to give the crude acid. The crude acid was purified by column chromatography using chloroform:methanol (95:5) as mobile phase and silica gel (100 to 200 mesh) as stationary phase to afford the pure product [15-17].

4-Methyl-2-oxo-6-phenylhexahydropyrimidine-5-carboxylic acid (2a): Colorless solid, Yield 35%. Mp. 217°C to 219°C. (Lit. [18] Mp. 210°C). R_f 0.26 (Chloroform: methanol (9:1)). IR (KBr) cm^{-1}: 3,431 (O-H str.), 3,225 (N-H str.), 1,645 (C = O str.), 1,705 (C = O str.).

4-(4-Fluorophenyl)-6-methyl-2-oxohexahydropyrimidine-5-carboxylic acid (2b): Colorless solid, Yield 36%. Mp. 200°C to 202°C. R_f 0.28 (Chloroform:methanol (9:1)). IR (KBr) cm^{-1}: 3,442 (O-H str.), 3,227 (N-H str.), 1,705 (C = O str.).

4-(4-Chlorophenyl)-6-methyl-2-oxohexahydropyrimidine-5-carboxylic acid (2c): Colorless solid, Yield 38%. Mp. 207°C to 209°C (Lit. [18] Mp. 199°C to 200°C). R_f 0.24 (Chloroform:methanol (9:1)). IR (KBr) cm^{-1}: 3,439 (O-H str.), 3,238 (N-H str.), 1,643 (C = O str.).

4-(2-Chlorophenyl)-6-methyl-2-oxohexahydropyrimidine-5-carboxylic acid (2d): Colorless solid, Yield 37%. Mp. 212°C to 214°C. R_f 0.27 (Chloroform:methanol (9:1)). IR (KBr) cm^{-1}: 3,444 (O-H str.), 3,238 (N-H str.), 1,708 (C = O str.), 1,645 (C = O str.). ^{1}H NMR (500 MHz, CD_3OD): δ 7.42 to 7.40 (dd, 2 H, *J* = 7.5 and 1.5 Hz), 7.36 to 7.34 (dd, 1 H, *J* = 8 and 2 Hz), 7.32 to 7.30 (dd, 1 H, *J* = 7.5 and 1.5 Hz), 7.27 to 7.26 (d, 1 H, *J* = 1.5 Hz), 5.83 (s, 1 H), 2.18 (s, 3 H). ESI-MS, 266.5 $[M]^+$.

General method for the preparation of compounds 3a to 3 l

A mixture of compounds 2a to 2d was added to tetramethyluronium tetraflouroborate (TBTU) (1.5 eq.) and diisopropylethylamine (2 eq.) in 2 mL dimethylformamide under nitrogen atmosphere. The mixture was stirred for 2 min at 25°C, and then, pyrrolidine/piperidine/morpholine (1.5 eq., 0.068 mL) was added to it. Another 2 equivalents of diisopropylethylamine (DIPEA) was again added to it. The reaction mixture was stirred for 10 min. The reaction was monitored by TLC using chloroform:methanol (9:1). The reaction mixture was poured into 50 mL ice-cold water and was extracted with dichloromethane (3 × 20 mL). The extract was purified by column chromatography using chloroform:methanol (97:3) and silica gel (100 to 200 mesh) as stationary phase to afford the desired product [19,20].

6-Methyl-4-phenyl-5-(pyrrolidine-1-carbonyl)-3,4-dihydropyrimidin-2(1 H)-one (3a): White solid, Yield 81%. Mp. 258°C to 260°C. Rf: 0.46 (Chloroform:methanol (9:1)). IR (KBr) cm^{-1}: 3,224, 3,145 (N-H str.), 1,696 (C = O str.), 2,881 (C-H str.). ^{13}C NMR (400 MHz, DMSO-d_6): δ 166.34 (C = O), 161.83 (C = O), 140.42 to 124.32 (6 C, aromatic), 151.74 (=C-NH), 25.32 to 23.96 (4 C, aliphatic), 15.56 (CH_3). ^{1}H NMR (400 MHz, $CDCl_3$): 7.26 to 7.24 (m, 5 H), 6.38 (br s, 1 H), 5.41 (s, 1 H), 5.11 (s, 1 H), 3.26 to 2.10 (m, 8 H), 1.73 (s, 3 H). MS (EI): 285 $[M]^+$, 270 $[M\text{-}CH_3]^+$, 214 $[M\text{-}C_5H_{10}N]^+$, 187 $[M\text{-}C_6H_{10}NO]^+$, 172 $[M\text{-}CH_3\text{-}C_6H_{10}NO]^+$, 132 $[M\text{-}C_9H_{14}N_2O]^+$.

6-Methyl-4-phenyl-5-(piperidine-1-carbonyl)-3,4-dihydropyrimidin-2(1 H)-one (3b): White solid, Yield 83%. Mp. 266°C to 268°C. R_f 0.49 (Chloroform:methanol (9:1)). IR (KBr) cm^{-1}: 3,223, 3,095 (N-H str.), 1,681 (C = O str.), 2,858 (C-H str.). ^{13}C NMR (400 MHz, DMSO-d_6):

165.88 (C = O), 162.28 (C = O), 141.56 to 125.56 (6 C aromatic), 152.26 (=C-NH), 104.48, 56.24 (CH), 26.32 to 23.80 (5 C, aliphatic), 15.78 (CH_3). ^1H NMR (400 MHz, $CDCl_3$): δ 8.44 (br s, 1 H), 7.35 (s, 1 H, aromatic H), 7.33 (d, 1 H, *J* = 0.8 Hz), 7.31 (t, 1 H, *J* = 2.4 Hz), δ 7.26 (m, 1 H), 7.19 (d, 1 H, *J* = 0.8 Hz), 7.17 (s, 1 H), 2.95 (s, 4 H), 1.34 (s, 2 H), 1.10 (d, 4 H, *J* = 2 Hz). MS (EI): 299 $[M]^+$, 284 $[M\text{-}CH_3]^+$, 214 $[M\text{-}C_5H_{10}N]^+$, 187 $[M\text{-}C_6H_{10}NO]^+$, 172 $[M\text{-}CH_3\text{-}C_6H_{10}NO]^+$, 133 $[M\text{-}C_9H_{14}N_2O]^+$.

4-Methyl-5-(morpholine-4-carbonyl)-6-phenyltetrahydropyrimidin-2(1 H)-one (3c): White solid, Yield 83%. Mp. 233°C to 234°C. R_f 0.52 (Chloroform:methanol (9:1)). IR (KBr) cm^{-1}: 3,240 (N-H str.), 1,695 (C = O str.), 2,858 (C-H str.). ^{13}C NMR (400 MHz, DMSO-d_6): 166.68 (C = O), 162.28 (C = O), 142.28 to 126.23 (6 C, aromatic), 152.38 (=C-NH), 103.76, 56.22 (CH), 30.42 to 26.68 (4 C, aliphatic), 15.32 (CH_3). ^1H NMR (400 MHz, $CDCl_3$): δ 7.35 to 7.31(m, 5 H) 7.21 (d, 1 H, *J* = 1.6 Hz) 5.49 (s, 1 H), 5.30 (s, 1 H), 3.22 to 3.05 (m, 6 H) 1.27 to 1.29 (m, 2 H). MS (EI): 301 $[M]^+$, 286 $[M\text{-}CH_3]^+$, 214 $[M\text{-}C_4H_8NO]^+$, 186 $[M\text{-}C_5H_8NO_2]^+$, 172$[M\text{-}CH_3\text{-}C_5H_8NO_2]^+$, 132 $[M\text{-}C_8H_{12}N_2O_2]^+$.

4-(4-Fluorophenyl)-6-methyl-5-(pyrrolidine-1-carbonyl)-3,4-dihydropyrimidin-2(1 H)-one (3d): White solid, Yield 80%. Mp. 242°C to 244°C. R_f 0.48 (Chloroform:methanol (9:1)). IR (KBr) cm^{-1}: 3,242, 3,142 (N-H str.), 1,689, 1,660 (C = O str.), 2,954 (C-H str.). ^{13}C NMR (400 MHz, DMSO-d_6): δ 166.57 (C = O), 160.15 (C = O), 162.15 to 114 (6 C aromatic), 152.58 (=C-NH), 105.79, 55.6 (CH), 25.11 to 23.80 (4 C, aliphatic), 15.96 (CH_3). ^1H NMR (400 MHz, $CDCl_3$): 7.26 to 6.29 (m, 4 H), 6.87 (br s, 1 H), 5.41 (s, 1 H), 5.23 (s, 1 H), 3.26 to 2.59 (m,4 H), 1.67 (s, 3 H), 1.66 to 1.18 (m, 4 H). MS (EI): 303 $[M]^+$, 288 $[M\text{-}CH_3]^+$, 233 $[M\text{-}C_4H_8NO]^+$, 205 $[M\text{-}C_5H_8NO_2]^+$, 190 $[M\text{-}CH_3\text{-}C_5H_8NO_2]^+$, 150 $[M\text{-}C_8H_{12}N_2O]^+$.

4-(4-Fluorophenyl)-6-methyl-5-(piperidine-1-carbonyl)-3,4-dihydropyrimidin-2(1 H)-one (3e): White solid, Yield 82%. Mp. 264°C to 266°C. R_f: 0.53 (Chloroform:methanol (9:1)). IR (KBr) cm^{-1}: 3,240 (N-H str), 1,691 (C = O str), 1,658 (amide C = O str). ^{13}C NMR (400 MHz, DMSO-d_6): δ 165.76 (C = O), 160.52 (C = O), 163.18 to 113.32 (6 C, aromatic), 153.26 (=C-NH), 106.72, 55.4 (CH), 26.52 to 23.20 (5 C, aliphatic), 15.40 (CH_3). ^1H NMR (400 MHz, $CDCl_3$): δ 7.55 (s, 1 H), 7.35 to 7.30 (m, 2 H,), 7.05 to 7.01 (m, 2 H), 5.45 (s, 1 H), 5.43 (s, 1 H), 3.86 to 3.04 (m, 4 H), 1.76 (s, 3 H), 1.60 to 1.55 (m, 2 H), 1.46 to 1.41 (m, 2 H), 1.29 to 1.24(m, 2 H). MS (EI): 317 $[M]^+$, 302 $[M\text{-}CH_3]^+$, 233 $[M\text{-}C_5H_{10}N]^+$, 222 $[M\text{-}C_6H_4F]^+$, 205 $[M\text{-}C_6H_{10}NO]^+$, 193 $[M\text{-}CH_3\text{-}C_6H_{10}NO]^+$, 150 $[M\text{-}C_9H_{14}N_2O]^+$.

4-(4-Fluorophenyl)-6-methyl-5-(morpholine-4-carbonyl)-3,4-dihydropyrimidin-2(1 H)-one (3f): White solid, Yield 82%. Mp. 230°C to 232°C. R_f 0.51 (Chloroform:methanol (9:1)). IR (KBr) cm^{-1}: 3,248, 3,150 (N-H str.), 1,681, 1,608 (C = O str.), 2,875 (C-H str.). ^{13}C NMR (400 MHz, DMSO-d_6): δ 166.22 (C = O), 161.36 (C = O), 162.78 to 113.76 (6 C, aromatic), 152.64 (=C-NH), 105.63, 55.28 (CH), 29.22 to 24.46 (4 C, aliphatic), 15.63 (CH_3). ^1H NMR (400 MHz, $CDCl_3$): 7.27 to 6.96 (m, 4 H), 6.41 (s,1 H), 5.42 (s, 1 H), 5.10 (s, 1 H), 3.25 to 3.027 (m, 4 H), 1.72 (s, 3 H), 1.48 to 1.18 (m, 4 H). 319 $[M]^+$, 303 $[M\text{-}CH_3]^+$, 232 $[M\text{-}C_4H_8NO]^+$, 205 $[M\text{-}C_5H_8NO_2]^+$, 190 $[M\text{-}CH_3\text{-}C_5H_8NO_2]^+$, 150 $[M\text{-}C_8H_{12}N_2O_2]^+$.

4-(4-Chlorophenyl)-6-methyl-5-(pyrrolidine-1-carbonyl)-3,4-dihydropyrimidin-2(1 H)-one (3 g): White solid, Yield 84%. Mp. 260°C to 262°C. R_f 0.42 (Chloroform: methanol (9:1)). IR (KBr) cm^{-1}: 3,227, 3,151(N-H str.), 1,676, 1,608 (C = O str.), 2,862 (C-H str.). ^{13}C NMR (400 MHz, DMSO-d_6): δ 165.82 (C = O), 162.28 (C = O), 139.70 to 115.92 (6 C, aromatic), 153.72 (+C-NH), 103.02, 56.75 (CH), 24.78 to 23.20 (4 C, aliphatic), 15.34 (CH_3). ^1H NMR (400 MHz, $CDCl_3$): δ 7.55 (br s, 1 H), 7.32 to 7.29 (m, 2 H,), 7.28 to 7.26 (m, 2 H), 5.44 (s, 1 H), 5.46 (s, 1 H), 3.33 (s, 2 H), 3.02 (s, 1 H), 2.68 (s, 1 H), 1.80 (s, 3 H), 1.72 to 1.61 (m, 4 H). ESI-MS: 320 $[M]^+$, 249 $[M\text{-}C_5H_8N]^+$, 303 $[M\text{-}CH_4]^+$, 207 $[M\text{-}C_6H_5Cl]^+$.

4-(4-Chlorophenyl)-6-methyl-5-(piperidine-1-carbonyl)-3,4-dihydropyrimidin-2(1 H)-one (3 h): White solid, Yield 86%. Mp. 253°C to 255°C. R_f 0.48 (Chloroform:methanol (9:1)). IR (KBr) cm^{-1}: 3,227, 3,151(N-H str.), 1,676, 1,608 (C = O str.), 2,862 (C-H str.). ^{13}C NMR (400 MHz, DMSO-d_6): δ 166.25 (C = O), 161.48 (C = O), 138.78 to 116.26 (6 C, aromatic), 152.58 (=C-NH), 103.38, 56.53 (CH), 25.20 to 23.64 (5 C, aliphatic), 15.62 (CH_3). ^1H NMR (400 MHz, $CDCl_3$): δ 7.70 (br s, 1 H), 7.32 to 7.24 (m, 4 H), 3.48 to 3.02 (m, 4 H), 1.79 (s, 3 H), 1.66 to 1.25 (m, 6 H). MS (EI): 333$[M\text{-}1]^+$, 318 $[M\text{-}CH_3]^+$, 249 $[M\text{-}C_4H_8NO]^+$, 221 $[M\text{-}C_5H_8NO_2]^+$, 206$[M\text{-}CH_3\text{-}C_5H_8NO_2]^+$, 166 $[M\text{-}C_9H_{14}N_{20}]^+$.

4-(4-Chlorophenyl)-6-methyl-5-(morpholine-4-carbonyl)-3,4-dihydropyrimidin-2(1 H)-one (3i): White solid, Yield 84%. Mp. 228°C to 230°C. R_f 0.44 (Chloroform:methanol (9:1)). IR (KBr) cm^{-1}: 3,264, 3,102 (N-H str.), 1,681, 1,624 (C = O str.), 2,858 (C-H str.). ^{13}C NMR (400 MHz, DMSO-d_6): 165.62 (C = O), 162.36 (C = O), 139.28 to 116.44 (6 C, aromatic), 152.76 (=C-NH), 104.28, 56.24 (CH), 29.76 to 24.38 (4 C, aliphatic), 15.78 (CH_3). ^1H NMR (400 MHz, $CDCl_3$): 7.28 to 7.20 (m, 4 H), 7.04 (br s, 1 H), 5.41 (s, 1 H), 5.27 (s, 1 H), 3.25 to 3.03 (m, 6 H), 2.22 to 2.10 (m, 2 H), 1.72 (s, 3 H). MS (EI): 335$[M]^+$, 320 $[M\text{-}CH_3]^+$, 249 $[M\text{-}C_4H_8NO]^+$, 221$[M\text{-}C_5H_8NO_2]^+$, 207 $[M\text{-}CH_3\text{-}C_5H_8NO_2]^+$, 166$[M\text{-}C_8H_{12}N_2O_2]^+$.

4-(2-Chlorophenyl)-6-methyl-5-(pyrrolidine-1-carbonyl)-3,4-dihydropyrimidin-2(1 H)-one (3j): White solid, Yield 83%. Mp. 223°C to 224°C. R_f 0.53 (Chloroform:methanol (9:1)). IR (KBr) cm^{-1}: 3,221, 3,095 (N-H str.), 1,686 (C = O str.), 2,877 (C-H str.). ^{13}C NMR (400 MHz, DMSO-d_6): 166.24 (C = O), 162.36 (C = O), 150.25 (=C-NH), 143.66 to 121.54 (6 C, aromatic), 105.65, 53.44 (CH), 26.28 to 23.93 (4 C, aliphatic), 15.65 (CH_3). ^1H NMR (400 MHz, $CDCl_3$): δ 7.52 to 7.50 (dd, 1 H, $J = 7.6$ and 1.6 Hz), 7.34 to 7.32 (dd, 1 H, $J = 7.6$ and 1.2 Hz,), 7.30 to 7.23 (dd, 1 H, $J = 7.6$ and 1.6 Hz), 7.22 to 7.20(dd, 1 H, $J = 7.6$ and 1.6 Hz,), 6.91 (br s, 1 H), 5.76 (d, 1 H, $J = 1.2$ Hz), 5.36 (s, 1 H), 3.37 to 3.20 (m, 4 H), 1.89 (d, 4 H, $J = 0.4$ Hz), 1.79 (s, 3 H). MS (EI): 319 $[M]^+$, 304 $[M\text{-}CH_3]^+$, 284 $[M\text{-}Cl]^+$, 249 $[M\text{-}C_4H_8N]^+$, 221 $[M\text{-}C_5H_8NO]$, 206 $[M\text{-}CH_3\text{-}C_5H_8NO]^+$, 166 $[M\text{-}C_8H_{12}N_2O]^+$.

4-(2-Chlorophenyl)-6-methyl-5-(piperidine-1-carbonyl)-3,4-dihydropyrimidin-2(1 H)-one (3 k): White solid, Yield 80%. Mp. 240°C to 242°C. R_f 0.52 (Chloroform:methanol (9:1)). IR (KBr) cm^{-1}: 3,222, 3,109 (N-H str.), 1,685 (C = O str.), 2,949 (C-H str.). ^{13}C NMR (400 MHz, DMSO-d_6): 166. 38 (C = O), 161.72 (C = O), 141.56 to 122.38 (6 C, aromatic), 151.36 (=C-NH), 104.72, 54.46 (CH), 25.92 to 23.80 (5 C, aliphatic), 15.55 (CH_3). ^1H NMR (400 MHz, $CDCl_3$): 7.49 to 7.48 (d, 1 H, $J = 7.2$ Hz), 7.43 (s, 1 H), 7.35 to 7.33 (d, 1 H, $J = 6.8$ Hz), 7.28 (t, 1 H, $J = 3.6$ Hz), 7.24 to 7.22 (dd, 1 H, $J = 1.6$ and 7.6 Hz), 5.74 (s, 1 H), 5.40 (s, 1 H), 3.35 to 3.21 (m, 4 H), 1.84 (s, 3 H), 1.49 to 1.33 (m, 6 H). MS (EI): 333 $[M\text{-}1]^+$, 318 $[M\text{-}CH_3]^+$, 298 $[M\text{-}Cl]^+$, 249 $[M\text{-}C_5H_{10}N]^+$, 221 $[M\text{-}C_6H_{10}NO]^+$, 207 $[M\text{-}CH_3\text{-}C_6H_{10}NO]^+$.

4-(2-Chlorophenyl)-6-methyl-5-(morpholine-4-carbonyl)-3,4-dihydropyrimidin-2(1 H)-one (3 l): White solid, Yield 80%. Mp. 240°C to 242°C. R_f 0.52 (Chloroform:methanol (9:1)). IR (KBr) cm^{-1}: 3,240, 3,099 (N-H str.), 1,685(C = O str.), 2,860 (C-H str.). ^{13}C NMR (400 MHz, DMSO-d_6): 165.42 (C = O), 161.56 (C = O), 140.49 to 121.25 (6 C, aromatic), 153.25 (=C-NH), 104.72, 54.72 (CH), 28.56 to 24.78 (4 C, aliphatic), 15.45 (CH_3). ^1H NMR (400 MHz, $CDCl_3$): 7.47 (br s, 1 H), 7.40 to 7.38 (dd, 1 H, $J = 1.6$ and 7.6 Hz), 7.31 to 7.18 (dd, 1 H, $J = 1.6$ and 7.6 Hz), 7.24 to 7.22 (dd, 1 H, $J = 1.6$ and 7.2 Hz), 7.20 to 7.18 (m, 2 H), 3.22 to 2.77 (m, 8 H), 1.77 (s, 3 H). 335$[M]^+$, 320 $[M\text{-}CH_3]^+$, 249 $[M\text{-}C_4H_8NO]^+$, 221$[M\text{-}C_5H_8NO_2]^+$, 207 $[M\text{-}CH_3\text{-}C_5H_8NO_2]^+$, 166$[M\text{-}C_8H_{12}N_2O_2]^+$.

Cytotoxicity studies

In order to assess the *in vitro* cytotoxicity potential of these monastrol mimics, 3-(4,5-dimethylthiazol-2-yl)-2,5-diphenyltetrazolium bromide (MTT) assay on HepG2 and HeLa cell lines was performed. Exponentially growing cell lines were harvested from 25 cm^2. Tissue culture flasks and a stock cell suspension (1×10^5 cell/mL) were prepared. A 96-well flat-bottom tissue culture plate was seeded with 1×10^4 cells in 0.1 ml of MEM and DMEM mediums supplemented with 10% FBS and allowed to attach for 24 h. Test compounds were prepared just prior to the experiment in 0.5% DMSO and serially diluted with medium to get the working stock of 500, 250, 125 and 62.5 μg/mL solution. After 24 h of incubation, cells were treated with 20 μL of test solutions from the respective top stocks, 80 μL of fresh medium was added, and the cells were incubated for 48 h. The cells in the control group received only the medium containing 0.5% DMSO. Each treatment was performed in triplicates. After the treatment, the drug-containing media was removed and washed with 200 μL of phosphate buffered saline (PBS). To each well of the 96-well plate, 100 μL of MTT reagent (stock, 1 mg/mL in PBS) was added and incubated for 4 h at 37°C. After 4 h of incubation, the plate was inverted on tissue paper to remove the MTT reagent. To solubilize formazan crystals in the wells, 100 μL of 100% DMSO was added to each well. The optical density was measured by an enzyme-linked immunosorbent assay plate reader at 540 nm [21].

Molecular modeling

Molecular modeling studies were performed using a flexible docking method with the Glide version 2010 as described by Yan *et al.* [22] and Garcia-Saez et al. [23]. The X-ray crystal structure of Eg5 complexed with monastrol (Protein Data Bank ID: 1Q0B) was retrieved from the Protein Data Bank. The three-dimensional structures of the DHPM derivatives were constructed with the Chemdraw Ultra 8.0. Energy minimizations were performed by Ligprep using OPLS-2004 force field. The binding affinity of the inhibitors to the protein was then evaluated by the total glide docking energies. The physicochemical properties of the compounds, such as molecular weight, log P, hydrogen bond acceptors/donors, polar surface area (PSA) and number of rotatable bonds of the synthesized compounds, were calculated using QuikPro (Schrodinger-2010).

Results and discussion

Chemistry

The dihydropyrimidinones in this study were prepared by the Biginelli reaction [24] of the substituted benzaldehyde, urea and ethylacetoacetate depicted in Scheme 1. Interestingly, the hydrolysis of DHPM was much slower and stalled at less than 10% conversion. A substantial amount of decarboxylated product was formed during hydrolysis, similar to the earlier reports [7]. Since a simultaneous decarboxylation accompanied the formation of acid, it was found that the temperature and reaction time played a crucial role in the productivity of the reaction.

Since mild hydrolyzing agent could prevent the extent of decarboxylation, lithium hydroxide with different solvent combinations (methanol/THF/dioxane) [25] was used for hydrolysis. The reaction was found to proceed slowly, along with the formation of lesser decarboxylated product, but also resulted in low yields of acid (>20%).

Earlier literature reports of DHPM esters hydrolysis in ethyl acetate and sodium hydroxide (25°C to 27°C, 2 h) [26] also failed to form the acid. The ester did not proceed to form the acid even after refluxing with ethyl acetate for 12 h.

Acid hydrolysis using concentrated HCl and TFA (25°C/reflux) also failed to yield any acid. Refluxing with KOH and ethanol led to decarboxylation due to higher refluxing temperature (around 80°C). These observations propelled us to use a solvent with a lower boiling point.

Studies also reported that refluxing in methanol in the presence of aqueous NaOH (10%) led to hydrolysis and consequent decarboxylation [16,17]. Hence, the optimized method for hydrolysis involved heating the ester in methanol with aqueous NaOH at 60°C to 62°C for 8 h. Prolongation of the reaction time or increase in temperature resulted in decarboxlyation. However, it was observed that higher quantities of NaOH did not affect the decarboxylation process.

The synthesis of compounds 3a to 3 l with a stable amide linker between DHPMs and cyclic amines was achieved via TBTU/DIPEA-promoted coupling reaction, which was quick and high yielding. The physical data of all the synthesized compounds are summarized in Table 1. The mass, proton and carbon NMR spectra of some of the final compounds synthesized can be found in Additional files 1, 2, 3, 4, 5, 6, 7 and 8.

Cytotoxicity studies

The data obtained from *in vitro* cytotoxicity assay suggest that compounds 3 g and 3 h were found to be the most potent against the HepG2 cell lines with IC_{50} 124.46 and 120.62 μg/mL, respectively. However, most of the compounds exhibited weak activity (IC_{50} 200 μg/mL) against HeLa cell lines. Hence, it was anticipated that substitution of electron-withdrawing substituents, such as chlorine, at the para position may be essential for the ligand-receptor interaction. Structure-activity relationship (SAR) analysis revealed that compounds with weakly basic pyrrolidine and piperidine substitution in the side chain attenuate the anticancer activity. In contrast, morpholine was not tolerated at the side chain of DHPMs and hence resulted in decreased IC_{50}. Molecular modeling studies showed the absence of hydrogen bonding interactions with Glu-118, which could be attributed to the missing

Table 1 Structural details and percentage yield of compounds 3a to 3 l

Compound code	R	R_1	Yield (%)	Compound code	R	R_1	Yield (%)
3a	H	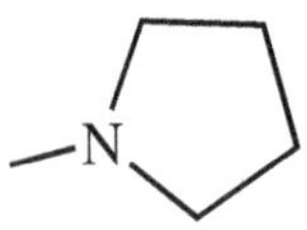	82	3 g	4-Cl	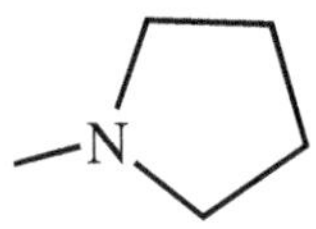	81
3b	H	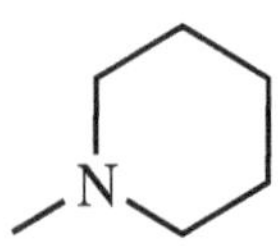	80	3 h	4-Cl	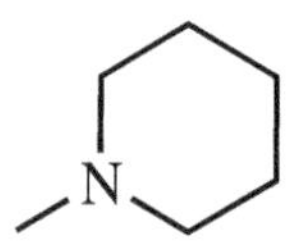	83
3c	H	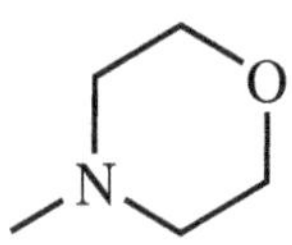	82	3i	4-Cl	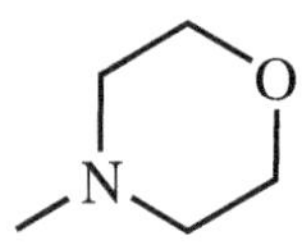	83
3d	4-F	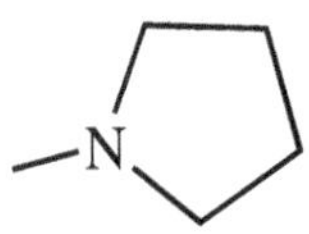	84	3j	2-Cl	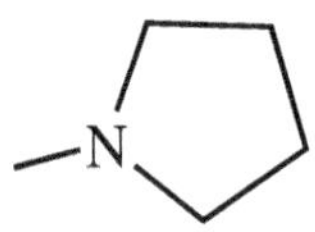	83
3e	4-F	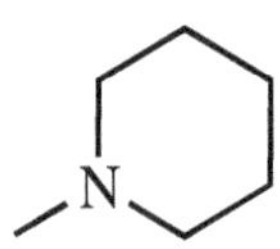	86	3 k	2-Cl	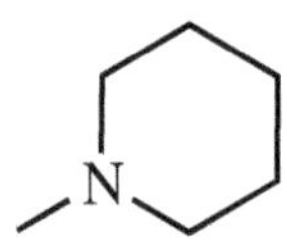	80
3f	4-F	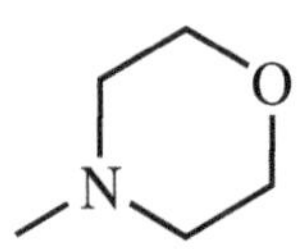	84	3 l	2-Cl	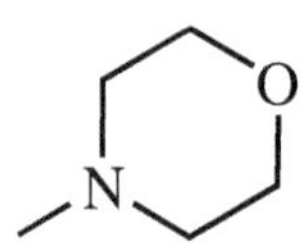	86

R, substitution on the phenyl ring; R_1, substituted cyclic amine (as depicted in Scheme 1).

Table 2 IC_{50} of compounds 3a-l by MTT assay

Compound code	IC^{a}_{50} (μg/mL)	
	HepG2	HeLa
3a	180	216
3b	166	189
3c	207	240
3d	178	229
3e	194	-
3f	269	346
3 g	124	187
3 h	120	217
3i	218	374
3j	192	261
3 k	191	398
3 l	218	374

[a]50% inhibitory concentration. HepG2, human hepatocellular carcinoma; HeLa, human epithelial carcinoma.

hydrogen bond donor on the phenyl ring. Hydrogen bonding interactions of water molecules with the oxygen atom of morpholine in compounds 3c, 3f, 3i and 3 l proved to be fatal for anticancer activity. *In vitro* data for these compounds are summarized in Table 2. Figure 1 shows the schematic view of the contacts of S-monastrol and compound 3 h with the residues of Eg5 inhibitor-binding pockets with in 3 Å, and hydrogen bonds are depicted by dashed lines.

Structure-activity relationship

To determine the SAR, functionality modification was carried out on the phenyl ring, while different cyclic amines were introduced at the side chain of DHPMs. Unsubstituted compounds (3a, 3b and 3c) which displayed IC_{50} of 180.92, 166.96 and 207.45 μg/mL and 216, 189 and 240 μg/mL against HePG2 and HeLa cell lines, respectively, served as the template for cytotoxicity potential comparison. Replacement of the protons in compounds 3a, 3b and 3c with fluorine at the para position of the phenyl ring did not improve the cytotoxicity against both cell lines. However, compound 3d showed a better IC_{50} (178 μg/mL) than its analog 3a against HepG2 cell lines. Encouraged by this result, fluorine was replaced by chlorine at the same position on the phenyl ring in compounds 3d, 3e and 3f to afford compounds 3 g, 3 h and 3i. Surprisingly, compound 3 g and 3 h significantly inhibited the proliferations of HepG2 cell lines with IC_{50} of 124.46 and 120.62 μg/mL. The anticancer activities of these two compounds against HeLa cell lines were equally frustrating like the previous results. The possibility to change the position of chlorine from para to ortho in the phenyl ring was then explored. Interestingly, this modification proved detrimental, and compounds 3j, 3 k and 3 l displayed IC_{50} of 190 μg/mL.

Molecular modeling

In order to further investigate the relationships between the virtual receptor-ligand binding interaction and physicochemical properties of the new compounds with their anticancer activity, molecular modeling studies were performed. Docking analysis revealed that hydrogen bond formation and hydrophobic interactions were the key factors affecting inhibitory action of the compounds. The Glu-116, Gly-117, Glu-118, Ar-119, Trp-127, Pro-137, Tyr-211 and Leu-214 of Eg5 protein were found to be directly interacting with the synthesized DHPMs. Most of the synthesized compounds showed hydrogen bonding interaction with Glu-116 as monastrol. However, the unsubstituted compounds, except 3c (Figure 2),

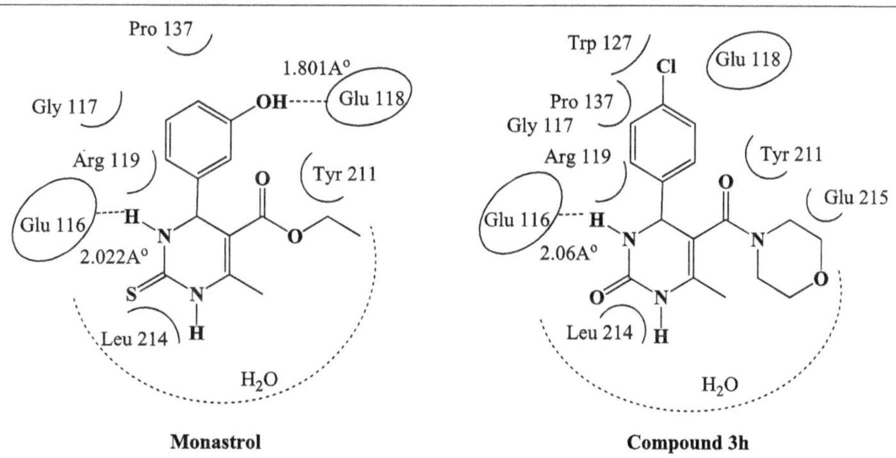

Figure 1 S-monastrol and compound 3 h.

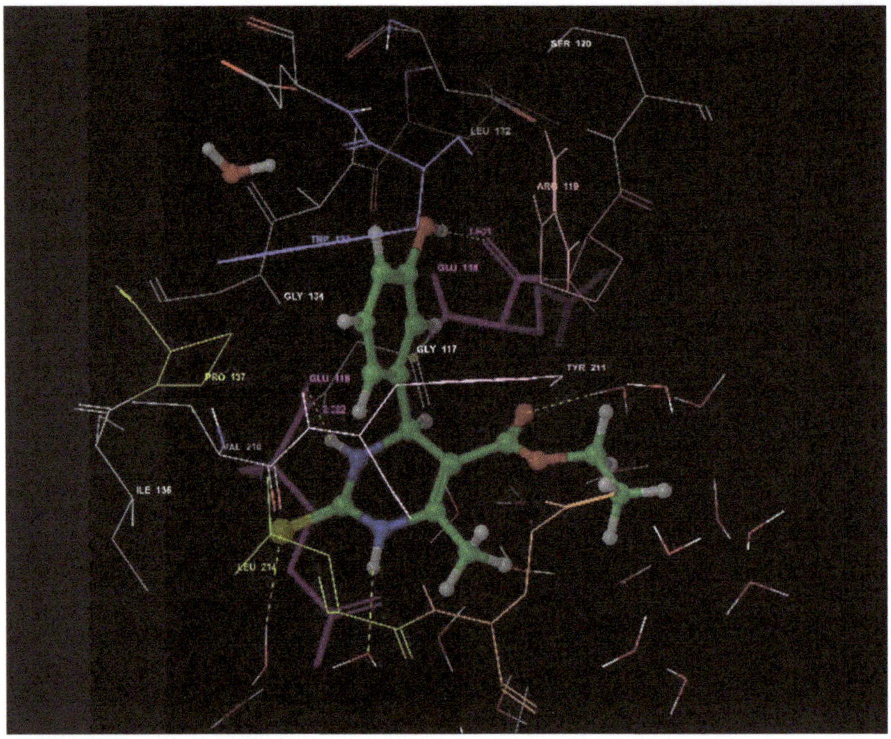

Figure 2 Compound 3c with Eg5 protein (1Q0B).

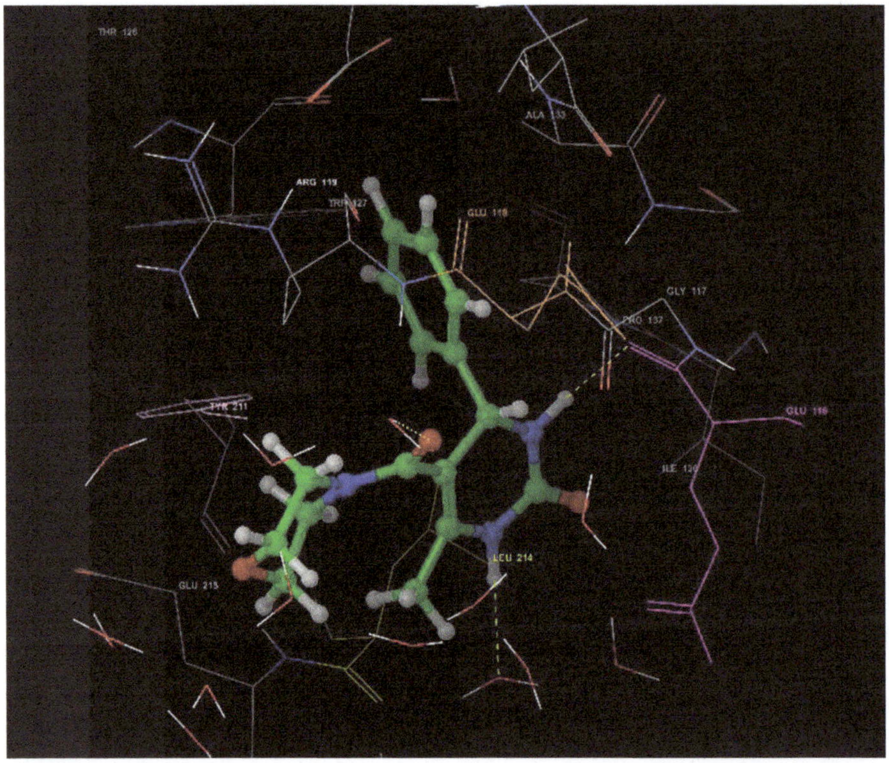

Figure 3 Monastrol with Eg5 protein (1Q0B). The yellow dotted lines represent hydrogen bonding interaction.

Table 3 *In silico* docking results

Compound	Docking score[a]	H-bonding with Glu-116		H-bonding with Glu-118	
		Distance (Å)	Energy (Kcal/mol)	Distance (Å)	Energy (Kcal/mol)
Monastrol	−9.780843	2.022	−0.25495	1.800922	−0.25495
3a	−4.623578	1.794177	0	1.91532	0
3b	−4.099871	2.087333	0	2.437469	0
3c	−7.66649	2.184935	−0.155458	2.543947	0
3d	−3.518203	2.579143	−0.092150	2.579143	0
3e	−7.396385	2.231526	−0.123687	2.472871	0
3f	−3.336005	2.365419	−0.097571	2.477461	0
3 g	−8.667402	2.226021	−0.076754	2.496712	0
3 h	−7.541568	1.947079	−0.215195	2.240761	0
3i	−6.983773	2.04085	−0.226944	2.243988	0
3j	−7.419477	2.224107	−0.171504	2.25015	0
3 k	−6.988692	2.242662	−0.124171	2.197052	0
3 l	−6.8606	2.266054	−0.068286	2.199539	0

[a]Grid scoring from flexible docking (kcal/mol).

lack the hydrogen-bonding interactions, which are weakly active to inhibit proliferation of cancer cell lines.

None of the compounds showed hydrogen bonding interaction with Glu-118. This may be attributed to the absence of hydrogen bond donors on the phenyl ring of DHPMs. Bioisosteric replacement of thiourea 'S' with urea 'O' in the synthesized compounds appeared to be oriented in similar fashion and retained similar interactions as monastrol. Co-crystallized S-monastrol when redocked in the active site of KSP attained a score of −9.78 kcal/mol. It displayed vital H-bonding interactions (−0.25495 kcal/mol) with the residues Glu-116 and Glu-118 (Figure 3).

The most active compounds, 3 h against HepG2 (Figure 1) and compound 3 g against HeLa, fitted best in the active site of Eg5 inhibitor protein and attained the score of −7.541568 kcal/mol and −8.667402 kcal/mol, respectively. It retained all the prime interactions to anchor well in the active sites of the receptor, except the missing hydrogen bonding with Glu-118. Moreover, hydrophobic interactions were observed to be involved in the binding of the most active compounds. All active compounds (compounds 3b, 3d, 3 g and 3 h) of the DHPM series were oriented in the active site of the protein in a way that places the aromatic ring into the pocket comprising the residues Glu-118, Arg-119, Trp-127, Pro-137 and Tyr-211. On the other hand, the ethyl group of S-monastrol and the cyclic amine substituents of DHPMs were almost pointed towards aqueous environment (Table 3).

The virtual physicochemical parameters of the synthesized compounds were benchmarked against standard monastrol, and none of the descriptors were found to violate the optimal range of the parameters required for anticancer drugs. All the compounds validated Lipinski's rule of five, which extends the scope of performance in the *in vivo* studies. This shows the potential of the compounds to bind with the enzyme effectively and inhibit cell proliferation with minimized toxic effects. Optimal pharmacokinetic properties such as lipophilicity and absorption were established by the QLogP values and polar surface areas, which correlated with the number of hydrogen bond donors/acceptors (Table 4).

Table 4 *In silico* physicochemical properties prediction[a]

Compound	Mol. Wt.	Log P	H donor	H acceptor	Rot. bonds	PSA (Å2)
Monastrol	292.352	3.31	1	3.25	3	85.118
3a	285.345	3.406	0	3	1	78.312
3b	299.372	3.681	0	3	1	77.135
3c	301.344	2.533	0	4.7	1	86.394
3d	303.335	3.67	0	3	1	78.367
3e	319.335	2.818	0	3	1	77.133
3f	317.362	3.919	0	4.7	1	86.585
3 g	319.79	3.925	0	3	1	78.307
3 h	333.817	4.092	0	3	1	76.989
3i	335.789	3.083	0	4.7	1	86.586
3j	319.79	3.761	0	3	1	77.458
3 k	333.817	3.812	0	3	1	75.797
3 l	335.789	2.897	0	4.7	1	86.938

[a]QikProp v3.4 (Schrodinger-2010). H donor, hydrogen bond donor; H acceptor, hydrogen bond acceptor; Mol. Wt., molecular weight; Rot. bonds, number of rotational bonds; PSA, polar surface area in Å^2.

Conclusion

Eg5 represents a promising target, and designing Eg5 inhibitors would offer a novel approach to develop potent anticancer agents. A series of 12 novel monastrol analogs based on Biginelli reaction were synthesized with IC_{50} in the range of 120 to 398 μg/mL against HeLa and HepG2 cell lines. This new series consisted of pyrrolidine, piperidine and morpholine as privileged structures attached to the side chain of Biginelli dihydropyrimidinones through amide bond to improve the metabolic stability. SAR analysis and molecular modeling studies revealed that the positioning of a hydrogen bond donor/acceptor on the phenyl ring of the dihydropyrimidinone plays a crucial role in the inhibition of Eg5 enzyme to exhibit anticancer activity. Although the new compounds were found to have moderate to weak activity against cancer cell lines, the reported results are expected to contribute toward deeper insight into structure-activity relationship and could be helpful in further designing dihydropyrimidinones as potential anticancer agents.

Additional files

Additional file 1: Proton NMR spectrum of compound 1d.
Additional file 2: Mass spectrum of compound 1d.
Additional file 3: Carbon NMR spectrum of compound 3f.
Additional file 4: Mass spectrum of compound 3f.
Additional file 5: Proton NMR spectrum of compound 3 g.
Additional file 6: Mass spectrum of compound 3 g.
Additional file 7: Proton NMR spectrum of compound 3j.
Additional file 8: Mass spectrum of compound 3j.

Abbreviations

DHPM: dihydropyrimidinones; HeLa: human hepatocellular carcinoma; HepG2: human epithelial carcinoma; MTT: 3-(4,5-dimethylthiazol-2-yl)-2, 5-diphenyltetrazolium bromide; HCl: hydrochloric acid; TBTU- O: (Benzotriazol-1-yl)-N,N,N',N'- tetramethyluronium tetraflouroborate; DIPEA: diisopropylethylamine; IC_{50}: concentration at 50% inhibition; SAR: structure activity relationship; Glu: glutamic acid; Gly: glycine; Arg: arginine; Trp: tryptophan; Tyr: tyrosine; Pro: proline; Leu: leucine.

Competing interests

The authors declare that they have no competing interests.

Acknowledgments

We thank Mr. Balaji of the Department of Pharmacology for his support at the PSG College of Pharmacy, Coimbatore (Tamilnadu) for molecular modeling studies. We are also grateful for the financial assistance of Manipal University, Manipal.

Author details

[1]Department of Pharmaceutical Chemistry, Manipal College of Pharmaceutical Sciences, Manipal University, Manipal, Karnataka 576104, India. [2]Department of Pharmaceutical Biotechnology, Manipal College of Pharmaceutical Sciences, Manipal University, Manipal, Karnataka 576104, India.

References

1. DeBonis S, Skoufias DA, Indorato R-L, Liger F, Marquet B, Laggner C, Benoît J, Kozielski F (2008) Structure activity relationship of S-Trityl-L-Cysteine analogues as inhibitors of the human mitotic kinesin Eg5. J Med Chem 51:1115–1125
2. Matsuno K, Sawada J, Sugimoto M, Ogo N, Asai A (2009) Bis(hetero)aryl derivatives as unique kinesin spindle protein inhibitors. Bioorg Med Chem Lett 19:1058–1061
3. Mayer TU, Kapoor TM, Haggarty SJ, King RW, Schreiber SL, Mitchison TJ (1999) Small molecule inhibitor of mitotic spindle bipolarity identified in a phenotype-based screen. Science 286:971–974
4. Maliga Z, Kapoor TM, Mitchison T (2002) Evidence that monastrol is an allosteric inhibitor of the mitotic kinesin Eg5. J Chem Biol 9:989–996
5. Haque SA, Hasaka TP, Brooks AD, Lobanov PV, Baas PW (2004) Monastrol, a prototype anticancer drug that inhibits mitotic kinesin, induces rapid bursts of axonal outgrowth from cultured postmitotic neurons. Cell Motil Cytoskeleton 58:10–16
6. Yoon SY, Choi JE, Huh JW, Hwang O, Lee HS, Hong HN, Kim D (2005) Monastrol, a selective inhibitor of mitotic kinesin Eg5, induces a distinctive growth profile of dendrites and axons in primary cortical neuron cultures. Cell Motil Cytoskeleton 60:181–190
7. Klein E, DeBonis S, Thiede B, Skoufias DA, Kozielski F, Lebeau L (2007) New Chemical tools for investigating human mitotic kinesin Eg5. Bioorg Med Chem 15:6474–6488
8. Russowsky D, Canto RFS, Sanches SAA, D'Oca MGM, de Fátima A, Pilli RA, Kohn LK, De Antônio MA, Carvalho JE (2006) Synthesis and differential antiproliferative activity of Biginelli compounds against cancer cell lines: monastrol, oxo-monastrol and oxygenated analogues. Bioorganic Chemistry 34:173–182
9. Horton D, Bourne GT, Smythe ML (2003) The combinatorial synthesis of bicyclic privileged structures or privileged substructures. Chem Rev 103:893–930
10. Tu S, Xiao-Tong Z, Fang F, Xiao-Jing Z, Song-Lei Z, Tuan-Jie L, Da-Qing S, Xiang-Shan W, Shun-Jun J (2003) One pot synthesis of 3,4-dihydropyrimidin-2(1 H)- ones using boric acid as catalyst. Tetrahedron Lett 44:6153–6155
11. Wang Y, Yu J, Miao Z, Chen R (2011) Bifunctional primary amine- thiourea-TfOH (BPAT·TfOH) as a chiral phase-transfer catalyst: the asymmetric synthesis of dihydropyrimidines. Organic & Bimolecular Chemistry 9(8):3050–3054
12. Ma Y, Qian C, Wang L, Yang M (2000) Lanthanoid triflate catalyzed Biginelli reaction- one-pot synthesis of dihydropyrimidinones under solvent-free conditions. Journal of Organic Chemistry 65(12):3864–3868
13. Murata H, Ishitani H, Iwamoto M (2010) Synthesis of Biginelli dihydropyrimidinone derivatives with various substituents on aluminium- planted mesoporous silica catalyst. Organic & Biomolecular Chemistry 8(5):1202–1211
14. Litvić M, Večenaj I, Mikuldaš LZ, Lovrić M, Vinković V, Filipan-Litvić M (2010) First application of hexaaquaaluminium(III) tetrafluoroborate as a mild, recyclable, non-hygroscopic acid catalyst in organic synthesis: a simple and efficient protocol for the multigram scale synthesis of 3,4-dihydropyrimidinones by Biginelli reaction. Tetrahedron 66(19):3463–3471
15. Barrow JC, Nantermet PG, Selnick HG, Glass KL, Rittle KE, Gilbert KF, Steele TG, Homnick CF, Freidinger RM, Ransom RW, Kling P, Reiss D, Broten TP, Schorn TW, Chang RSL, Malley SSO, Olah TV, Ellis JD, Barrish A, Kassahun K, Leppert P, Nagarathnam D, Forray C (2000) In vitro and in vivo evaluation of dihydropyrimidinone C-5 amides as potent and selective r1A receptor antagonists for the treatment of benign prostatic hyperplasia. J Med Chem 43 (14):2703–2718
16. Shutalev AD, Aksionov AN (2005) Simple synthesis of 4-aryl-6-styryl-1,2,3,4-tetrahydropyrimidin-2-ones by the alkaline hydrolysis of Biginelli compounds. Mendeleev Comm 15:73–75
17. Steele TG, Coburn CA, Patane MA, Bock MG (1998) Expedient synthesis of 5-unsubstituted-3,4-dihydropyrimidin-2(1 H)-ones. Tetrahedron Lett 39:9315–9318
18. Desai B (2006) Microwave-assisted solution phase synthesis of dihydropyrimidine C5 amides and esters. Tetrahedron 62(19):4651–4664
19. Movassagh B, Balalaie S, Shaygan P (2007) A new and efficient protocol for preparation of thiol esters from carboxylic acids and thiols in the presence of 2-(1 H- benzotriazole-1-yl)-1,1,3,3-tetramethyluronium tetraflouroborate (TBTU). ARKIVOC 13:47–52
20. Balalaie S, Mahdidoust M, Eshaghi-Najafabadi R (2007) 2-(1 H-benzotriazole-1-yl)- 1,1,3,3-tetramethyluronium tetraflouroborate as an efficient coupling reagent for the amidation and phenylhydrazation of carboxylic acids at room temperature. J Iran Chem Soc 4(3):364–369

21. Mosmann T (1983) Rapid colorimetric assay for cellular growth and survival: application to proliferation and cytotoxicity assays. J Immunol Methods 65 (1–2):55–63
22. Yan Y, Sardana V, Xu B, Homnick C, Halczenko W, Buser CA, Schaber M, Hartman GD, Huber HE, Kuo LC (2004) Inhibition of a mitotic motor protein: where, how, and conformational consequences. J Mol Biol 335:547–554
23. Garcia-Saez I, DeBonis S, Lopez R, Trucco F, Rousseau B, Thuery P, Kozielski F (2007) Structure of human Eg5 in complex with a new monastrol-based inhibitor bound in the *R* configuration. J Bio Chem 282(13):9740–9747
24. Hu EH, Sidler DR, Dolling U-H (1998) Unprecedented catalytic three component one-pot condensation reaction: an efficient synthesis of 5-alkoxycarbonyl-4-aryl-3,4- dihydropyrimidin-2(1 H)-ones. J Org Chem 63:3454–3457
25. Dayal B, Salen G, Toome B, Tint GS, Shefer S, Padia J (1990) Lithium hydroxide/aqueous methanol: mild reagent for the hydrolysis of bile acid methyl esters. Steroid 55(5):233–237
26. Kumar R, Mittal A, Ramachandran U (2007) Design and synthesis of 6-methyl-2-oxo- 1,2,3,4-tetrahydropyrimidine-5-carboxylic acid derivatives as PPAR activators. Bioorg Med Chem 17(16):4613–4618

12

Chemical composition of ethanol extract of *Macrotyloma uniflorum* (Lam.) Verdc. using GC-MS spectroscopy

Sneha Das, Neeru Vasudeva* and Sunil Sharma

Abstract

Background: *Macrotyloma uniflorum* Linn (Fabaceae) is a herbaceous plant with annual branches. It is used in kidney stones, inflamed joints, fever, musculoskeletal disorders, sinus wounds and localized abdominal tumors. It is reported as an antioxidant and nutraceutical (forage and food). GC-MS analysis of ethanol extract has led to identification of twenty-eight compounds from *M. uniflorum* by comparison of their retention indices and mass spectra fragmentation patterns with those stored on the GC-MS computer library.

Results: The main constituents identified were mome inositol, ethyl alpha-d-glucopyranoside, n- hexadecanoic acid, linoleic acid (9, 12-octadecadienoic acid), its esters and ethyl derivatives, Vitamin E, stigmasterol and 3-beta-stigmast-5-en-3-ol.

Conclusions: The extracts are rich in linoleic acid and its esters, mome inositol and ethyl alpha-d-glucopyranoside; therefore, this plant can be medicinally beneficial as an antioxidant, in diabetes and its related disorders.

Keywords: GC-MS; *Macrotyloma uniflorum*; Chemical constituents; Retention indices

Background

Macrotyloma uniflorum (synonym: *Dolichos biflorus* Linn.) belonging to the family Fabaceae is commonly known as Kulthi in Hindi and horse gram in English. It is a herbaceous plant with annual branches, sub-erect or twining, leaflets of 2.5 to 5 cm. Its seed is 6 to 8 mm long and 3 to 4 mm broad. The seeds are trapezoidal oblong or somewhat rounded in shape and pale to dark reddish brown or orange brown or all black in colour. The genus *Macrotyloma* comprises about 25 species, most of which are restricted to Africa of which four have been identified as *M. uniflorum, M. stenocarpum, M. verrucosum* and *M. benadirianum* [1]. Traditionally, it has been widely used in the treatment of kidney stones, inflamed joints, fever, musculoskeletal disorders, sinus wounds and localized abdominal tumors [2,3]. Experimentally, the seeds are reported as hepato-protective, diuretic and antioxidant [4-6]. To the best of the authors' knowledge, no published literature exists about the chemical contents of the ethanol extract of *M. uniflorum.* Thus it was planned to carry out GC-MS analysis of ethanol extract of the seeds of *M. uniflorum.*

Methods

Preparation of crude extract

The seeds (1 Kg) were coarsely powdered and defatted with petroleum ether (60°C to 80°C) for 7 days by cold maceration. The fat-exhausted drug was further extracted with ethanol (95% *v*/*v*) by soxhlation for 72 h. The extract was concentrated in a rotary vacuum evaporator to yield 25.0% *w*/*w* of dark-brown-coloured extract. The ethanol extract of seeds was diluted with ethanol and filtered with Whatman No. 42 to obtain a particle-free extract for analysis by GC-MS.

GC-MS analysis

The extract was directly used for the analysis. GC-MS was carried out on a GCMS-QP2010 Plus (Shimadzu, Kyoto, Japan) system with head space sampler (AOC-20s) and auto injector (AOC-20i), equipped with mass selective detector, having ion source temperature of 230°C, interface temperature of 260°C, a solvent cut time of 2.50 min threshold of 1,000 eV and mass range of 40 to 650 m/z.

* Correspondence: neeruvasudeva@gmail.com
Department of Pharmaceutical Sciences, Guru Jambheshwar University of Science and Technology, Hisar, Haryana 125001, India

Compounds were separated using a Rtx 5 MS capillary column (Restek Company, Bellefonte, USA: crossbond 5% diphenyl/ 95% dimethyl polysiloxane) having dimensions 30 m (length) × 0.25 mm (diameter) × 0.25 μm (film thickness). The split mode was used at a ratio of 10:1. The temperature of the injector was initialized to 250°C, having a split injection mode. The temperature was programmed from 100°C (3 min), then further increased to 280°C at a ramp rate of 10°C/min (19 min hold).

Helium (>99.999%) was used as the carrier gas at a linear flow velocity of 40.9 cm/s. The debit of gas (helium) vector was fixed to 16.3 mL/min, with a total flow of 1. 21 mL/min. The volume of injected sample was 1.0 μL of ethanol extract. The components were identified by comparison of their retention indices (RI) relative to homologous alkane series (purchased from Sigma, St. Louis, USA) and by comparison of their mass spectral fragmentation patterns with those data provided in WILEY8.LIB, NIST08.LIB, NIST08s.LIB and NIST.LIB. Identification was assumed when a good match of mass spectrum and RI was achieved.

Results and discussion

The seeds were purchased from Bhagalpur district, Bihar, India, and identified by Dr. K. C. Bhatt, NBPGR, New Delhi. A voucher specimen (PGS-13-02) has been deposited in the Department of Pharmaceutical Sciences (Pharmacognosy Division), Guru Jambheshwar University of Science and Technology, Hisar, Haryana, India.

Chemical composition

GC-MS analysis of ethanol extract led to the identification of twenty-eight compounds from *M. uniflorum* (Table 1, Figure 1). The main constituents identified were two

Table 1 Chemical composition of ethanol extract of *M. uniflorum* seed

Peak	Retention time	Retention indices	Area%	Name
1	3.645	1,056	0.67	Benzeneacetaldehyde
2	4.465	1,116	0.51	Benzeneethanamine
3	10.051	1,499	0.27	L-Phenylalanine, ethyl ester
4	11.076	1,580	0.53	2-(1-methyl-2-propenyl)bicyclo[2.2.1]heptane
5	11.331	1,602	0.39	1H-Pyrrole, 2-(2,4,6-cycloheptatrienyl)
6	12.007	1,660	11.14	Ethyl .alpha.-d-glucopyranoside
7	13.027	1,750	23.24	Mome inositol
8	15.312	1,971	2.76	n-Hexadecanoic acid
9	15.568	1,996	0.49	Heptadecanoic acid, ethyl ester
10	17.015	2,151	19.79	9,12-Octadecadienoic acid (Z,Z)
11	17.176	2,169	1.61	Ethyl (9Z,12Z)-9,12-octadecadienoate
12	18.319	2,300	0.12	Heptadecane, 3-methyl
13	18.543	2,327	1.88	Octanamide, N-(2-hydroxyethyl)
14	19.678	2,465	3.18	3-Cyclopentylpropionic acid, 2-dimethylaminoethyl ester
15	19.833	2,484	0.60	(R)14-Methyl-8-hexadecyn-1-ol
16	20.158	2,526	1.77	Hexadecanoic acid, 2-hydroxy-1-(hydroxymethyl)ethyl ester
17	21.207	2,662	1.27	1-Cyclohexyldimethylsilyloxybutane
18	21.483	2,698	0.22	Eicosane
19	21.607	2,712	19.49	9,12-Octadecadienoic acid (Z,Z)-, 2,3-dihydroxypropyl ester
20	22.342	2,798	0.50	Heneicosane
21	22.414	2,805	0.33	9-Methyl-10,12-hexadecadien-1-ol acetate
22	23.334	2,897	0.19	Hexatriacontane
23	26.396	3,116	2.42	i-Propyl 9,12-octadecenadienoate
24	26.966	3,154	0.72	Vitamin E
25	27.432	3,181	1.76	Tricyclo[20.8.0.0(7,16)]triacontane, 1(22),7(16)-diepoxy
26	29.695	3,290	0.97	Stigmasterol
27	31.064	3,355	2.42	Stigmast-5-en-3-ol, (3 beta)
28	32.328	3,413	0.74	(−)-Isolongifolol, acetate

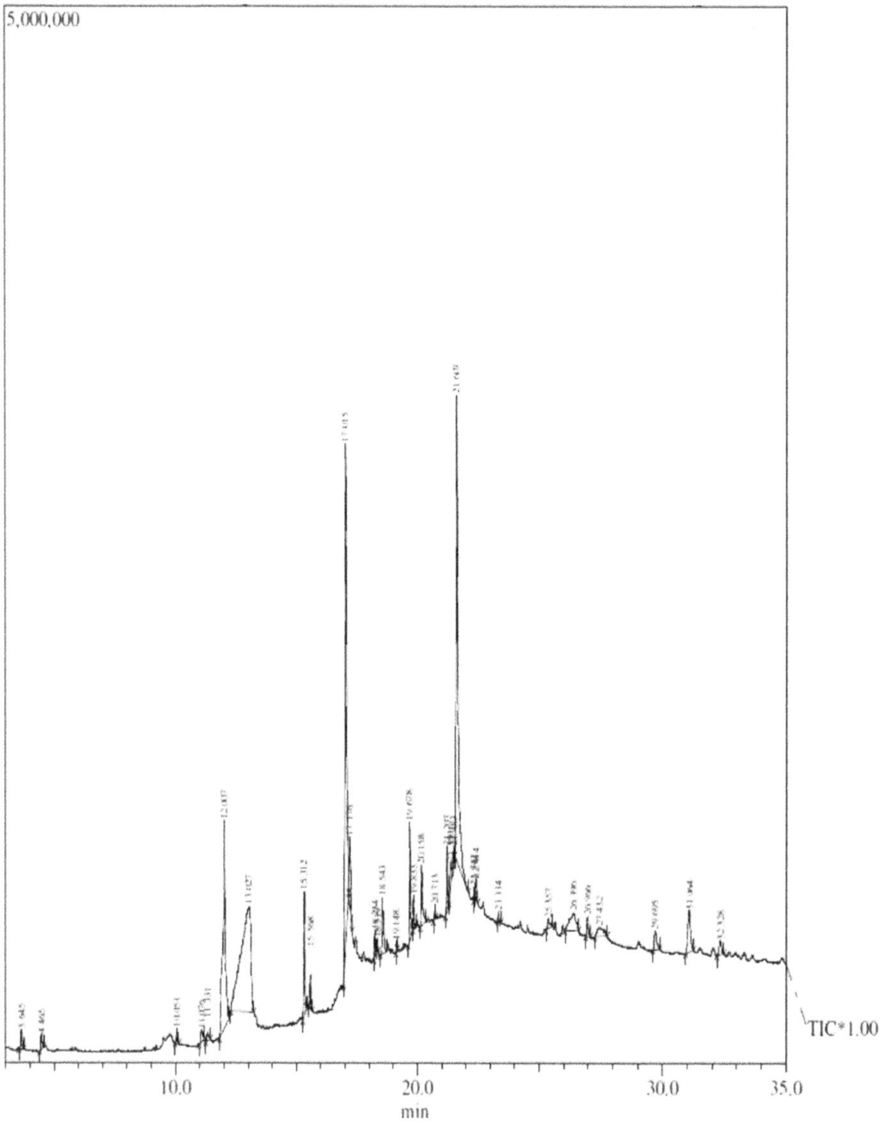

Figure 1 A typical GC-MS chromatogram of the constituents of ethanol extract of seeds of *M. uniflorum*.

polysaccharides namely mome inositol and ethyl alpha-d-glucopyranoside. A number of fatty acids and their esters have also been identified; they were n- hexadecanoic acid, 9, 12-octadecadienoic acid and its esters. Phytosterols, namely stigmasterol and 3-β-stigmast-5-en-3-ol, were present in traces. Other compounds present were 3-cyclopentylpropionic acid, 2-dimethylaminoethyl ester, heneicosane and vitamin E. literature survey showed that Dolichin A and B and pyroglutaminylglutamine along with some flavonoids were isolated from this plant. Seeds of *M. uniflorum* contain lectins, glycoprotein, agglutinin, an anti-A phytoagglutinin, four glycosidase enzymes, allantoinase and a strong diuretic dipeptide, pyroglutamylglutamine. The seeds are rich source of the enzyme urease and also contain β-sitosterol [7].

Conclusions

Mome inositol, one of the major components of extract of *M. uniflorum*, is reported as anti-alopecic, anti-cirrhotic, anti-neuropathic, cholesterolytic, lipotropic and a sweetener. n-hexadecanoic acids act as a 5-alpha-reductase inhibitor, a hemolytic agent and an antioxidant [8]. (3β)-stigmast-5-en-3-ol has shown an insulin-like effect, that is, stimulating glucose transport apart from its existing cholesterol-lowering efficacy. Therefore, it can play a beneficial role as an antidiabetic agent [9]. Animal studies have revealed that linoleic acid is converted to gamma linoleic acid in the body and can prevent chemically induced diabetes while restoring normal antioxidant status in tissues [10]. It can also prevent diabetic neuropathy, a painful condition resulting from exposure of nerves to high glucose levels [11]. Hence, the plant can be utilized as a natural sweetener, anti-alopecic, anti-cirrhotic, anti-neuropathic, cholesterolytic, lipotropic, antioxidant and antidiabetic.

Competing interests

The authors declare that they have no competing interests.

Authors' contributions

SD has carried out all practical work and wrote the manuscript. NV and SS supervised all the work including the designing and drafting of the manuscript. All authors read and approved the final manuscript.

Authors' information

Sneha Das is PhD research scholar pursuing her doctorate under supervision of Professor Neeru Vasudeva and Professor Sunil Sharma at Department of Pharmaceutical Sciences, Guru Jambheshwar University of Science and Technology, Hisar, Haryana, India, 125001.

Acknowledgements

We are grateful to Department of Science and Technology, New Delhi, India, under the Ministry of Science and Technology, New Delhi, India, and the Department of Pharmaceutical Sciences, Guru Jambheshwar University of Science and Technology, Hisar, Haryana, for providing fellowship and infrastructure, respectively to Sneha Das for carrying out the research. Also we would like to thank Dr. Ajay Kumar, scientist at AIRF, JNU, Delhi, for helping us perform GC-MS.

References

1. Mehra A, Upadhyaya M (2013) *Macrotyloma uniflorum* Lam traditional crop of kumaun himalaya and ethnobotanical perspectives. Int J Agric Food Sci 3(4):148–150
2. Muthu AK, Sethupathy S, Manavalan R, Karar PK (2005) Hypolipidemic effect of methanolic extract of *Dolichos biflorus* Linn in high fat diet fed rats. Ind J Exp Biol 43:522
3. Muthu AK, Sethupathy S, Manavalan R, Karar PK (2006) Antioxidant potential of methanolic extract of *Dolichos biflorus* Linn. in high fat diet fed rabbits. Ind J Pharmacol 38:131
4. Parmar HB, Das SK, Gohil KJ (2012) Hepatoprotective activity of *Macrotyloma uniflorum* seed extract on paracetamol and d-galactosamine induced liver toxicity in Albino rats. IJPR 2(2):86–91
5. Ravishankar K, Priya PSVV (2012) Evaluation of diuretic effect of ethanolic seed extracts of *Macrotyloma uniflorum* and *Cucumis melo* in rats. Int J Pharm Bio Sci 3(3):251–255
6. Ravishankar K, Priya PSVV (2012) In vitro antioxidant activity of ethanolic seed extracts of *Macrotyloma uniflorum* and *Cucumis melo* for therapeutic potential. IJRPC 2(2):442–445
7. Ghani A (2003) Medicinal Plants of Bangladesh with Chemical Constituents and Uses. Asiatic Society of Bangladesh, Dhaka, Bangladesh, p 181
8. Kumar NR, Reddy JS, Gopikrishna G, Solomon KA (2012) GC-MS determination of bioactive constituents of *Cycas beddomei* cones. Int J Pharm Bio Sci 3(3):344–350
9. Sujatha S, Anand S, Sangeetha KN, Shilpa K, Lakshmi J, Balakrishnan A, Lakshmi BS (2010) Biological evaluation of (3β)-STIGMAST-5-EN-3-OL as potent anti-diabetic agent in regulating glucose transport using in vitro model. Int J Diabetes Mellitus 2:101–109
10. Suresh Y, Das UN (2003) Long-chain polyunsaturated fatty acids and chemically induced diabetes mellitus: effect of omega-6 fatty acids. Nutrition 19(2):93–114
11. Pitel S, Raccah D, Gerbi A, Pieroni G, Vague P, Coste TC (2007) At low doses, a gamma-linolenic acid-lipoic acid conjugate is more effective than docosahexaenoic acid-enriched phospholipids in preventing neuropathy in diabetic rats. J Nutr 137(2):368–372

13

The potential of anti-malarial compounds derived from African medicinal plants: an *in silico* evaluation of drug metabolism and pharmacokinetics profiling

Pascal Amoa Onguéné[1†], Fidele Ntie-Kang[2,3†], James Ajeck Mbah[2], Lydia Likowo Lifongo[2], Jean Claude Ndom[1], Wolfgang Sippl[3] and Luc Meva'a Mbaze[1*]

Abstract

Background: Malaria is an endemic disease affecting many countries in Tropical regions. In the search for compound hits for the design and/or development of new drugs against the disease, many research teams have resorted to African medicinal plants in order to identify lead compounds. Three-dimensional molecular models were generated for anti-malarial compounds of African origin (from 'weakly' active to 'highly' active), which were identified from literature sources. Selected computed molecular descriptors related to absorption, distribution, metabolism, excretion and toxicity (ADMET) of the phytochemicals have been analysed and compared with those of known drugs in order to access the 'drug-likeness' of these compounds.

Results: In the present study, more than 500 anti-malarial compounds identified from 131 distinct medicinal plant species belonging to 44 plant families from the African flora have been considered. On the basis of Lipinski's 'Rule of Five', about 70% of the compounds were predicted to be orally bioavailable, while on the basis of Jorgensen's 'Rule of Three', a corresponding >80% were compliant. An overall drug-likeness parameter indicated that approximately 55% of the compounds could be potential leads for the development of drugs.

Conclusions: From the above analyses, it could be estimated that >50% of the compounds exhibiting anti-plasmodial/ anti-malarial activities, derived from the African flora, could be starting points for drug discovery against malaria. The 3D models of the compounds have been included as an accompanying file and could be employed in virtual screening.

Keywords: Africa; Malaria; Medicinal plants; Metabolism; Natural products; Pharmacokinetics

Background

Malaria is an endemic disease which affects vast proportions of the populations of most Tropical countries (covering Africa, Asia and Latin America) [1,2]. The disease condition is caused by protozoans of the *Plasmodium* genus, mostly *Plasmodium falciparum* [3]. Statistics show that about half of the world's population is at risk of contracting malaria and that 1 to 2 million annual deaths (mostly amongst African children) can be attributed to malaria alone [2-4]. In addition, the spread of the disease has been enhanced by the development of resistance in the anopheline vector against standard insecticides, amongst other factors, which have not unfortunately been put under check [5].

One promising way to fight malaria is to search for vaccines and new drugs, since no vaccine has yet been put in the market and the disease-causing parasites have developed resistant strains against existing chemotherapies [5-7]. It should however be mentioned that the process of discovering a drug is quite timely and costly [8]. One of the current approaches for shortening the time required and cutting down the cost for the discovery of lead

* Correspondence: lmbazze@yahoo.fr
[†]Equal contributors
[1]Department of Chemistry, Faculty of Science, University of Douala, 00237, P. O. Box 24157 Douala, Cameroon
Full list of author information is available at the end of the article

compounds which potentially inhibit or modulate known drug targets is to incorporate computer-based methods like docking techniques, pharmacophore-based searches and neural networking [9-13]. Computer-based methods have also been incorporated in the prediction of likely metabolic pathways of drug molecules, as well as predict their pharmacokinetic profiles [14-17]. The absorption, distribution, metabolism, excretion and toxicity (ADMET) profile of a potential drug molecule should be known if it has to stand the chances of entering the market. Hence, assessing such information for lead compounds early enough would help eliminate molecules with predicted uninteresting profiles and eventually cut down the price of drug discovery [8].

With the accumulation of 'wet lab' biodata on drug metabolism and pharmacokinetics (DMPK) by the close of the 1990s, pharmaceutical companies are increasingly switching over to the use of statistical and knowledge-based methods, implemented in computer software, in the prediction of ADMET/DMPK properties of drug leads, in contrast to the former approach which is more costly and time consuming [14-17]. In our quest to assess the potential of natural products (NPs) derived from African medicinal plants for the development of anti-malarial drugs [18,19], an *in silico* approach based on computed molecular descriptors has been carried out, in comparison with those of known drugs, as previously described in the literature [20-24]. In this paper, we present a computer-based DMPK analysis of >500 anti-malarial compounds, which have been previously isolated from the African flora.

Methods

Data sources

The plant sources, geographical collection sites, chemical structures of pure compounds as well as their spectroscopic data were retrieved from literature sources comprising of MSc theses, PhD theses, textbook chapters and journal articles, with references ranging from 1971 to 2013. A full list of journals consulted is given in the supplementary material (Additional file 1). By convention, activities were categorized into 'very potent', 'good', 'good to moderate', 'weak', 'very weak' and 'inactive'. Following the criteria used by Mahmoudi et al. [25] and Wilcox et al. [26], a pure compound was considered highly active if $IC_{50} < 0.06$ μM, being active with $0.06\ \mu M \leq IC_{50} \leq 5\ \mu M$, weakly active when $5\ \mu M \leq IC_{50} \leq 10\ \mu M$, and compounds with IC50 > 10 μM were considered inactive. The following inhibition percentages were proposed for *in vivo* activity of anti-malarial extracts at a fixed dose of 250 mg kg^{-1} day^{-1}: 100% to 90% (very good activity), 90% to 50% (good to moderate), 50% to 10% (moderate to weak) and 0% (inactive) [27].

Generation of 3D models, optimization and correction of protonation states

The 2D structures of the compounds were retrieved from the literature sources, and all 3D molecular models were generated using the graphical user interface (GUI) of the MOE software [28] running on a Linux workstation with a 3.5 GHz Intel Core2 Duo processor. The 3D structures were generated using the builder module of MOE, and energy minimization was subsequently carried out using the MMFF94 force field [29] until a gradient of 0.01 kcal mol^{-1} was reached. The 3D structures of the compounds were then saved as .mol2 files subsequently treated with LigPrep [30]. This implementation was carried out with the GUI of the Maestro software package [31], using the optimized potentials for liquid simulations (OPLS) forcefield [32-34]. Protonation states at biologically relevant pH were correctly assigned (group I metals in simple salts were disconnected, strong acids were deprotonated, strong bases protonated, while topological duplicates and explicit hydrogens were added). The generated 3D models have been included in the supplementary material (Additional file 2).

Calculation of molecular descriptors

A set of ADMET-related properties (a total of 46 molecular descriptors) were calculated by using the QikProp program [35] running in normal mode. QikProp generates physically relevant descriptors and uses them to perform ADMET predictions. An overall ADME-compliance score - drug-likeness parameter (indicated by #stars) - was used to assess the pharmacokinetic profiles of the compounds. The #stars parameter indicates the number of property descriptors computed by QikProp that fall outside the optimum range of values for 95% of known drugs. The methods implemented were developed by Jorgensen and Duffy [36-38]. Some of the computed ADMET descriptors are shown in Additional file 3: Table S1, along with their significance in DMPK profiling and the recommended ranges for 95% of known drugs.

Results and discussion

Plant families and compound types

From this survey, 511 anti-malarial compounds were identified from 131 plant species belonging to 45 families, a majority being isolated from the Loganiaceae family (10.6%). Significant proportions were also identified from the Guttiferae, Zingiberaceae, Rutaceae, Asteraceae, Ancistrocladaceae, Annonaceae, Clusiaceae, Meliaceae, Sapindaceae, Lamiaceae, Moraceae, Dioncophyllaceae, Cyperaceae, Asphodelaceae, Leguminosae, Periplocaceae and Bignoniaceae families, with respective percentage compound counts of 8.0%, 7.1%, 6.9%, 6.4%, 4.3%, 4.0%, 3.6%, 3.6%, 3.6%, 3.5%, 3.5%, 2.8%,

2.6%, 2.4%, 2.4%, 2.1% and 2.1% of identified anti-malarials (Figure 1). Less than 2% of the anti-malarials were isolated from each of the remaining plant families. A majority of the compounds were terpenoids (30.7%), followed by alkaloids, flavonoids, quinones and xanthones, respectively representing 27.7%, 12.9%, 4.5% and 4.5% by compound count (Figure 2). Only 20 compounds were identified with *in vivo* anti-malarial activities, while 278 compounds showed *in vitro* activities from moderate to very high activities. These have been discussed in our previous review articles in this series [18,19].

Significance of selected computed molecular descriptors

Selected molecular descriptors, along with the recommended range of values for 95% of known drugs, as computed by the QikProp program [35], have been shown in Additional file 3: Table S1. According to Lipinski's 'Rule of Five', a compound is likely to be orally available when the molecular weight (MW) <500, the logarithm of the octan-1-ol/water partition coefficient (log P) < 5, the number of hydrogen donors (HBD) ≤5 and the number of hydrogen bond acceptors (HBA) ≤10 [39]. Compounds which comply with this rule are considered to be drug-like. Moreover, Jorgensen's 'Rule of Three' has often been used as a criterion to predict oral availability of drugs [40]. According to this rule, a compound will more likely be orally available when all or some of the rules, the logarithm of the predicted aqueous solubility (log S_{wat}) > −5.7, the predicted Caco-2 permeability (BIP_{Caco-2}) >22 nm s^{-1} and the number of primary metabolites <7, are respected. The solubility calculation procedure implemented depends on the similarity property space between the given molecule and its most similar analogue within the experimental training set used to develop the model implemented in QikProp; i.e., if the similarity is <0.9, then the QikProp predicted value is taken, otherwise, the predicted property, P_{pred}, is adjusted such that

$$P_{pred} = SP_{exp} + (1-S)P_{QP} \quad (1)$$

where S is the similarity, and P_{exp} and P_{QP} are the respective experimental and QikProp predictions for the most similar molecule within the training set. In Equation 1, if $S = 1$, then the predicted property is equal to the measured experimental property of the training set compound. The predicted apparent Caco-2 cell permeability, BIP_{Caco-2} (in nm s^{-1}), models the permeability of the gut-blood barrier (for non-active transport), even though this parameter is not often correctly predicted computationally [41]. Moreover, a molecule's size, its capacity to make hydrogen bonds, its overall lipophilicity, and its shape and flexibility are important properties to consider when determining permeability. Molecular flexibility has been seen as a parameter which is dependent on the number of rotatable bonds (NRB), a property which influences bioavailability in rats [42].

The overall drug-likeness of a molecule is often determined by the #stars parameter, which depends on 24 computed parameters (descriptors) of a molecule with respect to the recommended range for 95% of known drugs (Additional file 3: Table S1). A #star = 0 corresponds to an ideally drug-like molecule, while #stars = n indicates that a given molecule has n non-compliant descriptors (values fall outside the recommended range for 95% of known drugs). The solubility of a drug, evaluated by the model of Jorgensen and Duffy [36,37], determines

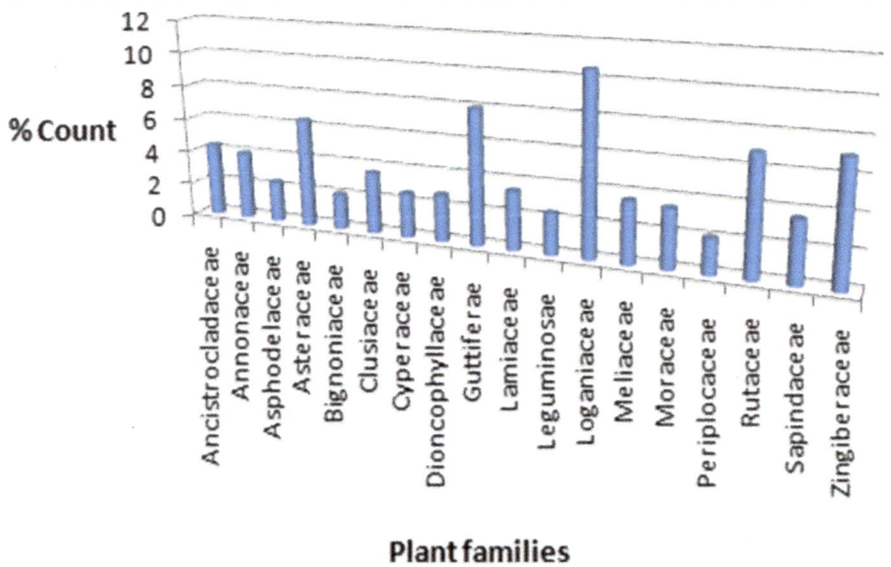

Figure 1 Bar chart showing the distribution of the 511 anti-malarial compounds by plant family of origin.

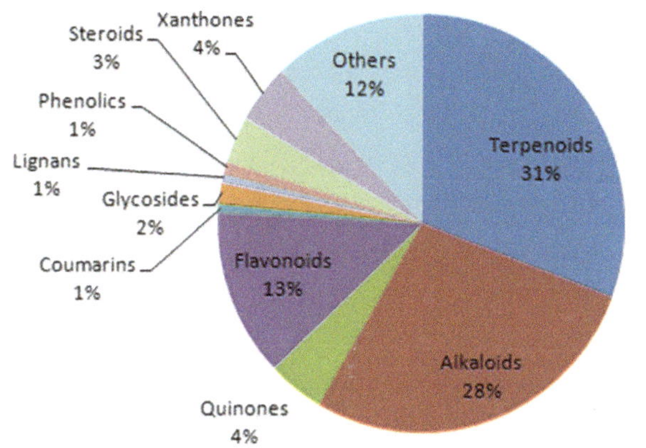

Figure 2 Pie chart showing the classification by compound types.

the bioavailability of a drug to an extent, since the bioavailability of a compound depends on the processes of absorption and liver first-pass metabolism [43]. Absorption in turn depends on the solubility and permeability of the compound, as well as interactions with transporters and metabolizing enzymes in the gut wall.

The computed blood/brain partition coefficients (log *B*/*B*) of drug molecules are often used as indicators to predict access to the central nervous system (CNS). This is because too polar drugs do not cross the blood/brain barrier (BBB). In addition, Madin-Darby canine kidney (MDCK) monolayers are widely used to make oral absorption estimates, the reason being that these cells also express transporter proteins but only express very low levels of metabolizing enzymes [42]. They are also used as an additional criterion to predict BBB penetration. Thus, our calculated apparent MDCK cell permeability could be considered to be a good mimic for the BBB (for non-active transport). The predicted skin permeability parameter (log K_p) is another important parameter for drug distribution [44,45]. The predicted maximum transdermal transport rates, J_m (in μ cm^{-2} h^{-1}), were computed from the aqueous solubility (S_{wat}) and skin permeability (K_p), using the relation (2), also expresses the efficiency of drug distribution:

$$J_m = K_p \times MW \times S_{wat} \quad (2)$$

The efficiency and distribution of a drug may be affected by the degree to which it binds to the proteins within blood plasma. When a drug binds to plasma proteins (like human serum albumin, lipoprotein, glycoprotein, α, β, and γ globulins), the quantity of the drug in general blood circulation is greatly reduced and hence the less bound a drug is, the more efficiently it can traverse cell membranes. The predicted plasma-protein binding has been estimated by the prediction of binding to human serum albumin; the log K_{HSA} parameter (recommended range is −1.5 to 1.5 for 95% of known drugs). The number of metabolic steps (#metab) also determines whether the molecules can easily gain access to the target site after entering the blood stream.

The toxicity parameter is often predicted by the logarithm of IC_{50} values for blockage of the human ether-a-go-go related gene (HERG). HERG encodes a potassium ion (K^+) channel that is implicated in the fatal arrhythmia known as *torsade de pointes* or the long QT syndrome [46]. The HERG K^+ channel is best known for its contribution to the electrical activity of the heart that coordinates the heart's beating. It therefore appears to be the molecular target responsible for the cardiac toxicity of a wide range of therapeutic drugs [47]. HERG has also been associated with modulating the functions of some cells of the nervous system and with establishing and maintaining cancer-like features in leukemic cells [48]. Thus, HERG K^+ channel blockers are potentially toxic and the predicted IC_{50} values often provide reasonable predictions for cardiac toxicity of drugs in the early stages of drug discovery [49].

Lipinski's criteria for evaluation of oral bioavailability

Lipinski's 'rule' was extracted from chemical libraries from the World Dug Index (WDI) as a criterion to evaluate likely oral bioavailability [39,50]. This rule did not take NPs into consideration initially, since Lipinski had postulated that the Rule of Five was not respected by NPs. However, NP libraries have been previously analysed comparatively using this rule in order to have a rough idea of the extent of 'drug-likeness' of a compound library to be used in virtual screening [20-22,51,52]. In summary, 352 of the 511 compounds analysed showed no violations of Lipinski rules, while 435 compounds showed <2 violations. The maximum number of violations was 3 and the average number was 0.5 (Table 1). This implies that the anti-malarial compounds from the African flora could generally be categorized as 'drug-like' up to approximately 70%. Considering the individual parameters, it was observed that for the MW, 432 out of the 511 compounds analysed complied with

Table 1 Minimum, maximum and mean values for computed Lipinski parameters

Lipinski parameter	Minimum	Mean	Maximum
MW (Da)	78.1	394.1	1084.7
log P	−5.1	3.2	16
HBA	0	6.4	28
HBD	0	1.8	17
NRB	0	5.9	32
LV	0	0.5	3

LV, Lipinski violations.

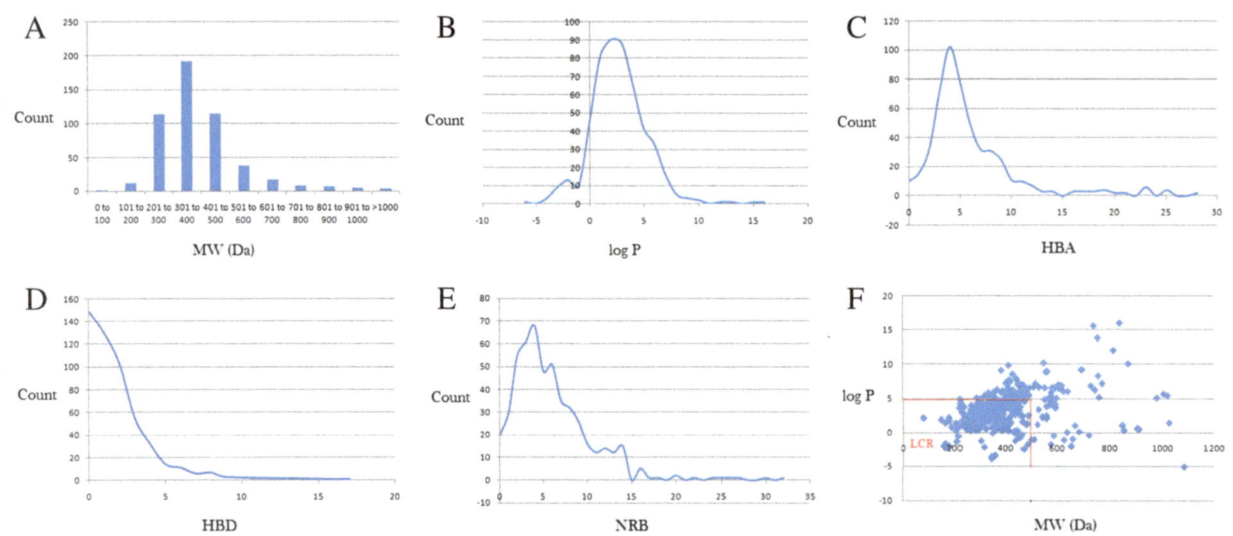

Figure 3 Graph distribution of Lipinski determinant of 'drug-likeness'. (A) Bar chart showing distribution of MW. **(B, C, D and E)** Distribution curves of the log P, HBA, HBD and NRB respectively for the 511 anti-malarial compounds from the African flora. **(F)** Scatter plot of MW against log P. For (B), the *x*-axis label is the lower limit of binned data, e.g., 0 is equivalent to 0.00 to 0.99.

Lipinski's criterion (MW < 500 Da), constituting 84.5%. Meanwhile, the greatest proportion of the molecules had MW in the interval 301 ≤ MW ≤ 400, Figure 3A. The log P curve showed a Gaussian-shape, centred on a peak value of 1.5 log P units, with approximately 88% of the compounds complying to Lipinski's criterion (log P < 5), Figure 3B. The graphs of the HBA, HBD and NRB have been shown in Figure 3C,D,E. The number of HBA rose rapidly to a peak value of 4 acceptors, comprising 102 compounds, then fell off rapidly to 28 acceptors for the most complex NPs in this study. The curve for the HBD had a maximum at 0 donors (for 149 of the compounds) and fell off to 1 compound having as many as 17 donors. The distribution for the NRB gave a rugged curve with a peak value at 4 rotatable bonds (RBs), comprising 68 compounds and as many as 32 RBs for the most flexible compound. A scatter plot of MW against log P showed that the region of maximum density of points lay in the interval MW ≤ 500 ∩ log P ≤ 5, defined as Lipinski's compliance region (LCR). A similar trend was seen in the pairwise scatter plots of the other parameters (results not shown).

Jorgensen's criteria for assessment of oral bioavailability

In the assessment of oral bioavailability, 279 compounds showed no violation of the Rule of Three, while 422 compounds violated this rule only once, indicating that >80% of the compounds are predicted to be orally bioavailable. Regarding the individual parameters, the solubility parameter showed a significant performance, with about 80% of the compounds complying with the recommended range for 95% of known drugs ($-6 \leq \log S_{wat} \leq 0.5$). In accordance to Jorgensen's ro3, 77.3% of the compounds had $\log S_{wat} > 5.7$, while 91% complied with the $BIP_{Caco-2} > 22$ nm s^{-1} criterion. The percentage of compounds complying with each of the other DMPK parameters has been shown in Table 2. The distribution curves of both parameters are shown in Figure 4A,B, along with the histogram for the human oral absorption (HOA) parameter. It was estimated that 312 compounds

Table 2 Mean values and percentage compliances of selected ADMET-related descriptors for 511 anti-malarial compounds from African medicinal plants

Property[a]	Mean value	Percentage compliance
log *B/B*	−1.0	93.3
BIP_{Caco-2} (nm s^{-1})	1,139.0	14.1
S_{mol} (Å^2)	641.5	95.1
$S_{mol,\ hfob}$ (Å^2)	350.0	95.5
V_{mol} (Å^3)	1,202.3	94.5
log S_{wat} (*S* in mol L^{-1})	−4.3	79.3
log K_{HSA}	0.3	83.6
MDCK	627.8	54.0
Ind_{coh}	0.012	95.3
Glob	0.9	92.8
QP_{polz}	39.6	94.1
logHERG	−4.6	57.3
log K_p	−3.2	93.3
#metab	5.4	84.5

[a]The descriptors (entries in the first column and the recommended ranges for 95% of drugs) are defined in Additional file 3: Table S1.

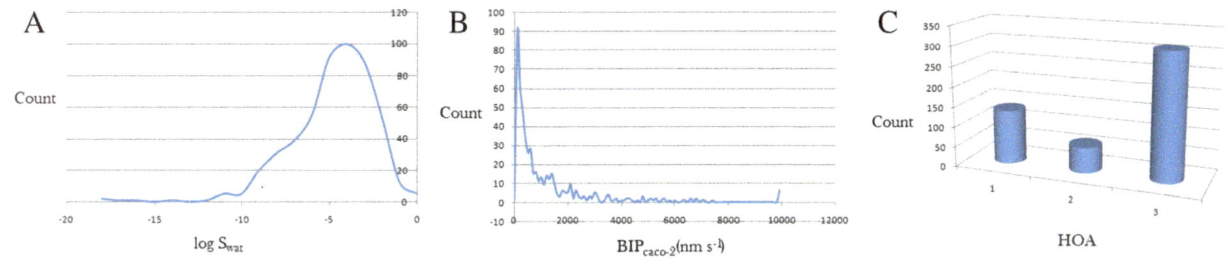

Figure 4 Distribution of parameters for oral bioavailability and human oral absorption. (A) log S_{wat}, **(B)** BIP_{Caco-2} and **(C)** HOA. For the HOA parameter (C), 1, low absorption; 2, medium absorption; 3, high absorption.

could have high HOA (attributed to a value of 3 on Figure 4C), while 64 compounds were estimated to have medium HOA (attributed to a value of 2) and 135 compounds were estimated to have low absorption. Estimations of the percentage of human oral absorption (PHOA) showed that 38.1% of the compounds could be absorbed at 100%, while 52.2% could be absorbed at >90% and 69.9% were estimated to have high PHOA (i.e., absorbed at >80%).

Assessment of the overall DMPK compliance by the drug-likeness parameter

The #stars parameter was also used to evaluate the overall drug-likeness of the anti-malarial compounds from African flora. The distribution curve for this parameter has been shown in Figure 5. The graph started with 0 violations of drug-likeness indicators (corresponding to a maximum number of 282 compounds) and went up to 15 violations. The steepness of the curve, however, showed that the compounds had an overall interesting drug-likeness. Additionally, 79.2% of the compounds violated only ≤2 out of the recommended range of values for the 24 essential descriptors of drug-likeness computed by QikProp in this study.

Prediction of drug distribution and binding to human serum albumin and dermal penetration parameters

The distribution of the compounds was simulated by calculation of binding affinities to human serum albumin (HSA). The distribution of log K_{HSA} gave a smooth Gaussian-shaped curve with a peak value at 0.5 log K_{HSA} units (Figure 6A), with 83.6% of the compounds falling within the required range for 95% of drugs. This is an indication that a significant proportion of the compounds are likely to circulate freely in the blood stream and hence reach the drug target sites.

The skin permeability parameter showed 93.3% compliance with 95% of drugs. The distribution curve was a Gaussian-shape centred on −2.5 log K_p units (Additional file 3: Figure S1), while the predicted maximum transdermal transport rates, J_m (in μ cm^{-2} h^{-1}), were estimated to vary from 0 to about 1,640 units, with only five compounds having predicted value of $J_m > 100$ μ cm^{-2} h^{-1}.

Prediction of blood/brain barrier penetration and activity in the central nervous system

Access to the central nervous system was simulated by the log *B*/*B* parameter, while activity in the central nervous system was estimated by the CNS parameter (on the −2 =

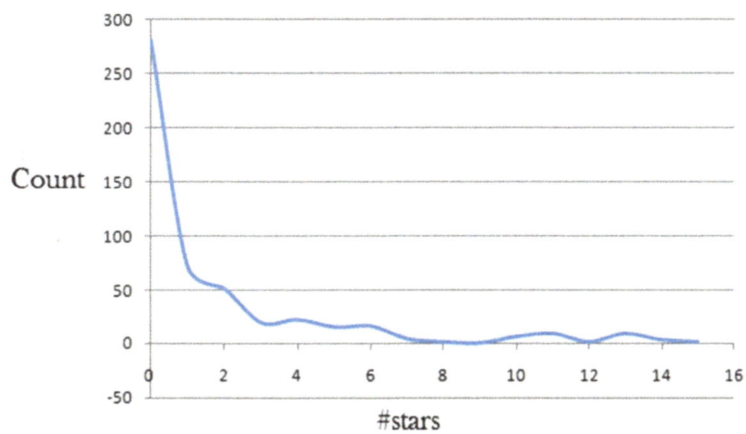

Figure 5 Distribution curves for #stars for 511 anti-malarial compounds derived from African medicinal plants.

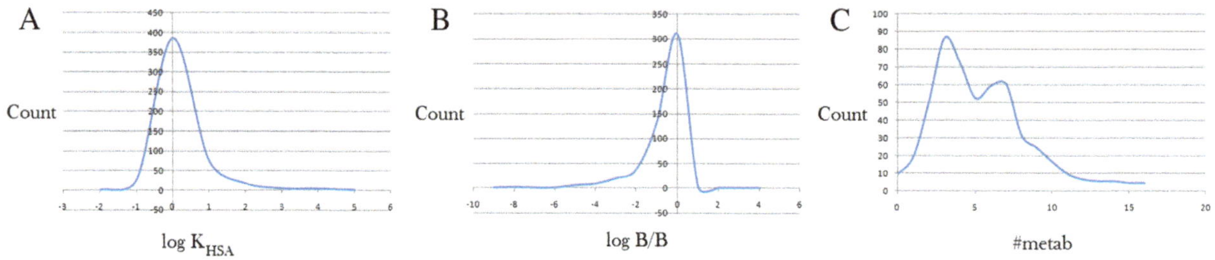

Figure 6 Plot of the physicochemical descriptors used to predict DMPK. (A) Predicted log K_{HSA} against count, **(B)** Predicted log *B/B* against count and **(C)** Predicted # metab against count.

inactive and +2 = active scale). The log *B/B* plot (Figure 6B) showed a sharp peak at 0.5 log *B/B* units, with 93.3% compliance with 95% of drugs. On the other hand, only 3.5% of the compounds were estimated to have an activity in the central nervous system.

Prediction of number of likely metabolic reactions

The number of likely metabolic steps was also computed by QikProp and plotted against the counts (Figure 6C). This parameter is often used to assess the likelihood of a molecule to easily gain access to the target site after entering the blood stream. The average estimated number of possible metabolic reactions was between 5 and 6, even though some of the compounds are likely to undergo as many as up to 16 metabolic reactions due to the complexity of some of the plant secondary metabolites. About 84% of the compounds are predicted to undergo the recommended number of metabolic steps (1 to 8 reactions),

Prediction of toxicity by blockage of HERG K^+ channel

In this study, the estimated or predicted IC_{50} values for blockage of the HERG K^+ channel have been used to model the drug toxicity *in silico*. The recommended range for predicted log IC_{50} values for blockage of HERG K^+ channels (logHERG) is > −5. A distribution curve for the variation of the predicted logHERG is shown in Figure 7, which is a left-slanted Gaussian-shaped curve, with a peak at −5.5 logHERG units. It was observed that in general, this parameter is predicted to fall within the recommended range for about 57% of the compounds.

Conclusions

In this study, the calculated physicochemical properties and indicators of drug-likeness have been used in the assessment of the ADMET/DMPK profiles of >500 compounds isolated from medicinal plants in Africa, which have exhibited from weak to high *in vitro* and/or *in vivo* anti-plasmodial/anti-malarial activity. The overall estimate gave good compliance with the computed parameters for 95% of known drugs, as well as with Lipinski' drug-likeness criteria. The results give good reason for further investigation of the suitability of anti-malarial compounds derived from African flora to be directly employed as drugs or as lead compounds from which

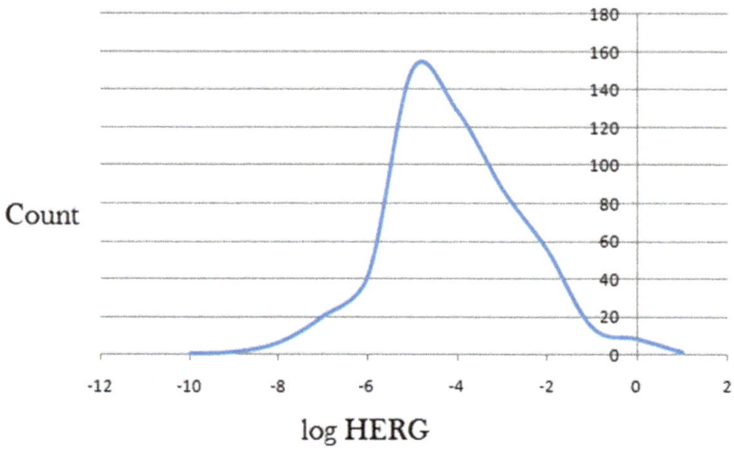

Figure 7 A plot of predicted logHERG values for 511 anti-malarial compounds derived from the African flora.

new anti-malarial drugs could be developed. The generated 3D structures of the compounds have been included as a supplementary file (Additional file 2), while enquiries for the availability of compounds for screening purposes could be addressed to the p-ANAPL consortium [52], which has the mandate to collect compound samples from African flora for biological screening purposes.

Additional files

Additional file 1: List of journals consulted in the literature search.

Additional file 2: The 3D structures of the anti-malarial compounds isolated from African medicinal plants in this survey. This file is saved in .sdf format (which can be viewed using a wide range of software, including MOE, LigandScout, Discovery Studio, and Maestro).

Additional file 3: Table S1. Selected computed ADMET-related descriptors and their recommended ranges for 95% of known drugs. **Figure S1.** Distribution curves for the predicted skin permeability parameter.

Abbreviations

3D: three-dimensional; ADMET: absorption, distribution, metabolism, excretion and toxicity; DMPK: drug metabolism and pharmacokinetics; HBA: hydrogen bond acceptors; HBD: hydrogen bond donors; log P: logarithm of the octan-1-ol/water partition coefficient; MDCK: Madin-Darby canine kidney; MW: molecular weight; NP: natural product; NRB: number of rotatable bonds.

Competing interests

The authors declare no competing interests.

Authors' contributions

FNK, LLL, JAM, JCN and LMM conceived the idea. FNK, LLL and PAO participated in the data collection and molecular simulation experiments. FNK, JAM and PAO contributed in the data analysis, the discussion of results and the conception of the paper under the supervision of LMM, WS, LLL and JCN. FNK and PAO wrote the first draft of the paper, and all authors agreed on the final version before submission. This work is part of the PhD of PAO. All authors read and approved the final manuscript.

Acknowledgements

Financial support is acknowledged from Lhasa Ltd, Leeds, UK through the Chemical and Bioactivity Information Centre (CBIC), University of Buea, Cameroon. Schrodinger Inc. is acknowledged for the academic license.

Author details

[1]Department of Chemistry, Faculty of Science, University of Douala, 00237, P. O. Box 24157 Douala, Cameroon. [2]Department of Chemistry, Faculty of Science, Chemical and Bioactivity Information Centre, University of Buea, 00237, P. O. Box 63 Buea, Cameroon. [3]Department of Pharmaceutical Sciences, Martin-Luther University of Halle-Wittenberg, Wolfgang-Langenbeck Str. 4, Halle (Saale) 06120, Germany.

References

1. Malaria atlas project (MAP). http://www.map.ox.ac.uk. Accessed 2 August 2013
2. WHO - World Health Organization (2012) World malaria report 2012. Geneva, Available from http://who.int/malaria/publications/world_malaria_report_2012/wmr2012_no_profiles.pdf. Accessed 2 August 2013
3. Vogel G (2010) Infectious disease - new map illustrates risk from the 'other' malaria. Science 329:618–618
4. Hoffman SL, Subramanian GM, Collins FH, Venter JC (2002) *Plasmodium*, human and *Anopheles* genomics and malaria. Nature 415:702–709
5. White NJ (2004) Antimalarial drug resistance. J Clin Invest 113:1084–1092
6. Anthony MP, Burrows JN, Duparc S, Moehrle J, Wells TNC (2012) The global pipeline of new medicines for the control and elimination of malaria. Malar J 11:316
7. Wongsrichanalai C, Pickard AL, Wernsdorfer WH, Meshnick SR (2002) Epidemiology of drug-resistant malaria. Lancet Infect Diseases 2:209–218
8. DiMasi JA, Hansen RW, Grabowsk HG (2003) The price of innovation: new estimates of drug development costs. J Health Econ 22:151–185
9. Sullivan DJ Jr, Kaludov N, Martinov MN (2011) Discovery of potent, novel, non-toxic anti-malarial compounds via quantum modelling, virtual screening and *in vitro* experimental validation. Malar J 10:274
10. Singh N, Cheve G, Avery MA, McCurdy CR (2007) Targeting the methyl erythritol phosphate (MEP) pathway for novel antimalarial, antibacterial and herbicidal drug discovery: inhibition of 1-deoxy-*D*-xylulose-5-phosphate reductoisomerase (DXR) enzyme. Curr Pharm Des 13:1161–1177
11. Griffith R, Chanphen R, Leach SP, Keller PA (2002) New anti-malarial compounds from database searching. Bioorg Med Chem Lett 12(4):539–542
12. Bhattacharjee AK, Geyer JA, Woodard CL, Kathcart AK, Nichols DA, Prigge ST, Li Z, Mott BT, Waters NC (2004) A three-dimensional *in silico* pharmacophore model for inhibition of *Plasmodium falciparum* cyclin-dependent kinases and discovery of different classes of novel *Pf*mrk specific inhibitors. J Med Chem 47(22):5418–5426
13. Jacq N, Salzemann J, Jacq F, Legré Y, Medernach E, Montagnat J, Maaß A, Reichstadt M, Schwichtenberg H, Sridhar M, Kasam V, Zimmermann M, Hofmann M, Breton V (2008) Grid-enabled virtual screening against malaria. Journal of Grid Computing 6(1):29–43
14. Hecht D, Cheung M, Fogel GB (2008) QSAR using evolved neural networks for the inhibition of mutant *Pf*DHFR by pyrimethamine derivatives. Biosystems 92(1):10–15
15. Darvas F, Keseru G, Papp A, Dormán G, Urge L, Krajcsi P (2002) *In silico* and *ex silico* ADME approaches for drug discovery. Top Med Chem 2:1287–1304
16. Hodgson J (2001) ADMET – turning chemicals into drugs. Nat Biotechnol 19:722–726
17. Cronin MTD (2003) Computer-assisted prediction of drug toxicity and metabolism in modern methods of drug discovery. In: Hilgenfeld R, Hillisch A (eds) Modern methods of drug discovery. Birkhäuser, Basel
18. Amoa Onguéné P, Ntie-Kang F, Lifongo LL, Ndom JC, Sippl W, Mbaze LM (2013) The potential of anti-malarial compounds derived from African medicinal plants, part I: a pharmacological evaluation of alkaloids and terpenoids. Malar J 12:449
19. Ntie-Kang F, Amoa Onguéné P, Lifongo LL, Ndom JC, Sippl W, Mbaze LM (2014) The potential of anti-malarial compounds derived from African medicinal plants, part II: a pharmacological evaluation of non-alkaloids and non-terpenoids. Malar J 13:81
20. Ntie-Kang F, Mbah JA, Mbaze LM, Lifongo LL, Scharfe M, Ngo Hanna J, Cho-Ngwa F, Amoa Onguéné P, Owono LC, Megnassan E, Sippl W, Efange SMN (2013) CamMedNP: building the Cameroonian 3D structural natural products database for virtual screening. BMC Complement Altern Med 13:88
21. Ntie-Kang F, Onguéné PA, Scharfe M, Owono LCO, Megnassan E, Mbaze LM, Sippl W, Efange SMN (2014) ConMedNP: a natural product library from central African medicinal plants for drug discovery. RSC Adv 4:409–419
22. Ntie-Kang F, Zofou D, Babiaka SB, Meudom R, Scharfe M, Lifongo LL, Mbah JA, Mbaze LM, Sippl W, Efange SMN, AfroDb (2013) A select highly potent and diverse natural product library from African medicinal plants. PLOS ONE 8(10):e78085
23. Ntie-Kang F, Mbah JA, Lifongo LL, Owono LCO, Megnassan E, Mbaze LM, Judson PN, Sippl W, Efange SMN (2013) Assessing the pharmacokinetic profile of the CamMedNP natural products database: an *in silico* approach. Org Med Chem Lett 3:10
24. Ntie-Kang F, Lifongo LL, Mbah JA, Owono LCO, Megnassan E, Mbaze LM, Judson PN, Sippl W, Efange SMN (2013) *In silico* drug metabolism and pharmacokinetic profiles of natural products from medicinal plants in the Congo basin. In Silico Pharmacology 1:12
25. Mahmoudi N, de Julian-Ortiz JV, Cicerone L, Galvez J, Mazier D, Danism M, Derouin F, Garcia-Domenech R (2006) Identification of new antimalarial drugs by linear discriminant analysis and topological virtual screening. J Antimicrob Chemother 57:489–497
26. Willcox M, Bodeker G, Rasanaivo P (2004) Traditional medicinal plants and malaria. CRC, Paris

27. Rasoanaivo P, Oketch-Rabah H (1998) Preclinical considerations on anti-malarial phytomedicines: part II, efficacy evaluation. Institut Malgache des Recherches Appliquées, Antananarivo
28. Chemical Computing Group Inc (2010) Molecular operating environment software. Chemical Computing Group Inc, Montreal
29. Halgren TA (1996) Merck molecular forcefield. J Comput Chem 17:490–641
30. Schrödinger (2011) LigPrep software, version 2.5. LLC, New York
31. Schrödinger (2011) Maestro, version 9.2. LLC, New York
32. Shivakumar D, Williams J, Wu Y, Damm W, Shelley J, Sherman W (2010) Prediction of absolute solvation free energies using molecular dynamics free energy perturbation and the OPLS force field. J Chem Theory Comput 6:1509–1519
33. Jorgensen WL, Tirado-Rives J (1988) The OPLS [optimized potentials for liquid simulations] potential functions for proteins, energy minimizations for crystals of cyclic peptides and crambin. J Am Chem Soc 110(6):1657–1666
34. Jorgensen WL, Maxwell DS, Tirado-Rives J (1996) Development and testing of the OPLS all-atom force field on conformational energetics and properties of organic liquids. J Am Chem Soc 118(45):11225–11236
35. Schrödinger (2011) QikProp, version 3.4. LLC, New York
36. Jorgensen WL, Duffy EM (2000) Prediction of drug solubility from Monte Carlo simulations. Bioorg Med Chem Lett 10:1155–1158
37. Jorgensen WL, Duffy EM (2002) Prediction of drug solubility from structure. Adv Drug Deliv Rev 54:355–366
38. Duffy EM, Jorgensen WL (2000) Prediction of properties from simulations: free energies of solvation in hexadecane, octanol, and water. J Am Chem Soc 122:2878–2888
39. Lipinski CA, Lombardo F, Dominy BW, Feeney PJ (1997) Experimental and computational approaches to estimate solubility and permeability in drug discovery and development settings. Adv Drug Delivery Rev 23:3–25
40. Schrödinger (2011) QikProp 3.4 user manual. LLC, New York
41. Tetko IV, Bruneau P, Mewes H-W, Rohrer DC, Poda GI (2006) Can we estimate the accuracy of ADMET predictions? Drug Discov Today 11:700–707
42. Veber DF, Johnson SR, Cheng HY, Smith BR, Ward KW, Kopple KD (2002) Molecular properties that influence the oral bioavailability of drug candidates. J Med Chem 45:2615–2623
43. Van de Waterbeemd H, Gifford E (2003) ADMET *in silico* modelling: towards prediction paradise? Nat Rev Drug Discov 2:192–204
44. Potts RO, Guy RH (1992) Predicting skin permeability. Pharm Res 9:663–669
45. Potts RO, Guy RH (1995) A predictive algorithm for skin permeability: the effects of molecular size and hydrogen bond activity. Pharm Res 12:1628–1633
46. Hedley PL, Jørgensen P, Schlamowitz S, Wangari R, Moolman-Smook J, Brink PA, Kanters JK, Corfield VA, Christiansen M (2009) The genetic basis of long QT and short QT syndromes: a mutation update. Hum Mutat 30:1486–1511
47. Vandenberg JI, Walker BD, Campbell TJ (2001) HERG K^+ channels: friend or foe. Trends Pharmacol Sci 22:240–246
48. Chiesa N, Rosati B, Arcangeli A, Olivotto M, Wanke E (1997) A novel role for HERG K^+ channels: spike-frequency adaptation. J Physiol 501:313–318
49. Aronov AM (2005) Predictive *in silico* modeling for hERG channel blockers. Drug Discov Today 10:149–155
50. Lipinski CA (2000) Drug-like properties and the causes of poor solubility and poor permeability. J Pharmacol Toxicol Methods 44:235–249
51. Quinn RJ, Carroll AR, Pham MB, Baron P, Palframan ME, Suraweera L, Pierens GK, Muresan S (2008) Developing a drug-like natural product library. J Nat Prod 71:464–468
52. Ntie-Kang F, Amoa Onguéné P, Fotso GW, Andrae-Marobela K, Bezabih M, Ndom JC, Ngadjui BT, Ogundaini AO, Abegaz BM, Mbaze LM (2014) Virtualizing the p-ANAPL library: a step towards drug discovery from African medicinal plants. PLoS ONE 9:e90655

Pyrimidine containing furanose derivative having antifungal, antioxidant, and anticancer activity

Rupesh Dudhe[1,2*], Pramod Kumar Sharma[2] and Prabhakar Kumar Verma[3]

Abstract

Background: A series of 6-(substituted aldehyde)-3,4-dihydro-1-(tetrahydro-3,4-dihydroxy-5-(hydroxymethyl) furan-2-yl)-4-phenylpyrimidine-2(1H)-one derivative (**6A-6P**) was synthesized from the 6-(substituted aldehyde)-4-phenylpyrimidine-2(1H)-one derivative **(5A-5P)** through following reaction mechanisms Claisen-Schmidt, Cyclization, and Satos fusion. The structures of the synthesized compounds were elucidated by I.R.,^{1}H-NMR, elemental analysis, and mass spectroscopic techniques.

Result: The synthesized compounds were screened for *in vitro* antifungal activity at 25, 50, 100, and 200 μg/ml concentrations. Among them, compounds **6P, 6D,** and **6M** exhibited significant antifungal activity that was carried out by cup plate method against fungal strain which was collected from IMTECH Chandigarh, India, against standard drug fluconazole. Compounds have been further evaluated by measuring zone of inhibition and percent inhibition. The synthesized compounds were screened for *in vitro* antioxidant activity using the DPPH assay, based on the AAI and antioxidant activity unit (AAU), using a combination relation between DPPH concentration and absorbance. The antioxidant strength of compounds was compared against ascorbic acid. Among them, compounds **6K, 6F, 6E, 6G, 6H,** and **6M** exhibited significant antioxidant activity and **6J** have less active compound. The data of these synthesized compounds were submitted to the National Institute of Health, USA, under the drug discovery program of National Cancer Institute (NCI) and screened for anticancer activity at a single high dose (10^{-5} M) in full NCI 60 cell lines. The selected compounds have shown potent significant anticancer activity in the NCI 60 cell line screening.

Conclusion: A new series of pyrimidine analogues that contain furanose moiety were synthesized by Satos fusion and characterized. The synthesized compounds screened for their *in vitro* antioxidant, antifungal activity, as well as anticancer activity given by the derivative which has chloro, methoxy, nitro, and chloro substitution having furanose contain pyrimidine derivative that showed the most potent activity.

Keywords: Pyrimidine; Anticancer; Antifungal; Antioxidant

Background

Pyrimidine is a six-member heterocyclic compound that contains two nitrogen atoms at positions 1 and 3. Pyrimidines, being an integral part of DNA and RNA impart to diverse pharmacological properties as effective bactericide and fungicides [1], nitrogen containing heterocyclic ring such as pyrimidine is a promising structural moiety for drug designing. Pyrimidine derivatives form a component in a number of useful drugs and are associated with many biological and therapeutically activities [2]. Condensed furanose pyrimidine derivatives have been reported as antioxidant [3], antimicrobial [4], analgesic [5], antiviral [6], anti-inflammatory [7], anti-HIV [8], antitubercular [9], antitumor [10], antineoplastic [11], and antimalarial [12]. The condensed furanose pyrimidine derivative has the power to accept free radical during different abovementioned diseases due to the presence of NH and OH molecule in ring.

Free radicals are well known for playing a dual role in our body, deleterious as well as beneficial. It includes metabolic pathway for its generation [13]. It mainly explores the formation and the scavenging of free radicals, as well as the damage caused by free radicals in

* Correspondence: rdudhe121@rediffmail.com
[1]Uttarakhand Technical University, Dehradun, Uttarakhand 284007, India
[2]Department of Pharmacy, SMAS, Galgotias University, Greater Noida, Uttar Pradesh 201306, India
Full list of author information is available at the end of the article

biological system. Oxidative stress in our body occurs due to excessive generation of free radical and reduced level of antioxidant, but at low concentration, these radicals performs normal physiological functions of body. Scientific evidence suggests that antioxidants reduce the risk for chronic diseases including cancer and heart disease [14].

About 13% deaths of human beings throughout the world are caused by cancer, which is characterized by uncontrolled cell growth, metastasis, and invasion [13]. Although the risk of cancer increases with age, people of all ages, even fetuses, can be affected by the disease. The most occurring fatal cancers are lung, stomach, liver, colon, and breast cancer. Therefore, continuous search for new anticancer agents should be an active work in the research field at various laboratories. Among potential anticancer agents, heterocyclic compounds represent an outstanding type of anticancer drug moiety (Figure 1).

Free radical may be defined as the atoms, molecules, or ions with unpaired electrons in an open shell configuration. Sometime, free radicals may contain positive, negative, or zero charge [15]. Free radicals play an important role in combustion, atmospheric chemistry, polymerization, plasma chemistry, and many other chemical processes [16]. The large generation of free radicals particularly reactive oxygen species and their high activity plays an important role in the progression of great number of pathological disturbances such as inflammation [17], atherosclerosis [18], cancer [19], parkinsonism [20], and Alzheimer's disease [21]. Inflammation is mostly caused through excessive generation of free radical in the body (Figure 2).

Methods

Chemistry

All the reagents and solvents used were laboratory grade and obtained from the supplier (Sigma-Aldrich, St. Louis, MO, USA; CDH, Beijing, China; and Rankem, Faridabad, India) or recrystallized/redistilled as necessary. The purity of compounds synthesized, commercial reagents used, and monitor of reaction was done by thin layer chromatography (TLC) plates (silica gel G). Two solvent systems: toluene/ethyl acetate/formic acid (5:4:1) and ethyl acetate/n-hexane (3:7) were used to run TLC. The spots were located under iodine vapors and UV light. The melting points of the products were determined by open capillaries method and are uncorrected. Infrared (IR) spectra (KBr) were recorded on FTIR spectrophotometer (Shimadzu FTIR 8400 S, 4,000 to 400 cm^{-1}, Kyoto, Japan). The elemental analysis was carried out using Heraus CHN rapid analyzer (Hanau, Germany) [1].H-NMR spectra were recorded on a JEOL AL300 FTNMR 300 MHz spectrometer (Akishima-shi, Japan) in dimethyl sulfoxide (DMSO) using TMS as an internal standard, with [1] H resonance frequency of 300 MHz chemical shift values are expressed in δ ppm. The activity was performed on instrument UV-visible spectrophotometer UV-1800 Pharmaspec Shimadzu.

Screening of compounds

Antifungal activity

All the synthesized compound were screened *in vitro* for their antifungal activity *Candida inconspicua* (Microbial Type culture collection (MTCC)-1074, American Type Culture Collection (ATCC)-16783), *Candida viswanathii* (MTCC-1629, ATCC-22981), *Candida albicans* (MTCC-227, ATCC-10231), *Candida tropicalis* (MTCC-230, ATCC-20336), *Candida glabrata* (MTCC-3019, ATCC-90030) against standard drug fluconazole [19]. The incubation time was 48 h at 37°C for fungal strain. All the screened compounds were found to possess moderate to good antifungal activity. The cup plate test was performed using agar medium and dextrose agar medium, and the medium was autoclaved at 15 lbs pressure (121°C) for 15 min then immediately cooled to 50°C to 55°C in a water bath after removing it from autoclave. The cooled medium was poured into sterile petri plates to a uniform depth of 4 mm or 25 ml in a 90-mm plate. Once the medium had solidified, then the culture was

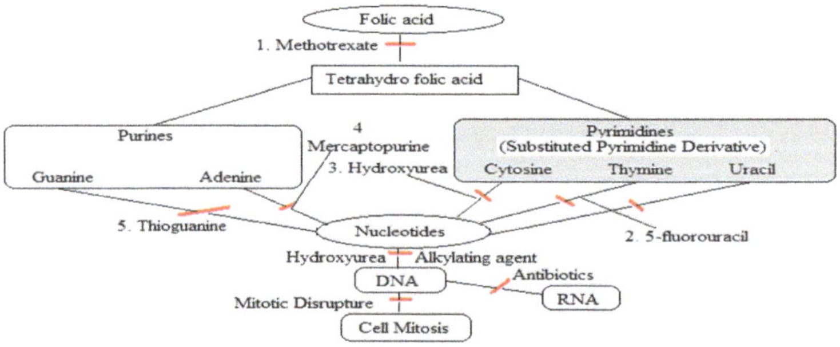

Figure 1 Mechanism of anticancer compound.

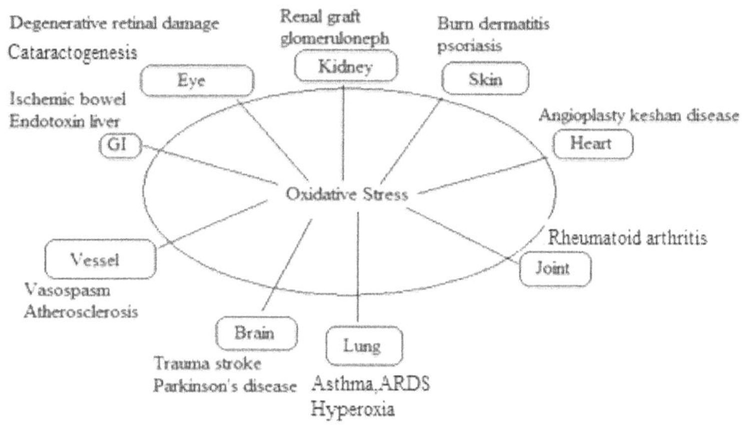

Figure 2 Effect of free radical in the body parts.

inoculated on the medium by a sterile swab that was dipped into the fungus suspension or inoculated with 1 ml of the organism suspension. Sterillized 9-mm cork borer was used to make agar wells, than placed 25, 50, 100 and 200 μg/ml diluted test compound as well as standard compound were placed into each wells and DMSO as a control. The plate were inoculate for 48 h at 37°C for fungal strain and measure zone of inhibition in mm and the percentage (%) of inhibition was calculated by using the formula [17] (Tables 1, 2, 3, 4 and 5) (Figures 3, 4, 5, 6 and 7).

$$\%\,\text{of inhibition} = \frac{\text{Diameter of the inhibition zone in mm}}{\text{Diameter of the petri plates in mm (90)}}$$

Free radical scavenging method by DPPH assay

Various concentrations of test compound 10 to 200 μg/ml were prepared in the methanol and 1 ml of each concentration was added to 1 ml of 0.1 mM solution of DPPH [3]. The mixture was shaken vigorously and allowed to stand for 30 min in dark place; absorbance at 517 nm was determined by UV spectrometer, and the percentage scavenging activity was calculated. A blank solution of DPPH was prepared, and ascorbic acid was used as reference compound. All the compounds were tested and analyzed by their absorbance. The equation used to measure free radical scavenging is as follows (Equation 1, Figure 8, Scheme 1):

A lower value of mean inhibitory concentration shows a higher free radical scavenging activity.

$$\%\,\text{Scavenging} = \frac{\text{Absorbance of control} - \text{Absorbance of test compounds/Std.}}{\text{Absorbance of control}} \times 100$$

AAU equation

The free radical scavenging fitting curve equation ($y = BX + D$) when combined with theoretical value of DPPH concentration and absorbance ($y = KX$) to assume the index antioxidant activity unit (AAU), it is defined as 'one mole of DPPH free radical was completely scavenged to consume amount (mole number) of the scavenger'. The lower the value of AAU, the stronger the antioxidant ability of compound (Table 6) (Figure 9).

$$\text{AAU} = 394.32 \times \frac{R}{B \times C \times Mr},$$

where R = solution volume ratio of sample to solution volume of DPPH for each sample, B = slope of fitting equation of free radical scavenging ratio, C = initial concentration of DPPH solution observed, and Mr = molecular weight of sample.

Anticancer screening

Pharmacological evaluation of the anticancer activity was performed on the compounds inconvertibly selected by the National Institute of Health, Bethesda, USA, under the drug discovery program of National Cancer Institute (NCI) [13]. All the finally synthesized 20 compounds have been registered on its website, and from those, only 13 compounds have been selected. All the selected compounds have been given a unique NCI number [19].

Methodology of the *in vitro* cancer screening

The human tumor cell lines of the cancer screening panel are grown in RPMI 1640 medium containing 5% fetal bovine serum and 2 μL glutamine. The cells are

Table 1 Antifungal activity for MTCC-230 strain

Compounds	% Inhibition at µg/ml MTCC-230			
	25	50	100	200
Standard	21.11	22.89	25.33	27.56
6B	19.11	22	24	26.44
6C	17.11	20	21.7	22.24
6E	26	27.33	28	28.66
6F	20.22	22.26	23.55	24
6G	17.11	18	22	22.04
6I	19.11	20.66	22.66	21.2
6K	20.4	22.22	24	26.66
6M	20.44	21.7	23.55	25.2
6P	15.33	20.66	26.66	29.1

inoculated into 96-well microtiter plates in 100 µL at plating densities ranging from 5,000 to 40,000 cells/well depending on the doubling time of individual cell lines. After cell inoculation, the microtiter plates are incubated at 37°C in the presence of 5% CO_2, 95% air, and 100% relative humidity for 24 h prior to addition of experimental drugs. After 24 h, two plates of each cell line are fixed *in situ* with TCA to represent a measurement of the cell population for each cell line at the time of drug addition (Tz). Experimental drugs are solubilized in dimethyl sulfoxide at desired final maximum test concentration and stored frozen prior to use. At the time of drug addition, an aliquot of frozen concentrate is thawed and diluted to twice the desired final maximum test concentration with complete medium containing 50 µg/ml gentamicin. Additional 4-, 10-fold, or ½ log serial dilutions are made to provide a total of five drug concentrations plus control. Aliquots of 100 µl of these different drug dilutions are added to the appropriate microtiter

Table 2 Antifungal activity for MTCC-3019

Compounds	% Inhibition at µg/ml MTCC-3019			
	25	50	100	200
Standard	14.00	16.44	19.56	22.00
6B	17.33	19.33	20	22.22
6C	0	0	12.22	13.11
6D	0	12.22	14.44	17.11
6E	0	0	13.11	13.77
6F	14.44	15.77	17.77	20.44
6G	16.88	18.88	20.04	21.33
6H	0	12.88	14.22	15.77
6J	0	0	12.44	14.44
6M	15.55	16.88	19.55	21.55
6n	13.33	15.77	17.55	19.11
6P	15.3	17.07	18.44	20.88

Table 3 Antifungal activity for MTCC-1074

Compounds	% Inhibition at µg/ml MTCC-1074			
	25	50	100	200
Standard	15.33	18.44	22.00	25.33
6C	0	17.77	20	21.33
6D	20.44	22.24	23.33	24.22
6E	15.55	17.55	19.11	22.66
6F	18.66	21.33	23.11	25.77
6G	0	0	13.77	15.88
6H	0	0	14.44	16.88
6I	15.33	16.88	18.22	20.97
6J	18.66	19.55	21.55	22.66
6K	20.22	22.22	25.55	27.77
6M	17.11	19.11	22	26
6P	16.66	19.11	20.44	23.77

wells already containing 100 µl of medium, resulting in the required final drug concentrations.

After the following drug addition, the plates are incubated for an additional 48 h at 37°C, 5% CO_2, 95% air, and 100% relative humidity. For adherent cells, the assay is terminated by the addition of cold TCA. Cells are fixed *in situ* by the gentle addition of 50 µl of cold 50% (*w*/*v*) TCA (final concentration, 10% TCA) and incubated for 60 min at 4°C. The supernatant is discarded, and the plates are washed five times with tap water and air dried. Sulforhodamine B (SRB) solution (100 µl) at 0.4% (*w*/*v*) in 1% acetic acid is added to each well, and plates are incubated for 10 min at room temperature. After staining, unbound dye is removed by washing five times with 1% acetic acid and the plates are air dried. Bound stain is subsequently solubilized with 10 mM trizma base, and the absorbance is read on an automated plate reader at a wavelength of 515 nm. For suspension cells, the methodology is the same except that the assay

Table 4 Antifungal activity for MTCC-227

Compounds	% Inhibition at µg/ml MTCC-227			
	25	50	100	200
Standard	16.44	19.33	23.33	27.33
6B	14	16	16.88	18.66
6C	16.88	18.22	19.55	20.44
6D	20.2	24	29.33	34.66
6E	15.77	18.66	21.55	26.22
6E	13.77	14.66	16.22	18
6G	13.11	14	14.66	15.33
6H	14.66	17.11	19.11	22.8
6J	0	13.77	15.11	16.88
6K	0	0	13.77	16.22

Table 5 Antifungal activity for MTCC-1629

Compounds	% Inhibition at µg/ml MTCC-1629			
	25	50	100	200
Standard	16.44	19.33	23.33	27.33
6C	13.11	14.66	16.22	18
6D	17.33	19.77	22.6	25.53
6F	23.55	26.22	28	30.44
6G	21.33	24	26.11	30.22
6I	14.66	16.44	18	21.55
6J	14.22	16.22	19.11	23.77
6K	21.55	23.55	27.33	31.55
6M	15.11	16.44	18	21.55
6P	21.77	23.77	25.77	28.66

is terminated by fixing settled cells at the bottom of the wells by gently adding 50 µl of 80% TCA (final concentration, 16% TCA). Using the seven absorbance measurements (time zero, (Tz), control growth, (C), and test growth in the presence of drug at the five concentration levels (Ti)), the percentage growth is calculated at each of the drug concentrations levels. Percentage growth inhibition is calculated as:

$$[(Ti-Tz)/(C-Tz)] \times 100 \text{ for concentrations for which } Ti >/= Tz$$

$$[(Ti-Tz)/Tz] \times 100 \text{ for concentrations for which } Ti < Tz.$$

Three dose response parameters are calculated for each experimental agent. Growth inhibition of 50% (GI50) is calculated from $[(Ti - Tz)/(C - Tz)] \times 100 = 50$, which is the drug concentration resulting in a 50% reduction in the net protein increase (as measured by SRB staining) in control cells during the drug incubation. The drug concentration resulting in total growth inhibition (TGI) is calculated from $Ti = Tz$. The LC50 (concentration of drug resulting in a 50% reduction in the measured protein at the end of the drug treatment as compared to that at the beginning) indicating a net loss of cells following treatment is calculated from $[(Ti - Tz)/Tz] \times 100 = -50$. Values are calculated for each of these three parameters if the level of activity is reached; however, if the effect is not reached or is exceeded, the value for that parameter is expressed as greater or less than the maximum or minimum concentration tested. The compounds which reduce the growth of any one of the cell lines by 32% or less are passed on for further evaluation in the full panel of 60 cell lines (Table 7) (Figures 10, 11, 12 and 13).

General procedures for the synthesis of compounds

Synthesis of compounds (3A-3P)

Equimolar portions of the appropriately substituted aromatic aldehyde (10 mmol) and acetophenone (10 mmol) were dissolved in approximately in 15 ml of ethanol. The mixture was allowed to stir for several minutes at 5°C to 10°C. Then, 10 ml of 40% aq. NaOH solution was added dropwise to the reaction mixture in the conical flask. The reaction mixture then allowed stirring at room temperature for 4 h on stirrer and precipitate is allowed to stand overnight in refrigerator. Precipitate is formed which is collected by filtration and repeatedly washed with distilled water and finally recrystallized in ethanol. The solvent system was used for the TLC ethyl acetate/n-hexane (3:7) (Scheme 2).

Synthesis of 3-phenyl-1-phenylprop-2-en-1-one (chalcone) (3A): It was obtained by reaction of acetophenon with benzaldehyde. Molecular formula, $C_{17}H_{16}O_3$; molecular weight, 208; m.p., 58°C to 60°C; Rf. value (ethyl acetate/n-hexane, 3:7), 0.78; IR (KBr, cm^{-1}), 3,001.03(C-H stretch.), 1,660.60(conj. C = C), 1,604.66(Ar. C = C), 1,288.36(Ar. C-O), 688.54(Ar. C-H bend).

Synthesis of 3-(3,4-dimethoxyphenyl)-1-phenylprop-2-en-1-one (3B): It was obtained by reaction of acetophenon (2) with 3,4-dimethoxy benzaldehyde. Molecular formula, $C_{17}H_{16}O_3$; molecular weight, 268; m.p., 76°C to 78°C; Rf. value (ethyl acetate/n-hexane, 3:7), 0.80; I.R. (KBr, cm^{-1}), 2,939.31(C-H str.), 1,654.81(conj. C = C), 1,587.31(Ar. C = C), 1,255.57(Ar. C-O), 698.18(Ar. C-H bend).

Synthesis of 3-(2-methoxyphenyl)-1-phenylprop-2-en-1-one (3C): It was obtained by reaction of acetophenon with 2-methoxy benzaldehyde. Molecular formula,

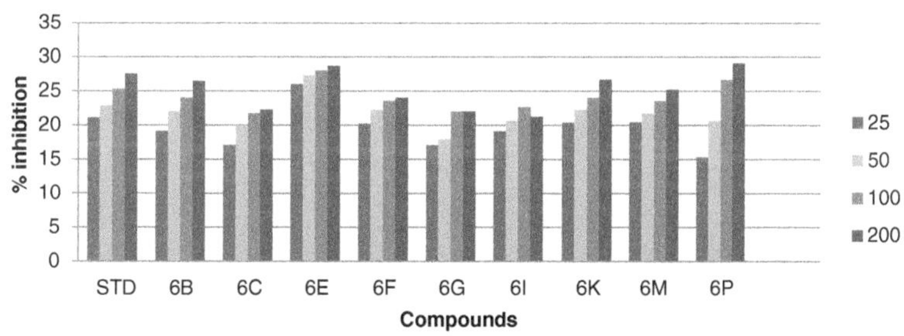

Figure 3 Antifungal activity of synthesized compound against *Candida tropicalis* (MTCC-230).

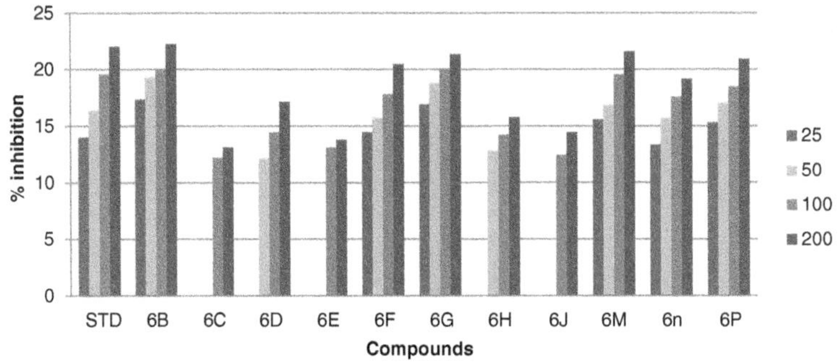

Figure 4 Antifungal activity of synthesized compound against *Candida glabrata* (MTCC-3019).

$C_{16}H_{14}O_2$; molecular weight, 238; m. p., 52°C to 54°C; Rf. value (ethyl acetate/n-hexane, 3:7), 0.72; I.R. (KBr, cm^{-1}), 1,670.44(conj. C = C), 1,602.74(Ar. C = C), 1,249.79(Ar. C-O), 692.40(Ar. C-H bend).

Synthesis of 3-(4-methoxyphenyl)-1-phenylprop-2-en-1-one (3D): It was obtained by reaction of acetophenon with 4-methoxy benzaldehyde. Molecular formula, $C_{16}H_{14}O_2$; molecular weight, 238; m. p., 72°C to 74°C; Rf. value (Ethyl acetate/n-hexane, 3:7), 0.76; I.R. (KBr, cm^{-1}), 1,656.74(conj. C = C), 1,600.81(Ar. C = C), 1,213.14(Ar. C-O), 688.54(Ar. C-H bend.).

Synthesis of 3-(2-chlorophenyl)-1-phenylprop-2-en-1-one (3E): It was obtained by reaction of acetophenon with 2-chloro benzaldehyde. Molecular formula, $C_{15}H_{11}ClO$; molecular weight, 242; m. p., 55°C to 57°C; Rf. value (ethyl acetate/n-hexane, 3:7), 0.78; I.R. (KBr, cm^{-1}), 2,956.67 (C-H str.), 1,660.60(conj. C = C), 1,577.66(Ar. C = C), 1,249.79(Ar. C-O), 752.19 (C-Cl), 692.40(Ar. C-H bend.).

Synthesis of 3-(4-chlorophenyl)-1-phenylprop-2-en-1-one (3F): It was obtained by reaction of acetophenon- with 4-chloro benzaldehyde. Molecular formula, $C_{15}H_{11}ClO$; molecular weight, 242; m. p., 80°C to 84°C; Rf. value (ethyl acetate/n-hexane, 3:7), 0.75; I.R. (KBr, cm^{-1}), 2,918.10(C-H, str.), 1,658.67(conj. C = C), 1,602.74 (Ar. C = C), 1,217.00(Ar. C-O), 775.33 (C-Cl), 690.47(Ar. C-H bend.).

Synthesis of 3-(2, 4-dichlorophenyl)-1-phenylprop-2-en-1-one (3G): It was obtained by reaction of acetophenon with 2,4-dichlorobenzaldehyde. Molecular formula, $C_{15}H_{10}Cl_2O$; molecular weight, 277; m. p., 70°C to 72°C; Rf. value (ethyl acetate/n-hexane, 3:7), 0.72; I.R. (KBr, cm^{-1}), 2,958.60(C-H str.), 1,662.52(conj. C = C), 1,608.52(Ar. C = C), 1,286.36(Ar. C-O), 713.61 (C-Cl), 684.68(Ar. C-H bend.).

Synthesis of 3-(2, 6-dichlorophenyl)-1-phenylprop-2-en-1-one (3H): It was obtained by reaction of acetophenon with 2,6-dichlorobenzaldehyde. Molecular formula, $C_{15}H_{10}Cl_2O$; molecular weight, 277; m. p., 76°C to 78°C; Rf. value (ethyl acetate/n-hexane, 3:7), 0.74; I.R. (KBr, cm^{-1}), 3,082.04(C-H str.), 1,660.60(conj. C = C), 1,612.38(Ar. C = C), 1,265.22(Ar. C-O), 719.40 (C-Cl), 696.25(Ar. C-H bend.).

Synthesis of 3-(2-fluorophenyl)-1-phenylprop-2-en-1-one (3I): It was obtained by reaction of acetophenon with 2-fluorobenzaldehyde. Molecular formula, $C_{15}H_{11}FO$; molecular weight, 226; m. p., 38°C to 40°C; Rf. value (ethyl acetate/n-hexane, 3:7), 0.78; I.R. (KBr, cm^{-1}), 3,028.03(C-H str.), 1,641.31(conj. C = C), 1,612.38(Ar. C = C), 1,384.79 (C-F), 1,244.36(Ar. C-O), 686.61(Ar. C-H bend.).

Synthesis of 3-(4-fluorophenyl)-1-phenylprop-2-en-1-one (3J): It was obtained by reaction of acetophenon with 4-flurobenzaldehyde. Molecular formula, $C_{15}H_{11}FO$; molecular weight, 226; m. p., 40°C to 42°C; Rf. value (ethyl acetate/n-hexane, 3:7), 0.80; I.R. (KBr, cm^{-1}), 1,696.60 (conj. C = C), 1,609.59(Ar. C = C), 1,382.87 (C-F), 1,213.14 (Ar. C-O), 688.54(Ar. C-H bend).

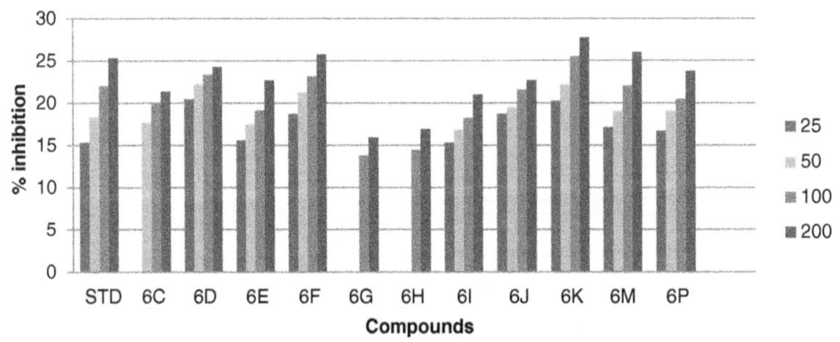

Figure 5 Antifungal activity of synthesized compound against *Candida inconspicua* (MTCC-1074).

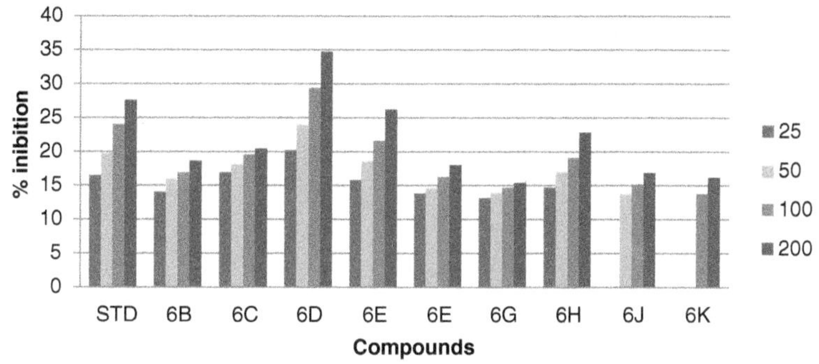

Figure 6 Antifungal activity of synthesized compound against *Candida albicans* (MTCC-227).

Synthesis of 3-(4-bromophenyl)-1-phenylprop-2-en-1-one (3K): It was obtained by reaction of acetophenon with 4-bromobenzaldehyde. Molecular formula, $C_{15}H_{11}BrO$; molecular weight, 287; m. p., 112°C to 114°C; Rf. value (ethyl acetate/n-hexane, 3:7), 0.72; I.R. (KBr, cm^{-1}), 3,056.96(C-H str.), 1,658.67(conj. C = C), 1,608.52(Ar. C = C), 1,332.72(Ar. C-O), 688.54(Ar. C-H bend), 532.32 (C-Br).

Synthesis of 3-(2-nitrophenyl)-1-phenylprop-2-en-1-one (3L): It was obtained by reaction of acetophenon with 2-nitrobenzaldehyde. Molecular formula, $C_{15}H_{11}NO_3$; molecular weight, 253; m. p., 78°C to 80°C; Rf. value (ethyl acetate/n-hexane, 3:7), 0.68; I.R. (KBr, cm^{-1}), 3,006.82(C-H str.), 1,631.67(conj. C = C), 1,382.87 (Ar-NO_2), 1,276.79(Ar. C-O), 686.88(Ar. C-H bend).

Synthesis of 3-(3-nitrophenyl)-1-phenylprop-2-en-1-one (3M): It was obtained by reaction of acetophenon with 3-nitrobenzaldehyde. Molecular formula, $C_{15}H_{11}NO_3$; molecular weight, 253; m. p., 68°C to 70°C; Rf. value (ethyl acetate/n-hexane, 3:7), 0.66; I.R. (KBr, cm^{-1}), 2,918.10 (C-H str.), 1,662.52(conj. C = C), 1,608.52(Ar. C = C), 1,529.45(Ar-NO_2), 1,218.93(Ar. C-O), 655.75(Ar. C-H bend.).

Synthesis of 3-(4-nitrophenyl)-1-phenylprop-2-en-1-one (3N): It was obtained by reaction of acetophenon with 4-nitrobenzaldehyde. Molecular formula, $C_{15}H_{11}NO_3$; molecular weight, 253; m. p., 62°C to 74°C; Rf. value (ethyl acetate/n-hexane, 3:7), 0.74; I.R. (KBr, cm^{-1}), 2,968.24(C-H str.), 1,629.74(conj. C = C), 1,595.02(Ar. C = C), 1,384.79 (Ar-NO_2), 1,218.93(Ar. C-O), 684.68 (Ar. C-H bend).

Synthesis of 3-(2,4-dinitrophenyl)-1-phenylprop-2-en-1-one (3O): It was obtained by reaction of acetophenon with 2,4-dinitrobenzaldehyde. Molecular formula, $C_{15}H_{10}N_2O_5$; molecular weight, 253; m. p., 92°C to 94°C; Rf. value (ethyl acetate/n-hexane, 3:7), 0.78; I.R. (KBr, cm^{-1}), 2,918.10(C-H str.), 1,631.67(conj. C = C), 1,531.37 (Ar-C-NO_2), 1,384.79 (Ar-NO_2), 1,218.93(Ar. C-O), 688.54(Ar. C-H bend.).

Synthesis of 3-(3, 4, 5-trimethoxyphenyl)-1-phenylprop-2-en-1-one (3P): It was obtained by reaction of acetophenon with 3,4,5-trimethoxybenzaldehyde. Molecular formula, $C_{18}H_{18}O_4$; molecular weight, 298.33; Rf. value (ethyl acetate/n-hexane; 3:7), 0.78; I.R. (KBr, cm^{-1}) 2,908.45(C-H str.), 1,662.52(conj. C = C), 1,232.43(Ar. C-O), 665.54(Ar. C-H bend.).

Synthesis of compounds (5A-5P): general procedure

A mixture of compound, i.e., substituted chalcone (0.01 M) (3A-3P), add 0.01 M of NaOH and urea (0.01 M) was refluxed in ethanol for 8 to 10 h after completion of reaction. The content was concentrated and poured into cold water. The product so obtained was washed with water repeatedly and recrystallized in ethanol.

Synthesis of 3,4-dihydro-4,6-diphenylpyrimidin-2 (1H)-one (5A): It was obtained by reaction of compound

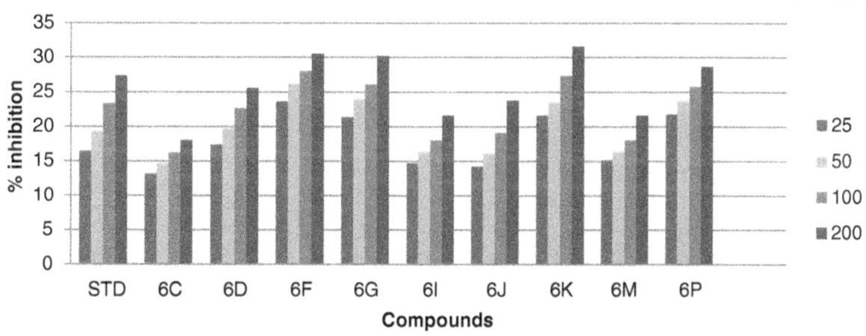

Figure 7 Antifungal activity of synthesized compound against *Candida viswanathii* (MTCC-1629).

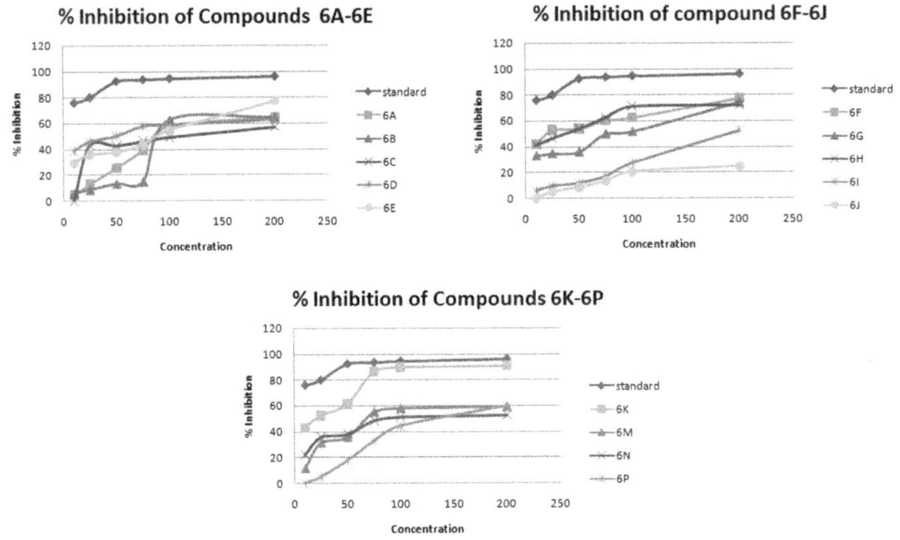

Figure 8 Percent inhibition for antioxidant activity of pyrimidine derivative.

3-phenyl-1-phenylprop-2-en-1-one(chalcone) (3A) (0.01 M), add 0.01 M of NaOH and urea (0.01 M). Molecular formula, $C_{16}H_{14}N_2O$; molecular weight, 250.2; m. p., 111°C to 113°C.; Rf. value (toluene/ethyl acetate/formic acid, 5:4:1), 0.64; I.R. value (KBr, cm^{-1}), 3,319.26(N-H), 3,001.03 (Ar C-H), 1,625.88(C = O), 1,579.59(C = C), 854.53(C-H bend.).

Synthesis of 3,4-dihydro-4-(2, 4-dimethoxyphenyl)-6-phenylpyrimidin-2(1H)-one (5B): It was obtained by reaction of compound 3-(2,4-dimethoxyphenyl)-1-phenylprop-2-en-1-one (3B) (0.01 M), add 0.01 M of NaOH and urea (0.01 M). Molecular formula, $C_{18}H_{18}N_2O3$; molecular weight, 310.32; m. p., 121°C to 123°C.; Rf. value (toluene/ethyl acetate/formic acid, 5:4:1), 0.68; I.R. value (KBr, cm^{-1}), 3,137.97(N-H), 3,008.75(Ar C-H), 1,670.24 (C = O), 1,544.88(C = C), 842.83(C-H bend.).

Synthesis of 3,4-dihydro-4-(2-methoxyphenyl)-6-phenylpyrimidin-2(1H)-one (5C): It was obtained by reaction of compound 3-(2-methoxyphenyl)-1-phenylprop-2-en-1-one (3C) (0.01 M), add 0.01 M of NaOH and urea (0.01 M). Molecular formula, $C_{17}H_{16}N_2O_2$; molecular weight, 380.32; m. p., 132°C to 134°C.; Rf. value (toluene/ethyl acetate/formic acid, 5:4:1), 0.76; I.R. value, 3,440.77 (N-H), 2,916.17(C-H str.), 1,645.17(C = O), 1,596.95(N-H bend.), 838.98(C-H bend.).

Synthesis of 3,4-dihydro-4-(4-methoxyphenyl)-6-phenylpyrimidin-2(1H)-one (5D): It was obtained by reaction of compound 3-(4-methoxyphenyl)-1-phenylprop-2-en-1-one (3D) (0.01 M), add 0.01 M of NaOH and urea (0.01 M). Molecular formula, $C_{17}H_{16}N_2O_2$; molecular weight, 380.32; Rf. value (toluene/ethyl acetate/formic acid, 5:4:1), 0.78; I.R. value, 3,470.67(N-H), 2,903.63(C-H str.), 1,684.70(C = O), 1,584.41(N-H bend.), 815.83(C-H bend.).

Synthesis of 4-(2-chlorophenyl)-3,4-dihydro-6-phenylpyrimidin-2(1H)-one (5E): It was obtained by reaction of compound 3-(2-chlorophenyl)-1-phenylprop-2-en-1-one (3E) (0.01 M), add 0.01 M of NaOH and urea (0.01 M). Molecular formula, $C_{16}H_{13}ClN_2O$; molecular weight, 284.74; m. p., 60°C to 62°C.; Rf. value (toluene/ethyl acetate/formic acid, 5:4:1),0.74; I.R. value, 3,415.70(N-H), 2,918.10(C-H str.), 1,618.17(C = O), 1,585.38(N-H bend.), 827.41(C-H bend.). m/e, 285.1, 268.0, 249.0, 223.1, 207.0, 192.0 (100%), 183.1.

Synthesis of 4-(4-chlorophenyl)-3,4-dihydro-6-phenylpyrimidin-2(1H)-one (5F): It was obtained by reaction of

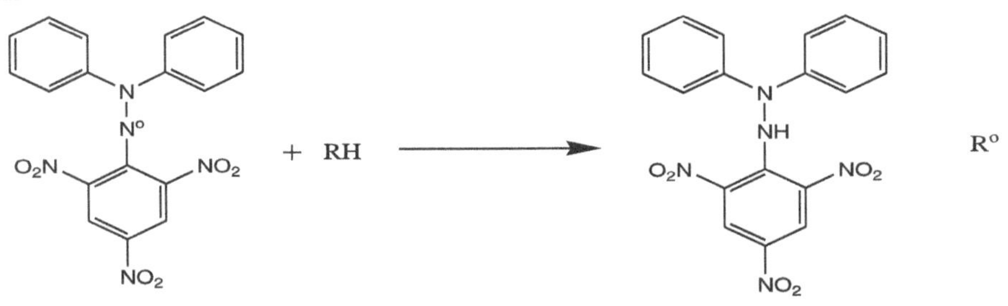

Scheme 1 Reaction of DPPH with compound having proton.

Table 6 AAU and IC50 value of synthesized pyrimidine derivatives

Sample number	Compound code	Slop	IC_{50}value µg/ml	r^2	AAU
1	6A	0.566	89	0.704	8.076
2	6B	0.835	94	0.322	8.13
3	6C	0.753	111	0.35	6.47
4	6D	0.764	50	0.257	9.43
5	6E	0.76	88.5	0.117	20.76
6	6F	0.912	28.5	0.312	7.69
7	6G	0.763	81	0.27	8.9
8	6H	0.891	45	0.293	8.15
9	6I	0.767	196	0.164	13.56
10	6J	0.984	0	0.249	10.05
11	6K	0.872	21.5	0.126	19.86
12	6M	0.775	68.5	0.368	5.9
13	6N	0.819	81.45	0.279	8.37
14	6P	0.761	212	0.209	11.19

compound 3-(4-chlorophenyl)-1-phenylprop-2-en-1-one (3 F) (0.01 M), add 0.01 M of NaOH and urea (0.01 M). Molecular formula, $C_{16}H_{13}ClN_2O$; molecular weight, 284.74; m. p., 104°C to 106°C.; Rf. value (toluene/ethyl acetate/formic acid, 5:4:1), 0.94; I.R. value, 3,442.70(N-H), 3,056.96(C-H str.), 1,635.59(C = O), 1,595.02(N-H bend.), 823.55(C-H bend.).

Synthesis of 4-(2,4-dichlorophenyl)-3,4-dihydro-6-phenylpyrimidin-2(1H)-one (5G): It was obtained by reaction of compound 3-(2,4-dichlorophenyl)-1-phenylprop-2-en-1-one (3G) (0.01 M), add 0.01 M of NaOH and urea (0.01 M). Molecular formula, $C_{16}H_{12}Cl_2N_2O$; molecular weight, 319.19; m. p., 143°C to 145°C.; Rf. value (toluene/ethyl acetate/formic acid, 5:4:1), 0.88; I.R. value, 3,421.48 (N-H), 2,916.17(C-H str.), 1,635.59(C = O), 1,581.52(N-H bend.), 830.65(C-H bend.).

Synthesis of 4-(2,6-dichlorophenyl)-3,4-dihydro-6-phenylpyrimidin-2(1H)-one (5H): It was obtained by reaction of compound 3-(2,6-dichlorophenyl)-1-phenylprop-2-en-1-one (3H) (0.01 M), add 0.01 M of NaOH and urea (0.01 M). Molecular formula, $C_{16}H_{12}Cl_2N_2O$; molecular weight, 319.19; m. p., 116°C to 118°C.; Rf. value (toluene/ethyl acetate/formic acid, −5:4:1), 0.96; I.R. value, 3,417.63 (N-H), 2,918.10(C-H str.), 1,683.74(C = O), 1,585.87(N-H bend.), 850.86(C-H bend.).

Synthesis of 4-(4-fluorophenyl)-3,4-dihydro-6-phenylpyrimidin-2(1H)-one (5I): It was obtained by reaction of compound 3-(2-fluorophenyl)-1-phenylprop-2-en-1-one (3I) (0.01 M), add 0.01 M of NaOH and urea (0.01 M). Molecular formula, $C_{16}H_{13}FN_2O$; molecular weight, 268.29; Rf. value (toluene/ethyl acetate/formic acid, 5:4:1), 0.78; I.R. value, 3,225.05(N-H), 2,920.03(C-H str.), 1,683.74 (C = O), 1,596.95(N-H bend.), 815.83(C-H bend.).

Synthesis of 4-(4-bromophenyl)-3,4-dihydro-6-phenylpyrimidin-2(1H)-one (5K): It was obtained by reaction of compound 3-(4-bromophenyl)-1-phenylprop-2-en-1-one (3 K) (0.01 M), add 0.01 M of NaOH and urea (0.01 M). Molecular formula, $C_{16}H_{13}FN_2O$; molecular weight, 268.29; Rf. value (toluene/ethyl acetate/formic acid, −5:4:1), 0.72; I.R. value, 3,415.70(N-H), 2,921.96 (C-H str.), 1,677.95(C = O), 1,589.23(N-H bend.), 831.26 (C-H bend.).

Synthesis of 3,4-dihydro-4-(3-nitrophenyl)-6-phenylpyrimidin-2(1H)-one (5M): It was obtained by reaction of compound 3-(3-nitrophenyl)-1-phenylprop-2-en-1-one (3 M) (0.01 M), add 0.01 M of NaOH and urea (0.01 M). Molecular formula, $C_{16}H_{13}N_3O_2$; molecular weight, 295.29; Rf. Value (toluene/ethyl acetate/formic acid, −5:4:1), 0.75; I.R. value, 3,417.63(N-H), 2,916.17(C-H str.), 1,677.95(C – O), 1,596.95(N-H bend.), 831.26(C-H bend.).

Synthesis of 3,4-dihydro-4-(4-nitrophenyl)-6-phenylpyrimidin-2(1H)-one (5N): It was obtained by reaction

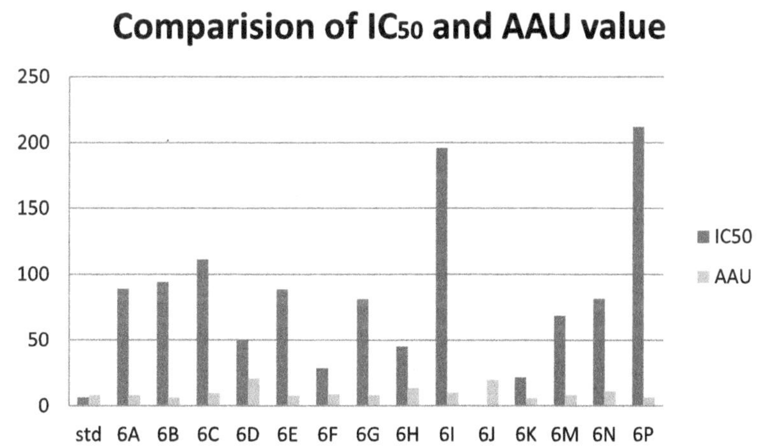

Figure 9 AAU and IC50 value.

Table 7 Growth percentage of synthesized compound against cancer cell line

Code number	Mean	Growth percent of cancer cells								
6E	102.27	92.25	103.34	105.00	102.40	103.21	102.66	101.33	109.04	103.00
6N	89.17	76.08	85.07	95.26	92.38	89.75	93.04	87.27	88.45	92.58
6P	95.90	93.62	91.55	100.10	96.00	94.52	97.92	97.16	96.96	96.27
6C	100.69	95.66	96.75	103.51	96.14	102.20	102.64	101.08	112.87	102.25

of compound 3-(4-nitrophenyl)-1-phenylprop-2-en-1-one (3 N) (0.01 M), add 0.01 M of NaOH and urea (0.01 M). Molecular formula, $C_{16}H_{13}N_3O_2$; molecular weight, 295.29; m. p., 143°C to 145°C.; Rf. value (toluene/ethyl acetate/formic acid, –5:4:1), 0.70; I.R. value, 3,415.70 (N-H), 2,918.10(C-H str.), 1,614.31(C = O), 1,598.88(N-H bend.), 696.25(C-H bend.).

Synthesis of 3,4-dihydro-4-(3,4,5-trimethoxyphenyl)-6-phenylpyrimidin-2(1H)-one (5P): It was obtained by reaction of compound 3-(3,4,5-trimethoxyphenyl)-1-phenylprop-2-en-1-one (3P) (0.01 M), add 0.01 M of NaOH and urea (0.01 M). Molecular formula, $C_{19}H_{20}N_2O_4$; molecular weight, 340.37; m. p., 66°C to 68°C; Rf. value, (toluene/ethyl acetate/formic acid, 5:4:1), 0.82; I.R. value, 3,325.05(N-H), 2,920.03(C-H str.), 1,643.76(C = O), 1,589.23(N-H bend.), 838.98(C-H bend.).

Synthesis of compounds (6A-6P): general procedure

To a solution of 5A-5P (0.01 mol) in ethanol, β-D-ribofuranose-1,2,3,5-tetra-o-acetate (0.01 mol) was added in the presence of TsOH and the content were refluxed under vacuum with stirring at 155°C to 160°C for 15 to 30 min. The vacuum was removed, and the reaction mixture was protected from moisture by fitting a guard tube. Stirring was further continued for 10 h and vacuum was applied for 10 min. at every hour. The viscous mass thus obtained was dissolved in sodium-containing methanol and boiled for 10 min then left for stirring overnight at room temperature. The reaction mixture was filtered, and the filtrate was evaporated to dryness. The viscous residue, thus obtained was dissolved in ether, filtered, concentrated, and kept in refrigerator overnight to get crystalline product.

Synthesis of 3,4-dihydro-1-(tetrahydro-3, 4-dihydroxy-5-(hydroxymethyl)furan-2-yl)-4, 6-diphenylpyrimidin-2 (1H)-one (6A): It was obtained from the reaction of 3,4-dihydro-6-(phenyl)-4-phenylpyrimidin-2(1H)-one (5A) (0.01 mol) in ethanol, β-D-ribofuranose-1,2,3,5-tetra-o-acetate (0.01 mol) was added in the presence of TsOH. Molecular formula, $C_{23}H_{26}N_2O_7$; molecular weight, 382.41; m. p., 121°C to 123°C; Rf. value (ethyl acetate/n-hexane. 3:7), 0.73; I.R. (KBr cm^{-1}), 3,542.99 (O-H, str.), 3,286.48(N-H str.), 3,006.82(C-H, str.), 1,613.67 (C = C), 1,380.94 (C = O), 1,114.78 (C-O-C), 744.47(C-H, bend.). 1H-NMR ($CDCl_3$-d, δ, ppm), 2.46 (s, 1H, NH), 3.22(s, 3H, OH), 3.81 to 3.95(d, 3H, CH_2, CH), 3.99 to 4.55 (m, 4H, CH), 5.28(d, 1H, CH), 6.41 to 7.259(m, 10H, Ar-CH). m/e, 382.15(M^+); elemental analysis calculated, C, 65.96; H, 5.80; N, 7.33.

Synthesis of 3,4-dihydro-1-(tetrahydro-3,4-dihydroxy-5-(hydroxymethyl)furan-2-yl)-6-(2,4-dimethoxyphenyl)-4-phenylpyrimidin-2(1H)-one (6B):It was obtained from the reaction of 3,4-dihydro-6-(2,4-dimethoxyphenyl)-4-phenylpyrimidin-2(1H)-one (5B) (0.01 mol) in ethanol, β-D-ribofuranose-1,2,3,5-tetra-o-acetate (0.01 mol) was added in the presence of TsOH. Molecular formula, $C_{23}H_{26}N_2O_7$; molecular weight, 442.17; m. p., 142°C to 144°C; Rf. value (ethyl acetate/n-hexane, 3:7); 0.80, IR (KBr cm^{-1}), 3,440.77(O-H, str.), 3,375.20(N-H, str.), 2,921.96(C-H, str.), 1,504.37 (C = C), 1,215.07 (C = O), 1,193.85 (C-O-C), 815.83(C-H, bend.). 1H-NMR (CDCl3-d, δ, ppm), 2.59(s, 1H, NH), 3.37(s, 3H, OH), 3.54 to 3.61 (d, 3H, CH_2, CH), 3.69(s, 6H, OCH_3), 4.23 to 4.55 (m, 4H, CH), 5.65 to 5.67(d, 1H, CH), 6.95 to 7.25 (m, 8H, Ar-CH). m/e, 442.2, 417.2, 343.2, 310.0, 288.0, 213.0(100%), 165.1, 135.1. Elemental analysis calculated, C, 62.43; H, 5.92; N, 6.33.

Synthesis of 3,4-dihydro-1-(tetrahydro-3, 4-dihydroxy-5-(hydroxymethyl)furan-2-yl)-6-(2-methoxyphenyl)-4-phenylpyrimidin-2(1H)-one(6C): It was obtained from the reaction of 3,4-dihydro-4-(2-methoxyphenyl)-6-phenylpyrimidine-2(1H)-one(5C) (0.01 mol) in ethanol, β-D-ribofuranose-1,2,3,5-tetra-o-acetate (0.01 mol) was added in the presence of TsOH. Molecular formula, $C_{22}H_{24}N_2O_6$; molecular weight, 412.5; m. p., 55°C to 57°C; Rf. value (toluene/ethyl acetate/formic acid, 5:4:1), 0.92; I.R.(KBr, cm^{-1}), 3,487.06 (O-H, str.), 3,307.69 (N-H, str.), 2,920.03 (C-H, Ar.), 1,596.95 (C = C), 1,091.63 (C-O-C), 827.41 (C-H, bend.); 1H-NMR, 1.556(s, 1H, NH), 3.330 to 3.338(s, 3H, OH), 3.343(s, 3H, OCH_3), 3.740 to 3.75(d, 2H, CH), 4.054 to 4.11(m, 4H, CH), 6.297 to 6.299(d, 2H, CH), 6.902to 7.954(m, 9H, Ar-CH); m/e, 412.23, 362.3 (100%), 359.5, 195. Elemental analysis calculated, C, 64.07; H, 5.87; N, 6.79.

Synthesis of 3,4-dihydro-1-(tetrahydro-3,4-dihydroxy-5-(hydroxymethyl)furan-2-yl)-6-(4-methoxyphenyl)-4-phenylpyrimidin-2(1H)-one (6D): It was obtained from the reaction of 3,4-dihydro-6-(4-methoxyphenyl)-4-phenylpyrimidin-2(1H)-one (5D) (0.01 mol) in ethanol, β-D-ribofuranose-1,2,3,5-tetra-o-acetate (0.01 mol) was added in the presence of TsOH. Molecular formula, $C_{22}H_{24}N_2O_6$; molecular weight, 412.44; m. p., 146°C to

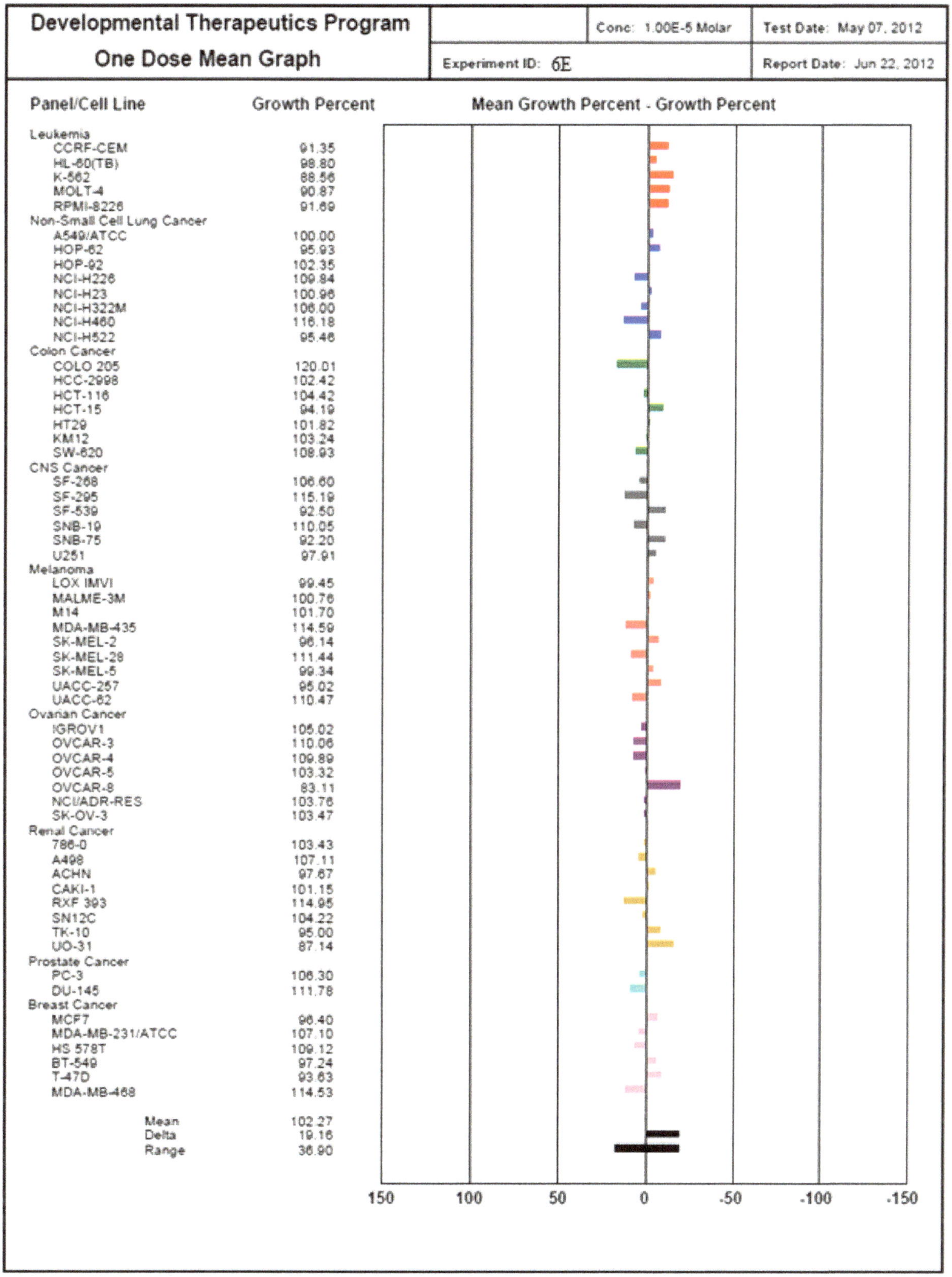

Figure 10 Growth percent of cancer cells of compound 6E.

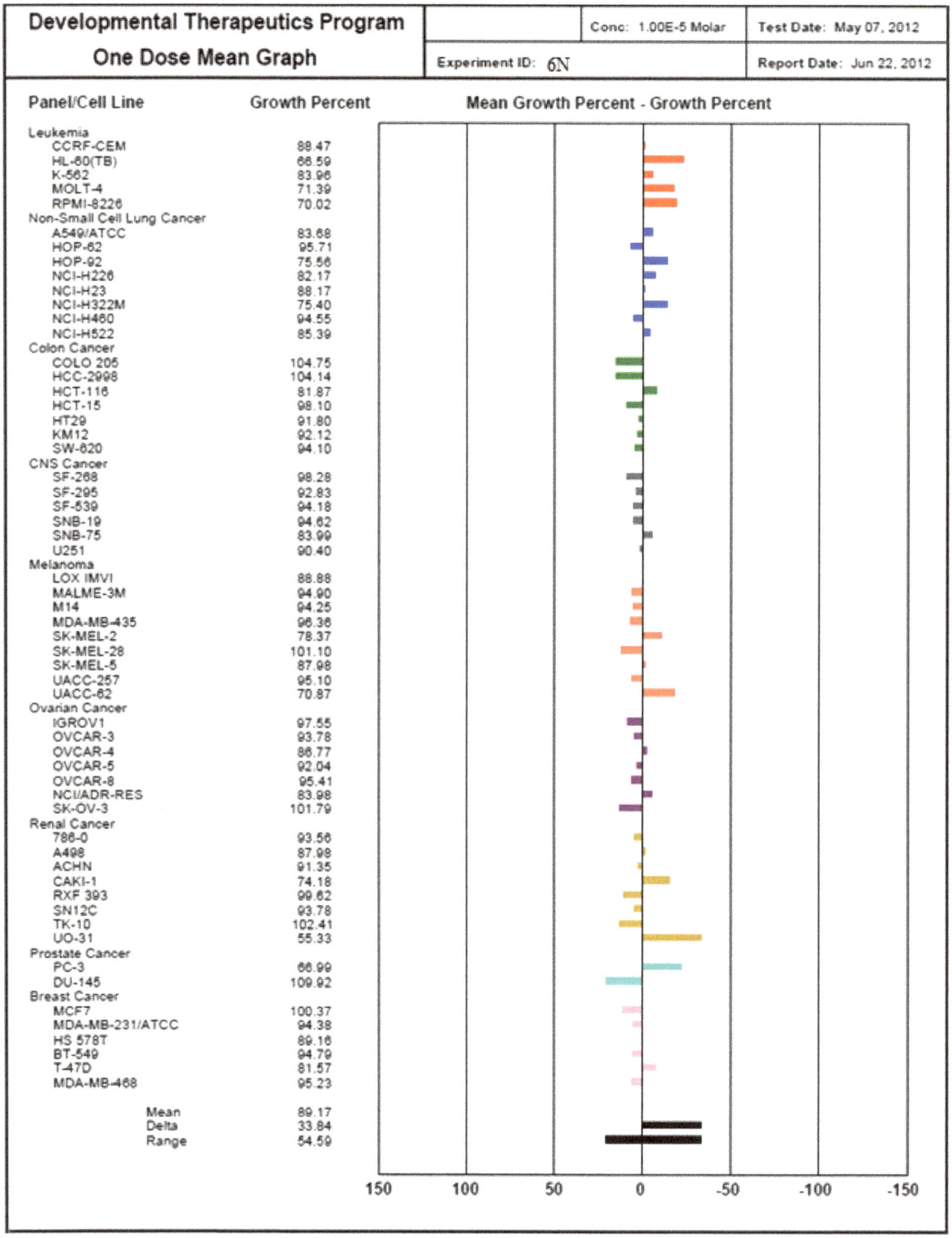

Figure 11 Growth percent of cancer cells of compound 6N.

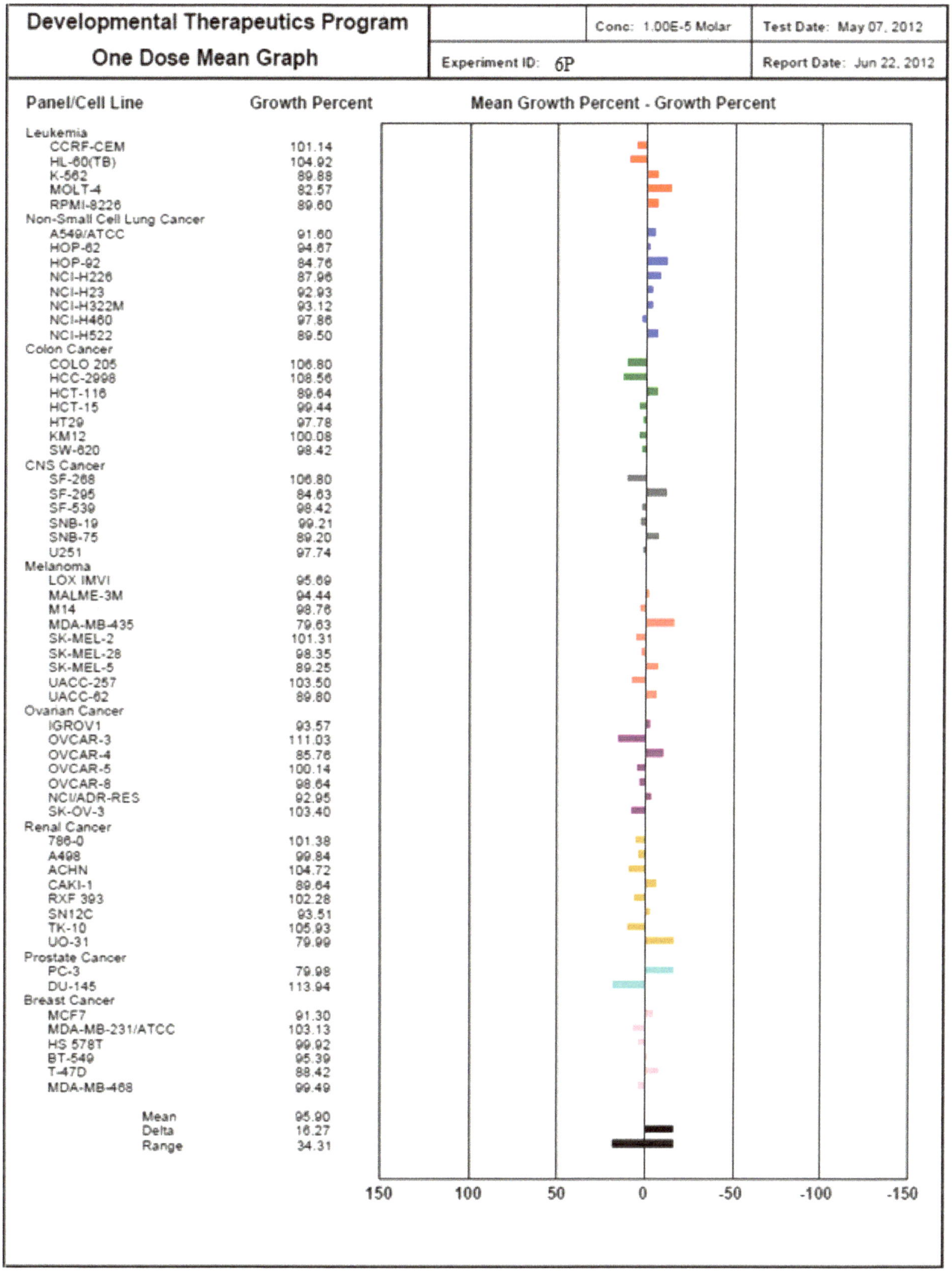

Figure 12 Growth percent of cancer cells of 6P.

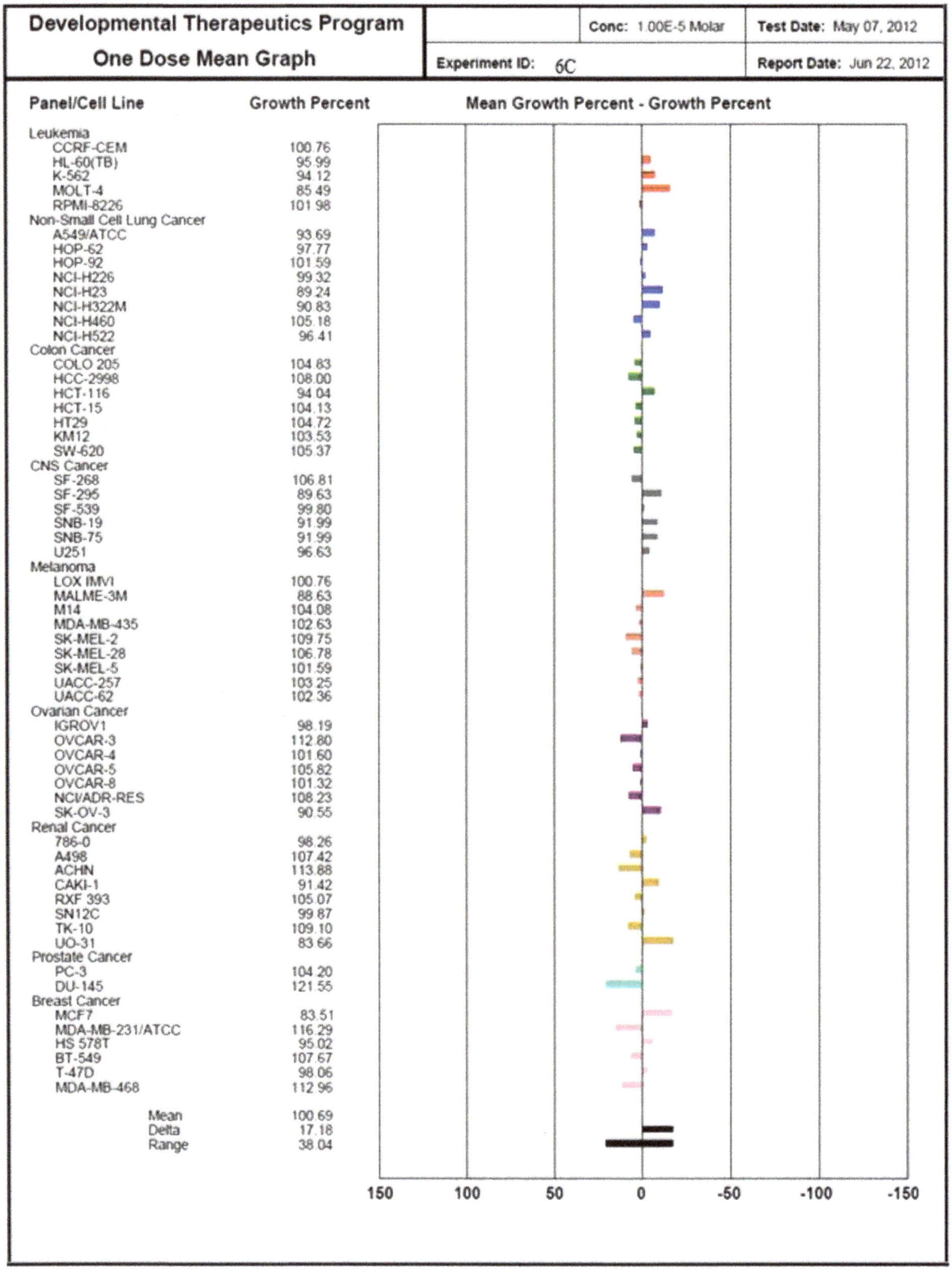

Figure 13 Growth percent of cancer cells of 6C.

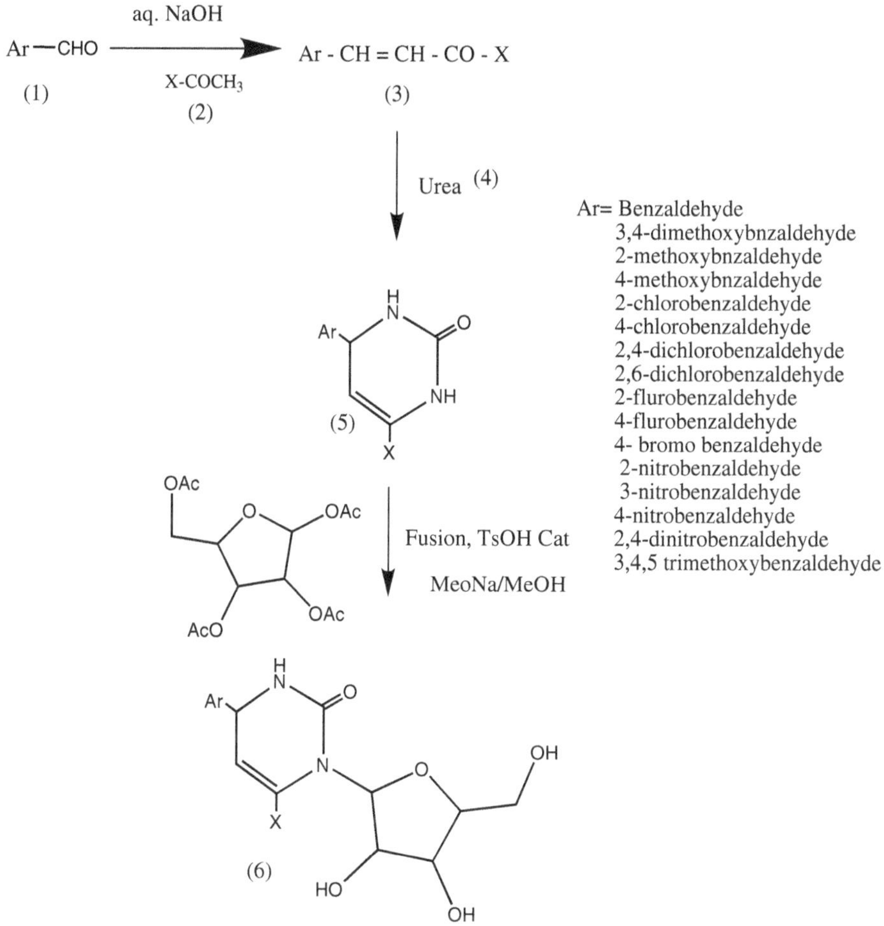

Scheme 2 Reaction scheme.

148°C; Rf. value (ethyl acetate/n-hexane, 3:7), 0.62; I.R. (KBr, cm^{-1}), 3,375.20 (O-H str.), 3,286.48 (N-H, str.), 2,918.10 (C-H, Ar.), 1,598.88 (C = C), 1,134.07 (C-O-C), 815.83(C-H, bend.); 1H-NMR ($CDCl_3$-d, δ, ppm), 2.507 (s, 1H, NH), 3.346 (s, 3H, OH), 3.607(s, 3H, OCH_3), 3.654 to 3.709 (m, 5H, CH,CH_2), 3.740 to 3.910(d, 3H, CH), 4.111 to 4.13(d, 1H, CH), 6.857-7.038(m, 9H, Ar-CH). m/e, 399.2, 365.1, 305.3, 294.0, 278.0, 249.2, 214.1 (100%). Elemental analysis calculated, C, 64.07; H, 5.87; N, 6.79.

Synthesis of*6-(2-chlorophenyl)-3,4-dihydro-1-(tetra-hydro-3, 4-dihydroxy-5-(hydroxymethyl) furan-2-yl)-4-phenylpyrimidin-2(1H)-one (6E):* It was obtained from the reaction of 4-(2-chlorophenyl)-3, 4-dihydro-6-phenylpyrimidine-2(1H)-one(5E) (0.01 mol) in ethanol, β-D-ribofuranose-1,2,3,5-tetra-o-acetate (0.01 mol) was added in the presence of TsOH. Molecular formula, $C_{21}H_{21}ClN_2O_5$; molecular weight, 416; m. p., 97°C to 99°C; Rf. value (toluene/ethyl acetate/formic acid, 5:4:1), 0.89; I.R. (KBr, cm^{-1}), 3,365.55(O-H, str.), 3,244.05(N-H, str.), 2,850.59(C-H, str.), 1,656.74(C = O), 1,596.95 (C = C), 1,132.14 (C-O-C), 815.83(C-H, bend.), 690.47(C-Cl). 1H-NMR ($CDCl_3$-d, δ, ppm), 0.880(d, 1H, CH), 1.254(d, 2H, CH_2), 2.591(s, 1H, NH), 3.293 to 3.479(s, 3H, OH), 3.899 to 3.982(m, 4H, CH), 6.297(d, 2H, CH), 7.257 to 8.690(m, 9H, Ar-CH). m/e, 416.13, 374.2, 360.2, 359.2 (100%), 258.9; elemental analysis calculated, C, 60.51; H, 5.08; N, 6.72.

Synthesis of 6-(4-chlorophenyl)-3,4-dihydro-1-(tetra-hydro-3,4-dihydroxy-5-(hydroxymethyl) furan -2-yl)-4-phenylpyrimidin-2(1H)-one (6F): It was obtained from the reaction of 3,4-dihydro-6-(4-chlorophenyl)-4-phenylpyrimidin-2(1H)-one (5F) (0.01 mol) in ethanol, β-D-ribofuranose-1,2,3,5-tetra-o-acetate (0.01 mol) was added in the presence of TsOH. Molecular formula, $C_{21}H_{21}ClN_2O_5$; molecular weight, 416.85; m. p., 65°C to 67°C; Rf. value (ethyl acetate/n-hexane, 3:7), 0.61. I.R. (KBr cm^{-1}), 3,475.49(O-H, str.), 3,380.98(N-H str.), 2,920.03(C-H, str.), 1,569.95 (C = C), 1,662.52 (C = 0), 1,134.07 (C-O-C), 775.33(C-Cl), 815.83(C-H, bend.). 1H-NMR, 2.034 (s, 1H, NH), 3.034 (s, 3H, OH), 3.325 to 3.412(m, 5H, CH, CH_2), 3.826 to 3.925(d, 3H, CH), 5.352(d, 1H, CH), 7.256 to 7.561(m, 8H, Ar-CH). m/e, 416.85(M^+). Elemental analysis calculated, C, 60.51; H, 5.08; N, 6.72.

Synthesis of 6-(2, 4-dichlorophenyl)-3, 4-dihydro-1-(tetrahydro-3, 4-dihydroxy-5-(hydroxymethyl)furan-2-yl)-4-phenylpyrimidin-2(1H)-one (6G): It was obtained from the reaction of (2,4-dichlorophenyl)-3,4-dihydro-6-phenylpyrimidin-2(1H)-one(5G) (0.01 mol) in ethanol, β-D-ribofuranose-1,2,3,5-tetra-o-acetate (0.01 mol) was added in the presence of TsOH. Molecular formula, $C_{21}H_{20}Cl_2N_2O_5$; molecular weight, 450.0; m. p., 72°C to 74°C; Rf. value (toluene/ethyl acetate/formic acid, 5:4:1), 0.77; I.R. (KBr, cm^{-1}), 3,460.06(O-H str.), 3,175.58(N-H, str.), 3,089.75(C-H, str.), 1,558.38 (C = C), 1,660.60 (C = O), 1,193.85 (C-O-C), 815.85(C-H, bend.), 688.54 (C-Cl). 1H-NMR ($CDCl_3$-d, δ, ppm), 1.253(s, 1H, CH), 1.286(d, 2H, CH_2), 2.034(s, 1H, NH), 3.826(s, 3H, OH), 5.352(d, 2H, CH), 7.256 to 7.561(m, 8H, Ar-CH); m/e, 450.2, 387.32, 369.42, 197.17(100%); elemental analysis calculated, C, 55.89; H, 4.47; N, 6.21.

Synthesis of 6-(2,6-dichlorophenyl)-3,4-dihydro-1-(tetrahydro-3,4-dihydroxy-5-(hydroxymethyl)furan-2-yl)-4-phenylpyrimidin-2(1H)-one (6H): It was obtained from the reaction of 3,4-dihydro-6-(2.6-dichlorophenyl)-4-phenylpyrimidin-2(1H)-one (5H) (0.01 mol) in ethanol, β-D-ribofuranose-1,2,3,5-tetra-o-acetate (0.01 mol) was added in the presence of TsOH. Molecular formula, $C_{21}H_{20}Cl_2N_2O_5$; molecular weight, 451.3; Rf. value (ethyl acetate/n-hexane,3:7), 0.65; I.R. (KBr cm^{-1}), 3,419.56(O-H, str.), 3,274.90(N-H, str.), 3,058.89(C-H, str.), 1,595.02 (C = C), 1,681.81 (C = 0), 1,178.43 (C-O-C),775.33(C-Cl), 821.62(C-H, bend.). 1H-NMR ($CDCl_3$-d, δ, ppm), 2.800(s, 1H, NH), 3.323 to 3.402(s, 3H, OH), 3.562 to 3.662(d, 3H, CH_2, CH), 3.677 to 4.685(m, 4H, CH), 5.29 to 5.31(d, 1H, CH), 6.910 to 7.645(m, 8H, Ar-CH). m/e, 451.3(M^+); elemental analysis calculated, C, 55.89; H, 4.47; N, 6.21.

Synthesis of 6-(2-fluorophenyl)-3,4-dihydro-1-(tetrahydro-3,4-dihydroxy-5-(hydroxymethyl)furan-2-yl)-4-phenylpyrimidin-2(1H)-one (6I): It was obtained from the reaction of 3,4-dihydro-4-(2-flurophenyl)-6-phenylpyrimidine-2(1H)-one(5I) (0.01 mol) in ethanol, β-D-ribofuranose-1,2,3,5-tetra-o-acetate (0.01 mol) was added in the presence of TsOH. Molecular formula, $C_{21}H_{21}FN_2O_5$; molecular weight, 400.14; m.p.,105°C to 107°C; Rf. value (ethyl acetate/n-hexane, 3:7), 0.52; I.R. (KBr, cm^{-1}), 3,363.62(O-H str.), 3,288.40 (N-H str.), 2,921.96 (C-H, Ar.), 1,600.81 (C = C), 1,134.07 (C-O-C), 815.83(C-H, bend.); 1H-NMR (CDC13-d, δ, ppm), 2.82(s, 1H, NH), 3.33 to 3.41(s, 3H, OH), 3.55 to 3.61(d, 3H, CH_2, CH), 3.671 to 4.681(m, 4H, CH), 5.51 to 5.31(d, 1H, CH), 7.11 to 7.645(m, 9H, Ar-CH). m/e, 400.14 (M^+); elemental analysis calculated, C, 62.43; H, 5.92; N, 6.33.

Synthesis of 6-(4-fluorophenyl)-3,4-dihydro-1-(tetrahydro-3,4-dihydroxy-5-(hydroxymethyl) furan-2-yl)-4-phenylpyrimidin-2(1H)-one (6J): It was obtained from the reaction of 3,4-dihydro-4-(2-flurophenyl)-6-phenylpyrimidine-2(1H)-one (5J) (0.01 mol) in ethanol, β-D-ribofuranose-1,2,3,5-tetra-o-acetate (0.01 mol) was added in the presence of TsOH. Molecular formula, $C_{21}H_{21}FN_2O_5$; molecular weight, 400.14; m. p., 94°C to 96°C; Rf. value (ethyl acetate/n-hexane, 3:7), 0.94; I.R. (KBr, cm^{-1}), 3,419.56 (O-H, str.), 3,380.98 (N-H, str.), 2,921.96 (C-H, Ar.), 1,596.95 (C = C), 1,132.14 (C-O-C), 815.83(C-H, bend.); 1H-NMR ($CDCl_3$-d, δ, ppm), 2.51(s, 1H, NH), 3.54 (s, 3H, OH), 3.51 to 3.60(d, 3H, CH_2, CH), 3.661 to 4.181 (m, 4H, CH), 5.55 to 5.61(d, 1H, CH), 7.01 to 7.345(m, 9H, Ar-CH). m/e, 400.11(M^+); elemental analysis calculated, C, 62.43; H, 5.92; N, 6.33.

Synthesis of 6-(4-bromophenyl)-3,4-dihydro-1-(tetrahydro-3, 4-dihydroxy-5-(hydroxymethyl) furan-2-yl)-4-phenylpyrimidin-2(1H)-one (6K): It was obtained from the reaction of 6-(4-bromophenyl)-3,4-dihydro-4-phenylpyrimidin-2(1H)-one (5K) (0.01 mol) in ethanol, β-D-ribofuranose-1,2,3,5-tetra-o-acetate (0.01 mol) was added in the presence of TsOH. Molecular formula, $C_{21}H_{21}BrN_2O_5$; molecular weight, 461.31; m. p., 68°C to 70°C; Rf. value. (ethyl acetate/n-hexane, 3:7), 0.81; I.R. (KBr, cm^{-1}), 3,442.70(O-H, str.), 3,346.27(N-H, str.), 3,064.68 (C-H, str.), 1,604.24(C = C), 1,670.24 (C = 0), 1,174.57 (C-O-C), 640.32(C-Cl), 829.33(C-H, bend.). m/e, 413.3, 381.2, 345.0, 305.3, 249.2, 181.0, 105.0(100%).1H-NMR ($CDCl_3$-d, δ, ppm), 2.087(s, 1H, NH), 2.506(s, 3H, OH), 3.357 to 3.399(m, 5H, CH, CH_2), 3.467 to 3.471 (d, 2H, CH), 5.566 (d, 1H, CH), 7.543 to 7.866 (m, 9H, Ar-CH); elemental analysis calculated, C, 54.68; H, 4.59; N, 6.07.

Synthesis of 3,4-dihydro-1-(tetrahydro-3,4-dihydroxy-5-(hydroxymethyl)furan-2-yl)-6-(3-nitrophenyl)-4-phenylpyrimidin-2(1H)-one (6M): It was obtained from the reaction of 3,4-dihydro-6-(3-nitrophenyl)-4-phenylpyrimidin-2(1H)-one (5M) (0.01 mol) in ethanol, β-D-ribofuranose-1,2,3,5-tetra-o-acetate (0.01 mol) was added in the presence of TsOH. Molecular formula, $C_{21}H_{21}N_3O_7$; molecular weight, 427.41; m.p., 112°C to 114°C; Rf. value (ethyl acetate/n-hexane, 3:7), 0.82; I.R. (KBr cm^{-1}), 3,411.84(O-H, str.), 3,319.26 (N-H, str.), 2,918.10(C-H, str.), 1,596.95(C = C), 1,658.69 (C = O), 1,174.57 (C-O-C), 1,386.72(NO2), 796.55(C-H, bend.). 1H-NMR ($CDCl_3$-d, δ, ppm), 2.41 (s, 1H, NH), 3.23 (s, 3H, OH), 3.61 to 3.65(d, 3H, CH_2, CH), 3.66 to 4.29 (m, 4H, CH), 5.51 to 5.61(d, 1H, CH), 7.13 to 7.445 (m, 9H, Ar-CH). Elemental analysis calculated, C, 59.01; H, 4.95; N, 9.83.

Synthesis of 3,4-dihydro-1-(tetrahydro-3,4-dihydroxy-5-(hydroxymethyl)furan-2-yl)-6-(4-nitrophenyl) -4-phenylpyrimidin-2(1H)-one (6N): It was obtained from the reaction of 3,4-dihydro-4-(4-nitrophenyl)-6-phenylpyrimidin-2(1H)-one(5N) (0.01 mol) in ethanol, β-D-ribofuranose-1,2,3,5-tetra-o-acetate (0.01 mol) was added in the presence of TsOH. Molecular formula, $C_{21}H_{21}N_3O_7$; molecular weight, 427.41; m. p., 96°C to

98°C; Rf. value (toluene/ethyl acetate/formic acid, 5:4:1), 0.89; I.R. (KBr, cm^{-1}), 3,448.49(O-H, str.), 3,024.18(N-H, str.), 2,918.10(C-H, str.), 1,602.74(C = O), 1,584.79 (C = C), 1,355.86 (O = N = O), 815.83 (C-H, bend.); 1H-NMR ($CDCl_3$-d, δ, ppm), 0.880 (d, 2H, CH_2), 1.255(s, 1H, CH), 3.321 to 3.703(s, 3H, OH), 3.841 to 3.993(m, 4H, CH), 6.022(d, 2H, CH), 6.724 to 7.947(m, 9H, Ar-CH). m/e, 427.5, 367.0 (100%), 245, 167; elemental analysis calculated, C, 59.01; H, 4.95; N, 9.83.

Synthesis of 3,4-dihydro-1-(tetrahydro-3,4-dihydroxy-5-(hydroxymethyl)furan-2-yl)-6-(3,4 5-trimethoxyphenyl)-4-phenylpyrimidin-2(1H)-one (6P): It was obtained from the reaction of 3,4-dihydro-4-(3, 4, 5-trimethoxyphenyl)-6-phenylpyrimidin-2(1H)-one(5P) (0.01 mol) in ethanol, β-D-ribofuranose-1,2,3,5-tetra-o-acetate (0.01 mol) was added in the presence of TsOH. Molecular formula, $C_{24}H_{28}N_2O_8$; molecular weight, 472; m. p., 64°C to 66°C; Rf. value (toluene/ethyl acetate/formic acid, 5:4:1), 0.67; I.R. (KBr, cm^{-1}), 3,460.06(O-H, str.), 3,175.58(N-H, str.), 3,071.43(C-H, str.), 1,570.80 (C = C), 1,650.13 (C = O), 1,192.89(C-O-C), 810.51(C-H, bend.). 1H-NMR ($CDCl_3$-d, δ, ppm), 0.885(s, 9H, CH_3), 0.878 (s, 1H, CH), 1.253(d, 2H, CH_2), 2.021(s, 1H, NH), 3.302 to 3.885 (s, 3H, OH), 6.126 (d, 2H, CH), 7.255(m, 7H, Ar-CH); m/e, 472.49, 338.3 (100%), 415.0, 167.07; elemental analysis calculated, C, 61.01; H, 5.97; N, 5.93.

Results and discussion

The scavenging effects of the synthesized compounds **6A-6P** on the DPPH radical was evaluated according to Leong and Shui et al. Various concentrations (10, 25, 50, 75, 100, and 200 μg/ml) of the test compounds in methanol were added to a 0.1-mM solution of DPPH radical in methanol. All the tests and analysis were undertaken on three replicates and the results averaged. The antioxidant activity of tested compounds revealed that the reaction with DPPH is a time-dependent fashion and the higher the concentration of the tested compounds showed the higher the radical scavenging activity as well as percent inhibition and AAU. However, Compounds **6K, 6F, 6E, 6G, 6H,** and **6M** exhibited potent activity compared by AAU and IC_{50} value. The profiles of the scavenging effect of synthesized compounds are comparable to that of the ascorbic acid as reference compound. The synthesized compounds were compounds **6P, 6D,** and **6M** which exhibited significant antifungal activity that was carried out by cup plate method against fungal strain on strains such as *Candida inconspicua* (MTCC-1074, ATCC16783), *Candida viswanathii* (MTCC-1629, ATCC-22981), *Candida albicans* (MTCC-227, ATCC-10231), *Candida tropicalis* (MTCC-230, ATCC-20336), and *Candida glabrata* (MTCC-3019, ATCC-90030) against standard drug fluconazole. The National Institute of Health, USA, under the drug discovery program of NCI and screened for anticancer activity at a single high dose (10^{-5} M) in full NCI 60 cell lines and the compound 6E, 6N, 6P, 6C showed anticancer activity. The introduction of bromo, chloro, dichloro (at 2, 4 and 2, 6 positions) group showed almost equivalent antioxidant activity as that of the ascorbic acid. Based on the structure activity relationships, it can be concluded that the presence of halogen group and methoxy group at the second, fourth, and sixth position exhibited potent activity.

Conclusions

A new series of compounds (6A-6P), i.e., pyrimidine analogues, were synthesized by urea and characterized. The synthesized compounds screened for their *in vitro* antioxidant activity by calculating percentage scavenging, AAU and IC_{50} value, antifungal activity, as well as anticancer activity given by the derivative which has chloro, methoxy, nitro, and chloro substitution having furanose contain pyrimidine derivative that showed the most potent activity.

Competing interests

The authors declare that they have no competing interests.

Author details

[1]Uttarakhand Technical University, Dehradun, Uttarakhand 284007, India. [2]Department of Pharmacy, SMAS, Galgotias University, Greater Noida, Uttar Pradesh 201306, India. [3]Department of Pharmaceutical Sciences, M. D. University, Rohtak, Haryana 124001, India.

References

1. Gursoy E, Guzeldemirci NU (2007) Synthesis and primary cytotoxicity evaluation of new imidazo[2,1-b]thiazole derivatives. Eur J Med Chem 42:320–326
2. Gorlitzer K, Herbig S, Walter RD (1997) Parallel synthesis of trisubstituted formamidines: a facile and versatile procedure. Pharmazie 52:670–679
3. Dudhe R, Sharma PK, Chaudhary A, Verma PK (2013) Synthesis and antioxidant activities of 6-aryl-3,4-dihydro-1-(tetrahydro-3,4-dihydroxy-5-(hydroxymethyl)-furan-2-yl)-4-phenylpyrimidine-2(1h)-thione derivatives. Eur Chem Bull 2:341–347
4. Jaen JC, Wise LD, Caprathe BW, Tecle H, Bergmeier S, Humblet CC (1990) 4-(1,2,5,6-tetrahydro-1-alkyl-3-pyridinyl)-2-thiazolamines: a novel class of compounds with central dopamine agonist properties. J Med Chem 33:311–317
5. Gupta JK, Sharma PK, Dudhe R, Chaudhary A, Singh A, Verma PK, Sambhu C, Yadav Rakesh Kumar M, Kashyap S (2012) Analgesic study of novel pyrimidine derivatives link with coumarin moiety. Med Chem Res 21:1625–1632
6. Kurono M, Hayashi M, Miura K, Isogawa Y, Sawai K (1988) One pot synthesis of pyrimidine and bispyrimidine derivatives and their evaluation for anti-inflammatory and analgesic activities. Chem Abstr 109:37832–37841
7. Patt WC, Hamilton HW, Taylor MD, Ryan MJ, Taylor DG, Connolly CJC (1992) Structure-activity relationships of a series of 2-amino-4-thiazole containing renin inhibitors. J Med Chem 35:2562–2572
8. Rudolph J, Theis H, Hanke R, Endermann R, Johannsen L, Geschke FU (2001) Seco-Cyclothialidines: new concise synthesis, inhibitory activity toward bacterial and human DNA topoisomerases, and antibacterial properties. J Med Chem 44:619–626
9. Sharma RN, Xavier FP, Vasu KK, Chaturvedi SC, Pancholi SS (2009) Synthesis of 4-benzyl-1,3-thiazole derivatives as potential anti-inflammatory agents: an analogue-based drug design approach. J Enz Inhib Med Chem 24:890–897

10. Tsuji K, Ishikawa H (1994) Synthesis and anti-pseudomonal activity of new 2-isocephems with a dihydroxypyridone moiety at C-7. Bioorg Med Chem Lett 4:1601–1606
11. Ukrainets IV, Tugaibei IA, Bereznykova NL, Karvechenko VN, Turov AV (2008) Analgesic, anticonvulsant and anti-inflammatory activities of some synthesized benzodiazipine, triazolopyrimidine and bis-imide derivatives. Chem Heterocycl Comp 5:565–573
12. Wagner E, Al-Kadasi K, Zimecki M, Sawka-Dobrowolska W (2008) Synthesis and pharmacological screening of derivatives of isoxazolo[4,5-d]pyrimidine. Eur J Med Chem 43:677–682
13. Dudhe R, Sharma PK, Singh VK, Chaudhary A, Kumar N, Verma PK (2013) Anticancer activity of ribose fused pyrimidine derivative by SRB assay method. Int J Pure Appl Chem 7:333–339
14. Bell FW, Cantrell AS, Hogberg M, Jaskunas SR, Johansson NG, Jordon CL (1995) Phenethylthiazolethiourea (PETT) compounds, a new class of HIV-1 reverse transcriptase inhibitors. Synthesis and basic structure-activity relationship studies of PETT analogs. J Med Chem 38:4929–4936
15. Badorc A, Bordes MF, De Cointet P, Savi P, Bernat A, Lale A (1997) New orally active non- peptide fibrinogen receptor (GpIIb-IIIa) antagonists: identification of ethyl 3-[N-[4-[4-amino[(ethoxycarbonyl)imino]methyl] phenyl]-1,3-thiazol-2-yl]-N-[1-(ethoxycarbonyl) methyl]piperid-4 yl]amino] propionate (SR 121787) as a potent and long-acting antithrombotic agent. J Med Chem 40:3393–3401
16. Ballell L, Field RA, Chung GAC, Young RJ (2007) New thiopyrazolo[3,4 d] pyrimidine derivatives as antimycobacterial agents. Bioorg Med Chem Lett 17:1736–1745
17. Carter JS, Kramer S, Talley JJ, Penning T, Collins P, Graneto MJ (1999) Synthesis and activity of sulfonamide-substituted 4,5-diaryl thiazoles as selective cyclooxygenase-2 inhibitors. Bioorg Med Chem Lett 9:1171–1174
18. Cordeu L, Cubedo E, Bandres E, Rebollo A, Saenz X, Chozas H, Victoria Dominguez M, Echeverria M, Mendivil B, Sanmartin C (2007) Biological profile of new apoptotic agents based on 2,4-pyrido[2,3-d]pyrimidine derivatives. Bioorg Med Chem 15:1659
19. Desai K, Patel R, Chikhalia K (2006) Design, synthesis and antimicrobial study of some pyrimidine derivatives. J Ind Chem 45:773–779
20. Ergenc N, Capan G, Gunay NS, Ozkirimli S, Gungor M, Ozbey S, Kendi E (1999) Synthesis and hypnotic activity of new 4-thiazolidinone and 2-thioxo-4, 5-imidazolidinedione derivatives. Arch Pharm Med Chem 332:343–347
21. Fujiwara N, Nakajima T, Ueda Y, Fujita H, Kawakami H (2008) Novel piperidinylpyrimidine derivatives as inhibitors of HIV-1 LTR activation. Bioorg Med Chem 16:9804–9814

Synthesis and antileishmanial evaluation of some 2,3-disubstituted-4(3*H*)-quinazolinone derivatives

Yihenew Simegniew Birhan[1*], Adnan Ahmed Bekhit[2] and Ariaya Hymete[3]

Abstract

Background: Leishmaniasis is a neglected tropical parasitic diseases affecting millions of people around the globe. Quinazolines are a group of compounds with diverse pharmacological activities. Owing to their promising antileishmanial activities, some 3-aryl-2-(substitutedstyryl)-4(3*H*)-quinazolinones were synthesized in good yields (65.2% to 86.4%).

Results: The target compounds were synthesized by using cyclization, condensation, and hydrolysis reactions. The structures of the synthesized compounds were determined using elemental microanalysis, infrared (IR), and proton nuclear magnetic resonance (^{1}H NMR). The *in vitro* antileishmanial activities of the synthesized compounds were evaluated using *Leishmania donovani* strain. All the synthesized compounds displayed appreciable antileishmanial activities (IC_{50} values, 0.0128 to 3.1085 μg/ml) as compared to the standard drug miltefosine (IC_{50} = 3.1911 μg/ml). (*E*)-2-(4-chlorostyryl)-3-*p*-tolyl-4(3*H*)-quinazolinone (**7**) is the compound with the most promising antileishmanial activities (IC_{50} = 0.0128 μg/ml) which is approximately 4 and 250 times more active than the standard drugs amphotericin B deoxycholate (IC_{50} = 0.0460 μg/ml) and miltefosine (IC_{50} = 3.1911 μg/ml), respectively.

Conclusions: The results obtained from this investigation indicate that the synthesized and biologically evaluated quinazoline compounds showed promising antileishmanial activities and are good scaffolds for the synthesis of different antileishmanial agents.

Keywords: Quinazolinones; Leishmania; Antileishmanial activities

Background

Leishmanisis is a neglected tropical disease resulting from infection of macrophages by obligate intracellular parasites of the genus *Leishmania* [1-3]. It is a public health problem in at least 88 countries with an estimated 350 million people at risk. The estimated global prevalence of all forms of the disease is 12 million. Every year, 1.5 to 2 million new cases and 70,000 deaths occur due to cutaneous leishmaniasis (CL). In addition, 500,000 new cases and 59,000 deaths from visceral leishmaniasis (VL) occur annually [4]. The number of cases of leishmaniasis is increasing globally due to *Leishmania*/HIV co-infection [5,6], international travel, and migration of immigrants and refugees from endemic regions [7,8].

The prophylactic treatment of leishmaniasis mainly rely on vector and reservoir control [9-11]. Control of reservoir host and vector is difficult due to high coast, operational difficulties, and frequent relapses in the host [12]. Although considerable effort has been made to produce vaccine candidates for the treatment of leishmaniasis, there is no vaccine against any form of human leishmaniasis yet [13-17].

Pentavalent antimonials (Sb^V) have been used for the treatment of leishmania infections. Unfortunately, in many parts of the world, the parasite has become resistant to Sb^V [18]. Treatment failure to sodium stibogluconate (SSG) is observed in Eastern Sudan [19] and in Tigray, Northern Ethiopia [20]. Recent reports showed that pentamidine also developed resistance as well as difficulties in treating patients with *Leishmania*/HIV co-infection [21].

Combination chemotherapy has improved prospects for decreasing the emergence of drug resistance, increasing activity, and reducing required doses and thereby toxic side effects. In the previous study, WR 279,396 (a topical formulation containing 15% paromomycin and 0.5% gentamicin) was found to be safe and effective against CL

* Correspondence: yihenews@gmail.com
[1]Department of Chemistry, Natural and Computational Science College, Debre Markos University, Debre Markos, Ethiopia
Full list of author information is available at the end of the article

caused by *Leishmania major* [22]. In addition, AmBisome-paromomycin is the most cost-effective combination among miltefosine-paromomycin and AmBisome-miltefosine [23]. So far, no combination chemotherapy has been used in treatment programs, except paromomycin/SSG [24].

Tremendous quinazoline derivatives are synthesized in the past two decades, using different synthetic pathways [25-30], due to their diverse pharmacological activities [31-36] including antileishmanial activities [37-40]. These reports indicate that several quinazolines were synthesized and tested for their antileishmanial activities, with the aim of discovering alternative chemotherapeutic agents for the development of new antileishmanials. Promising antileishmanial activities were observed in some 4-aminoquinazoline [37], indolo[2,1-*b*]quinazoline-6,12-dione [38], and 2,3-disubstituted-4(3*H*)-quinazolinone derivatives [39,40]. As part of the efforts to discover less toxic and more effective drug analogues for the treatment of leishmaniasis, we synthesized some 2,3-disubstituted-4(3*H*)-quinazolinones and tested their *in vitro* antileishmanial activities.

Methods

Chemicals and reagents

Anthranilic acid, acetic anhydride, aniline, *p*-toluidine, *o*-toluidine, acetone, dimethylsulfoxide, anhydrous zinc chloride, *p*-chlorobenzaldehyde, *p*-nitrobenzaldehyde, *p*-hydroxybenzaldehyde, chloroform, absolute ethanol, resazurin sodium salt, anhydrous petroleum ether, distilled water, iodine, HCl, and KOH were used in the study.

Instruments and apparatuses

Melting points were determined in open capillaries using electro-thermal 9100 melting point apparatus and were uncorrected. Infrared (IR) spectra in nujol were recorded with the SHIMADZU 8400SP FT-IR spectrophotometer (Shimadzu Corporation, Nakagyo-ku, Kyoto, Japan), and proton nuclear magnetic resonance (^{1}H NMR) spectral data were performed on Bruker Avance DMX400 FT-NMR spectrometer (Bruker, Billerica, MA, USA) using tetramethyl silane (TMS) as internal standard. Silica gel TLC plates of 0.25-mm thickness were used in the study.

Experimental animals and strains

Swiss albino male mice of weight 20 to 32 g and age 6 to 8 weeks (for acute toxicity test) were obtained from Biomedical Laboratory, Department of Biology, Faculty of Science, AAU. *Leishmania donovani* isolate used in this study was obtained from Leishmania Diagnosis and Research Laboratory (LDRL) culture bank, School of Medicine, AAU.

Culture medium and conditions

RPMI-1640, 10% heat-inactivated fetal calf serum (HIFCS), 1% penicillin-streptomycin, and 1% L-glutamine were supplied to make a complete culture medium. The *L. donovani* isolate was grown first on Novy-MacNeal-Nicolle (NNN) medium and then in tissue culture flasks containing RPMI-1640 medium supplemented with 10% HIFCS and 1% 100 IU penicillin/ml-100 μg/ml streptomycin solution at 22°C for promastigotes.

Reference drugs

Miltefosine/hexadecylphosphocholine (AG Scientific, San Diego, CA, USA) and amphotericin B deoxyhcholate (Fungizone®, ER Squibb, Middlesex, UK) were employed as reference drugs in the *in vitro* antileishmanial activity testing of the synthesized compounds.

Preparation of stock and working solutions

Stock solutions of 10 mg/ml of the synthesized compounds were prepared by dissolving each compound in DMSO. Stock solutions were diluted using complete RPMI to obtain aliquots of 10 μg/ml. Then, threefold serial dilution with complete RPMI gave the final six working concentrations (10, 3.33, 1.11, 0.37, 0.12, and 0.04 μg/ml) of each of the synthesized compounds. Amphotericin B deoxycholate and miltefosine, which were used as a positive control for comparison of the antileishmanial activities of the test compounds, were also made in threefold serial dilutions. All the prepared drugs were stored at −20°C and retrieved only during use [41].

In vitro antileishmanial activity

In a 96-well microtiter plate, 100 μl of each of the seven threefold serial dilutions of synthesized compounds were added in triplicate wells. Then, 100 μl of suspension of parasites (3.0×10^6 promastigotes/ml of *L. donovani*) was added in duplicate. Some of the wells contained only the parasites which served as a positive control. The media and DMSO alone acted as a negative control. The contents of the plates were then maintained in humidified atmosphere at 22°C under 5% CO_2.

After 68 h of incubation, 10 μl of fluorochrome resazurin solution (12.5 mg dissolved in 100 ml of distilled water) was added into each well. The fluorescence intensity was measured after a total incubation period of 72 h using Victor3 Multilabel Counter (PerkinElmer, Waltham, MA, USA), at an excitation wavelength of 530 nm and emission wavelength of 590 nm [42]. The IC_{50} values were evaluated from sigmoidal dose-response curves using GraphPad Prism 5.0 software (GraphPad Software, Inc., San Diego, CA, USA).

In vivo acute toxicity test

The oral acute toxicity of compound 7 that exhibited promising antileishmanial activity was investigated using male Swiss albino mice (approximately 20 g each) following reported methods [43]. The experimental animals were divided into six groups (containing six mice per group) and fasted overnight. Groups **1-5** received compound **7** suspended in a vehicle containing 1% gum acacia, in doses of 10, 50, 100, 200, and 300 mg/kg, respectively. The sixth group received vehicle containing 1% gum acacia (served as a control group) at a maximum dose of 1 ml/100 g of body weight by oral route. The mice were observed closely for 24 h with special attention to the first 4 h. Acute toxicity signs were checked in the test mice.

Statistical analysis

The IC_{50} values for *in vitro* promastigotes assay of synthesized compounds were evaluated from sigmoidal dose-response curves using computer software GraphPad Prism 5.0.

Results and discussion

Chemistry of the synthesized compounds

Synthesis of the target compounds involved the formation of **2-5** and **10** as intermediates. It was accomplished using nucleophilic reaction, nucleophilic with ring opening and closing, condensation reaction, and hydrolysis reactions. The target compounds are synthesized in a good yield, which ranged from 65.2% to 86.4% (Table 1). All the synthesized compounds were readily soluble in DMSO and chloroform except compound **12** which is readily soluble in acetone. Spectral data (IR and ^1H NMR) of the synthesized compounds were in full agreement with the proposed structures.

Biological activity testing results

In vitro antileishmanial activity of the synthesized compounds

The antipromastigote activities of the synthesized compounds and the standard antileishmanial drugs (amphotericin B deoxycholate and miltefosine) were evaluated using the clinical isolate of *L. donovani* strain. The IC_{50} of the synthesized and reference drugs were evaluated from fluorescence characteristic of AlamarBlue® (resazurin) (Trek Diagnostic Systems, Inc., Cleveland, OH, USA) which is soluble, stable in culture medium, non-toxic to cells, and does not affect the secretary abilities of cells [44]. The test works as a cell viability and proliferation indicator through the conversion of resazurin to resorufin via reduction. The amount of fluorescence produced is proportional to the number of living cells [45,46].

The quinazolinone derivatives synthesized were shown to have good antileishmanial activity which was in line with the previous reports [37-40]. All the tested compounds exhibited better antileishmanial activity than the standard drug miltefosine as shown in Table 2. Among them, compound **7** was found to have a very promising antileishmanial activity with an IC_{50} value of 0.0128 μg/ml which was 250 times superior than miltefosine (3.1911 μg/ml). Compounds **8** and **11** were 30 times more active than miltefosine. Compounds **6** and **12** were 10 times and twice more active than miltefosine, respectively. Compounds **9** and **13** were as active as miltefosine.

All the synthesized compounds except compound **7** displayed weak antileishmanial activities as compared to amphotericin B deoxycholate. Better antipromastigote activity was observed for (*E*)-2-(4-chlorostyryl)-3-*p*-tolyl-4(3*H*)-quinazolinone (**7**) with an IC_{50} value of 0.0128 μg/ml which is four times higher than the standard drug amphotericin B deoxycholate with an IC_{50} value of 0.0128 μg/ml. (*E*)-2-(4-chlorostyryl)-3-*p*-tolyl-4(3*H*)-quinazolinone (**7**) was found to be 4 times more active than amphotericin B deoxycholate and 250 times more active than miltefosine.

Oral acute toxicity study

Compound (*E*)-2-(4-chlorostyryl)-3-*p*-tolyl-4(3*H*)-quinazolinone (**7**) was observed to be devoid of any inherent acute toxicities at a maximum dose of 300 mg/kg.

Experimental

Synthesis of target compounds

The synthesis of target compounds, 3-aryl-2-(substitutedstyryl)-4(3*H*)-quinazolinones (**6-9** and **11-13**), was achieved using cyclization, condensation, and hydrolysis reactions. It involved the synthesis of acetanthranil (2-methyl-3,1-benzoxazin-4-one (**2**)) and 3-aryl-2-methyl-4

Table 1 Physical constants and percent yield of the synthesized compounds

Test compound	Molecular formula	Molecular weight (g/mol)	% yield	Melting point (°C)	R_f values [$CHCl_3$/C_6H_6 (9:1)]
6	$C_{22}H_{17}ClN_2O$	360.85	68.3	201 to 203	0.520
7	$C_{23}H_{19}ClN_2O$	374.87	65.2	189 to 191	0.577
8	$C_{23}H_{18}N_3O_3$	384.41	74.8	214 to 216	0.422
9	$C_{23}H_{18}N_3O_3$	384.41	76.2	235 to 237	0.642
11	$C_{26}H_{24}N_2O_4$	428.49	86.4	151 to 153	0.781
12	$C_{22}H_{18}N_2O_2$	342.40	80.3	298 to 300	0.524
13	$C_{24}H_{22}N_2O_3$	386.45	82.2	196 to 198	0.711

Table 2 Antipromastigote activity (IC_{50}) of the synthesized compounds

Test compounds	IC_{50} values (μg/ml)	IC_{50} values (ng/ml)
6	0.3014	301.40
7	0.0128	12.80
8	0.1085	108.50
9	2.7017	2,701.70
11	0.1086	108.60
12	1.6472	1,647.20
13	3.1085	3,108.50
Miltefosine	3.1911	3,191.10
Amphotericin B	0.0460	46.00

IC_{50}: effective concentration required to achieve 50% growth inhibition (in μg/ml).

(3*H*)-quinazolinones (**3-5**) as intermediates (Scheme 1). The details of each reactions and reaction conditions, the summarized characteristic stretching and bending IR vibration frequencies, the elemental microanalysis, and the ^1H NMR chemical shift data for each of the synthesized target compounds are given below.

General procedure for the synthesis of 2-methyl-3,1-benzoxazin-4-one (2)

A solution of anthranillic acid (**1**) (10 g, 0.073 mol) in acetic anhydride (25 ml) was heated under reflux for 1 h. The precipitate formed on cooling was filtered and the excess acetic anhydride was washed with anhydrous petroleum ether, where upon a solid mass is obtained. This solid mass (**2**), without purification, was used for subsequent reaction [47].

General procedure for the synthesis of 3-aryl-2-methyl-4(3H)-quinazolinones (3-5)

A mixture of 2-methyl-3,1-benzoxazin-4-one (**2**) (3 g, 0.017 mol) and equimolar amounts of aromatic amines (aniline, *p*-toluidine, and *o*-toluidine, respectively) was heated under reflux at 190°C for 5 h. The dark sticky mass formed were cooled and recrystallized from ethanol to yield compounds **3-5**, respectively [48].

General procedure for the synthesis of 3-aryl-2-(4-chlorostyryl)-4(3H)-quinazolinones (6 and 7)

To a solution of **3** or **4** (0.5 g each) in acetic anhydride (10 ml), an equimolar amount of *p*-chlorobenzaldehyde

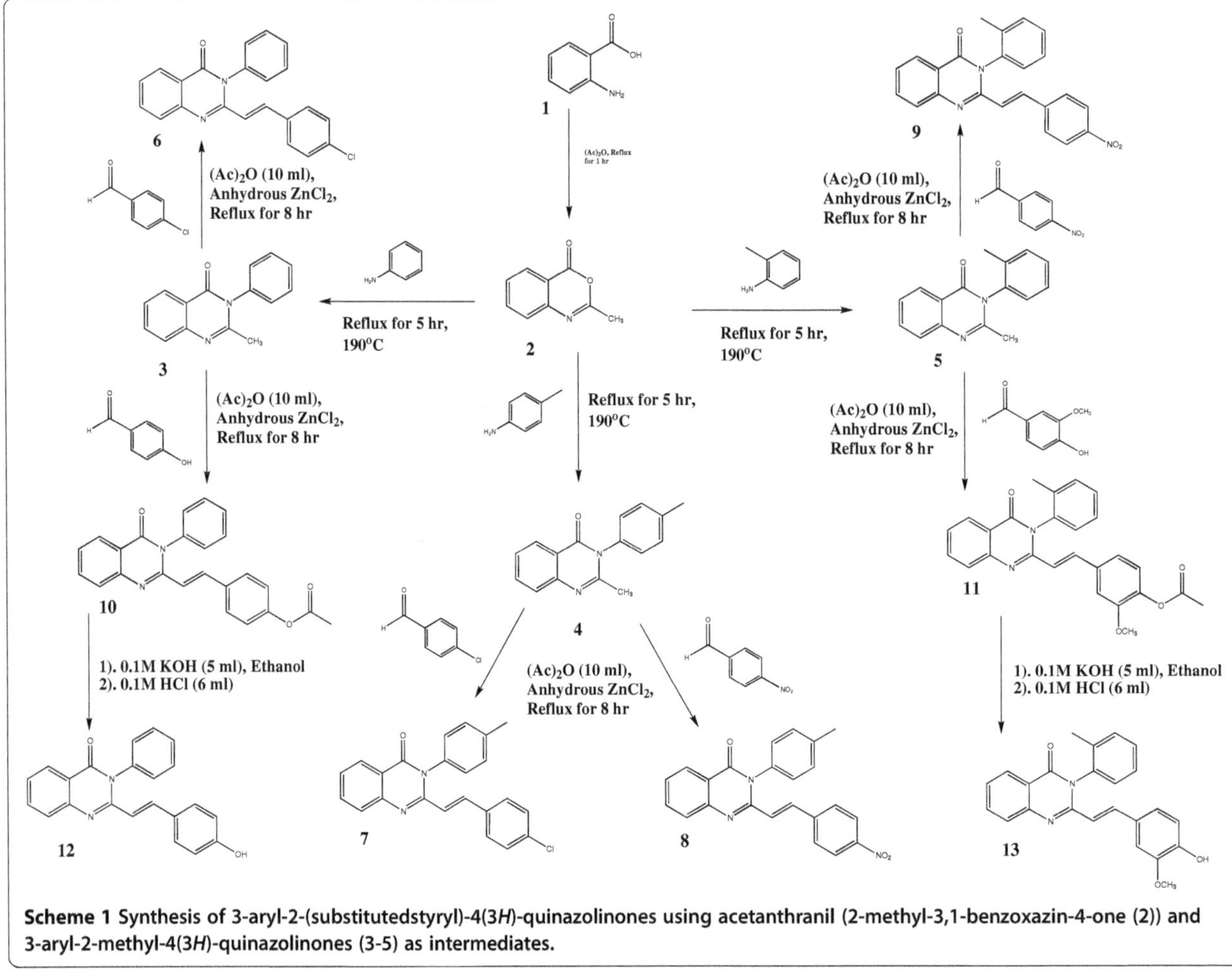

Scheme 1 Synthesis of 3-aryl-2-(substitutedstyryl)-4(3*H*)-quinazolinones using acetanthranil (2-methyl-3,1-benzoxazin-4-one (2)) and 3-aryl-2-methyl-4(3*H*)-quinazolinones (3-5) as intermediates.

was added in the presence of 10 mg of anhydrous zinc chloride as a catalyst. The reaction mixture was heated under reflux for 8 h, cooled, and poured into ice-cooled water. The solid products formed (**6** or **7**) were filtered, dried, and recrystallized from chloroform/ethanol (2:1) [49].

(E)-2-(4-chlorostyryl)-3-phenylquinazolin-4(3H)-one (6)

IR (Nujol) (cm^{-1}): 1,682 (C = O), 1,597 (C = N), and 1,224 (C-Cl). ^{1}H NMR ($CDCl_3$) δ (ppm): 6.33 (*d*, 1H, *J* = 15.49 Hz, vinyl-C_2 H), 7.23 (*d*, 2H, *J* = 8.53 Hz, 4-chlorophenyl $C_{3,5}$ H), 7.28 (*d*, 2H, *J* = 8.47 Hz, 4-chlorophenyl $C_{2,6}$ H), 7.34 (*d*, 2H, *J* = 6.82 Hz, phenyl $C_{2,6}$ H), 7.45 to 7.49 (*m*, 1H, quina-C_6 H), 7.58 to 7.63 (*m*, 3H, phenyl $C_{3,4,5}$ H), 7.75 to 7.79 (*m*, 2H, quina-$C_{7,8}$ H), 7.91 (*d*, 1H, *J* = 15.47 Hz, vinyl-C_1 H), 8.29 (*d*, 1H, *J* = 7.95 Hz, quina-C_5). Anal. calcd. for $C_{22}H_{17}ClN_2O$: C, 73.23; H, 4.75; Cl, 9.83; N, 7.76. Found: C, 73.64; H, 4.92; Cl, 10.22; N, 7.54.

(E)-2-(4-chlorostyryl)-3-p-tolylquinazolin-4(3H)-one (7)

IR (Nujol) (cm^{-1}): 1,682 (C = O), 1,597 (C = N), and 1,224 (C-Cl). ^{1}H NMR ($CDCl_3$) δ (ppm): 2.5 (*s*, 3H, *p*-tolyl CH_3), 6.42 (*d*, 1H, *J* = 15.70 Hz, vinyl-C_2 H), 7.21 (*d*, 2H, 4-chlorophenyl $C_{3,5}$ H), 7.26 to 7.32 (*m*, 4H, *p*-tolyl $C_{2,3,5,6}$ H), 7.40 (*d*, 2H, 4-chlorophenyl $C_{2,6}$ H), 7.47 to 7.51 (*m*, 1H, quina-C_6 H), 7.79 to 7.83 (*m*, 2H, quina-$C_{7,8}$ H), 7.93 (*d*, 1H, vinyl-C_1 H), 8.32 (*d*, 1H, quina-C_5 H). Anal. calcd. for $C_{23}H_{19}ClN_2O$: C, 73.69; H, 5.12; Cl, 9.46; N, 7.47. Found: C, 73.98; H, 5.38; Cl, 9.35; N, 7.21.

General procedure for the synthesis of 3-aryl-2-(4-nitrostyryl)-4(3H)-quinazolinones (8 and 9)

To a solution of **4** or **5** (0.5 g each) in acetic anhydride (10 ml), an equimolar amount of *p*-nitrobenzaldehyde was added in the presence of 10 mg of anhydrous zinc chloride as a catalyst. The reaction mixture was heated under reflux for 8 h, cooled, and poured into ice-cooled water. The solid products formed (**8** or **9**) were filtered, dried, and recrystallized from chloroform/ethanol (2:1) [49].

(E)-2-(4-nitrostyryl)-3-p-tolylquinazolin-4(3H)-one (8)

IR (Nujol) (cm^{-1}): 1,684 (C = O), 1,593 (C = N), 1,556 and 1,377 (NO_2). ^{1}H NMR ($CDCl_3$) δ (ppm): 2.5 (*s*, 3H, *p*-tolyl CH_3), 6.56 (*d*, 1H, *J* = 15.52 Hz, vinyl-C_2 H), 7.21 (*d*, 2H, *J* = 8.19 Hz, *p*-tolyl $C_{3,5}$ H), 7.41 (*d*, 2H, *J* = 7.97 Hz, *p*-tolyl $C_{2,6}$ H), 7.46 to 7.53 (*m*, 3H, 4-nitrophenyl $C_{2,6}$ and quina-C_6), 7.77 to 7.81 (*m*, 2H, quina-$C_{7,8}$), 8.00 (*d*, 1H, *J* = 15.52 Hz, vinyl-C_1), 8.19 (*d*, 2H, *J* = 8.74 Hz, 4-nitrophenyl $C_{3,5}$), 8.30 (*d*, 1H, *J* = 8.01 Hz, quina-C_5). Anal. calcd. for $C_{23}H_{18}N_3O_3$: C, 71.86; H, 4.72; N, 10.93. Found: C, 72.12; H, 4.35; N, 11.10.

(E)-2-(4-nitrostyryl)-3-o-tolylquinazolin-4(3H)-one (9)

IR (Nujol) (cm^{-1}): 1,682 (C = O), 1,593 (C = N), 1,556 and 1,377 (NO_2). ^{1}H NMR ($CDCl_3$) δ (ppm): 2.17 (*s*, 3H, *o*-tolyl CH_3), 6.47 (*d*, 1H, *J* = 15.66 Hz, vinyl-C_2 H), 7.25 (*d*, 1H, *J* = 7.91 Hz, *o*-tolyl C_3 H), 7.44 to 7.46 (*m*, 3H, 4-nitrophenyl $C_{2,6}$ and *o*-tolyl C_6 H), 7.47 to 7.58 (*m*, 3H, *o*-tolyl $C_{4,5}$ and quina-C_6 H), 7.82 to 7.89 (*m*, 2H, quina-$C_{7,8}$ H), 8.05 (*d*, 1H, *J* = 15.56 Hz, vinyl-C_1 H), 8.19 (*d*, 2H, *J* = 8.73 Hz, 4-nitrophenyl $C_{4,6}$ H), 8.36 (*d*, 1H, *J* = 8.25 Hz, quina-C_5 H). Anal. calcd. for $C_{23}H_{18}N_3O_3$: C, 71.86; H, 4.72; N, 10.93. Found: C, 71.68; H, 4.93; N, 11.24.

General procedure for the synthesis of 3-aryl-2-(4-acetylatedstyryl)-4(3H)-quinazolinones (10)

To a solution of **3** (0.5 g) in acetic anhydride (10 ml), an equimolar amount of *p*-hydroxybenzaldehyde was added. Anhydrous zinc chloride (10 mg) is added as a catalyst. The reaction mixture is heated under reflux for 8 h, cooled, and poured into ice-cooled water. The solid product formed (**10**) was filtered, dried, and recrystallized from ethanol [49].

General procedure for the synthesis of 3-aryl-2-(4-acetylatedstyryl)-4(3H)-quinazolinones (11)

To a solution of **5** (0.5 g) in acetic anhydride (10 ml), an equimolar amount of vanillin was added. Anhydrous zinc chloride (10 mg) is added as a catalyst. The reaction mixture is heated under reflux for 8 h, cooled, and poured into ice-cooled water. The solid product (**11**) was filtered, dried, and recrystallized from ethanol [49].

4-{(1E)-2-[-3,4-dihydro-3-(2-methylphenyl)-4-oxoquinazoline-2-yl)]vinyl}-2-methoxyphenyl acetate (11)

IR (Nujol) (cm^{-1}): 1,761 (C = O), 1,682 (C = O), 1,634 (C = N), 1,260 and 1,149 (C-O-C). ^{1}H NMR ($CDCl_3$) δ (ppm): 2.15 (*s*, 3H, phenylacetate CH_3), 2.33 (*s*, 3H, *o*-tolyl CH_3), 3.80 (*s*, 3H, methoxy -O-CH_3), 6.27 (*d*, 1H, *J* = 15.44 Hz, vinyl-C_2 H), 6.88 to 6.93 (*m*, 2H, 2-methoxyphenyl $C_{3,5}$ H), 6.98 (*d*, 1H, *J* = 8.12 Hz, 2-methoxyphenyl C_6 H), 7.24 (*d*, 1H, *J* = 7.52 Hz, *o*-tolyl C_3 H), 7.42 to 7.53 (*m*, 4H, *o*-tolyl $C_{4,5,6}$ H and quina-C_6 H), 7.82 to 7.83 (*m*, 2H, quina-$C_{7,8}$ H), 7.96 (*d*, 1H, *J* = 15.48 Hz, vinyl-C_1 H), 8.34 (*d*, 1H, *J* = 7.88 Hz, quina-C_5 H). Anal. calcd. for $C_{26}H_{24}N_2O_4$: C, 72.88; H, 5.65; N, 6.54. Found: C, 73.11; H, 5.89; N, 6.42.

General procedure for the synthesis of 3-aryl-2-(4-deacetylatedstyryl)-4(3H)-quinazolinones (12 and 13)

Subsequent treatment of **10** and **11** with 0.1 M alcoholic KOH (5 ml) in the presence of ethanol followed by 0.1 M HCl (6 ml) gave the corresponding 4-hydroxyl containing compounds **12** and **13** after recrystallization from ethanol [49].

(E)-2-(4-hydroxystyryl)-3-phenylquinazolin-4(3H)-one (12)

IR (Nujol) (cm^{-1}): 3,290 (OH), 1,652 (C = O), and 1,604 (C = N). ^{1}H NMR (acetone-d_6) δ (ppm): 6.24 (*d*, 1H, *J* = 15.39 Hz, vinyl-C_2 H), 6.80 (*d*, 2H, *J* = 8.64 Hz, 4-

hydroxyphenyl $C_{3,5}$ H), 7.24 (*d*, 2H, *J* = 8.62 Hz, 4-hydroxyphenyl $C_{2,6}$ H), 7.46 to 7.50 (*m*, 3H, phenyl $C_{3,4,5}$ H), 7.60 to 7.66 (*m*, 3H, quina-C_6, phenyl $C_{2,6}$ H), 7.73 (*d*, 1H, *J* = 8.07 Hz, quina-C_8 H), 7.81 to 7.85 (*m*, 1H, quina-C_7 H), 7.92 (*d*, 1H, *J* = 15.43 Hz, vinyl-C_1 H), 8.02 (*s*, 1H, 4-hydroxyphenyl -OH), 8.17 (*d*, 1H, *J* = 9.18 Hz, quina-C_5 H). Anal. calcd. for $C_{22}H_{18}N_2O_2$: C, 7.17; H, 5.23; N, 8.18. Found: C, 76.86; H, 5.02; N, 8.38.

(E)-2-(4-hydroxy-3-methoxystyryl)-3-o-tolylquinazolin-4(3H)-one (13)

IR (Nujol) (cm^{-1}): 3,400 (OH), 1,683 (C = O), 1,634 (C = N), 1,211 and 1,148 (C-O-C). ^1H NMR ($CDCl_3$) δ (ppm): 2.15 (*s*, 3H, *o*-tolyl CH_3), 3.80 (*s*, 3H, 4-hydroxy-2-methoxyphenyl -O-CH_3), 6.10 (*s*, 1H, 4-hydroxy-2-methoxyphenyl -OH), 6.27 (*d*, 1H, *J* = 15.44 Hz, vinyl-C_2 H), 6.88 to 6.93 (*m*, 2H, 4-hydroxy-2-methoxyphenyl $C_{3,5}$ H), 6.98 (*d*, 1H, *J* = 8.12 Hz, 4-hydroxy-2-methoxyphenyl C_6 H), 7.24 (*d*, 1H, *J* = 7.52 Hz, *o*-tolyl C_3 H), 7.42 to 7.53 (*m*, 4H, *o*-tolyl $C_{4,5,6}$ H and quina-C_6 H), 7.82 (*m*, 2H, quina-$C_{7,8}$ H), 7.96 (*d*, 1H, *J* = 15.48 Hz, vinyl-C_1 H), 8.34 (*d*, 1H, *J* = 7.884 Hz, quina-C_5 H). Anal. calcd. for $C_{24}H_{22}N_2O_3$: C, 74.59; H, 5.74; N, 7.23. Found: C, 74.28; H, 5.96; N, 7.56.

Conclusions

Some 3-aryl-2-(substitutedstyryl)-4(3*H*)-quinazolinone derivatives were synthesized and tested for their antileishamanial activities. Most of the synthesized compounds displayed better antileishmanial activities as compared to the standard drug miltefosine and lower antileishmanial activity as compared to amphotericin B deoxycholate except (*E*)-2-(4-chlorostyryl)-3-*p*-tolyl-4(3*H*)-quinazolinone (7). Compound 7 showed pronounced antileishmanial activities as compared to miltefosine and amphotericin B deoxycholate. Thus, 2,3-disubstituted-4(3*H*)-quinazolinones containing an aromatic substitution at 3-position and substituted styryl moiety at 2-position represent a promising matrix for the development of antileishmanial agents.

Competing interests

The authors declare that they have no competing interests.

Acknowledgements

The authors are thankful to Prof. Wondimagegn Mammo for his considerable support in running and interpreting the ^1H NMR data. The following were acknowledged: The Department of Pharmaceutical Chemistry, Faculty of Pharmacy, Alexandria University for performing the elemental microanalysis and providing some chemicals, Debre Markos University for granting study leave to Mr. Yihenew, and Addis Ababa University for financially supporting this research work.

Author details

[1]Department of Chemistry, Natural and Computational Science College, Debre Markos University, Debre Markos, Ethiopia. [2]Department of Pharmaceutical Chemistry, Alexandria University, Alexandria 21215, Egypt. [3]Department of Pharmaceutical Chemistry and Pharmacognosy, School of Pharmacy, Addis Ababa University, Addis Ababa, Ethiopia.

References

1. Renslo AR, McKerrow JH (2006) Drug discovery and development for neglected parasitic diseases. Nat Chem Biol 2:701–710
2. McConville MJ, Souza D, Saunders E, Likic VA, Thomas N (2007) Living in a phagolysosome; metabolism of *Leishmania* amastigotes. Trends Parasitol 23:368–375
3. Sharma U, Singh S (2008) Insect vectors of *Leishmania*: distribution, physiology and their control. J Vector Borne Dis 45:255–272
4. Manandhar KD, Yadav TP, Prajapati VK, Kumar S, Rai M, Dube A, Srivastava ON, Sundar S (2008) Antileishmanial activity of nano-amphotericin B deoxycholate. J Antimicrob Chemother 62:376–380
5. Nascimento ET, Moura MLN, Queiroz JW, Barroso AW, Araujo AF, Rego EF, Wilson ME, Pearson RD, Jeronimo SM (2011) The emergence of concurrent HIV-1/AIDS and visceral leishmaniasis in Northeast Brazil. Trans R Soc Trop Med Hyg 105:298–300
6. Cenderello G, Pasa A, Dusi A, Dentone C, Toscanini F, Bobbio N, Bondi E, Bono VD, Izzo M, Riccio G, Anselmo M, Giacchino R, Marazzi MG, Pagano G, Cassola G, Viscoli C, Ferrea G, De Maria A (2013) Varied spectrum of clinical presentation and mortality in a prospective registry of visceral leishmaniasis in a low endemicity area of Northern Italy. BMC Infect Dis 13:248
7. Herremans T, Pinelli E, Casparie M, Nozari N, Roelfsema J, Kortbeek L (2010) Increase of imported leishmaniasis in the Netherlands: a twelve-year overview (1996-2007). Int Health 2:42–46
8. Ignatius R, Loddenkemper C, Woitzik J, Schneider T, Harms G (2011) Localized leishmanial lymphadenopathy: an unusual manifestation of leishmaniasis in a traveler in southern Europe. Vector-Borne Zoonotic Dis 11(8):1213–1215
9. Bray DP, Hamilton JGC (2013) Insecticide-impregnated netting as a potential tool for long-lasting control of the leishmaniasis vector *Lutzomyia longipalpis* in animal shelters. Parasites Vectors 6:133
10. Mascari TM, Stout RW, Foil LD (2012) Laboratory evaluation of oral treatment of rodents with systemic insecticides for control of blood feeding sand flies (Diptera: Psychodidae). Vector-Borne Zoonotic Dis 12(8):699–704
11. Chaves LF, Calzada JE, Rigg C, Valderrama A, Gottdenker NL, Saldaña A (2013) Leishmaniasis sand fly vector density reduction is less marked in destitute housing after insecticide thermal fogging. Parasites Vectors 6:164
12. Thakur CP, Kumar K (1992) Post kala-azar dermal leishmaniasis: a neglected aspect of kala-azar control programmes. Ann Trop Med Parasitol 86:355–359
13. Topuzogullari M, Koc RC, Isoglu SD, Bagirova M, Akdeste Z, Elcicek S, Oztel ON, Baydar SY, Ates SC, Allahverdiyev AM (2013) Conjugation, characterization and toxicity of lipophosphoglycan-polyacrylic acid conjugate for vaccination against leishmaniasis. J Biomed Sci 20:35
14. Kaur J, Kaur T, Kaur S (2011) Studies on the protective efficacy and immunogenicity of Hsp70 and Hsp83 based vaccine formulations in *Leishmania donovani* infected BALB/c mice. Acta Trop 119:50–56
15. Abdian N, Gholami E, Zahedifard F, Safaee N, Rafati S (2011) Evaluation of DNA/DNA and prime-boost vaccination using LPG3 against *Leishmania major* infection in susceptible BALB/c mice and its antigenic properties in human leishmaniasis. Experimental Parasitol 127:627–636
16. Salazara MBM, Domíngueza JD, Estradaa JS, Bonillab CG, Becker I (2014) Vaccination with *Leishmania mexicana* LPG induces PD-1 in CD8+ and PD-L2 in macrophages thereby suppressing the immune response: a model to assess vaccine efficacy. Vaccine 32:1259–1265
17. Carrión J, Folgueira C, Soto M, Fresno M, Requena JM (2011) *Leishmania infantum* HSP70-II null mutant as candidate vaccine against leishmaniasis: a preliminary evaluation. Parasites Vectors 4:150
18. Ait-Oudhia K, Gazanion E, Oury B, Vergnes B, Sereno D (2011) The fitness of antimony-resistant *Leishmania* parasites: lessons from the field. Trends Parasitol 27:141–142
19. Adam GK, Abdulla MA, Ahmed AA, Adam I (2009) Maternal and perinatal outcomes of visceral leishmaniasis (kala-azar) treated with sodium stibogluconate in eastern Sudan. Int J Gynecol Obstet 107:208–210
20. Dorlo TPC, Kager PA (2010) Comment on: cutaneous and mucocutaneous leishmaniasis in Tigray, northern Ethiopia: clinical aspects and therapeutic concerns. Trans R Soc Trop Med Hyg 104:84–85
21. Bray PG, Barrett MP, Ward SA, Koning HP (2003) Pentamidine uptake and resistance in pathogenic protozoa: past, present and future. Trends Parasitol 19:232–239

22. Ben Salah A, Buffet PA, Morizot G, Ben Massoud N, Zaatour A, Ben Alaya N, Hamida NBH, El Ahmadi Z, Downs MT, Smith PL, Dellagi K, Grogl M (2009) WR279,396, a third generation aminoglycoside ointment for the treatment of *Leishmania major* cutaneous leishmaniasis: a phase 2, randomized, double blind, placebo-controlled study. PLoS Negl Trop Dis 3:e432
23. Sundar S, Sinha PK, Rai M, Verma DK, Nawin K, Alam S, Chakravarty J, Vaillant M, Verma N, Pandey K, Kumari P, Lal CS, Arora R, Sharma B, Ellis S, Strub-Wourgaft N, Balasegaram M, Olliaro P, Das P, Modabber F (2011) Comparison of short-course multidrug treatment with standard therapy for visceral leishmaniasis in India: an open-label, non-inferiority, randomised controlled trial. Lancet 377:477–486
24. Melaku Y, Collin SM, Keus K, Gatluak F, Ritmeijer K, Davidson RN (2007) Treatment of kala-azar in southern Sudan using a 17-day regimen of sodium stibogluconate combined with paromomycin: a retrospective comparison with 30-day sodium stibogluconate monotherapy. Am J Trop Med Hyg 77:89–94
25. Adib M, Ansari S, Mohammadi A, Bijanzadeh HR (2010) A novel, one-pot, solvent and catalyst-free synthesis of 2-aryl/alkyl-4(3*H*)-quinazolinones. Tetrahedron Lett 51:30–32
26. Kumar M, Sharma K, Sharma DK (2012) Diversity oriented one-pot three-component sequential synthesis of annulated benzothiazoloquinazolines. Org Med Chem Lett 2:10
27. Nouira I, Kostakis IK, Dubouilh C, Chosson E, Iannelli M, Besson T (2008) Decomposition of formamide assisted by microwaves, a tool for synthesis of nitrogen-containing heterocycles. Tetrahedron Lett 49:7033–7036
28. Ye C, You J, Li XF, You R, Weng Y, Li J, Wang Y (2010) Design, synthesis and anticoccidial activity of a series of 3-(2-(2-methoxyphenyl)-2-oxoethyl) quinazolinone derivatives. Pestic Biochem Physiol 97:194–198
29. Omar MA, Conrad J, Beifuss U (2014) Copper-catalyzed domino reaction between 1-(2-halophenyl)methanamines and amidines or imidates for the synthesis of 2-substituted quinazolinones. Tetrahedron 70:3061–3072
30. Safaei HR, Shekouhy M, Shafiee V, Davoodi M (2013) Glycerol based ionic liquid with a borone core: a new highly efficient and reusable promoting medium for the synthesis of quinazolinones. J Mol Liq 180:139–144
31. Fischer C, Shah S, Hughes BL, Nikov GN, Crispino JL, Middleton RE, Szewczak AA, Munoz B, Shearman MS (2011) Quinazolinones as γ-secretase modulators. Bioorg Med Chem Lett 21:773–776
32. Manivannan E, Chaturvedi SC (2011) Analogue-based design, synthesis and molecular docking analysis of 2,3-diarylquinazolinones as non-ulcerogenic anti-inflammatory agents. Bioorg Med Chem 19:4520–4528
33. Rhee H-K, Yoo JH, Lee E, Kwon YJ, Seo H-R, Lee Y-S, Choo H-YP (2011) Synthesis and cytotoxicity of 2-phenylquinazolin-4(3*H*)-one derivatives. Eur J Med Chem 46:3900–3909
34. Jagani CL, Sojitra NA, Vanparia SF, Patel TS, Dixit RB, Dixit BC Microwave promoted synthesis and antimicrobial activity of 3-thiazole substituted 2-styryl-4(3H)-quinazolinone derivatives. J Saudi Chem Soc doi:10.1016/j.jscs.2011.02.001
35. Shivananda MK, Holla BS (2011) Antifungal activity studies of some quinazolinone derivatives. J Chem Pharm Res 3:83–86
36. Špulák M, Pourová J, Vopršálová M, Mikušek J, Kuneš J, Vacek J, Ghavre M, Gathergood N, Pour M (2014) Novel bronchodilatory quinazolines and quinoxalines: synthesis and biological evaluation. Eur J Med Chem 74:65–72
37. Berman JD, King M, Edwards N (1989) Antileishmanial activities of 2,4-diaminoquinazoline putative dihydrofolate reductase inhibitors. Antimicrobial Agents Chemother 33:1860–1863
38. Bhattacharjee AK, Skanchy DJ, Jennings B, Hudson TH, Brendle JJ, Werbovetz KA (2002) Analysis of stereoelectronic properties, mechanism of action and pharmacophore of synthetic indolo [2,1-*b*]quinazoline-6,12-dione derivatives in relation to antileishmanial activity using quantum chemical, cyclic voltammetry and 3-D-QSAR catalyst procedures. Bioorg Med Chem 10:1979–1989
39. Arfan M, Khan R, Khan MA, Anjum S, Choudhary MI, Ahmad M (2010) Synthesis and antileishmanial and antimicrobial activities of some 2,3-disubstituted 3*H*-quinazolin-4-ones. J Enzyme Inhib Med Chem 25:451–558
40. Fleita DH, Mohareb RM, Sakka OK (2013) Antitumor and antileishmanial evaluation of novel heterocycles derived from quinazoline scaffold: a molecular modeling approach. Med Chem Res 22:2207–2221
41. Lara O, Raquel E, María A, Juan J, Francisco B, José M (2007) In vitro effect of new formulations of amphotericin B on amastigote and promastigote forms of *Leishmania infantum*. Int J Antimicrob Agents 30:325–329
42. Tariku Y, Hymete A, Hailu A, Rohloff J (2010) Essential-oil composition, antileishmanial and toxicity study of *Artemisia abyssinica* and *Satureja punctata ssp. punctata* from Ethiopia. Chem Biodivers 7:1013–1016
43. Lorke D (1983) A new approach to practical acute toxicity test. Arch Toxicol 54:275–286
44. Nakayama GR, Caton MC, Nova MP, Parandoosh Z (1997) Assessment of the Alamar Blue assay for cellular growth and viability *in vitro*. J Immunol Methods 204:205–208
45. Al-Nasiry S, Geusens N, Hanssens M, Luyten C, Pijnenborg R (2007) The use of Alamar Blue assay for quantitative analysis of viability, migration and invasion of choriocarcinoma cells. Hum Reprod 25:1–6
46. Shimony O, Jaffe CL (2006) Rapid fluorescent assay for screening drugs on *Leishmania* amastigotes. J Microbiol Methods 75:196–200
47. Kumar A, Sharma S, Bajaj K, Sharma S, Panwar H, Singh T, Srivastava VK (2003) Some new 2,3,6-trisubstituted quinazolinones as potent anti-inflammatory, analgesic and COX-II inhibitors. Bioorg Med Chem 11:5293–5299
48. Errede LA (1976) Acylanthranils 1. The pathway of quinazolone formation in the reaction of acylanthranils with anilines. J Org Chem 41:1763–1765
49. Raffa D, Edler MC, Daidone G, Maggio B, Merickech M, Plescia S, Schillaci D, Bai R, Hamel E (2004) Synthesis, cytotoxicity, and inhibitory effects on tubulin polymerization of a new 3-heterocyclo substituted 2-styrylquinazolinones. Eur J Med Chem 39:299–304

16

Synthesis and evaluation of substituted diphenyl-1,3,4-oxadiazole derivatives for central nervous system depressant activity

Poonam Singh[1*], Pramod Kumar Sharma[1], Jitendra Kumar Sharma[2], Anshu Upadhyay[1] and Nitin Kumar[1]

Abstract

Background: Substituted 1,3,4-oxadiazoles are of considerable pharmaceutical interest. 2,5-Substituted diphenyl-1,3,4-oxadiazoles are associated with diverse biological activities by the virtue of -N = C-O- grouping. In the view of wide range of biological properties associated with 1,3,4-oxadiazole, we have synthesized substituted derivatives of 1,3,4-oxadiazole (**XIII-XXII**), a versatile hydrophobic molecule possessing preliminary CNS properties, with the hope to potentiate the biological activities with lesser or limited amount of toxicities.

Method: The synthesis was based on ester substitution of substituted benzohydrazide in presence of hydrazine hydrate followed by cyclization in presence of phosphorus oxychloride. All the synthesized compounds were evaluated for their potential CNS depressant activities. Statistical analysis of the anticonvulsant, antidepressant, and antianxiety activity of the synthesized compounds on animals was evaluated using one-way analysis of variance (ANOVA).

Results: Two compounds 5-(4-nitrophenyl)-2-(4-chlorophenyl)-1,3,4-oxadiazole (**XIV**) and 5-(4-nitrophenyl)-2-(4-nitrophenyl)-1,3,4-oxadiazole (**XV**) were found to be the most promising compounds of the series in antidepressant, anticonvulsant and antianxiety activity with no neurotoxicity when compared with standard.

Conclusions: Among the synthesized compounds, it was found that incorporation of electron withdrawing group at C2 and C5 position of the oxadiazole ring led to high degree of pharmacological activity. Thus compounds 5-(4-nitrophenyl)-2-(4-chlorophenyl)-1,3,4-oxadiazole **(XIV)** and 5-(4-nitrophenyl)-2-(4-nitrophenyl)-1,3,4-oxadiazole **(XV)** showed excellent CNS depressant activities. The result of the present investigation may encourage us to develop and/or improve similar other related compounds and it may be assumed that further modifications may produce compounds of better activity with lesser side effects.

Background

Epilepsy is one of the most common neurological disorders responsible for substantial morbidity and mortality. It is a chronic neurological disorder characterized by paroxysmal, excessive, and hyper-synchronous neuronal activity in the brain affecting around 1-2% of the world population [1,2]. 75-80% of the epileptic patients may be provided with adequate seizure control with the help of conventional antiepileptic drugs. Despite the development of several new anticonvulsants, the treatments of epilepsy still remain inadequate. However, over 30% of people with epilepsy do not have seizure control even with the best available medications [3].

Most people with epilepsy have a normal emotional and cognitive life, however neurobehavioral problems can be found in a large number of patients. Higher rates of psychopathology have been reported in people with epilepsy compared with the general population and in people with chronic non-neurological disorders [4]. Depression and anxiety are the most frequent types of psychiatric disorders identified in patients with epilepsy [5]. There are numerous studies reporting that the severity of anxiety and depression in epileptic patients is higher than normal controls [6-8].

* Correspondence: poonamsingh048@gmail.com
[1]Department of Pharmaceutical Technology, Meerut Institute of Engineering & Technology, NH-58, Baghpat By-pass Crossing, Delhi-Haridwar Highway, Meerut-250005, India
Full list of author information is available at the end of the article

The comorbidity of major depressive disorder or anxiety is associated with medical, psychiatric, and social problems. A bidirectional relationship between epilepsy and depression is supposed to exist and studies suggested that depression and epilepsy may share common pathogenic mechanisms and the occurrence of one may facilitate the development of the other and vice versa [9,10]. Multiple factors are implicated in the development of depression in epilepsy including clinical (seizure frequency, seizure type or foci, epilepsy duration, age at onset, antiepileptic drugs) and psychosocial ones (life stressors, employment, marital status, quality of life) [11]. Here we have selected an *in-vivo* efficacy approach using maximal electroshock seizure (MES) model, spontaneous motor activity using actophotometer and elevated plus maze model. Benzodiazepines (BZDs) are the most frequently prescribed synthetic drugs for variety of conditions particularly anxiety, depression, epilepsy, and insomnia. But these psychoneural drugs have many side effects including addictive potential and frequent development of tolerance. BZDs have limited utility for long-term treatment. Therefore our strategy was to find drugs which are effective in all these models and are better tolerated than the BZDs and other conventional drugs.

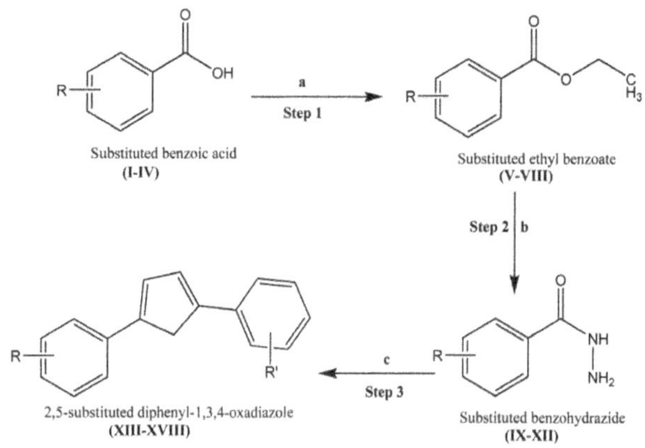

Scheme 1 (a) Conc. H2SO4, Ethanol, Reflux 4hr; (b) Hydrazine Hydrate, Ethanol, Reflux 8 hr; (c) Substituted benzoic acid (R=p-OH, p-NH2, p-Cl, p-NO2, o-Br), Phosphorous Oxychloride, Reflux 2-3 hr.

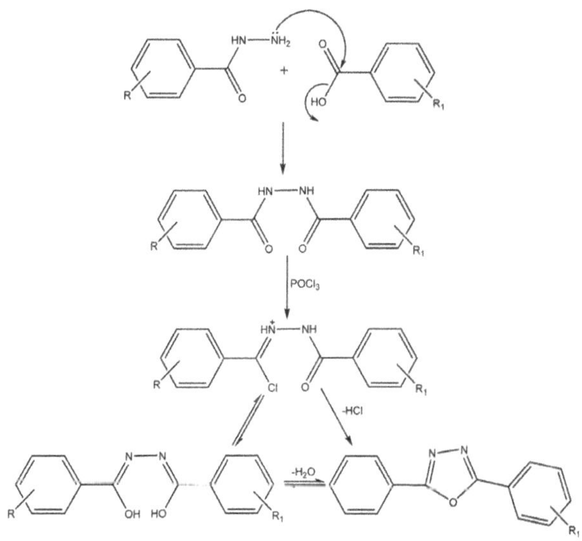

Scheme 2 Proposed mechanism for the cyclization of substituted benzohydrazide 2,5-substituted diphenyl-1,3,4-oxadiazole derivatives.

Results and discussion

Chemistry

Although various methods have been reported for the synthesis of oxadiazole derivatives [12] but these methods requires high reaction temperature, long reaction, time and expensive reagents. In present described experimental conditions the heterocyclization reaction reached completion with a relative simple operation giving high yield (65-95%) at shorter time (1.5-3.0 h) compared to the other reported cyclization methods for 1,3,4-oxadiazole ring. The synthetic route of the designed 1,3,4-oxadiazole derivatives 2,5-substituted diphenyl-1,3,4-oxadiazole (**XIII-XXII**) was outlined in Scheme 1. The possible mechanism of the final step involved in formation of target compounds was shown in Scheme 2. The presence of electron donating groups (-NH2, -OH) decreases the yield of the final compound (50-75%) with low reaction time (1.5-2.0 h) whereas the presence of electron withdrawing groups (-NO2, -Cl, -Br) increases the yield of the final compound thereby increasing the reaction time (2.5-3.0 h). The structures of the compounds were assigned on the basis of elemental analysis, IR, ^{1}H NMR, and mass spectra. The structures of newly synthesized compounds were confirmed by spectral and analytical data.

In general, the IR spectra of synthesized compounds showed a C = N stretching band around 1533-1684 cm^{-1}, C = O absorption band at around 1010-1091 cm^{-1}, and C-O-C absorption band at around 1239-1282 cm^{-1} indicating formation of the 1,3,4-oxadiazole ring. In ^{1}H NMR spectra, the signals of respective protons of newly synthesized compounds showed the peaks for -NH, -OH, and Ar-H near δ 3.8-4.9, 4.3-5.6, and 6.52-8.61, respectively. Further evidence for the formation of 2,5-substituted diphenyl-1,3,4-oxadiazole was obtained by recording the mass spectra. The general mass fragmentation pattern for the compound XIII showed the molecular ion peak at 272.69 which is in conformity with the molecular formula C14H9ClN2O2 (Scheme 3). Both analytical and spectral data (IR, ^{1}H NMR, and mass) of all the synthesized compounds were in full agreement with the proposed structures.

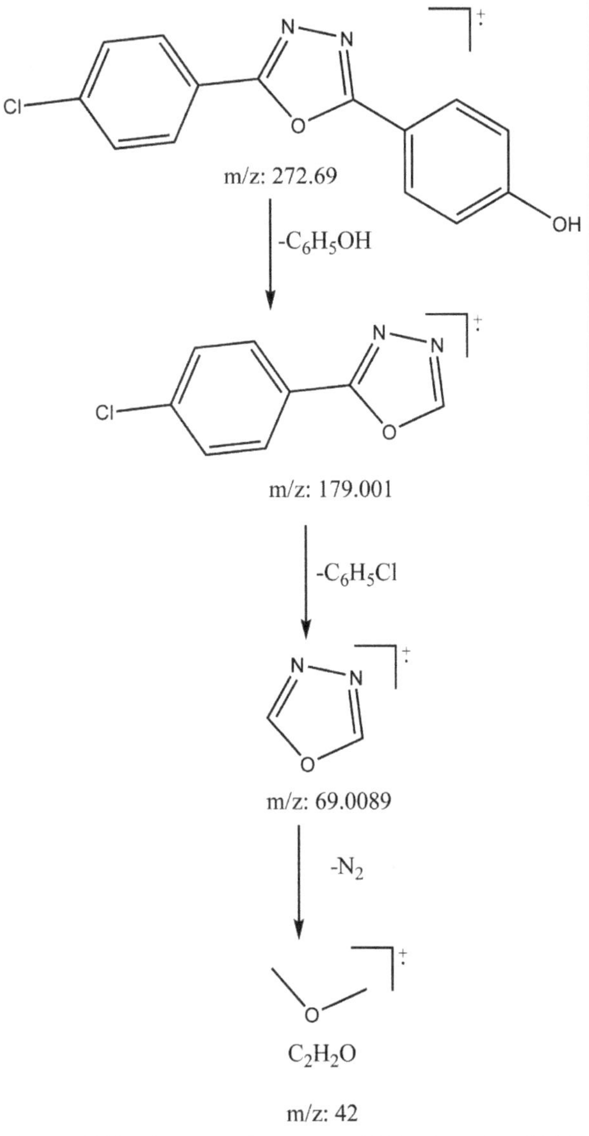

Scheme 3 Mass Fragmentation pattern of 5-(4-hydroxyphenyl)-2-(4-chlorophenyl)-1,3,4-oxadiazole (XIII).

Pharmacology

Among the compounds synthesized (**XIII-XXII**), few compounds were selected (**XIII-XVII**) and evaluated for CNS depressant activities such as antidepressant, anticonvulsant, antianxiety, and neurotoxicity activity. The pharmacological data indicated that among all the compounds being screened, compounds **XIV** and **XV** showed highly significant anticonvulsant activity (***$p \leq$ 0.001) and compound **XVI** showed less significant activity when compared to the standard (Table 1 and Figure 1). The % potency showing the mean convulsive threshold of the synthesized compounds was shown in Figure 2. In antidepressant screening, compounds **XIV**, **XV**, and **XVII** decreased the locomotor activity significantly (***$p \leq 0.001$) whereas, compounds **XVI** (**$p \leq 0.01$) and **XIII** (*$p \leq 0.05$) did not showed a significant reduction in the locomotor activity when compared to standard fluoxetine (Table 2 and Figure 3). In antianxiety screening, the number of entries and the mean time spent in open arm has been shown in (Table 3, Figures 4 and 5) and compounds, **XIII** and **XV** significantly increases the time spent in open arm thus showing higher activity when compared to the standard diazepam. Whereas another remarkable point is that compound having nitro group (electron withdrawing groups) at both position 2 and 5 of the 1,3,4-oxadiazole ring, i.e., 5-(4-nitrophenyl)-2-(4-nitrophenyl)-1,3,4-oxadiazole (**XV**) exhibited greater anticonvulsant, antidepressant, and antianxiety activity as compared to the other compounds of the series. Whereas compound 5-(4-nitrophenyl)-2-(4-chlorophenyl)-1,3,4-oxadiazole (**XIV**) showed highly significant anticonvulsant and antidepressant activity but less significant antianxiety activity. In the neurotoxicity screen, all the compounds being screened passed the neurotoxicity testing, i.e., not showing neurological deficit (Table 4). From the overall result it is evident that compound **XIV** and **XV** could be identified as the most biologically active member within this study with good anticonvulsant, antidepressant, and antianxiety activity.

Conclusions

This preliminary investigation showed the cyclization of -NH-NH2 group of benzohydrazide in presence of carboxylic group of benzoic acid into 1,3,4-oxadiazole with the objective to develop molecules with excellent yield and less reaction time. Addition of -NH2, -OH group as substituents enhances the yield of the prepared

Table 1 Anticonvulsant activity of synthesized compounds

Number	Compound	Dose (mg kg^{-1})	Hind limb extensor (mean ± S.E.M)	Hind limb convulsion (mean ± S.E.M)	% Potency
1.	Control	30	27.50 ± 0.42	6.5 ± 0.47	-
2.	Standard	30	15.25 ± 0.17	6.25 ± 0.30	-
3.	XIII	30	11.50 ± 0.15**	8.16 ± 0.30	130.672
4.	XIV	30	17.33 ± 0.33***	24.33 ± 0.42**	389.28
5.	XV	30	16.83 ± 0.20*	25.83 ± 0.54***	413.28
6.	XVI	30	15.83 ± 0.27*	10.83 ± 0.30***	173.28
7.	XVII	30	11.00 ± 0.30	7.33 ± 0.33	117.32

Values are mean ± SEM of six animals in each group. Statistical significance versus standard (***$p \leq 0.001$, **$p \leq 0.01$, *$p \leq 0.05$)

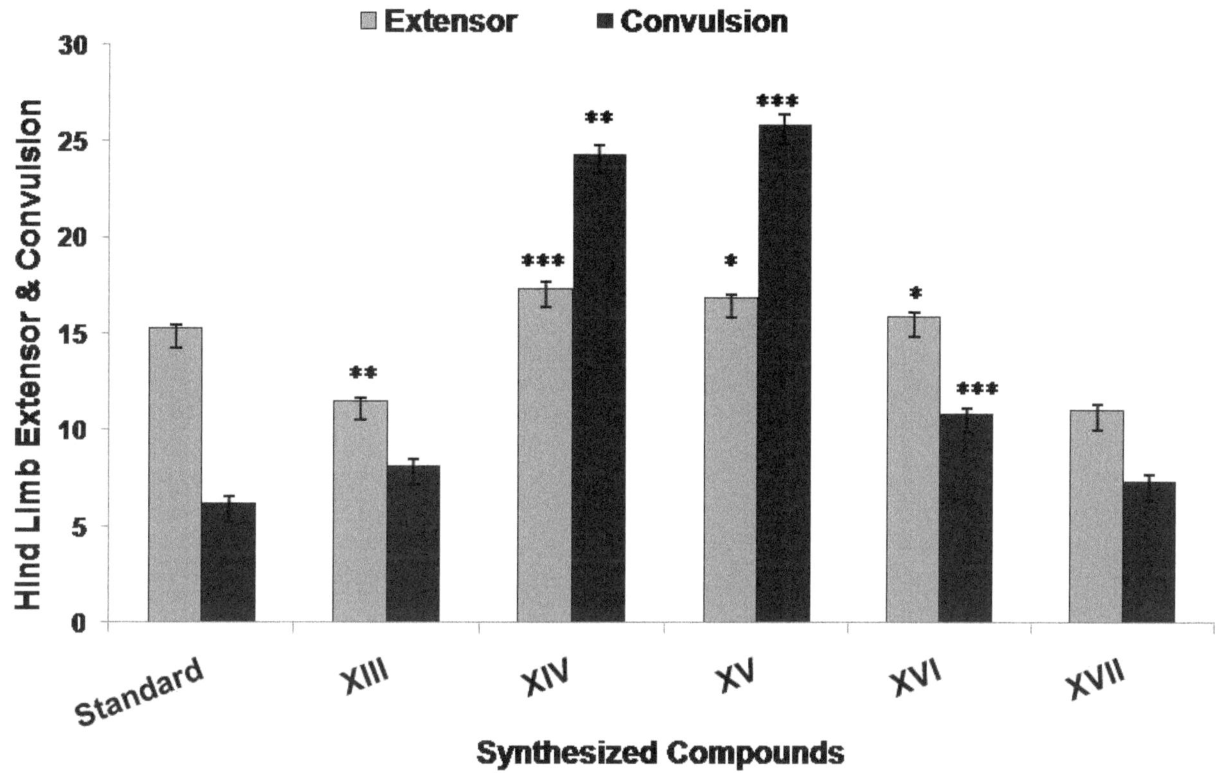

Figure 1 **Anticonvulsant activity of synthesized compounds at the dose (30 mg kg^{-1}, p.o.) in female albino mice for single administration**.

compounds. Among the synthesized compounds, those with electron withdrawing substituents: 5-(4-nitrophenyl)-2-(4-chlorophenyl)-1,3,4-oxadiazole **(XIV)** and 5-(4-nitrophenyl)-2-(4-nitrophenyl)-1,3,4-oxadiazole (**XV**) showed excellent anticonvulsant activity, antidepressant, and antianxiety activity with no neurotoxicity. The result of the present investigation may encourage us to develop and/or improve similar other related

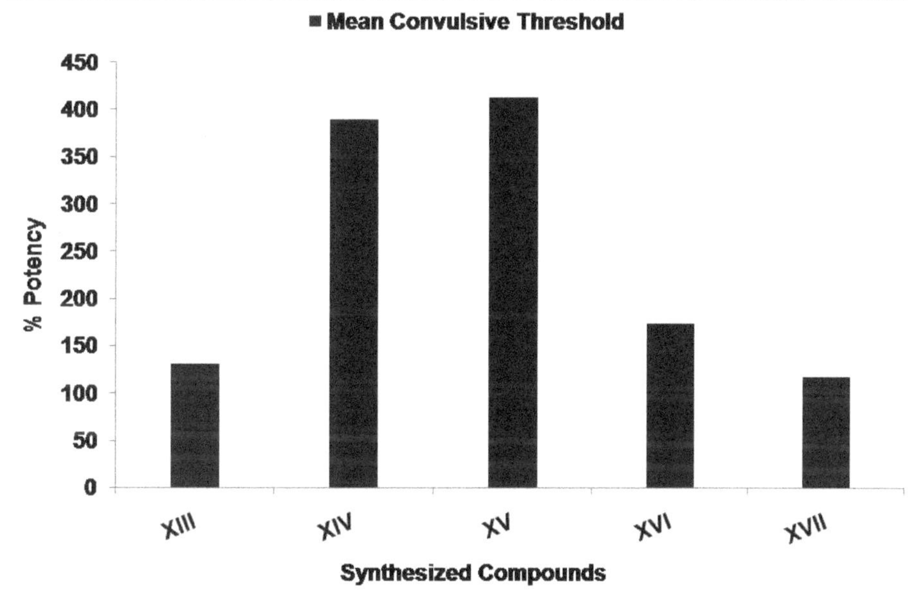

Figure 2 **%Potency of synthesized compounds at the dose (30 mg kg^{-1}, p.o.) in female albino mice for single administration**. All the values were expressed as mean convulsive threshold.

Table 2 Antidepressant activity of synthesized compounds

Number	Compound	Dose (mg kg^{-1})	0 h (mean ± S.E.M)	1 h (mean ± S.E.M)
1.	Control	10	345.83 ± 0.27	303.21 ± 0.42
2.	Standard	10	411.16 ± 0.30	91.33 ± 0.21
3.	XIII	10	401.50 ± 0.22*	85.16 ± 0.47*
4.	XIV	10	502.83 ± 0.47 ***	196.66 ± 0.42***
5.	XV	10	431.16 ± 0.30***	124.16 ± 0.40**
6.	XVI	10	455.83 ± 0.47*	89.16 ± 0.30**
7.	XVII	10	511.50 ± 0.42***	207.00 ± 0.36***

Values are mean ± SEM of six animals in each group. Statistical significance versus standard (***$p \le 0.001$, **$p \le 0.01$, *$p \le 0.05$)

compounds and it may be assumed that further modifications may produce compounds of better activity with less side effects.

Experimental

Chemical synthesis

All the chemicals and reagents were obtained from Sigma (Germany) and CDH (India) and were recrystallized/redistilled as necessary. Melting points were determined by open capillary tube method and are uncorrected. Purity of the compounds were checked on thin layer chromatography (TLC) plates precoated with silica gel G using solvent system ethyl acetate: petroleum ether (**1**) (3:7 v/v) and benzene: methanol (**2**) (2:1 v/v). The spots were visualized under iodine vapours and UV light. IR spectra were recorded using KBr on a FTIR Shimadzu 8400S IR spectrophotometer (Japan). A JEOL AL300 FTNMR 300 MHz spectrometer was used to acquire ^{1}H NMR spectra with DMSO as solvent and tetra methyl silane (TMS) as internal standard. Chemical shift values are expressed in δ ppm. Mass spectra were obtained with a VG70-70H mass spectrometer. Elemental analyses were carried out with a Perkin Elmer model 240-C apparatus. The results of the elemental analysis (C, H, N) are within ± 0.4% of the calculated amounts.

General procedure for the synthesis of 2,5-substituted diphenyl-1,3,4-oxadiazoles

Step 1: Synthesis of substituted ethyl benzoate (**V-VIII**):

Compounds (**V-VIII**) was synthesized by refluxing a mixture of substituted benzoic acid (I-IV) (0.0587 mol) with absolute ethanol (12 ml) in presence of conc. sulphuric acid (0.5 ml) for 5 h at 40-50°C. Excess of alcohol was distilled off and allowed to cool in ice bath. Reaction was monitored by TLC. The residue thus obtained was separated and washed with water and recrystallized with ethanol [13]. The physico-chemical data of the synthesized compounds (V-VIII) are given in Table 5.

V: IR (KBr, cm^{-1}): 3581 (O-H stretch), 3040 (Ar-H stretch), 1661 (C = O stretch), 1170 (C-O stretch); ^{1}H NMR (300 MHz-DMSO-d6-ppm) δ: 7.78 (d, 2H, Ar-H), 6.84 (d, 2H, Ar-H), 5.2 (s, 1H, OH), 4.19 (m, 2H, CH2), 1.30 (m, 3H, CH3); MS (EI) m/z 166.08 [M^+].

VI: IR (KBr, cm^{-1}): 3048 (Ar-H stretch), 1651 (C = O stretch), 1192 (C-O stretch), 1550 (C-NO2 stretch); ^{1}H NMR (300 MHz-DMSO-d6-ppm) δ: 8.34 (d, 2H, Ar-H), 8.27 (m, 2H, Ar-H), 4.26 (m, 1H, CH2), 1.32 (m, 1H, CH3); MS (EI) m/z 195.07 [M^+].

VII: IR (KBr, cm^{-1}): 3370 (N-H stretch), 3035 (Ar-H stretch), 1643 (C = O stretch), 1214 (C-O stretch); ^{1}H NMR (300 MHz-DMSO-d6-ppm) δ: 7.75 (d, 2H, Ar-H),

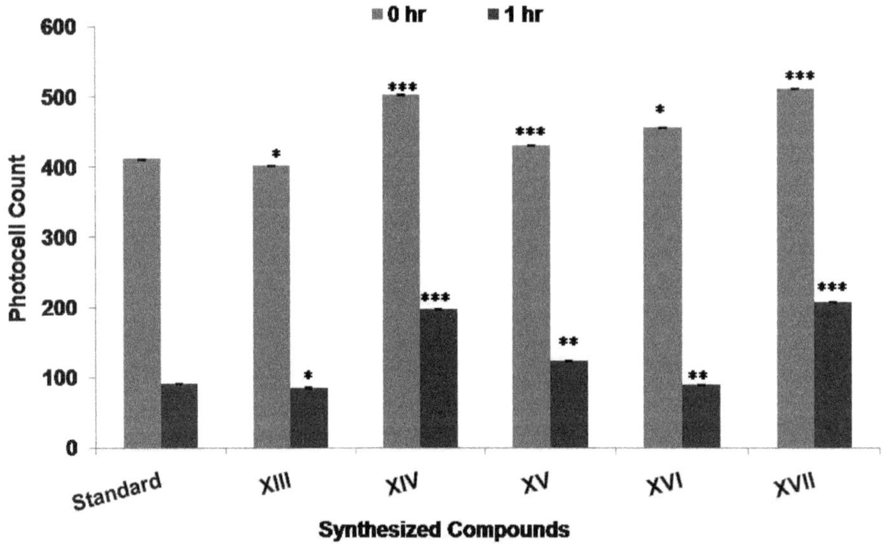

Figure 3 Antidepressant activity of synthesized compounds at the dose (10 mg kg^{-1}, p.o.) showing number of photocell count.

Table 3 Antianxiety activity of synthesized compounds

Number	Compound	Dose (mg kg^{-1})	Number of entries in open arms (Mean ± S.E.M)	Average time spent in open arms (Mean ± S.E.M)
1.	Control	10	2.10 ± 0.23	9.77 ± 0.27
2.	Standard	10	12.66 ± 0.33	32.66 ± 0.33
3.	XIII	10	13.33 ± 0.21***	68.00 ± 0.36***
4.	XIV	10	17.00 ± 0.36***	62.33 ± 0.21**
5.	XV	10	21.50 ± 0.42***	76.83 ± 0.30***
6.	XVI	10	8.83 ± 0.30***	45.83 ± 0.30**
7.	XVII	10	13.66 ± 0.42	52.66 ± 0.33*

Values are mean ± SEM of six animals in each group. Statistical significance versus standard (***$p \leq 0.001$, **$p \leq 0.01$, *$p \leq 0.05$)

6.51 (d, 2H, Ar-H), 4.35 (m, 1H, CH2), 3.97 (s, 1H, NH), 1.28 (m, 3H, CH3); MS (EI) m/z 165.03 [M^+].

VIII: IR (KBr, cm^{-1}): 30443 (Ar-H stretch), 1668 (C = O stretch), 1243 (C-O stretch), 748 (C-Cl stretch); ^1H NMR (300 MHz-DMSO-d6-ppm) δ: 7.94 (d, 2H, Ar-H), 7.35 (m, 2H, Ar-H), 4.27 (m, 2H, CH2), 1.26 (m, 2H, CH3); MS (EI) m/z 184.01 [M^+].

Step 2: Synthesis of substituted benzohydrazide (**IX-XII**):

Compounds **(IX-XII)** were synthesized by refluxing a mixture of substituted ethyl benzoate (**V-VIII**) (0.0602 mol) with hydrazine hydrate (5 ml) in absolute ethanol (12 ml) for 8 h at 30-40°C. The reaction mixture was cooled to room temperature and poured in ice with constant stirring. Reaction was monitored by TLC. The precipitate obtained was filtered, washed with water and recrystallized with ethanol to give crystalline product. The physico-chemical data of the synthesized compounds (**IX-XII**) are given in Table 6.

IX: IR (KBr, cm^{-1}): 3472 (O-H stretch), 3336 (N-H stretch), 3049 (Ar-H stretch), 1658 (amide C = O stretch); ^1H NMR (300 MHz-DMSO-d6-ppm) δ: 7.79 (m, 2H, Ar-H), 6.86 (m, 2H, Ar-H), 4.2 (s, 1H, OH), 3.21 (m, 2H, CH2), 2.17 (d, 2H, NH), 1.23 (m, 3H, CH3); MS (EI) m/z 180.01 [M^+].

X: IR (KBr, cm^{-1}): 3260 (N-H stretch), 3010 (Ar-H stretch), 1664 (amide C = O stretch), 1511 (C-NO2 stretch); ^1H NMR (300 MHz-DMSO-d6-ppm) δ: 8.35 (d, 2H, Ar-H), 8.19 (d, 2H, Ar-H), 3.25 (m, 2H, CH2), 1.90 (m, 2H, NH), 1.18 (m, 3H, CH3); MS (EI) m/z 209.05 [M^+].

XI: IR (KBr, cm^{-1}): 3368.71 (N-H stretch), 3030.95 (Ar-H stretch), 1642.31 (amide C = O stretch); ^1H NMR (300 MHz-DMSO-d6-ppm) δ: 7.68 (m, 2H, Ar-H), 6.62 (d, 2H, Ar-H), 3.98 (d, 2H, NH), 3.18 (m, 2H, CH2),

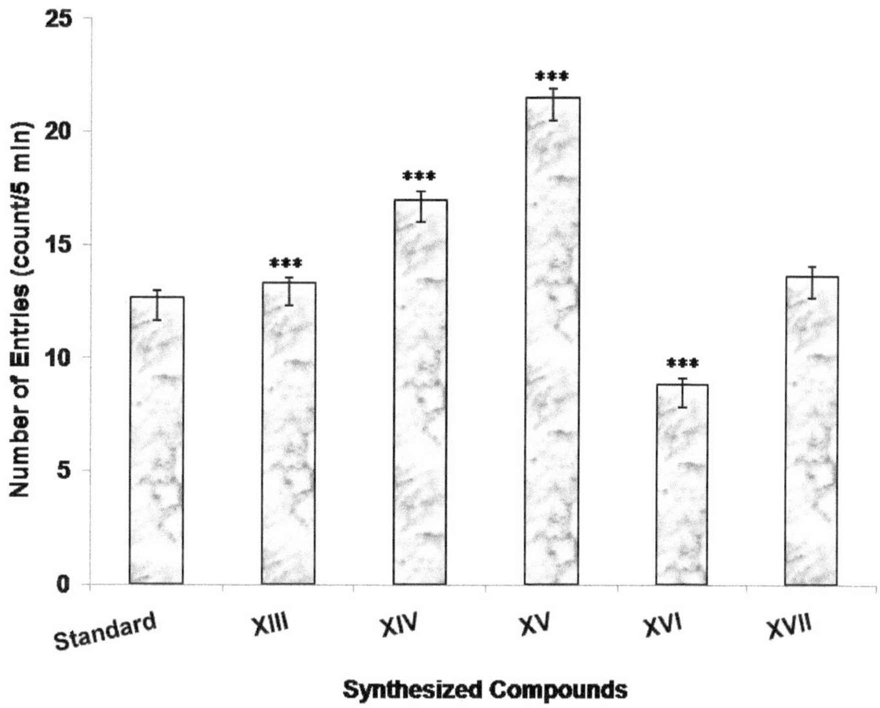

Figure 4 Antianxiety activity of synthesized compounds at the dose (2 mg kg^{-1}, p.o.) showing number of entries 5 min^{-1}.

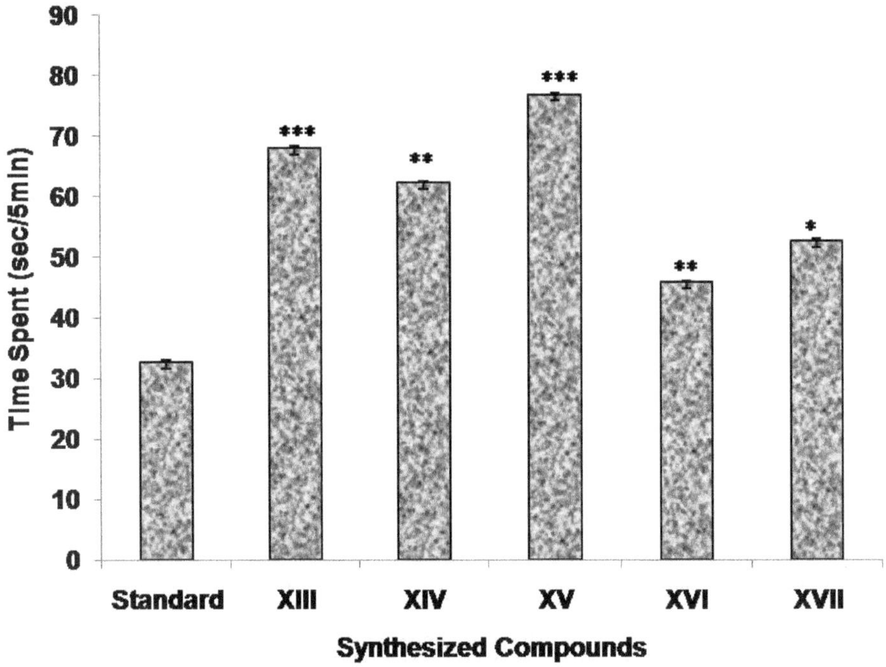

Figure 5 Antianxiety activity of synthesized compounds at the dose (2 mg kg^{-1}, p.o.) showing time spent by mouse in open arm.

1.81 (d, 2H, NH), 1.25 (m, 3H, CH3); MS (EI) m/z 179.15 [M^+].

XII: IR (KBr, cm^{-1}): 3279 (N-H stretch), 3047 (Ar-H), 1672 (amide C = O stretch), 727 (C-Cl stretch); ^{1}H NMR (300 MHz-DMSO-d6-ppm) δ: 7.84 (m, 2H, Ar-H), 7.44 (m, 2H, Ar-H), 3.26 (m, 2H, CH2), 2.35 (d, 2H, NH), 1.17 (m, 3H, CH3); MS (EI) m/z 198.63 [M^+].

Step 3: Synthesis of 2,5-substituted diphenyl-1,3,4-oxadiazole (**XIII-XXII**).

An equimolar mixture of substituted benzohydrazide (**IX-XII**) (0.0054 mol) with various substituted benzoic acids (0.0054 mol) was refluxed with phosphorus oxychloride (5 ml) for 2-3 h on water bath at 100°C. Reaction mixture was cooled to room temperature and poured in ice. The precipitate obtained was filtered off, washed with water and further purified by recrystallization with ethanol to give 2,5-substituted diphenyl-1,3,4-oxadiazole. The physico-chemical data of the synthesized compounds (**XIII-XXII**) are given in Table 7.

Table 4 Neurotoxic activity of the synthesized compounds

Compound	Dose (mg kg^{-1})	n	Result
Std. (Phenytoin)	30	6	X
XIII	30	6	-
XIV	30	6	X
XV	30	6	X
XVI	30	6	-
XVIII	30	6	X

n, number of mice = 6; X, does not show neurotoxicity; ROA, orally; -, neurotoxicity not checked.

XIII: IR (KBr, cm^{-1}): 3448 (O-H stretch), 3070 (Ar-H stretch), 2980 (C-H Ar. Stretch), 1593 (C = N stretch of 1,3,4-oxadiazole ring), 1417 (C = C ring stretching), 1275 (C-O-C stretch of 1,3,4-oxadiazole ring), 1016 (C-O stretch of oxadiazole ring), 852 (Ar. C-Cl); ^{1}H NMR (300 MHz-DMSO-d6-ppm) δ: 7.39 (d, 2H, Ar-H), 7.31 (m, 2H, Ar-H), 7.28 (m, 2H, Ar-H), 6.85 (d, 2H, Ar-H), 4.4-5.6 (s, 1H, OH); MS (EI) m/z 272.02 [M^+]; Anal. calcd. for C14H9ClN2O2 (%) C, 59.34; N, 9.52: O, 12.78.

XIV: IR (KBr, cm^{-1}): 3103 (Ar-H stretch), 2848 (Ar. C-H stretch), 1604 (C = N stretch of 1,3,4-oxadiazole ring), 1527 (C = C ring stretching), 1463 (C-H Bend), 1350 (N-O Assymetric stretch of C-NO2), 1242 (C-O-C stretch of 1,3,4-oxadiazole ring), 1010 (C-O stretch of oxadiazole ring), 865 (C-N stretch of Ar. C-NO2); 838 (Ar. C-Cl); ^{1}H NMR (300 MHz-DMSO-d6-ppm) δ: 8.16 (d, 2H, Ar-H), 7.71 (m, 2H, Ar-H), 7.46 (d, 2H, Ar-H), 7.30 (t, 2H, Ar-H); MS (EI) m/z 301.04 [M^+]; Anal. calcd. for C14H8ClN3O3 (%): C, 55.70; N, 12.73: O, 15.21.

XV: IR (KBr, cm^{-1}): 3038 (Ar-H stretch), 2941 (C-H Ar. stretch), 1533 (C = N stretch of 1,3,4-oxadiazole ring), 1409 (C = C ring stretching), 1359 (N-O stretch Assymetric N-O stretch of C-NO2), 1278 (C-O-C stretch of 1,3,4-oxadiazole ring), 1074 (C-O stretch of oxadiazole ring); ^{1}H NMR (300 MHz-DMSO-d6-ppm)

Table 5 Physico-chemical data of the synthesized compounds (V-VIII)

Compound	*R*	Molecular formula	Molecular weight	% Yield	m.p. (°C)	$Rf^{solvent\ system}$
V	4-OH	$C_9H_{10}O_3$	166.17	56.21	108-110	0.72[a]
VI	4-NO2	$C_9H_9NO_4$	195.17	85.25	114-116	0.78[a]
VII	4-NH2	$C_9H_{11}NO_2$	165.19	64.28	90-92	0.83[a]
VIII	4-Cl	$C_9H_9ClO_2$	184.62	87.16	127-129	0.76[a]

[a]Ethyl acetate: Petroleum ether (3:7 v/v);

δ: 7.79 (d, 4H, Ar-H), 8.32 (d, 4H, Ar-H); MS (EI) m/z 312.05 [M^+]; Anal. calcd. for C14H8N4O5 (%) C, 54.21; N, 18.03: O, 25.24.

XVI: IR (KBr, cm^{-1}): 3440 (O-H stretch), 3406 (N-H stretch), 2952 (C-H Ar. stretch), 1633 (C = N stretch of 1,3,4-oxadiazole ring), 1519 (C = C ring stretching), 1340 (N-O stretch Assymetric N-O stretch of C-NO2), 1249 (C-O-C stretch of 1,3,4-oxadiazole ring), 1072 (C-O stretch of 1,3,4-oxadiazole ring); 854 (C-N stretch of Ar. C-NO2); ^{1}H NMR (300 MHz-DMSO-d6-ppm) δ: 8.32 (d, 2H, Ar-H), 7.77 (d, 2H, Ar-H), 7.28 (d, 2H, Ar-H), 6.57 (t, 2H, Ar-H), 3.8-4.2 (d, 2H, NH); MS (EI) m/z 282.03 [M^+]; Anal. calcd. for C14H10N4O3 (%) C, 61.26; N, 18.87; O, 17.24.

XVII: IR (KBr, cm^{-1}): 3409 (N-H stretch), 3451 (O-H stretch), 2974 (C-H Ar. stretch), 1625 (C = N stretch of 1,3,4-oxadiazole ring), 1492 (C = C ring stretching), 1263 (C-O-C stretch of 1,3,4-oxadiazole ring), 1012 (C-O stretch of oxadiazole ring), ^{1}H NMR (300 MHz-DMSO-d6-ppm) δ: 7.37 (d, 2H, Ar-H), 7.28 (m, 1H, Ar-H), 6.91 (m, 1H, Ar-H), 6.75 (m, 2H, Ar-H), 6.62 (m, 1H, Ar-H), 6.47 (d, 1H, Ar-H), 4.3-5.5 (d, 1H, OH), 3.7-4.9 (d, 2H, NH); MS (EI) m/z 252.62 [M^+]; Anal calcd. for C14H11N3O2 (%) C, 66.35; N, 17.24: O, 10.35.

XVIII: IR (KBr, cm^{-1}): 3045 (Ar-H stretch), 1681 (C = N stretch of 1,3,4-oxadiazole ring), 1591 (C = C ring stretching), 1362 (Assymetric N-O stretch of C-NO2), 1247 (C-O-C stretch of 1,3,4-oxadiazole ring), 1087 (C-O stretch of 1,3,4-oxadiazole ring); 854 (C-N stretch of Ar. C-NO2); ^{1}H NMR (300 MHz-DMSO-d6-ppm) δ: 8.61 (m, 2H, Ar-H), 7.71 (m, 2H, Ar-H), 7.57 (m, 1H, Ar-H), 7.32 (m, 1H, Ar-H), 7.29 (m, 1H, Ar-H), 7.14 (m, 1H, Ar-H); MS (EI) m/z 344.89 [M^+]; Anal. calcd. for C14H8BrN3O3 (%) C, 50.27; N, 12.23; O, 13.58.

XIX: IR (KBr, cm^{-1}): 3448 (N-H stretch), 2924 (C-H Ar. stretch), 1685 (C = N stretch of 1,3,4-oxadiazole ring), 1593.09 (C = C), 1091 (C-O stretch of 1,3,4-oxadiazole ring), 837 (Ar. C-Cl); ^{1}H NMR (300 MHz-DMSO-d6-ppm) δ: 7.42 (m, 2H, Ar-H), 7.33 (m, 2H, Ar-H), 7.23 (m, 2H, Ar-H), 6.52 (m, 2H, Ar-H), 3.4-4.7 (m, 2H, NH); MS (EI) m/z 271.09 [M^+]; Anal. calcd. for C14H10ClN3O (%): C, 62.79; N, 14.37; O, 14.89.

XX: IR (KBr, cm^{-1}): 3402 (N-H stretch), 3110 (O-H stretch), 2987 (Ar. C-H stretch), 1608 (C = N stretch of 1,3,4-oxadiazole ring), 1525 (C = C ring stretching), 1350 (Assymetric N-O stretch of C-NO2), 1010 (C-O stretch of 1,3,4-oxadiazole ring); ^{1}H NMR (300 MHz-DMSO-d6-ppm) δ: 8.25 (m, 2H, Ar-H), 7.74 (m, 2H, Ar-H), 7.31 (m, 2H, Ar-H), 6.79 (m, 2H, Ar-H), 4.5-5.2 (s, 1H, OH); MS (EI) m/z 283.04 [M^+]; Anal calcd. for C14H9N3O4 (%) C, 60.24; N, 15.43; O, 21.75.

XXI: IR (KBr, cm^{-1}): 3457 (O-H stretch), 2996 (C-H Ar. stretch), 1632 (C = N stretch of 1,3,4-oxadiazole ring), 1578 (C = C ring stretching), 1213 (C-O-C stretch of 1,3,4-oxadiazole ring), 1075 (C-O stretch of 1,3,4-oxadiazole ring); ^{1}H NMR (300 MHz-DMSO-d6-ppm) δ: 7.57 (m, 1H, Ar-H), 7.36 (m, 1H, Ar-H), 7.28 (m, 2H, Ar-H), 7.21 (m, 1H, Ar-H), 7.09 (m, 1H, Ar-H), 6.81 (m, 2H, Ar-H), 4.9-5.4 (s, 1H, OH); MS (EI) m/z 315.98 [M^+]; Anal. calcd. for C14H9BrN2O2 (%) C, 54.24; N, 8.82; O, 10.94.

XXII: IR (KBr, cm^{-1}): 3051 (Ar-H stretch), 1618 (C = N stretch of 1,3,4-oxadiazole ring), 1519 (C = C ring stretching), 1282 (C-O-C stretch of 1,3,4-oxadiazole ring), 1059 (C-O stretch of 1,3,4-oxadiazole ring); 849 (C-N stretch of Ar. C-NO2); ^{1}H NMR (300 MHz-DMSO-d6-ppm) δ: 8.07 (m, 2H, Ar-H), 7.61 (m, 2H, Ar-H), 7.53 (m, 2H, Ar-H), 7.35 (m, 2H, Ar-H), 7.29 (m, 1H, Ar-H); MS (EI) m/z 267.06 [M^+]; Anal. calcd. for C14H9N3O3 (%) C, 62.26; N, 15.17; O, 17.74.

Pharmacology

Albino mice of either sex, weighing (25-30 g) were used for bioactivity studies. The animals were allowed food

Table 6 Physico-chemical data of the synthesized compounds (IX-XII)

Compound	*R*	Molecular formula	Molecular weight	% Yield	m.p. (°C)	$Rf^{solvent\ system}$
IX	4-OH	$C_7H_8N_2O_2$	152.1	35.96	132-134	0.74[a]
X	4-NO2	$C_7H_7N_3O_3$	181.15	58.01	148-150	0.82[a]
XI	4-NH2	$C_7H_9N_3O$	151.17	29.16	142-144	0.75[a]
XII	4-Cl	$C_7H_7ClN_2O$	170.60	53.13	156-158	0.77[a]

[a]Ethyl acetate: Petroleum ether (3:7 v/v);

Table 7 Physico-chemical data of the synthesized compounds (XIII-XXV)

Compound	*R*	*R'*	Molecular formula	Molecular weight	% Yield	m.p. (°C)	$Rf^{solvent\ system}$
XIII	4-OH	4-Cl	$C_{14}H_9ClN_2O_2$	272.69	74.11	95-97	0.78[a]
XIV	4-NO2	4-Cl	$C_{14}H_8ClN_3O_3$	301.68	82.22	165-167	0.75[a]
XV	4-NO2	4-NO2	$C_{14}H_8N_4O_5$	312.24	95.24	127-129	0.67[a]
XVI	4-NO2	4-NH2	$C_{14}H_8ClN_3O_3$	301.68	78.59	178-180	0.75[a]
XVII	4-OH	4-NH2	$C_{14}H_{11}N_3O_2$	253.26	65.26	106-108	0.61[b]
XVIII	4-NO2	2-Br	$C_{14}H_8BrN_3O_3$	346.14	86.01	120-122	0.82[a]
XIX	4-NH2	4-Cl	$C_{14}H_{10}ClN_3O$	271.7	78.06	175-177	0.55[b]
XX	4-NO2	4-OH	$C_{14}H_9N_3O_4$	283.24	64.79	104-107	0.66[b]
XXI	4-OH	2-Br	$C_{14}H_9BrN_2O_2$	317.14	52.36	102-104	0.74[b]
XXII	4-NO2	H	$C_{14}H_9N_3O_3$	267.24	81.79	104-106	0.81[a]

[a]Ethyl acetate: Petroleum ether (3:7 v/v)
[b]Benzene: Methanol (2:1 v/v).

and water *ad libitum* except during the experiments. They were housed in a room at 25 ± 2°C and 50 ± 5% relative humidity. Animals were obtained from Animal House Facility, Meerut Institute of Engineering and Technology, Meerut. All the test compounds and reference drug were administered orally, suspended in 1% (w/v) carboxymethyl cellulose (CMC) suspension.

Anticonvulsant activity (MES)

The synthesized compounds were evaluated for their anticonvulsant activity using MES method. The animals were randomly allocated into three groups (standard, control, and test) of six animals each and were fasted for 24 h before the experiment with free access to water. Control group received only 1% (w/v) carboxymethyl cellulose suspension. Standard drug phenytoin was administered orally at a dose of 30 mg kg^{-1}. The test compounds were administered orally at an equimolar oral dose relative to 30 mg kg^{-1} phenytoin. Test compounds and standard drug were administered orally as suspension in carboxymethyl cellulose in water (1% w/v). Supramaximal electroshock of current intensity 50 mA, 60 Hz was given for duration of 0.2 s after the administration of test and standard drug. The anticonvulsant activity was assessed after 30 min of administration. The abolition of hind limb tonic extensor spasm was recorded as a measure of anticonvulsant activity [14]. The results of anticonvulsant activity were summarized in Table 1 and the graphs for anticonvulsant activity were presented in Figures 1 and 2.

Antidepressant activity (spontaneous motor activity using actophotometer)

The synthesized compounds were evaluated for their antidepressant activity using actophotometer. The animals were randomly allocated into three groups (standard, control, and test) of six animals each and were fasted for 24 h before the experiment with free access to water. Control group received only 1% (w/v) carboxymethyl cellulose suspension. Standard drug fluoxetine was administered orally at a dose of 10 mg kg^{-1}. The test compounds were administered orally at an equimolar oral dose relative to 10 mg kg^{-1} fluoxetine. Test compounds and standard drug were administered orally as suspension in carboxymethyl cellulose in water (1% w/v). In locomotor activity, the basal activity score for all animals and after 60 min of drug treatment for 10 min was recorded [15]. The results of antidepressant activity were summarized in Table 2 and the graph for antidepressant activity was presented in Figure 3.

Antianxiety activity (elevated plus maze model)

The synthesized compounds were evaluated for their antianxiety activity using actophotometer. The animals were randomly allocated into 3 groups (standard, control, and test) of 6 animals each and were fasted for 24 h before the experiment with free access to water. Control group received only 1% (w/v) carboxymethyl cellulose suspension. Standard drug diazepam was administered orally at a dose of 2 mg kg^{-1}. The test compounds were administered orally at an equimolar oral dose relative to 2 mg kg^{-1} diazepam. Test compounds and standard drug were administered orally as suspension in carboxymethyl cellulose in water (1% w/v). The plus maze apparatus consists of two open arms and two closed arms having an open roof, with the plus maze elevated from the floor was used to observe anxiolytic behavior in animals. Each mouse was placed at the center of the elevated plus maze with its head facing the open arms [16]. During this, the behavior of the mouse was recorded as:

(1) The number of entries into the open arms
(2) Average time spent by the mouse in the open arms

$$\text{Average time} = \frac{\text{Total time spent in open arms}}{\text{Number of entries in arms}}$$

The results of antianxiety activity were summarized in Table 3 and the graphs for antianxiety activity were presented in Figures 4 and 5, respectively.

Neurotoxicity studies (rotarod animal model)

The disruptive effects on motor coordination were assessed using the Rotarod Tread mill mouse method. The mice were trained to stay on an accelerating rotarod that rotates at 10 revolutions min^{-1} and 3.2 cm in diameter. Trained mice were given test compounds in dose of 30 mg kg^{-1} orally. Unimpaired mice can easily remain on a rod rotating at this speed. Neurological deficit, e.g., ataxia, sedation, hyperexcitability is indicated by the inability of the mice to maintain equilibrium on the rod for at least 1 min in each of three concurrent trails [17]. The results of neurotoxic activity measured by rotarod animal model were summarized in Table 6.

Statistical analysis

Statistical analysis of the anticonvulsant, antidepressant, and antianxiety activity of the synthesized compounds on animals was evaluated using a one-way analysis of variance (ANOVA). In all the cases, post-hoc comparisons of the means of individual groups were performed using Tukey's test. Differences with $^{***}p \leq 0.001$ between experimental groups at each point were considered statistically significant. All values were expressed as mean ± SEM (standard error of mean). For statistical analysis we use sigma stat 2.03 version. (Systat Software, Inc. Point. CA, USA).

Acknowledgements

Authors were thankful to the Department of Pharmaceutical Technology, M.I. E.T., Meerut, for providing laboratory facilities. The help rendered by CDRI Lucknow for spectral and elemental analysis was also gratefully acknowledged.

Author details

[1]Department of Pharmaceutical Technology, Meerut Institute of Engineering & Technology, NH-58, Baghpat By-pass Crossing, Delhi-Haridwar Highway, Meerut-250005, India [2]Faculty of Pharmacy, Dehradun Institute of Technology, Dehradun, Uttarakhand, India

Competing interests

The authors declare that they have no competing interests.

References

1. Siddiqui N, Rana A, Khan SA, Bhat MA, Haque SE (2007) Synthesis of benzothiazole semicarbazones as novel anticonvulsants–the role of hydrophobic domain. Bioorg Med Chem Lett 17:4178–4182. doi:10.1016/j.bmcl.2007.05.048.
2. Fisher R, van Emde Boas W, Blume W, Elger C, Genton P, Lee P, Engel J (2005) Epileptic seizures and epilepsy: definitions proposed by the International League against Epilepsy (ILAE) and the International Bureau for Epilepsy (IBE). Epilepsia 46:470–472. doi:10.1111/j.0013-9580.2005.66104.x.
3. Czapin'ski P, Blaszczyk B, Czuczwar SJ (2005) Mechanisms of action of antiepileptic drugs. Curr Topics Med Chem 5:3–14. doi:10.2174/1568026053386962.
4. Lambert MV, Robertson MM (1999) Depression in epilepsy: etiology, phenomenology, and treatment. Epilepsia 40:21–47
5. Kanner AM, Palac S (2002) Neuropsychiatric complications of epilepsy. Curr Neurol Neurosci Rep 2:365–372. doi:10.1007/s11910-002-0012-7.
6. Beyenburg S, Mitchell AJ, Schmidth D (2005) Anxiety in patients with epilepsy: Systematic review and suggestions for clinical management. Epilepsy Behav 7:161–171. doi:10.1016/j.yebeh.2005.05.014.
7. Oguz A, Kurul S, Dirik E (2002) Relationship of epilepsy-related factors to anxiety and depression scores in epileptic children. J Child Neurol 17:37–40. doi:10.1177/088307380201700109.
8. Ott D, Caplan R, Guthrie D (2001) Measures of psychopathology in children with complex partial seizures and primary generalized epilepsy with absence. J Am Acad Child Adolesc Psychiatry 40:907–914. doi:10.1097/00004583-200108000-00012.
9. Hesdorffer DC, Hauser WA, Olafsson E, Ludvigsson P, Kjartansson O (2006) Depression and suicide attempt as risk factors for incident unprovoked seizures. Ann Neurol 59:35–41. doi:10.1002/ana.20685.
10. Kanner A, Balabanov A (2002) Depression and epilepsy: How closely related are they? Neurology 58:27–39
11. Titlic M, Basic S, Hajnsek S, Lusic I (2009) Comorbidity psychiatric disorders in epilepsy: a review of literature. Bratisl Lek Listy 110:105–109
12. Bhattacharya J, Pate K, Tailor P, Karthikeyan C, Moorthy NSHN, Trivedi P (2010) Design, synthesis and characterization of novel 1,3,4-oxadiazole dimmers from benzoic acids. Inter J Chem Tech Res 2:2055–2062
13. Furniss BS, Hannaford AJ, Rogers V, Smith PW, Tatchell AR Vogel's Textbook of Practical Organic Chemistry. John Wiley & Sons, New York
14. Patil VM, Sinha R, Masand N, Jain J (2009) Synthesis and anticonvulsant activities of small *N*-Substituted 2,5-dimethyl pyrrole and bipyrrole. Digest J Nanomat Biostr 4:471–477
15. Abid M, Hrishikeshavan HJ, Asad M (2006) Pharmacological evaluation of pachyrrhizus erosus (l) seeds for central nervous system depressant activity. Indian J Physiol Pharmacol 50:143–151
16. Madaan R, Sharma A (2011) Evaluation of anti-anxiety activity of *Actaea spicata* Linn., Inter. J Pharm Sci Drug Res 3:45–47
17. Clerci F, Pocar D (2001) Synthesis of 2-Amino-5-sulfanyl-1,3,4-thiadiazole derivatives and evaluation of their antidepressant and anxiolytic activity. J Med Chem 44:931–936. doi:10.1021/jm001027w.

17

Pathways of ion–molecular interactions of nucleogenic phenyl cations with the nucleophilic centers of picolines

Nadezhda E Shchepina[1*], Viktor V Avrorin[2], Gennady A Badun[3], Nikolay A Bumagin[4], Scott B Lewis[5] and Sergey N Shurov[6]

Abstract

Background: The nuclear-chemical method brought unique opportunity for synthesis of unknown and hardly available organic compounds. Presence of tritium labeling allows one-step preparation of radioactive markers for the investigation of chemical and biological processes.

Methods: The ion–molecular reactions of nucleogenic phenyl cations with 4-picoline have been carried out. The phenyl cations were generated by spontaneous tritium β-decay within the tritium-labeled benzene. Both additions to the nitrogen and substitutions about the aromatic ring were able to be studied simultaneously.

Results: Unusual substitutions on both the α- and β-positions of the ring system have been revealed.

Conclusion: By unknown direct phenylation of nitrogen atom tritium-labeled *N*-phenylpicolinium derivatives, perspective biological markers have been synthesized.

Keywords: nucleogenic phenyl cations, picoline, tritium-labeled biological markers

Background

The pyridine ring itself is a part of many natural and synthetically prepared pharmaceuticals [1,2]. In addition, the pyridine moiety plays a significant role in many biological processes [3,4]. Methyl-substituted pyridines, i.e., picolines, are not the exception in the list of important biologically active substances [5]. The observed increase of biological activity with the introduction of methyl group into the heterocyclic pyridine ring inspires synthetic chemists to find new methods for the preparation of derivatives with picoline fragment [6-11], and biologists for the detail investigations of biological mechanisms with the use of tritium markers [12-14]. Elaborated nuclear-chemical method opens the horizons for synthesis of unknown and hardly available organic compounds. Presence of tritium labeling allows one-step preparation of radioactive markers for the investigation of chemical and biological processes.

* Correspondence: neshchepina@mail.ru
[1]Laboratory of Radiochemistry, Natural Sciences Institute of Perm State University, 4 Genkel St, Perm 614990, Russia
Full list of author information is available at the end of the article

Methods

Previously, we have used the elaborated nuclear-chemical method for the detailed investigations of the ion–molecular reactions of pyridine and quinoline derivatives [15-17]. By these investigations it was shown that with the application of nucleogenic phenyl cations (cations generated by the processes of tritium β-decay), unusual direct phenylation of nitrogen atom in pyridine ring might be realized. Since by the classical methods of chemistry *N*-phenylpicolinium derivatives could not be prepared by phenylation reaction [18,19] and simultaneously syntheses of such compounds with the fixed tritium label are hardly available; our special interest was focused on prolongation of nuclear-chemical method on methyl-substituted pyridines and detail investigation of the pathways of ion–molecular interactions of nucleogenic phenyl cations with the 4-picoline nucleophilic centers.

Free phenyl cations generated by tritium β-decay in *p*-ditritiated benzene (double labeled benzene is necessary since the second tritium atom is a radioactive tracer) immediately attack the existed nucleophilic centers of the picoline molecule. As it was seen with pyridine, addition to the nitrogen atom to produce *N*-phenylpicolinium salts or substitution on the ring to produce phenyl picolines should be possible. In methylpyridines, also the substitution of hydrogen in methyl group with the formation of benzyl derivative may take place. Projected outcomes for the ion–molecular reactions in the case of 4-picoline are presented in Scheme 1.

The ion–molecular reactions of the 4-picoline with the tritium-labeled benzene were carried out in sealed glass ampoules. The ampoules also contained a large excess of a stabilizing salt (KBF_4). The tritiated benzene used in this study was synthesized from *p*-dibromobenzene by catalytic exchange [15]. After an appropriate accumulation time for the determination of products by radioactivity (approximately 1 month) the reaction mixtures were subjected to TLC analysis. Radiochromatography of tritium-labeled compounds and comparison with the reference compounds allowed determination of the yields for the products. For identification of the products, in the case of 4-picoline, we have undertaken the synthesis of reference compounds. Methods of synthesis and characterization of these compounds: *N*-phenyl-4-methylpyridinium tetrafluoroborate, 3-phenyl-4-picoline (proposed major substitution isomer), and 2-phenyl-4-picoline are presented in the "Experimental" section.

A typical radiochromatogram of the obtained tritiated products from the ion–molecular reactions of tritiated benzene with 4-picoline is presented in Figure 1. From the peak shapes and analysis of the chromatographic peaks with the help of the program "Fityk", it was possible to confirm that each obtained peak describes the chromatographic behavior of only one substance, not a mixture of substances.

Tritium β-radioactivity has been measured by liquid scintillation counter. Relative yields of ion–molecular reaction products were determined as the ratio of the radioactivity of an individual substance toward the sum of all tritium-labeled products.

Results and discussion

The radiochemical yields of the addition and substitution products from the reactions of the picoline derivative with the phenyl cations are presented in Table 1.

It was shown that methyl group in pyridine accents the direction of the interactions from the electrophilic addition of phenyl cations with the unshared electron pair of nitrogen atom toward the electrophilic substitution. And that causes the decrease in the yield of pyridinium salt (the yield in the case of unsubstituted pyridine was about 60%). The methyl group on the picoline is known to stabilize azaarene ions by being an electron donor [20,21]. This stabilization of the azaarene ion can make substitution on to the ring a more favorable process than even addition to the nitrogen atom. The data presented in Table 1 bear this out. We have found that 3-substitution by the phenyl cation was the preferential substitution product (41%). The compound 2-phenyl-4-picoline was produced in approximately 20%. These results fall well in line with the results published for the reactions of pyridine with phenyl cations, in which all three substituted isomers were discovered [22].

Explanation of this noncoincidence with the results of classic chemistry may have several explanations. Since nucleogenic phenyl cations are free, steric effects (especially from offending solvent molecules) become unimportant. We have observed this fact in our synthesis of

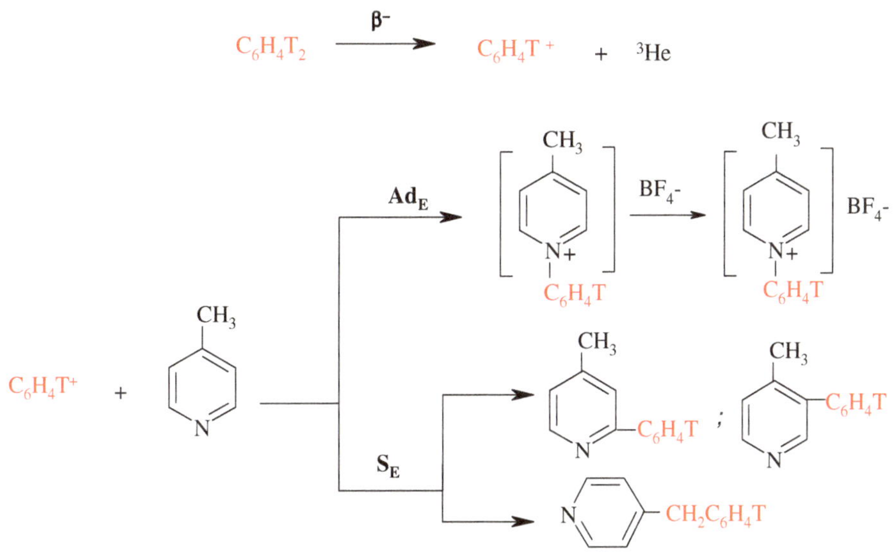

Scheme 1 Proposed ion-molecular reactions of nucleogenic phenyl cations with 4-picoline.

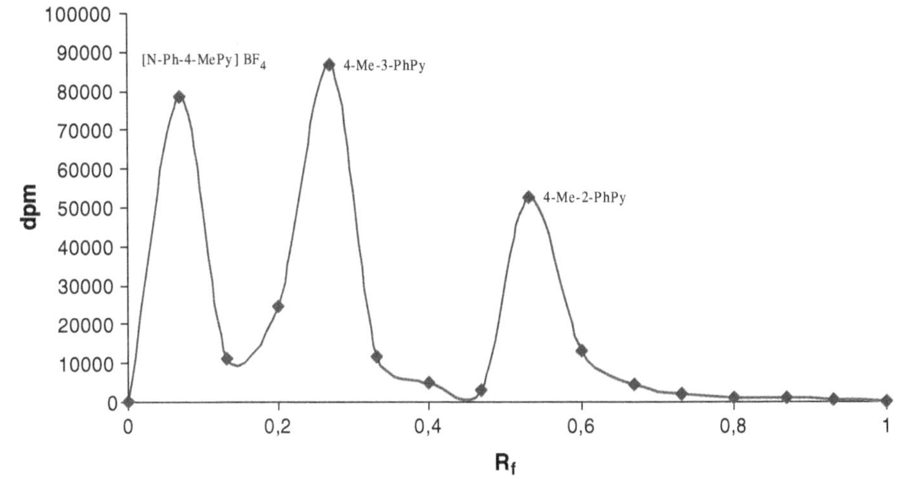

Figure 1 **Radioactivity distribution of tritium-labeled products on the chromatographic plates for the reaction of nucleogenic phenyl cations with 4-picoline.**

previously unknown tetraphenylammonium compounds [23]. Moreover, during classical electrophilic reaction on heterocyclic system deactivation of pyridine ring takes place due to the protonation of nitrogen atom by strong acids used for these reactions [24]. Such process does not exist in the ion–molecular reactions with the nucleogenic phenyl cations.

Formation of some amount of the unidentified products probably may refer to possibility of the interaction of phenyl cations with the methyl group of the heterocyclic ring.

Experimental

General experimental for nuclear-chemical synthesis: All ion–molecular reactions were carried out in sealed glass ampoules containing the source of the phenyl cations (tritiated benzene), the nucleophile of interest (4-picoline) and filled with an inorganic salt to serve as a stabilizing anion (KBF_4). The molar ratio for benzene and substrate was about 1:1000 (1 μL of hexane solution of tritium double-labeled benzene 4 Cu/sm^3 and 5.3 μL of the picoline). The ampoules were sealed cold and kept at 0–5°C during accumulation time (about 1 month). After this period, the radioactivity of the obtained products is enough for the detection. The ampoules were opened, solvent added (acetone), and the mixture subjected to TLC analysis on glass plates (Reverse phase C18 silica, fluorescent indicator, CH_3CN). Radioactivity of the sorbent layer was measured using a scintillation spectrometer RackBeta 1215 (LKB Wallac, Finland).

Table 1 Radiochemical yields of products from the addition and electrophilic substitution reactions with 4-methylpyridine

Substrate	Yield, % (Ad_E)	Yield, % (S_E)		
4-Methylpyridine	25 ± 2.0	Σ 72 ± 1.0		
		o-	*m*-	Unidentified products
		22 ± 3.0	41 ± 2.0	9.0 ± 2.0

Synthetic preparation of *p*-ditritiobenzene

The reaction of catalytic substitution of halogen atoms by tritium in a molecule of *p*-dibromobenzene serves as a basis for synthesis of tritium double-labeled benzene: from 5 mg of dibromobenzene, 6.5 μL thriethylamine diluted in 0.5 mL of hexane (addition of triethylamine is necessary for binding of the formed hydrogen bromide) and 5 Cu of gaseous tritium by hydrogenation at room temperature on 5% $Pd/BaSO_4$ catalyst during 1 h the solution of tritium double-labeled benzene has been obtained. The chemical purity was not less than 99%. The volume specific activity of the synthesized benzene came to 4 Cu/cm^3.

Synthesis of *N*-phenyl-4-picolinium tetrafluoroborate

N-phenyl-4-picolinium tetrafluoroborate was synthesized by a two-step method [25]. The first step was the reaction of 2,4-dinitrobromobenzene with 4-picoline resulting in *N*-(2,4-dinitrophenyl)-4-picolinium salt formation. The last one was converted to *N*-phenyl-4-picolinium tetrafluoroborate by reaction with aniline. *N*-phenyl-4-picolinium tetrafluoroborate was obtained as yellow–orange crystals, m.p. 68–70°C.

General procedure for the synthesis of 2(or 3)-phenyl-4-picoline

A 20-mL Schlenk tube was charged with 2(or 3)-bromo-4-methylpyridine (0.172 g, 1 mmol), phenylboronic acid

(0.146 g, 1.2 mmol), K_2CO_3 (0.276 g, 2 mmol), dioxane (7 mL), water (3 mL), and $PdCl_2(PPh_3)_2$ (0.0071 g, 0.01 mmol, 1 mol% of Pd) under argon. The reaction mixture was placed in a pre-heated oil bath at 150°C and stirred under reflux for 1 h. After this time, the reaction mixture was diluted with 20-mL H_2O and extracted with Et_2O (2 × 10 mL). The combined organic layers were washed with 5% KOH (2 × 5 mL), H_2O (2 × 5 mL), brine (2 × 5 mL), dried over Na_2SO_4 and filtrated through a pad of silica gel. The solvent was removed by evaporation in vacuum.

2-Phenyl-4-picoline

A pale yellow oil was obtained. Yield: 0.156 g (92%). ^1H NMR (acetone-d_6, 400 MHz): 2.39 (s, 3H), 7.12 (d, J = 4.80 Hz, 1H), 7.40 (t, 1H), 7,46 (t, 2H), 7.74 (s, 1H), 8.11 (d, J = 8.08 Hz, 2H), 8.50 (d, J = 4.80 Hz, 1H); Anal. Calcd for $C_{12}H_{11}N$: C, 85.17; H, 6.55; N, 8.28. Found: C, 85.21; H, 6.62; N, 8.17.

3-Phenyl-4-picoline

A pale yellow oil was obtained. Yield: 0.162 g (96%). ^1H NMR (acetone-d_6, 400 MHz): 2.26 (s, 3H), 7.25 (d, J = 4.55 Hz, 1H), 7.37 (d, 2H), 7,40 (t, 1H), 7.47 (t, 2H), 8.37 (s, 1H), 8.41 (d, J = 4.80 Hz, 1H); Anal. Calcd for $C_{12}H_{11}N$: C, 85.17; H, 6.55; N, 8.28. Found: C, 85.26; H, 6.48; N, 8.26.

Conclusions

With the use of nucleogenic phenyl cations, the direct phenylation of nitrogen atom in 4-methylpyridine followed by the formation of tritium-labeled biological marker, i.e., *N*-phenylpicolinium salt has been realized. Investigations of the pathways of ion–molecular interactions of nucleogenic phenyl cations with the nucleophilic centers of 4-picoline have been revealed the unusual electrophilic substitution on both the α- and β-positions of the heterocyclic ring system.

Competing interests

The authors declare that they have no competing interests.

Authors' contributions

All authors have contributed equally to this wok. All authors read and approved the final manuscript.

Acknowledgment

The study was carried out under the support of RFBR, grant number 10-03-00685-a.

Author details

[1]Laboratory of Radiochemistry, Natural Sciences Institute of Perm State University, 4 Genkel St, Perm 614990, Russia. [2]Chemistry Department, St-Petersburg State University, 26 Universitetsky Pr, St-Petersburg, Petrodvorets 198504, Russia. [3]Radiochemistry Department, M. V. Lomonosov Moscow State University, Leninskie Gory, Moscow 119992, Russia. [4]Department of Organic Chemistry, M. V. Lomonosov Moscow State University, Leninskie Gory, Moscow 119992, Russia. [5]Department of Chemistry, James Madison University, Harrisonburg, VA 22807, USA. [6]Department of Organic Chemistry, Perm State University, 15 Bukirev St, Perm 614990, Russia.

References

1. Joule J, Mills K (2000) Heterocyclic chemistry, 4th edn. Blackwell Science, London
2. Katritzky AR, Pozharski AF (2000) Handbook of heterocyclic chemistry. Pergamon, Amsterdam
3. Lukevits E (1995) Pyridine derivatives in the drug arsenal (150 years of pyridine chemistry). Chem Heterocyc Comp 31(6):639–650
4. Pozharskii AF, Soldatenkov AT, Katritzky AR (1997) Heterocycles in life and society. Wiley, New York
5. Tuyun AF, Uslu H (2011) Investigation of picolinic acid extraction by trioctylamine. Int J Chem React Eng 9:A29
6. Hameed S, Saeed M, Khan A, Ahmed M, Nizami SS, Kazmi MH (1994) Synthesis and antibacterial activity of picoline derivatives. J Islamic Acad Sci 7(1):26–29
7. Barbour LJ, Macgillivray LR, Atwood JL (1996) Structural consequences of M-Cl. . .H-N hydrogen bonds in substituted pyridinium salts of the cobalt(II) tetrachloride anion isolated from liquid clathrate media. Supramol Chem 7 (2):167–169
8. Sundararajan C, Falvey DE (2004) C – O bond fragmentation of 4-picolyl- and -methyl-4-picolinium esters triggered by photochemical electron transfer. J Org Chem 69(17):5547–5554
9. Przewloka T, Chen S, Xia Z, Li H, Zhang S, Chimmanamada D, Kostik E, James D, Koya K, Sun L (2007) Application of DMF–methyl sulfate adduct in the regioselective synthesis of 3-acylated indolizines. Tetrahedron Lett 48 (33):5739–5742
10. Darwish ES (2008) Facile synthesis of heterocycles via 2-picolinium bromide and antimicrobial activities of the products. Molecules 13:1066–1078
11. Chen S, Xia Z, Nagai M, Lu R, Kostik E, Przewloka T, Song M, Chimmanamada D, James D, Zhang S, Jiang J, Ono M, Koya K, Sun L (2011) Novel indolizine compounds as potent inhibitors of phosphodiesterase IV (PDE4): structure–activity relationship. Med Chem Commun 2(3):176–180
12. Alptuzun V, Parlar S, Tash H, Erciyas E (2009) Synthesis and antimicrobial activity of some pyridinium salts. Molecules 14:5203–5215
13. Dwoskin LP, Wooters TE, Sumithran SP, Siripurapu KB, Joyce BM, Lockman PR, Manda VK, Ayers JT, Zhang S, Deaciuc AG, McIntosh JM, Crooks PA, Bardo MT (2008) N, N-alkane-diyl-bis-3-picoliniums as nicotinic receptor antagonists: inhibition of nicotine-evoked dopamine release and hyperactivity. JPET 326(2):563–576
14. Grinevich VP, Crooks PA, Sumithan SP, Haubner AJ, Ayers JT, Dwoskin LP (2003) *N-n*-alkylpyridinium analogs, a novel class of nicotinic receptor antagonists: selective inhibition of nicotine-evoked [^{3}H] dopamine overflow from superfused rat striatal slices. JPET 306(3):1011–1020
15. Shchepina NE, Avrorin VV, Badun GA, Lewis SB, Fedoseev VM, Ukhanov SE (2009) The reaction of direct phenylation by nucleogenic cations as a method of synthesis of unknown or complicated tritium labeled compounds. Moscow Univ Chem Bull 64(5):244–248
16. Shchepina NE, Avrorin VV, Badun GA, Alexandrova GA, Ukhanov SE, Fedoseev VM, Boiko II (2009) Preparation of *N*-phenyl-substituted quinolinium derivatives labeled with tritium by chemonuclear synthesis. Chem Heterocyc Comp 45(7):796–801
17. Shchepina NE, Avrorin VV, Badun GA, Fedoseev VM, Lewis SB (2010) New method for the synthesis of difficultly available sterically hindered tritium-labeled pyridinium derivatives. Chem Heterocyc Comp 46:547–552
18. Pausacker KH (1958) Arylation of aromatic compounds. VI Benzoyl peroxide with pyridine and quinoline. Aust J Chem 11(2):200–210
19. Barnes RA, Brody F, Ruby PR (1960) Pyridine and its derivatives. In: Weissberger A, Klingberg A (eds) The chemistry of heterocyclic compounds, V. 1. Interscience Publishers, New York
20. Katritzky AR, Taylor R (1990) Electrophilic substitution of heterocycles: quantitative aspects: Part I. Adv Heterocycl Chem 47:1–75
21. Katritzky AR, Fan WO (1992) Mechanisms and rates of the electrophilic substitution reactions of heterocycles. Heterocycles 34:2179–2229
22. Shchepina NE, Nefedov VD, Toropova MA, Avrorin VV, Gembitzky DS, Lewis SB, Mattson B (1999) Ion molecule reactions of pyridine with free tritiated

phenyl cations generated by the nuclear chemical method. Radiochem (Russ) 41(6):562–565

23. Shchepina NE, Nefedov VD, Toropova MA, Avrorin VV, Lewis SB, Mattson B (2000) Ion-molecular reactions of free phenylium ions, generated by tritium β-decay with group V-VII elements. Tetrahedron Lett 41:5303–5306
24. Traven VF (2004) Organic chemistry: textbook for schools V. 2 Akademkniga, Moscow
25. Coe BJ, Horris JA, Asselbeighs J, Kloys K (2002) Quadratic nonlinear optical properties of *N*-aryl Stilbazolium dyes. Adv Funct Mater 12(2):110–116

2D, 3D-QSAR and docking studies of 1,2, 3-thiadiazole thioacetanilides analogues as potent HIV-1 non-nucleoside reverse transcriptase inhibitors

Shailesh V Jain[1*], Manjunath Ghate[1], Kamlendra S Bhadoriya[2], Sanjaykumar B Bari[2], Amar Chaudhari[2] and Jayshri S Borse[2]

Abstract

Background: The discovery of clinically relevant inhibitors of HIV-RT for antiviral therapy has proven to be a challenging task. To identify novel and potent HIV-RT inhibitors, the quantitative structure–activity relationship (QSAR) approach became very useful and largely widespread technique forligand-based drug design.

Methods: We perform the two- and three-dimensional (2D and 3D) QSAR studies of a series of 1,2,3-thiadiazole thioacetanilides analogues to elucidate the structural properties required for HIV-RT inhibitory activity.

Results: The 2D-QSAR studies were performed using multiple linear regression method, giving $r^2 = 0.97$ and $q^2 = 0.94$. The 3D-QSAR studies were performed using the stepwise variable selection *k*-nearest neighbor molecular field analysis approach; a leave-one-out cross-validated correlation coefficient $q^2 = 0.89$ and a non-cross-validated correlation coefficient $r^2 = 0.97$ were obtained. Docking analysis suggests that the new series have comparable binding affinity with the standard compounds.

Conclusions: This approach showed that hydrophobic and electrostatic effects dominantly determine binding affinities which will further useful for development of new NNRTIs.

Keywords: 1,2,3-Thiadiazole thioacetanilides, QSAR, Docking, HIV-RT inhibitors;*k*-nearest neighbor molecular field analysis (kNN-MFA)

Background

Acquired immunodeficiency syndrome (AIDS), caused by human immunodeficiency virus (HIV) infection, is still one of the most important challenges for the chemotherapy of the early 21st century [1]. The status of the HIV/AIDS epidemic has evolved with time and by many estimates the global adult prevalence of HIV has stabilized at slightly less than 1% of the world population [2]. The number of people living with HIV worldwide continued to grow in 2010, reaching an estimated 33.4 million. The total number of people living with the virus in 2010 was more than 20% higher than the number in 2000, and the prevalence was roughly threefold higher than in 1990. There are about 2.7 million adult and children are newly infected by HIV and about 2 million are died by AIDS [3].

HIV reverse transcriptase (RT) is a DNA polymerase enzyme that converts single-stranded viral genomic RNA into double-stranded DNA. HIV RT is one of the three key enzymes in the HIV life cycle and the primary target of numerous anti-viral drug discovery efforts [4]. Due to the essential role of the HIV RT in the viral replication, the inhibition of RT is regarded as one of the most attractive targets in the anti-HIV chemotherapy [5]. Current anti-AIDS therapy is based on drugs that belong either to the class of nucleoside/nucleotide (NRTIs/NtRTIs) and non-nucleoside reverse transcriptase inhibitors (NNRTIs), protease, or entry inhibitors. NNRTIs are

* Correspondence: shal.jain2007@gmail.com
[1]Institute of pharmacy, Nirma University, Ahmedabad, Gujarat 382481, India
Full list of author information is available at the end of the article

a structurally diverse group of compounds which interact with a specific allosteric non-substrate binding pocket site of HIV-1 RT (non-nucleoside inhibitor binding pocket), leading to a non-competitive inhibition of the enzyme [6]. Association of an NNRTI with the reverse transcriptase is thought to inhibit chain elongation by altering the motions of the protein residues that interact with the nucleic acid chain [7]. NNRTIs are an important part of the successful combination therapy for HIV-1 known as highly active anti-retroviral therapy [8].

Among the structurally diverse HIV-1 NNRTIs, substituted azole-thioacetanilide scaffolds have been of much interest for the development of novel NNRTIs because of their high potency and low toxicity against HIV-1 wild-type and resistant strains. It is worth noting that halogenated phenyl rings were regarded as ubiquitous moieties in numerous NNRTI molecules, and the substitution pattern of halogens has a significant influence on the overall protein–ligand binding affinity and anti-HIV activity [9].

The quantitative structure–activity relationship (QSAR) approach became very useful and largely widespread for the prediction of biological activities, particularly in drug design. This approach is based on the assumption that the variations in the properties of the compounds can be correlated with changes in their molecular features [10].

Thisstudy aimed to elucidate the structural features of 1,2,3-thiadiazole thioacetanilides derivatives required for HIV-RT inhibition and to obtain predictive two- and three-dimensional QSAR (2D- and 3D-QSAR) models. Further, the binding mode of the active molecule with the active site amino acid residues of reverse transcriptase enzyme was performed by docking using Glide XP. It is expected that such 3D-QSARs and ligand–receptor-based molecular docking studies of 1,2,3-thiadiazole thioacetanilides derivatives will provide better tools for rational design of promising HIV-1 NNRT inhibitors having greater therapeutic safety and efficacy.

Experimental methods

All molecular modeling studies (2D and 3D) were performed using the Molecular Design Suite (VLife MDS software package, version 3.5; from VLife Sciences, Pune, India) [11]. Docking studies were carried out using Schrodinger molecular modeling user interface implemented on Acer PC with a Pentium IV processor and Windows XP operating system. The structures of all compounds were sketches in Chem sketch version 12.0 [12]. All structures are cleaned and 3D optimized. Energy minimization and geometric optimization were conducted using the Merck molecular force field method with the root mean square-gradient set to 0.01 kcal/molÅ, and the iteration limit to 10,000. The conformers for all structures are generated and selected the low energy conformer for each compound and used for further study.

2D-QSAR study

Dataset and molecular modeling for 2D-QSAR

The effective concentration data on 1,2,3-thiadiazole thioacetanilides derivatives (Table 1) were taken from the literature [13]. The total set of compounds was divided into a training set (12 compounds) for generating 2D-QSAR models and a test set (10 compounds) for validating the quality of the models. Selection of molecules in the training set and test is a key and important feature of any QSAR model. Therefore, the care was taken in such a way that biological activities of all compounds in test lie within the maximum and minimum value range of biological activities of training set of compounds. The Uni-Column Statistics of test and training sets further reflected the correct selection of test and training sets. A Uni-Column statistics for training set and test set were generated to check correctness of selection criteria for trainings and test set molecules (Table 2).

Table 1 Molecular structures of compounds and their NNRT inhibitory activity

ID	R^1	R^2	X	Y	EC_{50}(μM)	pEC_{50}
7a1	H	H	Cl	H	26.11	4.58
7a4	H	H	Br	H	22.42	4.64
7a5[a]	H	H	Br	CH_3	13.73	4.86
7a6[a]	H	H	Br	$CO_2C_2H_5$	5.21	5.28
7a7	H	H	Br	CO_2CH_3	5.1	5.29
7b1[a]	H	OMe	Cl	H	2.63	5.58
7b2	H	OMe	NO_2	H	0.99	6
7b4[a]	H	OMe	Br	H	3.19	5.49
7b5[a]	H	OMe	Br	CH_3	5.06	5.29
7b6	H	OMe	Br	$CO_2C_2H_5$	3.01	5.52
7b7[a]	H	OMe	Br	CO_2CH_3	2	5.69
7c1	F	F	Cl	H	1.23	5.91
7c2	F	F	NO_2	H	4.14	5.38
7c3[a]	F	F	F	H	5.45	5.26
7c4	F	F	Br	H	2.26	5.64
7c5[a]	F	F	Br	CH_3	1.45	5.83
7d1[a]	Cl	Cl	Cl	H	0.12	6.92
7d2	Cl	Cl	NO_2	H	0.06	7.22
7d3	Cl	Cl	F	H	0.14	6.86
7d4	Cl	Cl	Br	H	0.15	6.82
7d5[a]	Cl	Cl	Br	CH_3	0.2	6.69
7d6	Cl	Cl	Br	$CO_2C_2H_5$	0.1	7

[a]Test compounds set.

Table 2 Uni-column statistics of the training and test sets for QSAR models

Data set	Column name	Average	Max.	Min.	SD	Sum
2D-QSAR						
Training	pEC_{50}(μM)	5.9092	7.2300	4.5800	0.9019	70.9100
Test	pEC_{50}(μM)	5.6940	6.9300	4.8600	0.6500	56.9400
3D-QSAR						
Training	pEC_{50}(μM)	5.8417	7.2300	4.5800	0.7859	105.1500
Test	pEC_{50}(μM)	5.6750	6.9300	4.8600	0.8967	22.7000

The maximum and minimum value in training and test set were compared in a way that:

1 The maximum value of pEC_{50} of test set should be less than or equal to maximum value of pEC_{50} of training set.
2 The minimum value of pEC_{50} of test set should be higher than or equal to minimum value of pEC_{50} of training set.

This observation showed that test set was interpolative and derived within the minimum–maximum range of training set. The mean and standard deviation of pEC_{50} values of sets of training and test provide insights to the relative difference of mean and point density distribution (along mean) of the two sets. *In vitro* effective concentrations (EC_{50}) of the molecules were converted into corresponding pEC_{50} values (Table 1) and used as dependent variables in 2D QSAR calculations.

Descriptor calculation

The basis of energy minimization is that the drug binds to effectors/receptors in the most stable form, i.e., the minimum energy form. 2D-QSAR study requires the calculation of molecular descriptors. A large number of theoretical 2D individual descriptors such as Mol. Wt., Volume, XlogP, smr; physiochemical such as Estate Numbers, Estate contributions, Polar Surface Area, Element Count, Dipole moment, Hydrophobicity XlogpA, Hydrophobicity SlogpA; topological such as T_2_Cl_6, T_C_Cl_6, T_T_S_7, T_T_Cl_7 type have been computed for these geometrically optimized structures from the chemical structures of the compounds referred to above with a view to develop structure–activity relationship of 1,2,3thiadiazole thioacetanilides derivatives against the HIV. A total of 938 descriptors were calculated by QSARPlus module within VLife Sciences Molecular Design Suite. The descriptors having the same value or almost same value or highly correlated with other descriptors were removed initially, as they do not contribute to the QSAR. The reduced set of descriptors was then treated by Forward Stepwise Variable Selection for further reduction of non-significant descriptors and finally the optimum models with four significant descriptors were considered in our 2D-QSAR analysis.

Statistical analysis

The 2D-QSAR model was generated by Multiple Linear Regression (MLRmethod by using V-Life Molecular Design Suite (MDS). It relates the dependent variable $\hat{\mathbf{y}}$ (biological activity) to a number of independent variables x_i (molecular descriptor) by using linear equations. This method of regression estimates the values of the regression coefficients by applying least square curve fitting method. MLR is the traditional and standard approach for multivariate data analysis. Multivariate analysis is the analysis of multidimensional data metrices by using statistical methods. Such data metrices can involve dependent and/or independent variables. For getting reliable results, parameters were set such that the regression equation should generate number of independent variables (descriptors) 5 times less than that of compounds or molecules.

The multiple regression equation takes the form as mentioned in Equation(1)

$$\hat{y} = b_o + b_1x_1 + b_2x_2 + b_px_p \quad (1)$$

where $\hat{y}$ = calculated dependent variable (biological activity pEC_{50})the b_1 to b_p are regression coefficients [contribution of respective descriptors that is x_1 to x_3, x_1 to x_p are independent variables (descriptors) and b_o is a regression constant or intercept].

The program computes the best model on the basis of squared correlation coefficient r^2, crossed validated q^2, which is relative measure of quality of fit, Fischer's value *F*-test which represents *F*-ratio between the variance of calculated and observed activity and pred_r^2. The calculated value of *F*-test when compared with tabulated value of *F*-test shows the level of statistical significance (99.99%) of the QSAR model. The low standard error of pred_r^2 se, q^2_se, and r^2_se shows absolute quality of fitness of the model. The generated QSAR model was validated for predictive ability inside the model by using cross validation (leave-one-out—LOO) for q^2 and external validation, which is more robust alternative method by dividing the data into training set & test set and calculating pred_r^2. The high pred_r^2 and low pred_r^2 se were showed high predictive ability of the model.

The statistical significance of selected 2D-QSAR model was further supported by the 'fitness plot' obtained, this is a plot of observed versus predicted activity of training and test set compounds and provides an idea about how well the model was trained & how well it predicts the activity of the external test set (Figure 1). The contribution chart for the significant model is presented in

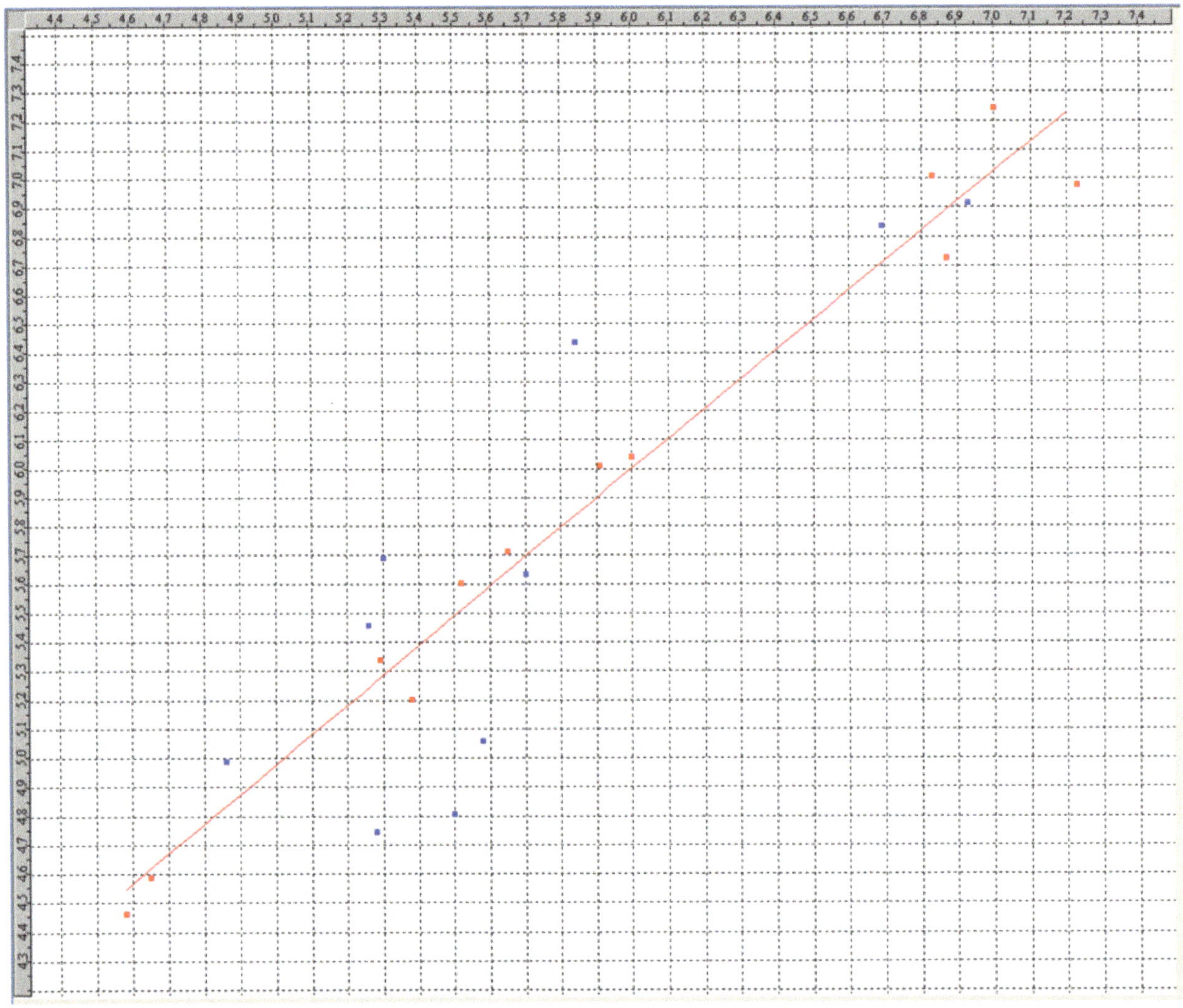

Figure 1 Comparison of observed activity versus predicted activity for training set & test set compounds according to 2D-QSAR model.

Figure 2, which gives the percentage contribution of the descriptors used in deriving the model.

3D-QSAR studies

Data set and molecular modeling for 3D-QSAR

The total set of compounds was divided into a training set (18 compounds) for generating 3D-QSAR models and a test set (4 compounds) for validating the quality of the models. Optimal training and test set were generated using the sphere exclusion (SE) algorithm. The SE method was adopted for division of training and test data set comprising of 18 and 4 molecules, respectively, with dissimilarity value of 13.4 where the dissimilarity value gives the SE radius. The SE method employs the following algorithm: (i) select a point and include it in the training set; (ii) build a sphere with radius *R* with a center in this point; (iii) include all points within the sphere, except for the center, in the test set; (iv) discard all points in the sphere from the initial set; (v) if no points are left, stop, otherwise go to step (i). The most active compound in the dataset is selected as the starting point for building a sphere. Four compounds, namely, 7d1, 7c3, 7a5, and 7c4, were used as test set while the remaining molecules were used as the training set (Table 3). The uni-column statistics of the training and test sets are reported in Table 2.

Alignment procedure

Molecular alignment is a crucial step in 3D-QSAR study to obtain meaningful results. This method is based on moving of molecules in 3D space, which is related to the conformational flexibility of molecules. Energy minimized and geometry optimized structure of molecules were aligned by the template based. In general, geometric similarity should exist between the modeled structures and the bioactive conformation for 3D-QSAR. The

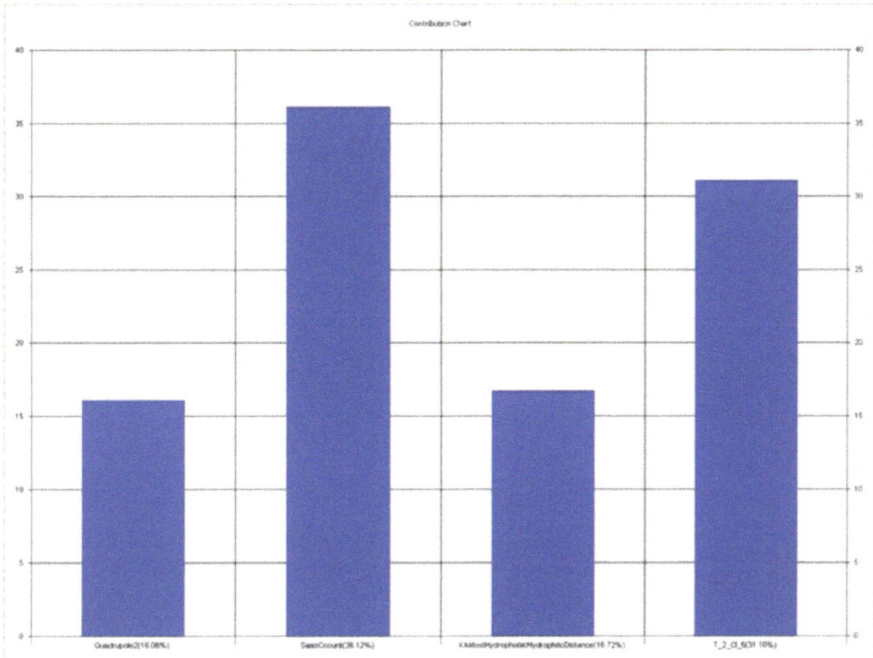

Figure 2 Contribution of descriptors for biological activity developed using MLR equation.

spatial alignment of compounds under study is thus one of the most sensitive and determining factor in obtaining a reliable model. The alignments define the putative pharmacophore for the series of ligands. Alignment of all 22 compounds was done using the template-based alignment by using the most active molecule as reference and 1,2,3-thiadiazole thioacetanilides as a template in MDS; the aligned structures were used for the study. In the template-based alignment, a template structure was defined and used as a basis for alignment of a set of molecules. These aligned conformations were used to generate the predictive QSAR model. Multiple conformation of each molecule was generated using Monte Carlo conformation search method. It is a random search method for finding the conformations of molecules which uses the metropolis condition to accept or discard generated conformers [14].

Descriptors calculation

Using Tripos force field [15] and Gasteiger and Marsili charge type [16] electrostatic, steric and hydrophobic field descriptors were calculated. The dielectric constant was set to 1.0, considering the distance-dependent dielectric function probe setting was carbon atom with charge 1.0. This resulted in calculation of 5,040 field descriptors (1,680 for each electrostatic, steric, and hydrophobic) for all the compounds in separate columns. QSAR analysis was performed after removal of all the invariable columns, as they do not contribute to the QSAR.

3D-QSAR studies were carried out by kNN method using Forward Stepwise Variable Selection as variable selection method. The kNN methodology relies on a simple distance learning approach whereby an unknown member is classified according to the majority of its kNNsin the training set. The nearness is measured by an appropriate distance metrics (e.g., a molecular similarity measure calculated using field interactions of molecular structures). The standard kNN MFA method was implemented simply as follows

1. Calculated distances between an unknown object (u) & all the objects in the training set
2. Select k objects from the training set most similar to object u, according to the calculated distances; and
3. Classify object u with the group to which the majority of the k objects belong. An optimal k value is selected by optimization through the classification of a test set of samples or by leave-one out cross-validation.

The variables and optimal k values were chosen using stepwise variable selection method. This method employs a stepwise variable selection procedure combined with kNN to optimize.

1. The number of nearest neighbors (k) and
2. The selection of variables from the original pool.

The step-by-step search procedure begins by developing a trial model with a single independent variable and

Table 3 Descriptors used in 2D & 3D-QSAR models with values

ID	2D-QSAR descriptors				3D-QSAR descriptors	
	Saas C count	Quadrupole2	T_2_Cl_6	XA most hydrophobic hydrophilic distance	H_171	E_587
7a1	5	16.12701	0	4.951941	0.337546	0.088079
7a4	5	22.34026	0	5.241149	0.340001	0.109635
7a5[a,b]	6	16.34572	0	4.63805	0.353856	0.057851
7a6[a]	6	3.079616	0	4.141958	0.342394	0.136266
7a7	6	−26.8322	0	7.462867	0.334305	0.117725
7b1[a]	6	10.24981	0	5.100435	0.350985	0.049167
7b2	6	30.74947	0	8.220488	0.332967	0.027609
7b4[a]	6	−38.4946	0	5.790629	0.345013	0.141681
7b5[a]	7	12.74566	0	5.113997	0.369819	−0.030558
7b6	7	−41.4985	0	6.625907	0.358049	0.154737
7b7[a]	7	−17.1541	0	5.913619	0.345649	0.196553
7c1	7	−13.5687	0	7.263344	0.368474	−0.008455
7c2	7	−46.9851	0	5.258711	0.329492	−0.064939
7c3[a,b]	7	−13.251	0	5.105986	0.335960	−0.034363
7c4[b]	7	−10.3413	0	5.992268	0.369205	0.042498
7c5[a]	8	−5.89083	0	6.29995	0.398119	0.028883
7d1[a,b]	7	−6.89132	2	6.834099	0.463411	0.019026
7d2	7	18.5915	2	6.196837	0.428789	−0.072705
7d3	7	−9.69926	2	6.197515	0.429396	−0.019153
7d4	7	36.29885	2	5.712653	0.437677	−0.026282
7d5[a]	8	−24.2613	2	4.75547	0.497335	−0.003169
7d6	8	−12.1663	2	5.933494	0.478959	−0.006141

[a]The compounds considered in the test set in 2D QSAR.
[b]The compounds considered in the test set in 3D QSAR.

adds independent variables, one step at a time, examining the fit of the model at each step (using weighted kNN cross-validation procedure). The method continues until there are no more significant variables remaining outside the model. Once the training and test sets are generating, kNN methodology is applied to the descriptors generated over the grid. The steric, electrostatic, and hydrophobic energies are computed at the lattice points of the grid using a methyl probe of charge +1. These interaction energy values are considered for relationship generation and utilized as descriptors to decide the nearness between molecules.

k-Nearest neighbor molecular field analysis (kNN-MFA) models were developed using the Forward Stepwise Variable Selection method with cross-correlation limit set of 1.0 and the term selection criteria as r^2. *F*-test 'in' was set to 4.0. As some additional parameters, variance cutoff was set at 0.000 kcal/molÅ and scaling to none; additionally, kNN parameter setting was done within the range of 2–5 and the prediction method was selected as the distance-based weighted average.

Crossvalidation

The standard LOO procedure was implemented that is a molecule in the training set was eliminated and its biological activity was predicted as the weighted average activity of the *k* most similar molecules (Equation 2)

$$\hat{y}_i = \sum w_i y_i \qquad (2)$$

The similarities were evaluated as the inverse of Euclidean distance between molecules (Equation 3) using only the subset of descriptors

$$v_n$$

$$d_{i,j} = \left[\sum (X_{i,k} - X^2{}_{j,k})\right]^{1/2} \qquad (3)$$

$$k = 1$$

This step was repeated until every molecule in the training set has been eliminated and its activity predicted once. The cross-validation r^2 (q^2) value was calculated using Equation(4) where y_i and $\hat{y}_i$ are the actual and the predicted activities of the ith molecule, respectively, and y_{mean} is the mean of observed activity of all molecules in training set. Both summations are over all molecules in the training set.

$$q^2 = 1 - \frac{\sum(y_i - \hat{y}_i)^2}{\sum(y_i - y_{mean})^2} \quad (4)$$

Since the calculation of the pairwise molecular similarities and hence the prediction was based upon current training set, the q^2 value obtained (0.89) is the indicative power of the current kNN-MFA model. The above steps were repeated for $k = 1$ to 18 (upper limit of k is the total number of molecules in the dataset). The optimum value of k for our training set was found to be 2 (this value led to the highest q^2 value, 0.89).

External validation

The external validation that is predicted r^2 (pred_r^2) value was calculated using the following equation where y_i and $\hat{y}_i$ are the actual and the predicted activities of the ith molecule in the test set, respectively, and y_{mean} is the observed activity of all molecules in training set.

$$pred_{r^2} = 1 - \frac{\sum(y_i - \hat{y}_i)^2}{\sum(y_i - y_{mean})^2} \quad (5)$$

Both the summations are over all the molecules in the test set. The pred_r^2 value is indicative of all the predictive power of the current kNN-MFA model for external test set. The pred_r^2 value of our 3D model was found to be 0.97.

Randomization test

To evaluate the statistical significance of the QSAR model for an actual dataset, we have employed a one-tail hypothesis testing. The robustness of the QSAR models for experimental training sets was examined by comparing these models to those derived for random datasets. Random sets were generated by rearranging biological activities of the training set molecules. The significance of the models hence obtained was derived on calculated Z score [17,18].

Evaluation of model

Developed quantitative model was evaluated using following statistical measures: N, number of observations (molecules) in the training set; Number of nearest neighbors, number of k-nearest neighbor in the model; q^2, cross-validated r^2 (by LOO) which is relative measure of quality of fit; pred_r^2, r^2 for external test set; q^2_se, standard error of cross-validation and pred_r^2 se, standard error of external test set prediction.

The low standard error of pred_r^2 se and q^2_se shows absolute quality of fitness of the model. The high pred_r^2 and low pred_r^2 se were showed high predictive ability of the model.

The q^2 and pred_r^2 values were used as deciding factors in selecting the optimal models.

Docking studies

These studies helped to sort out the designed compounds with good binding affinity against RT enzyme. The molecular docking tool, GLIDE (Schrodinger Inc., USA) software, was used for studying binding modes of the designed compounds in to the binding pocket of RT enzyme. To further understand the binding mode between 1,2,3-thiadiazole thioacetanilides analogs and HIV-1 NNRT, these compounds were docked to the core domain of NNRT. Fine 3D structure with a resolution of 2.65 Å of NNRT was retrieved from the Protein Data Bank (*PDB ID: 1KLM*). Before docking, the protein is prepared by using the protein preparation wizard, removing the water molecules and cofactors from the proteins, optimizing hydrogen bonding and deleting the ligand present in crystal structure.

Results and discussion

2D-QSAR

The various 2D-QSAR models were developed using MLR method. 2D-QSAR equations were selected by optimizing the statistical results generated along with variation of the descriptors in these models. The fitness/pattern plots were also generated for evaluating the dependence of the biological activity on various different types of the descriptors. The frequency of use of a particular descriptor in the population of equations indicated the relevant contributions of the descriptors.

The best regression equation obtained is represented in Equation(6):

$pEC_{50} = 0.607826$ SaasCcount + 0.00878695 Quadrupole2 + 0.478468 T_2_Cl_6 + 0.257279 XAMostHydrophobicHydrophilicDistance + 0.00652846 (6)

The equation explains 97% ($r^2 = 0.97$) of the total variance in the training set. It also has an internal (q^2) and external (pred_r^2) predictive ability of approximately 94 and 62%, respectively. The F-test = 60.77 shows the statistical significance of 99.99% of the model which means that probability of failure of the model is 1 in 10,000. In addition, the randomization test shows confidence of approximately 99.9% that the generated model is not random and hence it is chosen as the QSAR model (Table 4).

The plot of observed versus predicted activity provides an idea about how well the model was trained and how

Table 4 Observed, predicted activity, and residual values of statistically significantly models obtained by MLR & kNN-MFA

ID	Observed activity pEC_{50}	Predicted activity pEC_{50} by MLR	Residual values of pEC_{50} by MLR	Predicted activity of pEC_{50} by kNN-MFA	Residual values of pEC_{50} by kNN-MFA
7a1	4.58	4.46	0.12	4.97	−0.39
7a4	4.64	4.59	0.5	4.94	−0.30
7a5[a,b]	4.86	4.99	0.13	5.08	−0.15
7a6[a]	5.28	4.74	0.46	5.39	−0.11
7a7	5.29	5.33	0.4	4.96	0.33
7b1[a]	5.58	5.05	0.53	5.30	0.28
7b2	6	6.038	−0.38	5.74	0.26
7b4[a]	5.49	4.80	−0.31	5.40	0.9
7b5[a]	5.29	5.68	−0.39	5.65	−0.36
7b6	5.52	5.60	−0.8	5.39	0.13
7b7[a]	5.69	5.63	0.6	5.51	0.18
7c1	5.91	6.01	−0.10	5.57	0.34
7c2	5.38	5.20	0.18	5.60	−0.22
7c3[a,b]	5.26	5.45	0.19	5.34	−0.8
7c4[b]	5.64	5.71	−0.7	5.70	−0.6
7c5[a]	5.83	6.43	0.40	5.75	0.8
7d1[a,b]	6.92	6.92	0	6.84	0.8
7d2	7.22	6.97	0.25	6.85	0.37
7d3	6.86	6.73	0.13	6.91	−0.5
7d4	6.82	7	0.18	6.93	−0.11
7d5[a]	6.69	6.83	−0.14	6.92	−0.23
7d6	7	7.24	−0.24	6.76	0.24

[a]The compounds considered in the test set in 2D QSAR.
[b]The compounds considered in the test set in 3D QSAR.

well it predicts the activity of the external test set. From the plots it can be seen that the model is able to predict the activity of training set quite well (all points are close to regression line) as well as external test set up to 62% (only few points are relatively apart from the regression line) providing confidence in predictive ability of the model (Figure 1).

Interpretation of result

It is apparent from Equation (6) that the descriptor SaasCcount plays a pivotal role in determining activity. This descriptor (SaasCcount) signifies the total number of carbon connected with one single bond along with two aromatic bonds. Positive contribution of this descriptor revealed the increase of anti-HIV activity of 1,2,3-thiadiazole thioacetanilides with presence of more number of carbon connected with single bond along with two aromatic bonds (Figure 2). The positive coefficient of SaasCcount (36%) showed that increase in the values of this descriptor is beneficial for anti-HIV activity (like in compounds 7c1, 7c5, 7d1, 7d2, 7d3, 7d4, 7d5, and 7d6). The next most important factor governing variation in the activity is T_2_Cl_6 (approximately 31%) and is directly proportional to the anti-HIV activity. The descriptor T_2_Cl_6 indicates that the count of number of double-bonded atoms (i.e., any double-bonded atoms, T_2) separated from chlorine atom by six bonds. The descriptor T_2_Cl_6 reveals the importance of chlorine atom at R^2 position to be favorable for the activity. The positive coefficient of T_2_Cl_6 (approximately 31%) showed that increase in the values of this descriptor is beneficial for anti-HIV activity (like in compounds 7d1, 7d2, 7d3, 7d4, 7d5, and 7d6). As a positive contributing descriptor, XAMostHydrophobicHydrophilicDistance [signifies distance between most hydrophobic and hydrophilic point on the Vender Waals (vdW) surface] is also a physico-chemical descriptor influencing activity variation and is directly proportional to activity. The positive coefficient of XAMostHydrophobicHydrophilicDistance (17%) showed that increase in the values of this descriptor is beneficial for anti-HIV activity (like in compounds 7b2, 7c1, 7c5, 7d1, 7d2, and 7d3). The last

Table 5 Statistical results of 2D QSAR equation generated by MLR method and 3D QSAR models generated by forward stepwise variable selection kNN MFA method for 1,2,3-thiadiazole thioacetanilides derivatives

Serial number	Statistical parameter	Results	
		2D QSAR by MLR	3D QSAR by kNN
1	r^2	0.97	–
2	r^2_se	0.19	–
3	q^2	0.94	0.89
4	q^2_se	0.29	0.26
5	pred_r^2	0.62	0.97
6	pred_r^2se	0.43	0.15
7	*F*-test	60.77	–
8	*N*	12	18
9	Nearestneighbor	–	2
10	Degree of freedom	7	15
11	Contributing descriptors	SaasCcount (36.12%) Quadrupole2 (16.06%)T_2_Cl_6 (16.72%) XAMostHydrophobicHydrophilicDistance(31.10%)	H_171 (0.429396, 0.437677) E_587 (−0.026282, −0.019153)

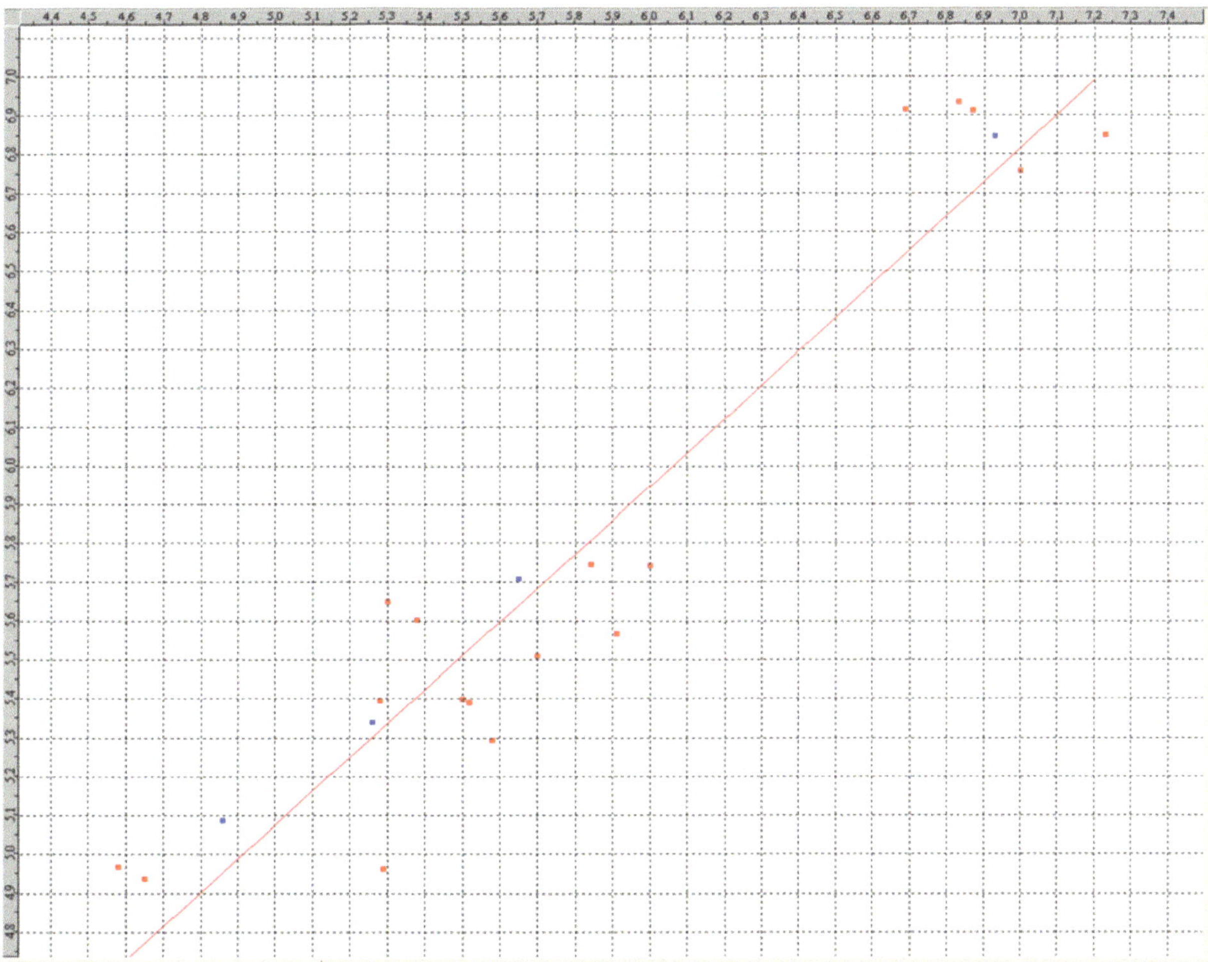

Figure 3 Comparison of observed activity versus predicted activity for training set and test set compounds according to 3D-QSAR model.

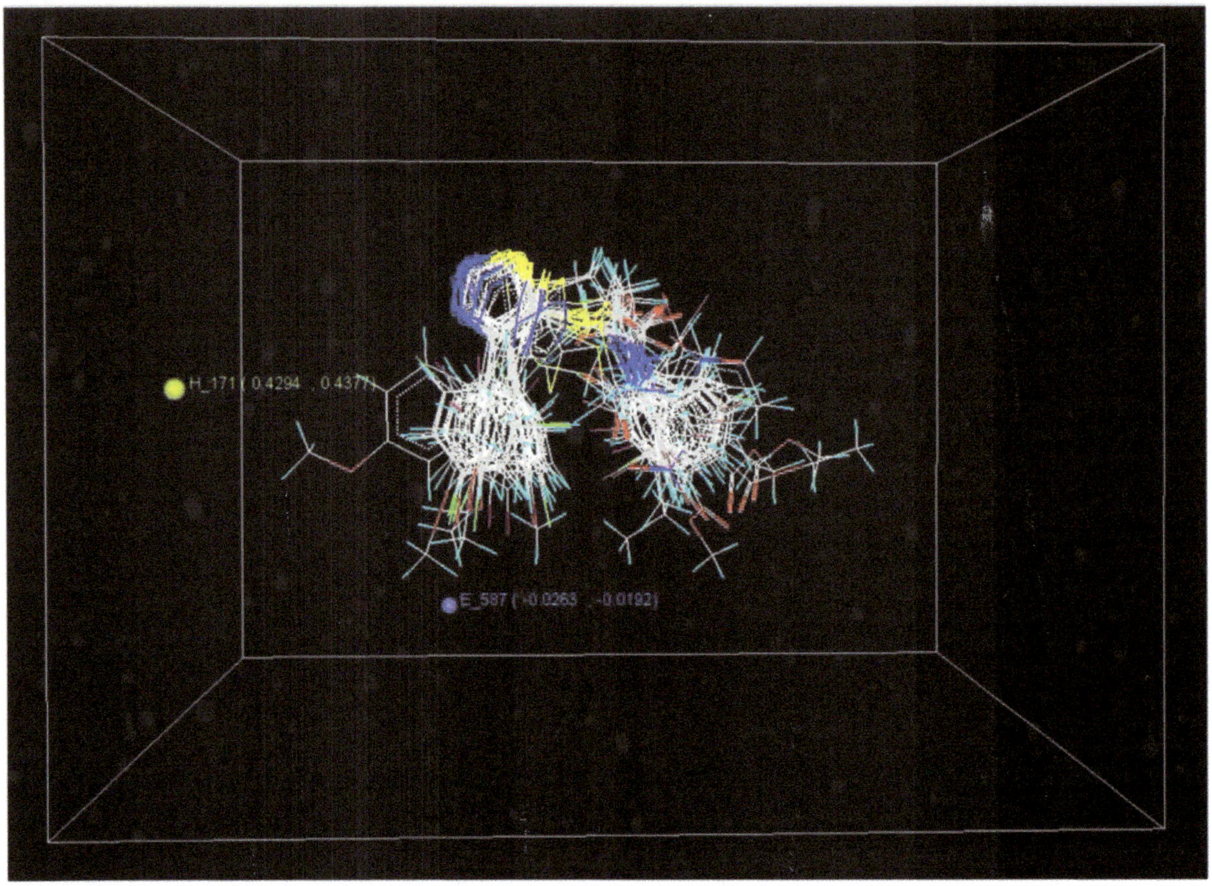

Figure 4 Stereo view of the molecular rectangular field grid around the superposed molecular units of 1,2,3-thiadiazole thioacetanilides series of compounds using SW-kNN MFA method.

descriptor is Quadrupole2 which shows the importance of magnitude. This descriptor is an individual descriptor that signifies magnitude of second tensor of quadrupole moments positively contributes to the biological activity (16%). The positive coefficient of Quadrupole2 showed that increase in the values of this descriptor is beneficial for anti-HIV activity (like in compounds 7b2, 7d2, and 7d4).

3D-QSAR

For 3D-QSAR, a kNN-MFA of 1,2,3-thiadiazole thioacetanilides derivatives with reported activities against HIV was prepared. Several 3D-QSAR models were generated using stepwise variable selection method resulted several statistically significant models, of which the corresponding best model is reported herein. 3D-QSAR model was selected based on the value of statistical parameters and the best kNN-MFA 3D-QSAR model with 18 training set compounds have a $q^2 = 0.89$ and $pred\_r^2 = 0.97$.

The kNN-MFA QSAR method explores formally the active analog approach which implies that compounds display similar profiles of pharmacological activities. In this method, the activity of each compound is predicted as average activity of k most chemically similar compounds from the dataset. The predictive ability of this Forward Stepwise Variable Selection kNN-MFA model was evaluated by predicting the biological activities of the test set molecules. Residuals values obtained by subtraction of predicted activities from biological activities were found near to zero. Therefore, it was concluded that the resultant QSAR model have good predictive ability. The actual, predicted activities,and residuals of both training and test sets molecules are given in Table 5. The plots of observed versus predicted activity of both training and test sets molecules helped in cross-validation of kNN-MFA QSAR model are depicted in Figure 3.

The model selection criterion is the value of q^2, the internal predictive ability of the model and that of $pred\_r^2$, the ability of the model to predict the activity of external test set. For anti-HIV activity, selected model was found to be statistically most significant, especially with respect to the internal predictive ability ($q^2 = 0.89$) of the model. As the cross-validated correlation coefficient (q^2) is used

Table 6 Results of molecular docking

Serial number	ID	G-Score	LipophilicEvdW	H-bond	Electro
1	7d1	−12.29	−7.22	−0.65	0.01
2	Efavirenz	−11.61	−5.59	−0.7	−0.21
3	7c5	−11.29	−6.7	−0.7	−0.36
4	7c4	−11.17	−6.53	−0.7	−0.35
5	7d3	−11.09	−7.6	−0.51	−0.11
6	7d4	−10.97	−7.99	0	−0.11
7	7c3	−10.95	−6.51	−0.7	−0.2
8	7d6	−10.9	−6.79	−0.7	−0.37
9	7c1	−10.83	−6.21	−0.7	−0.33
10	7b4	−10.81	−6.13	−0.68	−0.21
11	Zidovudine	−10.81	−3.68	−2.17	−0.47
12	7b1	−10.75	−6.03	−0.7	−0.25
13	7b2	−10.75	−6.77	−0.57	0.12
14	7d5	−10.6	−6.93	−0.7	−0.38
15	7b5	−10.46	−6.17	−0.6	−0.2
16	7b6	−10.38	−6.65	−0.7	−0.36
17	7a7	−10.33	−6.74	−0.7	−0.3
18	7b7	−10.15	−6.58	−0.7	−0.25
19	7a1	−10.15	−5.46	−0.61	−0.19
20	7c2	−10.13	−6.27	−0.67	−0.16
21	7a5	−10.05	−6.67	−0.7	−0.44
23	7a4	−9.98	−6.52	−0.7	−0.37
24	7a6	−9.92	−7.37	0	−0.11
25	Delavirdine	−9.89	−7.63	−1.27	−0.74
26	7d2	−9.47	−6.98	0	−0.05
27	Nevirapine	−6.59	−4.88	0	−0.1

as a measure of reliability of prediction, the correlation coefficient suggests that our model is reliable and accurate. A dataset of 4 compounds was selected as the test set from the original data of 22 compounds for the validation experiments. The predicted versus the experimental selectivity values for the training and test sets are depicted in Figure 3. The value of pred_r^2 was obtained for the test set and gave better results, with a value of 0.97, which means 97% predictive power for the external test set. Thus, our model displays good predictivity in regular crossvalidation (Table 4).

In 3D-QSAR studies, 3D data points generated 1,2,3-thiadiazole thioacetanilides pharmacophore were used to optimize the electrostatic and hydrophobic requirements of the 1,2,3-thiadiazole thioacetanilides nucleus for the anti-HIV activity. The range of property values in the generated data points helped for the design of NCEs. These ranges were based on the variation of the field values at the chosen points using the most active molecule and its nearest neighbor set. The points generated in SW-kNN MFA 3D-QSAR model are H_171 (0.429396, 0.437677) and E_587 (−0.026282, −0.019153) that is hydrophobic and electrostatic interaction field at lattice points 171 and 587, respectively (Figure 4). These points suggested the significance and requirement of hydrophobic and electrostatic properties as mentioned in the ranges in parenthesis for SAR and maximum biological activities of 1,2,3-thiadiazole thioacetanilides analogues.

From 3D-QSAR model, it is observed that electrostatic descriptor like E_587 (−0.026282, −0.019153) with negative values is near from R_2 position of the 1,2,3-thiadiazole thioacetanilides ring. This indicates that electronegative groups are favorable on this site and presence of electronegative groups increases the activity of 1,2,3-thiadiazole thioacetanilides analog. Most potent compounds (compounds 7d1, 7d2, 7d3, 7d4, 7d5, and 7d6) with higher activity having electronegative substitution (Cl) at the R_2 position of the 1,2,3-thiadiazole thioacetanilides ring strongly support the above statement. The negative values of electrostatic descriptors suggested the requirement of electronegative group like NO_2, SO_2R, CN, SO_2Ar, COOH, F, Cl, Br, I, COOR, OR, OH at the position of generated data point E_587 (−0.026282, −0.019153) around 1,2,3-thiadiazole thioacetanilides pharmacophore for maximum activity.

The presence of hydrophobic descriptor H_171 with positive values is also near from the R_1 position of the 1,2,3-thiadiazole thioacetanilides ring which indicates that more hydrophobic substituents are favorable on this site and presence of more hydrophobic substituents increases the anti-HIV activity of 1,2,3-thiadiazole thioacetanilides compounds. Therefore, more hydrophobic substituents such as $-C_6H_{11}$, $-C_6H_5$, $-C(CH_3)_3$, $-CF_3$,$-CH_3$, etc., were preferred at the position of generated data point H_171 around 1,2,3-thiadiazole thioacetanilides pharmacophore.

Molecular docking studies

The docking score in terms of G-Score (GLIDE Score), Emodel, and other results of docking studies of designed compounds of TTA series are presented in Table 6.

G-score

The scoring function of GLIDE docking program is presented in the G-score form. The G-score indicates the binding affinity of the new compound to the receptor/enzyme.

The G-score of the standard compound zidovudine and efavirenz was found to be −10 and −11.61, respectively. The G-score of the series compounds 7c5, 7c4, 7d3, 7d4, 7c3, 7d6, 7c1, 7b4 was found to be more than zidovudine,and the 7d1 having highest G-score −12.29 which is more than efavirenz. The close analysis of these

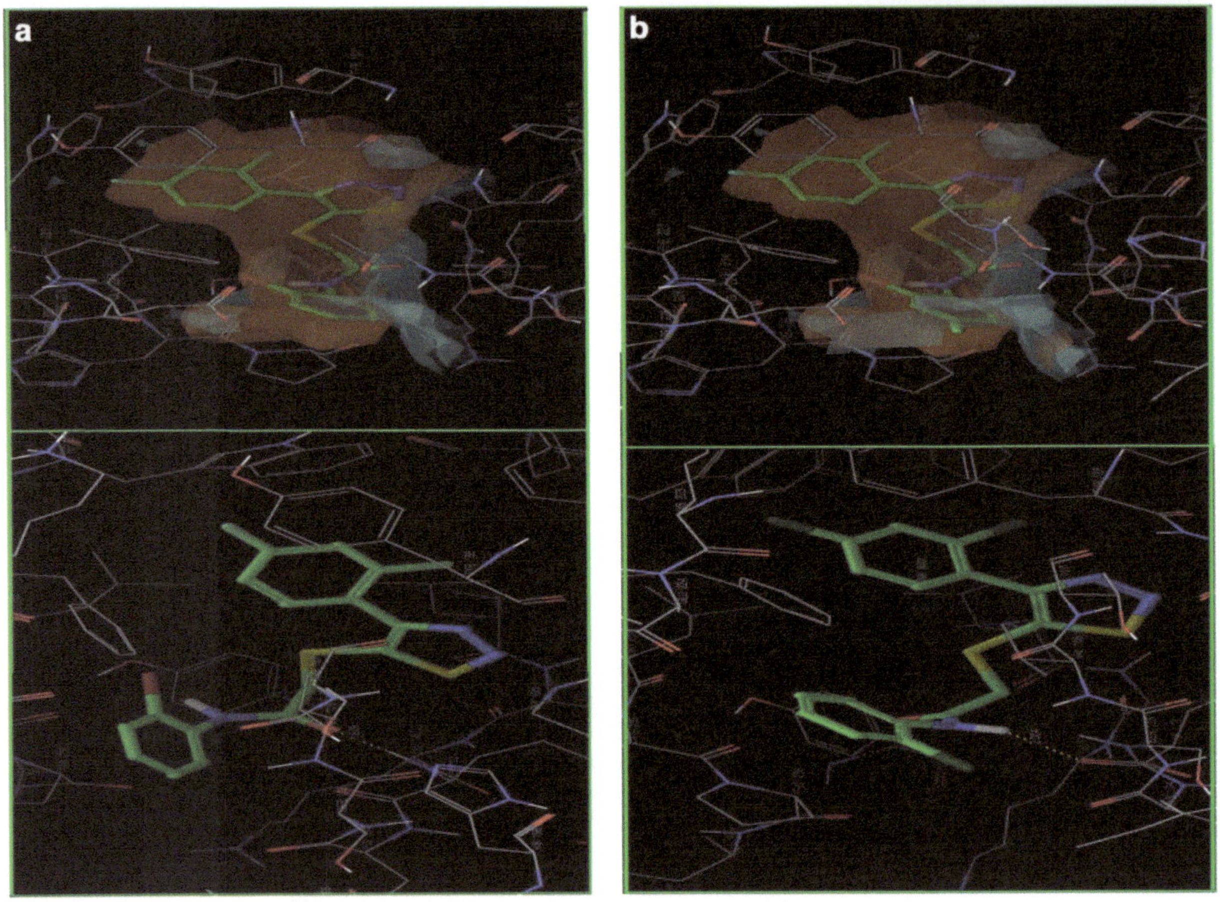

Figure 5 Binding interaction of compounds with NNRT receptors. (**a**) Compounds 7c4 interacting with NNRT receptor protein of PDB *1KLM*. (**b**) Compounds 7c5 interacting with NNRT receptor protein of PDB *1KLM*. Dotted yellow bond showing H-bond interactions with binding site residues. Grey surface showing lipophilic interaction and brown color showing electrostatic interactions.

results suggests that the new series have comparable G-score with the standard compounds.

H-bond

H-bond is one of the most widely used parameter for the evaluation of the docking results, as it is an influential parameter in the activity of the drug compound. The number of H-bond interactions in the standard compounds was compared with that of new series. The number of compounds shows a good H-bond interaction. Figure 5 has shown that compounds 7c5 and 7c4 show good H-bonding interaction with LYS102, LYS104, and LYS103 residues of NNRT, respectively.

vdWinteraction

The contacts are represented in the form of vdWinteraction.

- Good vdW interactions.
- Bad vdW interactions.
- Ugly vdW interactions.

The developed molecules show good number of vdW interaction. The molecule 7d1 shows highest lipophilic character −7.22 which is higher than standard compound efavirenz which show −5.59 only. The molecules 7c5,7c4, 7d3, 7d4, 7c3, 7d6, 7c1, 7b4 having optimum lipophilicity which is greater than standard compound zidovudine.

Conclusions

Our aim in this study was to biologically evaluate a series of analogs of 1,2,3-thiadiazole thioacetanilides by modifying systematically the molecule, in order to explore the SAR of these derivatives. In order to determine the better structural characteristics that were able to improve the anti-HIV-1 activity of this class of NNRTIs and to investigate the effects of different chemical modifications on the RT inhibition, an extensive SAR was examined by varying the nature and the position of the substituents both on the basic moiety. Positive values in hydrophobic field descriptor indicated the requirement of positive hydrophobic potential for enhancing the biological activity of 1,2,3-thiadiazole thioacetanilides analog. Series compounds 7c5, 7c4, 7d3, 7d4, 7c3, 7d6, 7c1, 7b4 showing good binding affinity as compared to standard drugs which revealed that the nature of the substituent and substitution pattern on the basic ring may have a considerable impact on the NNRTIs activity of the synthesized compounds.

Competing interests

The authors declare that they have no competing interests.

Acknowledgements

The authors are thankful to the principal of R. C. Patel Institute of Pharmaceutical Education & Research for providing the facilities to carry out the study.

Author details

[1]Institute of pharmacy, Nirma University, Ahmedabad, Gujarat 382481, India. [2]R. C. Patel Institute of Pharmaceutical Education and Research, Shirpur, Dhule District, Maharashtra 425405, India.

References

1. San-Felix A, Perez-Perez M, Gago F (2006) Dimerization inhibitors of HIV-1 reverse transcriptase, protease and integrase. Antiviral Res 71:260–267
2. Fader LD, Bethell R, Bonneau P, Bös M, Bousquet Y, Cordingley MG, Coulombe R, Deroy P, Faucher AM, Gagnon A, Goudreau N, Grand-Maître C, Guse I, Hucke O, Kawai SH, Lacoste JE, Landry S, Lemke CT, Malenfant E, Mason S, Morin S, O'Meara J, Simoneau B, Titolo S, Yoakim C (2011) Discovery of a 1,5-dihydrobenzo[b][1,4]diazepine-2,4-dione series of inhibitors of HIV-1 capsid assembly. Bioorg Med Chem Lett 21:398–404
3. AIDS Epidemic Update: November 2009, UNAIDS/WHO. http://www.unaids.org
4. Liu B, Lee Y, Zou J, Petrassi MH, Joseph RW, Chao W, Michelotti EL, Bukhtiyarova M, Springman EB, Dorsey BD (2010) Discovery and SAR of a series of 4,6-diamino-1,3,5-triazin-2-ol as novel non-nucleoside reverse transcriptase inhibitors of HIV-1. Bioorg Med Chem Lett 20:6592–6596
5. Sahlberg C, Zhou XX (2008) Development of non-nucleoside reverse transcriptase inhibitors for anti-HIV therapy. Anti-Inf Age Med Chem 7:101–117
6. Barreca ML, Rao A, De Luca L, Iraci N, Monforte AM, Maga G, Clercq ED, Pannecouque C, Balzarini J, Chimirri A (2007) Discovery of novel benzimidazolones as potent non-nucleoside reverse transcriptase inhibitors active against wild-type and mutant HIV-1 strains. Bioorg Med Chem Lett 17:1956–1960
7. Tang G, Kertesz DJ, Yang M, Lin X, Wang Z, Li W, Qiu Z, Chen J, Mei J, Chen L, Mirzadegan T, Harris SF, Villaseñor AG, Fretland J, Fitch WL, Hang JQ, Heilek G, Klumpp K (2010) Exploration of piperidine-4-yl-aminopyrimidines as HIV-1 reverse transcriptase inhibitors. N-phenyl derivatives with broad potency against resistant mutant viruses Bioorg Med Chem Lett 20:6020–6023
8. Zhan P, Liu XY, Li ZY, Fang ZJ, Pannecouque C, Clercq ED (2010) Synthesis and biological evaluation of a new series of 2-{[4-(3,4-Dichlorophenyl)-1,2,3-thiadiazol-5-yl]sulfanyl}acetanilides as HIV-1 inhibitors. Chem Biodivers 7:1717–1727
9. Zhan P, Liu X, Li Z, Fang Z, Li Z, Wang D, Pannecouque C, Clercq ED (2009) Novel 1,2,3-thiadiazole derivatives as HIV-1 NNRTIs with improved potency: synthesis and preliminary SAR studies. Bioorg Med Chem Lett 17:5920–5927
10. Darnag R, Mazouz ELM, Schmitzer A, Villemin D, Jarid A, Cherqaoui D (2010) Support vector machines: development of QSAR models for predicting anti-HIV-1 activity of TIBO derivatives. Eur J Med Chem 45:1590–1597
11. VLife MDS 3.5 (2004) Molecular Design Suite. Vlife Sciences Technologies Pvt. Ltd, Pune, India, www.vlifesciences.com
12. (2009) Advanced chemistry development inc./Chemsketch ver. 12.0
13. Zhan P, Liu X, Cao Y, Wang Y, Pannecouque C, Clercq ED (2008) 1,2,3-Thiadiazole thioacetanilides as a novel class of potent HIV-1 non-nucleoside reverse transcriptase inhibitors. Bioorg Med Chem Lett 18:5368–5371
14. Metropolis N, Rosenbluth AW, Rosenbluth MN (1953) Equation of state calculations by fast computing machines. J Chem Phys 21:1087–1092
15. Clark M, Cramer RD III, Van ON (1989) Validation of the general purpose tripos 5.2 force field. J Comput Chem 10:982–1012
16. Gasteiger J, Marsili M (1980) Iterative partial equalization of orbital electronegativity—a rapid access to atomic charges. Tetrahedron 36:3219–3228
17. Zheng W, Tropsha A (2000) Novel variable selection quantitative structure–property relationship approach based on the k-nearest-neighbor principle. J Chem Inf Comput Sci 40:185–194
18. Shen M, LeTiran A, Xiao Y, Golbraikh A, Kohn H, Tropsha A (2002) Quantitative structure–activity relationship analysis of functionalized amino acid anticonvulsant agents using k-nearest neighbor and simulated annealing PLS methods. J Med Chem 45:2811–2823

19

Cannabinoid receptor type 2 (CB2)-selective *N*-aryl-oxadiazolyl-propionamides: synthesis, radiolabelling, molecular modelling and biological evaluation

Thomas Rühl[1], Winnie Deuther-Conrad[1], Steffen Fischer[1], Robert Günther[1], Lothar Hennig[2], Harald Krautscheid[3] and Peter Brust[1*]

Abstract

Background: The endocannabinoid system is involved in many physiological and pathological processes. Two receptors (cannabinoid receptor type 1 (CB1) and type 2 (CB2)) are known so far. Many unwanted psychotic side effects of inhibitors of this system can be addressed to the interaction with CB1. While CB1 is one of the most abundant neuroreceptors, CB2 is expressed in the brain only at very low levels. Thus, highly potent and selective compounds for CB2 are desired. *N*-aryl-((hetero)aromatic)-oxadiazolyl-propionamides represent a promising class of such selective ligands for the human CB2. Here, a library of various derivatives is studied for suitable routes for labelling with ^{18}F. Such ^{18}F-labelled compounds can then be employed as CB2-selective radiotracers for molecular imaging studies employing positron emission tomography (PET).

Results: By varying the *N*-arylamide substructure, we explored the binding pocket of the human CB2 receptor and identified 9-ethyl-9*H*-carbazole amide as the group with optimal size. Radioligand replacement experiments revealed that the modification of the (hetero)aromatic moiety in 3-position of the 1,2,4-oxadiazoles shows only moderate impact on affinity to CB2 but high impact on selectivity towards CB2 with respect to CB1. Further, we could show by autoradiography studies that the most promising compounds bind selectively on CB2 receptors in mouse spleen tissue. Molecular docking studies based on a novel three-dimensional structural model of the human CB2 receptor in its activated form indicate that the compounds bind with the *N*-arylamide substructure in the binding pocket. ^{18}F labelling at the (hetero)aromatic moiety at the opposite site of the compounds via radiochemistry was carried out.

Conclusions: The synthesized CB2-selective compounds have high affinity towards CB2 and good selectivity against CB1. The introduction of labelling groups at the (hetero)aromatic moiety shows only moderate impact on CB2 affinity, indicating the introduction of potential labelling groups at this position as a promising approach to develop CB2-selective ligands suitable for molecular imaging with PET. The high affinity for human CB2 and selectivity against human CB1 of the herein presented compounds renders them as suitable candidates for molecular imaging studies.

Keywords: Cannabinoid receptors, Molecular modelling, Autoradiography, ^{18}F labelling, Molecular imaging, PET, Neuroimaging

* Correspondence: p.brust@hzdr.de
[1]Department of Neuroradiopharmaceuticals, Institute of Radiopharmacy, Research Site Leipzig, Helmholtz-Zentrum Dresden-Rossendorf e.V., Permoserstr. 15, Leipzig 04318, Germany
Full list of author information is available at the end of the article

Background

The role of the endocannabinoid system in specific CNS disorders is related to the regulation of the temporal dynamics of neurotransmitter release by the retrograde cannabinoid signalling network [1]. Mediated by the G protein-coupled cannabinoid receptors [2], the release of endogenous or the administration of exogenous ligands affects both the long-term synaptic plasticity as well as the short-term regulation of synaptic transmission [1,3]. Two types of specific cannabinoid receptors have been cloned so far, termed cannabinoid receptor type 1 (CB1) and type 2 (CB2) [2,4]. The existence of additional cannabinoid-binding receptors has been suggested [5,6]. In contrast to classical neurotransmitters, endocannabinoids function as retrograde synaptic messengers which are released from postsynaptic neurons, diffuse across synapses, activate CB1 on presynaptic axons and eventually suppress neurotransmitter release [7]. In addition, endocannabinoids and their receptors control the decision about survival or death of neuronal cells [8], such that the pharmacological manipulation of this system might provide either neuroprotective or pro-apoptotic effects. A therapeutic role of cannabinoids has also been suggested for mood disorders [9], traumatic brain injury [10,11] and tumour treatment [12,13]. The development of CB2-selective anticancer agents is regarded to be advantageous in light of unwanted central effects exerted by binding of those agents to CB1 [14].

CB1 is abundantly expressed in the central nervous system and has been thoroughly investigated on cellular [15] and functional levels [16,17] in the brain. In contrast to this, only few and, to some extent, ambiguous data are available regarding CB2 expression and function in the brain. Initial reports stated that CB2 is mainly expressed peripherally in the cells and organs of the immune system such as the B lymphocyte-enriched marginal zone of the spleen or the cortex of lymph nodes [4,18]. However, more recent studies have proven structural and functional CB2 expression in primed glial (as reviewed in [5]) or neural progenitor cells [19]. Moreover, CB2 mRNA was detected in mouse [20] and rat cerebellum [21]. It could be shown in immunostaining studies that CB2 protein is abundant under basal conditions in neuronal and glial processes in the cerebellum and hippocampus of mouse and rat [22-24]. As reviewed recently by Atwood and Mackie [25], a growing number of reports substantiate a neuronal expression of CB2 through immunohistochemical data. Thus, it has been described that the activation of microglia is paralleled by an increase in CB2 immunoreactivity in the injured brain [26]. For instance, significantly increased CB2 expression levels were observed in severe Alzheimer's disease [27]. This indicates that CB2 expressed in the cerebellum might be involved in the pathogenesis of various neurodegenerative disorders and therefore might represent an interesting target for the diagnostics and therapy of such diseases [14,28]. Consequently, detailed investigation of the functional changes of both receptor subtypes CB1 and CB2 is needed to achieve a better understanding of the endocannabinoid system and the effects of potential cannabinoid therapeutics in the normal and diseased human brain [29].

Despite numerous *in vitro* approaches to directly identify CB2 in the brain, a non-invasive and quantitative analysis of these receptors *in vivo* has not been reported to date, probably due to the lack of ligands applicable for molecular imaging approaches such as positron emission tomography (PET). Recently, in a microPET study in a rat model, Evens et al. [30] observed specific binding of the type 2 cannabinoid receptor PET tracer [^{11}C]NE40. In this model, hCB2 receptors were locally overexpressed in the brain after stereotactic injection of an adeno-associated viral vector (AAV2/7) encoding hCB2R with a point mutation (Asp80Asn) in the right striatum, yet the quantitative analysis of these receptors in native brain tissue remains a challenge.

Although CB2 has been already mentioned as a valuable biomarker of, e.g. neuroinflammation [30], the quantitative imaging of this target requires PET radioligands with superior affinity and specificity towards the low-abundance cerebral CB2 [31]. The [^{11}C]-methoxy-labelled potent inverse CB2 agonist Sch225336 [32] showed only poor brain uptake in mice under baseline conditions. Various ^{18}F-fluoroethoxy- [33] and [^{11}C]-methoxy-labelled [34] 2-oxoquinoline derivatives were suggested as CB2 PET radioligands too, yet unfavourable brain-to-plasma ratios reflect the need for further improvement(s) regarding CB2 imaging in the healthy brain as recently reviewed [35].

Methods

Here, we extend the synthesis of various CB2-binding [36] *N*-aryl-((hetero)aromatic)-oxadiazolyl-propionamides as potential PET imaging compounds. Guided by molecular docking studies employing a novel comparative model of the human CB2 receptor, the promising site for ^{18}F labelling was selected. *In vitro* binding experiments using human CB2-transfected Chinese hamster ovary (CHO) cells were performed. The obtained affinity data are in good agreement with predicted binding strength and could be verified by autoradiographic studies on mouse spleen slices.

Results and discussion

Synthesis of *N*-aryl-((hetero)aromatic)-oxadiazolyl-propionamides

The substituted 1,2,4-oxadiazolyl-propionamides synthesized in this study are compiled in Scheme 1.

As depicted in Scheme 2, the two-step synthesis starts from a properly substituted nitrile and hydroxylamine yielding the hydroxy-amidin derivative. Following the route described by Cheng at al. [36], the products were dried after dilution with methylene chloride, and succinic acid anhydride was added to give the 3-phenyl-subsituted 1,2,4-oxadiazole acids. To support the formation of the oxadiazole acids, 0.1 eq. KF was added except for the compound with R^1 = Br and R^2 = F. In this case, the free 3-phenyl-substituted 1,2,4-oxadiazol-5-yl propanoic acid was protected, employing (diazomethyl)trimethylsilane. Subsequently, Br was substituted with CN by addition of 4.2 eq. KCN. Deprotection with LiOH yielded then the product. In a final step, the so obtained differently substituted 3-((hetero)aromatic)-1,2,4-oxadiazol-5-yl-propanoic acids were coupled to various arylamides using standard (dimethylamino)-pyridine (DMAP)-catalysed carbodiimide chemistry. The obtained products were isolated either by semi-preparative high-performance liquid chromatography (HPLC) or crystallization (details can be found in the 'Experimental' section).

To suggest potential radiolabelling schemes of the compounds suitable for molecular imaging studies by PET, several strategies were evaluated, which are given in Scheme 3. For instance, **5e** was synthesized by methylation of **4e** with methyl iodide. This approach opens the way to introduce, for example, ^{11}C or ^{18}F by N-alkylation into the final compound. A further approach is the use of prosthetic groups, such as the introduction of fluorine-substituted alkyl chains via hydroxyl groups. In this study, **6k** was synthesized from **6j** by adding 1-fluoro-2-iodoethane. ^{18}F can then be introduced into the molecule by using ^{18}F-labelled alkylating agents. Another approach for the synthesis of ^{18}F-labelled compounds is the replacement of fluorine with ^{18}F via [2.2.2]cryptand chemistry, which is shown in this study as an example in the 'Radiochemistry' section.

Figure 1 shows the single-crystal X-ray structure of compound **6f**. As expected, the amide bond of this molecule (C5-N3 in Figure 1) is in *trans* configuration. Though several bonds in **6f** are freely rotatable, the structure is planar. Thus, the dihedrals of the planes defined by the ring systems are 8.16(9)° between rings A and B and 11.2(1)° between rings B and C.

In vitro binding studies

The specific binding of [^{3}H]CP55,940 towards cell membranes obtained from CHO cells stably transfected with

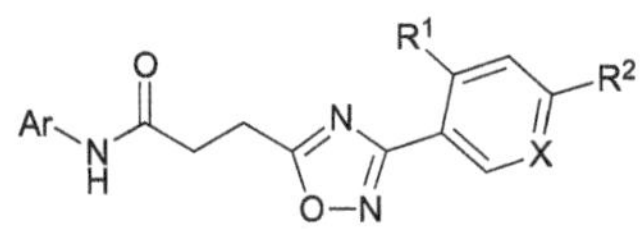

Compound	Ar	R¹	R²	X
1a	Y¹	CN	F	CH
1b	Y¹	CH	F	N
2a	Y²	CN	F	CH
2b	Y²	CH	F	N
2c	Y²	H	Br	N
3b	Y³	CH	F	N
4e	Y⁴ᵃ	Br	F	CH
5e	Y⁴ᵇ	Br	F	CH
6a	Y⁴ᶜ	CN	F	CH
6b	Y⁴ᶜ	CH	F	N
6c	Y⁴ᶜ	H	Br	N
6d	Y⁴ᶜ	F	NO_2	CH
6e	Y⁴ᶜ	Br	F	CH
6f	Y⁴ᶜ	CN	NO_2	CH
6g	Y⁴ᶜ	Br	NO_2	CH
6h	Y⁴ᶜ	F	F	CH
6i	Y⁴ᶜ	F	NH_2	CH
6j	Y⁴ᶜ	OH	F	CH
6k	Y⁴ᶜ	OCH_2CH_2F	F	CH
6l	Y⁴ᶜ	OCH_3	F	CH
6m	Y⁴ᶜ	Br	OCH_3	CH
7h	Y⁵	F	F	CH

Ar

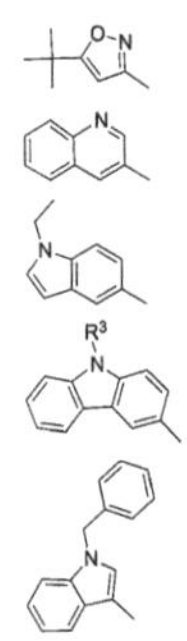

Y¹

Y²

Y³

Y⁴ᵃ R^3= H

Y⁴ᵇ R^3= CH_3

Y⁴ᶜ R^3= CH_2CH_3

Y⁵

Scheme 1 ***N*-aryl-((hetero)aromatic)-oxadiazolyl-propionamides synthesized in this study.**

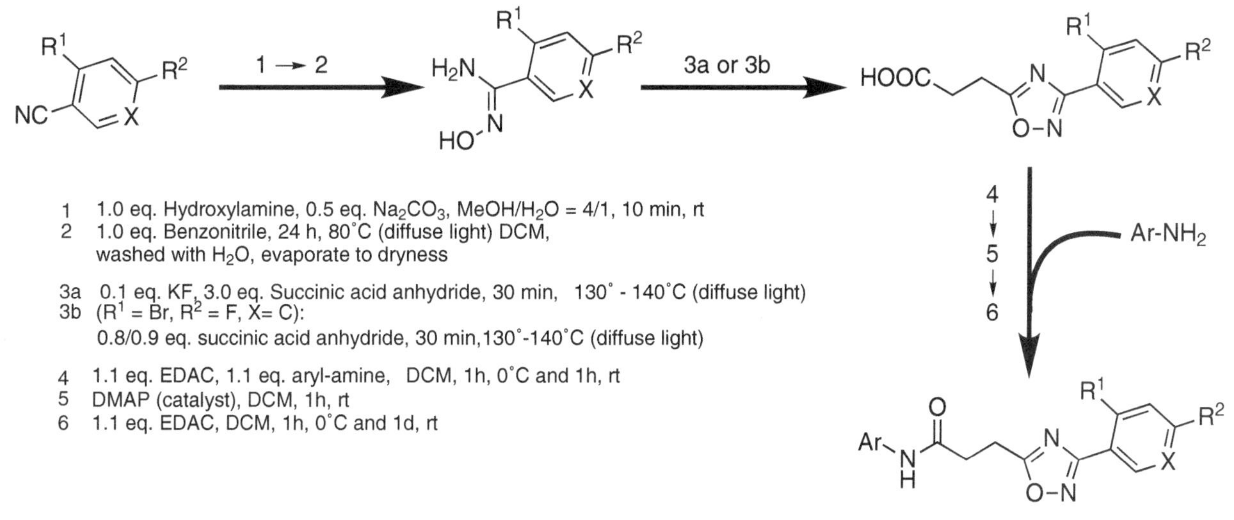

Scheme 2 Synthesis of *N*-aryl-((hetero)aromatic)-oxadiazolyl-propionamides.

human CB1 (hCB1-CHO) or CB2 (hCB2-CHO) hCB-CHO accounted for 40% to 50% of total binding. Non-specific binding was related mainly to binding to the glass fibre (data not shown). For the binding of [^{3}H]CP55,940 towards hCB1-CHO and hCB2-CHO cell membranes, K_D values of 2.43 ± 1.89 nM (n = 3) and 1.48 ± 0.88 nM (n = 4) were determined in competitive binding experiments, which correspond with recently published data [37,38]. Kinetic analysis of the binding of [^{3}H]CP55,940 towards hCB2-CHO cell membranes revealed the rate constants k_{on} = 0.266 × 10^9 M^{-1} min^{-1} and k_{off} = 0.196 min^{-1}. The accordingly estimated K_D value of 0.73 nM is consistent with the data obtained by saturation assay. The inhibition constants (K_i) for each of the human CB receptors are compiled together with reference compounds CP55,940, SR144528, and SR141716A in Table 1. In Figure 2, the inhibition curves of **6f** and **6h** on the hCB2-CHO cell homogenates obtained in the radioligand displacement experiments with [^{3}H]CP55,940 are given as examples.

The data on the hCB2 affinity and selectivity of the synthesized compounds are in good agreement with the results published by Cheng et al. [36] and are consistent with the therein reported potencies of similar compounds. For compound **6a** (compound 44 in [36]), very high potency with an EC50 value of 0.85 nM was obtained by functional cAMP assays. Taken together with the high affinity measured for **6a** (K_i = 6.98 nM), it is obvious that the efficacy of this compound is mainly caused by the strength of the direct physical interaction with CB2. Thus, the K_D values can be seen as a direct measure of the activity of the compounds under investigation.

As the data in Table 1 show, the variation of the arylamide moiety has a significant impact on the affinity

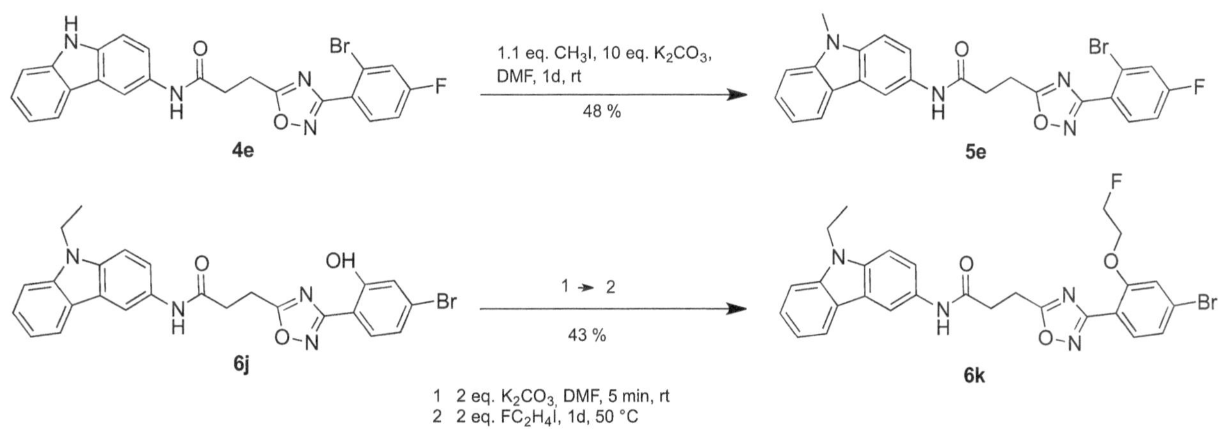

Scheme 3 Two strategies to introduce fluorine into the molecule, allowing labelling with ^{18}F.

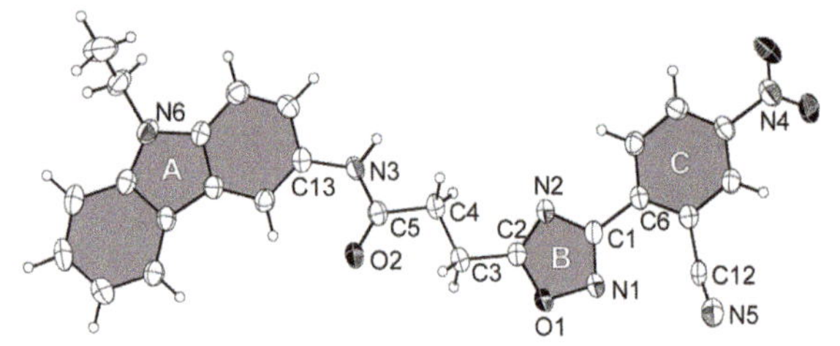

Figure 1 X-ray crystal structure of 6f (50% thermal ellipsoids). The planar ring systems have been noted by A, B and C and are highlighted in grey.

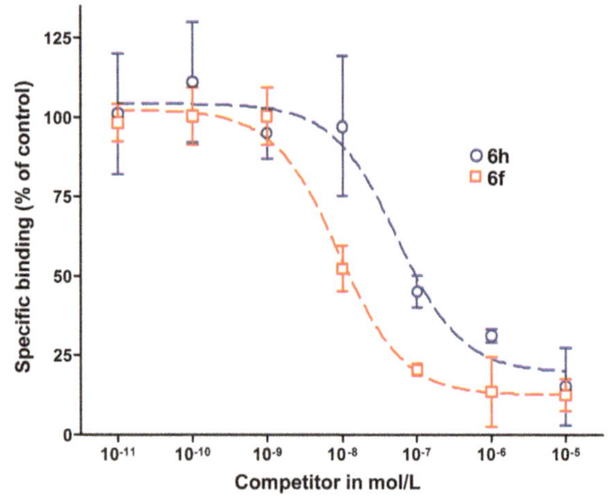

Figure 2 Radioligand displacement study of 6f and 6h against [^{3}H]CP55,940 on membrane homogenates of hCB2-CHO cells.

towards the cannabinoid receptors. The compounds with carbazolamides (Y^4 in Scheme 1) show, on average, the highest affinity to hCB2. The 5-*tert*-butyl-isoxazol-3-yl derivative **1a** shows high affinity too, while a quinoline substitution (Y^2 in Scheme 1) results in less favourable properties. The approximately 100-fold lower hCB2 affinity of the 3-substituted quinoline **2a** is in good agreement with published efficacy data, where a 6-substituted quinoline shows an approximately 50-fold lower [36] efficacy in comparison to **6a**. The situation is completely different for CB1. Here, replacement of the carbazole group with a smaller moiety results in a strong loss of affinity towards the hCB1 receptor. For compounds **2c**, **2b** and **2a**, binding on the hCB1 receptor could not be observed. Weak affinity towards hCB1 could be observed for **7h**, which bears a benzyl-substituted indole at the left-hand side. Remarkably, the affinity towards hCB2 is lost in comparison to **6h** despite the identical 2,4-diflourophenyl moieties at the 3-position of the oxadiazole ring. While the majority of the compounds bind to hCB2, those with an unsubstituted nitrogen in the ring system (aryles Y^1, Y^2, Y^{4a} in Scheme 1) show no binding to hCB1 at all. In general, the affinity of all compounds towards hCB1 is much lower than that towards hCB2. This might indicate a different binding mode of **6h** and **7h** at hCB2.

Table 1 Affinities in nM and selectivity of the tested compounds towards hCB1 and hCB2 expressed in CHO cells

Compound	hCB1	hCB2	Selectivity[a]
1a	>10^5	14.4	
1b	>10^5	>10^5	
2a	>10^5	722	
2b	>10^5	2,290	
2c	>10^5	>10^5	
3b	>10^5	>10^5	
4e	>10^5	>10^5	
5e	>10^5	250	
6a	>10^5	6.98	
6b	1,560	135	1.06
6c	>10^5	1,920	
6d	7,470	12.5	2.78
6e	>10^5	4.27	
6f	>10^5	5.89	
6g	397	2.38	2.22
6h	>10^5	39.4	
6i	>10^5	>10^5	
6j	>10^5	5,710	
6k	>10^5	3,190	
6l	>10^5	223	
6m	>10^5	>10^5	
7h	6,010	>10^5	
CP55,940	2.43	1.27	0.28
SR141716A	1.26	n.d.[b]	
SR144528	n.d.[b]	12.0	

[a]As calculated by pK_i (CB2) – pK_i (CB1) with pKi = -log (Ki); [b]., not determined.

Comparing the compounds with the highest affinity (**6g**) and the best specificity for hCB2 (**6e**), the cause of this seems to be encoded in the functional group at *para*-position of the phenyl group. In concordance with published data [36], a fluorine atom at this position increases the affinity and efficacy towards hCB2. Depending on its electronegativity, a second substituent at *ortho*-position shows a significant impact on the affinity as shown in Figure 3. While the introduction of -Br (**6e**) or -CN (**6a**) leads to a higher affinity, the $-OCH_3$ (**6l**) or $-OCH_2CH_2F$ (**6k**) substituents decrease the affinity. Interestingly, replacement of the methoxy group with a hydroxyl moiety (**6j**) results in a further loss of affinity.

Autoradiographic studies

For further investigation of the CB2 affinity of the test compounds, a preliminary autoradiographic investigation of the displacement potential of reference and test compounds on mouse spleen tissue co-incubated with [^{3}H]CP55,940 has been performed. Figure 4 shows representative autoradiograms of coronal mouse spleen sections incubated with 6 nM [^{3}H]CP55,940 in the presence of 1 μM of test compounds **6a**, **6e** and **6h**. For comparison, the autoradiograms for CP55,940, the CB1-selective antagonist SR141716A, and the CB2-selective antagonist SR144528 are shown in Figure 4b. As visible in Figure 4a, the distribution of [^{3}H]CP55,940 was heterogeneous within the coronal spleen sections, showing a pattern similar to that reported previously [18,39]. Accordingly, high-density (HD) and low-density (LD) regions were assumed to reflect binding sites in the white or the red pulp, respectively.

To estimate the displacement efficacy of the reference and test compounds, the intensity of the radioligand binding in the HD regions was chosen to assess total binding of [^{3}H]CP55,940. Specific binding of [^{3}H] CPCP55,940 was calculated by subtracting the intensity of the homogenous binding of [^{3}H]CP55,940 determined in the presence of 1 μM CP55,940 from the total binding values determined in the absence or presence of 1 μM compound. Accordingly, a high degree of specific binding of [^{3}H]CP55,940 in mouse spleen has been identified, which accounts for approximately 90% of total [^{3}H] CP55,940 binding. The density of specific binding sites of 6 nM [^{3}H]CP55,940 in mouse spleen, estimated by converting the photostimulated luminescence per square millimetre values to femtomoles per milligram wet weight using [^{3}H] standards, resembles, with 150 ± 25 fmol/mg wet weight, the values reported for the binding of 10 nM [^{3}H]CP55,940 in rat spleen (59 to 108 fmol/mg wet weight) [18]. The assignment of the [^{3}H]CP55,940 binding sites in mouse spleen to either CB1 or CB2 has been obtained by co-incubating the tissue with [^{3}H]CP55,940 and either the CB1-selective SR141716A or the CB2-selective SR144,528 antagonist. As visible in the panels of Figure 4, co-incubation with 1 μM SR144528 displaced 78% of the specific binding of 6 nM [^{3}H]CP55,940, while nearly no displacement has been detected in the presence of 1 μM SR141716A. In the latter, 94% of the specific CP55,940 binding remained. Thus, the basal binding of [^{3}H]CP55,940 in mouse spleen was identified to reflect mainly CB2 binding, and the experimental conditions in this autoradiographic study are suitable to assess the CB2 binding potential of the test compounds.

At 1 μM, **6a**, **6e**, and **6h** displaced 83%, 71%, and 66% of the specific binding of 6 nM [^{3}H]CP55,940 respectively, and these data correlate to the rank order of CB2 affinity obtained on hCB2-CHO cells (K_i = 4.27, 6.98 and 39.4 nM, respectively). However, the displacement potential of the three compounds in mouse spleen is slightly lower than that calculated according to the Gaddum equation, based on which a fractional occupancy of 98%, 97% and 83%, respectively, of [^{3}H]CP55,940 binding sites has been estimated (*cf.* 'Experimental' section). This difference between experimental and calculated data might reflect the previously reported non-significant variances between affinity values obtained on native tissue by *in vitro* autoradiography and in radioligand displacement studies using transfected cells [40]. Alternatively, as

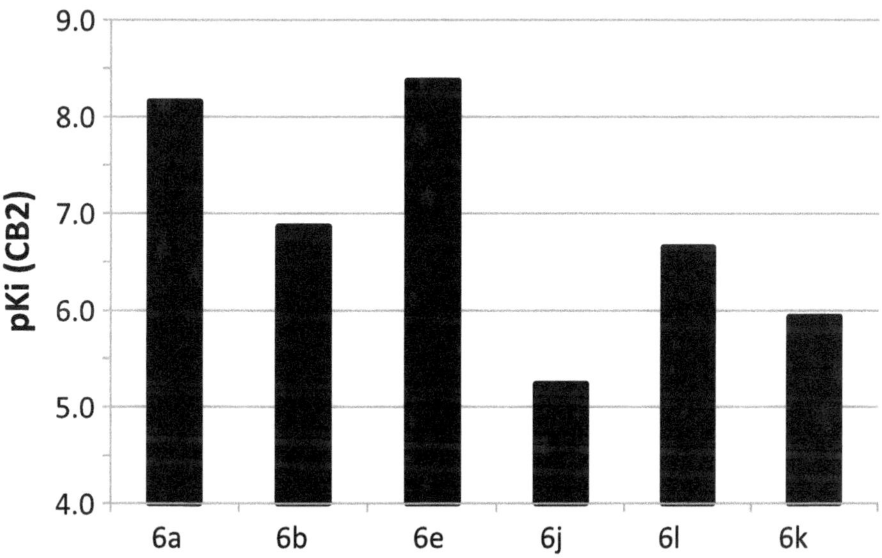

Figure 3 Influence of substitution at ring C (*cf.* Figure 1) on affinity towards hCB2. The pK_i values were calculated according to pK_i = −log (K_i). High pK_i values represent high affinity.

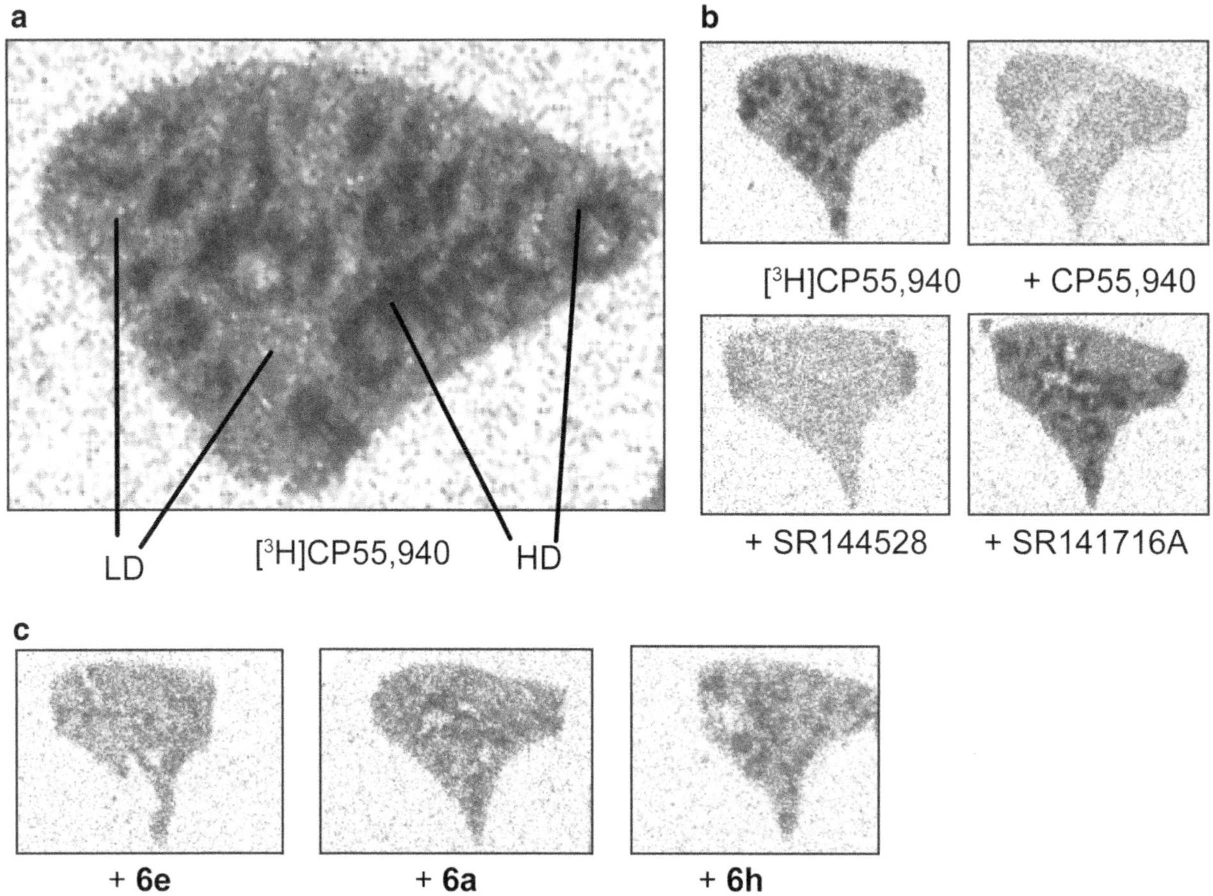

Figure 4 Autoradiogram of representative coronal sections of CD-1 mouse spleen tissue. (**a**) Incubated with 6 nM [^{3}H]CP55,940. HD binding and LD binding represent the white and the red pulp, respectively (*cf.* text). (**b**) Incubation with 1 μM selective antagonists for CB2 (SR144528) and CB1 (SR141716A). (**c**) Compounds **6e**, **6a** and **6h** compete at 1 μM with the binding of [^{3}H]CP55,940 on CB2 in good agreement with the determined binding data: **6e** > **6a** > **6h**.

shown for the binding of WIN55,212-2 towards [^{3}H] CP55,940-labelled mouse or human CB2, species differences might also explain the slightly distinct affinity of the studied compounds [41].

Molecular modelling

In order to gain more insight into the binding of the herein synthesized compounds towards hCB2, we performed molecular modelling studies. As no experimentally determined structures of cannabinoid receptors are available yet, we created a three-dimensional (3D) structure model of this G protein-coupled receptor (GPCR) by comparative modelling. Based on the results obtained by a sequence search with the BLAST server, the 3D structure of the human beta1-adrenergic receptor (bAR1) [PDB:2Y00] [42] was identified as the structure with the highest sequence similarity to the hCB2 sequence. However, during the course of this study, a GPCR structure with a bound agonist was published [43]. In comparison to the bAR1 structure [PDB:2Y00], which is crystalized with a bound inverse agonist, this novel structure is more opened and thus represents a better description of a GPCR in an active state. Thus, the X-ray structure of the human A2A adenosine receptor with UK-432097 ([PDB:3QAK]) [43] was chosen as the template for comparative modelling. The co-crystalized ligand of this structure was kept in place during the building process of the receptor model to ensure a state ready to host an agonist. Figure 5 shows the constructed 3D model of the human CB2 with the proposed binding pocket. In agreement with mutagenesis data compiled by Poso and Huffman [44], residues known to be involved in the binding of CP55,940 are accessible in our model.

The results of the docking of **6a**, **6e** and **6h** are shown in Figure 6. The pose with the lowest predicted binding energy is shown in green. In the majority of the predicted poses, the molecules are bent and deviated significantly from a planar structure, which was observed for

6f in the single crystal. However, the bound conformation of a ligand is not necessarily identical to that of the free molecule in solution or in a packed crystal. Moreover, due to thermal effects, several differently populated conformations might exist. Typically, molecular docking procedures deliver multiple suggestions for the binding geometry of a ligand in a protein-ligand complex. Identifying the native pose out of these suggestions is often challenging, especially, if no experimentally determined reference structure is available. By taking into account the computed binding energy, it is possible to weight the suggested poses employing Boltzmann statistics.

In Figure 6 this is illustrated by encoding the energy in the visibility of the molecule according to the method implemented in the program PostDock [45]. While for **6h** only one representative pose was predicted, for **6a** and **6e**, two and three lower populated binding modes were found, respectively. This is illustrated by the blue shades in Figure 6, which represent the less favourable poses of these compounds. Nevertheless, in all cases, the three compounds bind primarily with their arylamide moiety inside the binding pocket. A detailed analysis of the binding site revealed a hydrophobic microdomain at the bottom of the pocket. The comparison of **6a** with **5e** indicates that a substituent at the N atom of the ring system increases the affinity towards CB2. If such a substituent is missing like in **4e**, no binding at hCB2 could be observed (data not shown). However, a replacement with a longer or bulkier moiety reduces the binding affinity too, as it is visible from the data obtained for **7h**. As illustrated in Figure 7, the preferred binding of **7h** is with the arylamide moiety outside the binding pocket, which, together with the determined binding data, substantiates a different binding mode of this compound. Thus, the 9-ethyl-9*H*-carbazole group seems to have an optimal size for fitting into the CB2 binding pocket.

The low nanomolar affinity of **6a** (K_i = 6.98 nM), **6e** (K_i = 4.27 nM) and **6h** (K_i = 39.4 nM) towards the human CB2 and the more than 1,000-fold selectivity over hCB1 (K_i > 1 μM) make these fluorine-substituted analogues the currently most promising candidates for further development of PET imaging agents within the series investigated. A proposed labelling at *p*-position of the phenyl group at the right-hand site seems to be favourable, e.g. the replacement of fluorine by ^{18}F would allow applying these compounds for molecular imaging of CB2 receptors.

Radiochemistry

The labelling with ^{18}F was performed exemplarily on **6g**, yielding [^{18}F]-**6e**, since **6e** has been identified as highly selective for hCB2 with a high affinity of K_i = 4.27 nM (Scheme 4). ^{18}F was introduced by microwave-assisted nucleophilic substitution of the 4-NO_2 moiety employing [2.2.2]cryptand (Kryptofix®, VWR International GmbH, Darmstadt, Germany). The electron-withdrawing effect (–I effect) of the Br substituent in *meta*-position to the leaving group -NO_2 enables the nucleophilic attack.

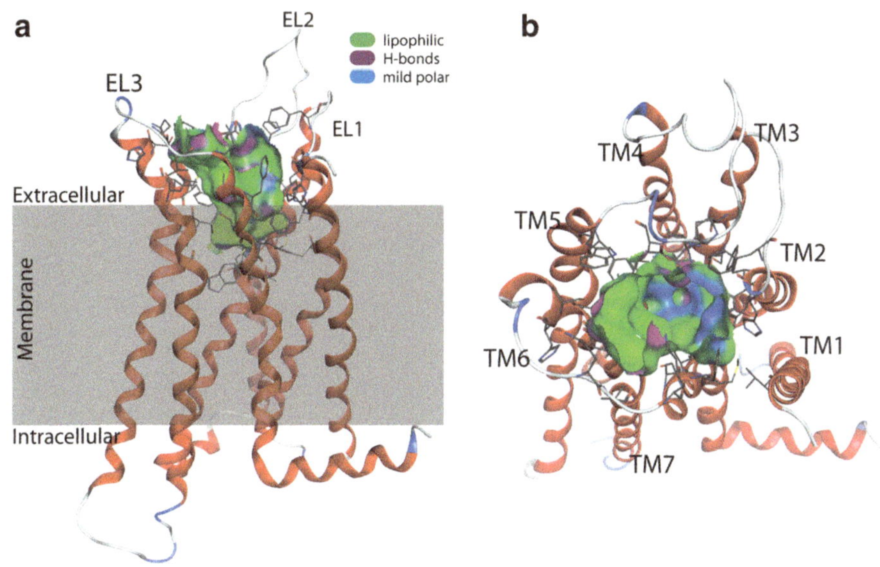

Figure 5 Model of the human cannabinoid receptor type 2. (**a**) Side view with the proposed transmembrane region shaded in grey. The protein is shown with the N-terminus at the top. (**b**) Top view from the extracellular space. The extracellular loops and the transmembrane helices are labelled to guide the reader. Only the residues forming the binding pocket are shown. The binding pocket identified by the Site Finder module of MOE (Chemical Computing Group Inc., Montreal, Canada) is shown as a surface with colour-coded features: H bonding (magenta), lipophilic (green), mild polar (blue).

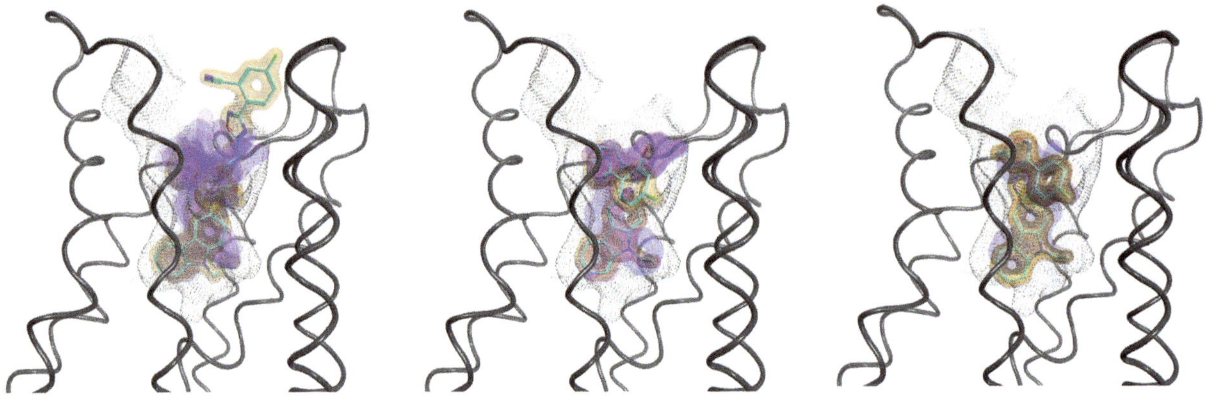

Figure 6 Predicted binding modes of 6e, 6a, 6h to human CB2 model after docking with GOLD. All compounds bind with their carbazole moiety (ring A, *cf.* Figure 1) in the binding pocket indicated by black dots. The figure was created with the software MOE (Chemical Computing Group Inc., Montreal, Canada) using the module PostDock [45]: The visibility of the surfaces is proportional to their binding energies based on Boltzman statistics. The surfaces are colour-coded with respect to the rmsd difference to the ligand with the lowest binding energy (from yellow to blue). As reference, the best-docked ligand is shown with cyan sticks.

However, this electron-withdrawing effect might not be strong enough as the reaction delivered only poor yields (3% radiochemical yield). An introduction of nitrogen into the aromatic ring should facilitate the nucleophilic substitution. Thus, the pyridine equivalent **6c** was labelled with ^{18}F under comparable conditions (Scheme 4). Though not supported by a further electron-withdrawing substituent, the radiochemical yield is significantly higher with 28%. Unfortunately, compounds with a pyridine moiety as ring C show only low affinity towards hCB2, as visible in Table 1 (compounds **1b, 2b, 2c, 3b, 6b, 6c**).

Experimental

Chemistry

All reagents were commercially obtained[a] and used without further purification unless otherwise stated. Anhydrous solvents were transferred via an oven-dried syringe or cannula. Flasks were oven-dried under vacuum and cooled under a constant stream of nitrogen. ^{1}H, ^{13}C, and ^{19}F nuclear magnetic resonance (NMR) spectra were recorded on VARIAN GEMINI 2000 (200 MHz for ^{1}H NMR, 50 MHz for ^{13}C NMR, 188 MHz for ^{19}F NMR; Palo Alto, CA, USA), VARIAN 'MERCURY plus' (300 MHz for ^{1}H NMR, 75 MHz for ^{13}C NMR, 228 MHz for ^{19}F NMR) and VARIAN 'MERCURY plus' and BRUKER DRX-400 (400 MHz for ^{1}H NMR, 100 MHz for ^{13}C NMR, 367 MHz for ^{19}F NMR; Billerica, MA, USA). The chemical shifts are reported relative to the residual solvent peak, which was used as an internal reference (chemical shifts in δ values, J in Hz). The following abbreviations were used to describe peak splitting patterns when appropriate: br = broad, s = singlet, d = doublet, t = triplet, q = quartet, m = multiplet, dd = doublet of doublet, ddd = triplet of doublet, pt = pseudo-triplet. High-resolution mass spectrometry (MS) was performed on a Bruker Daltonics APEX II FT-ICR, and low-resolved mass spectra (using electrospray ionization (ESI)) were recorded on a Bruker ESQUIRE. Reactions involving moisture-sensitive reactants were performed in oven-dried glassware under an atmosphere of nitrogen, reactants being added via a syringe. Flash column chromatography was performed on

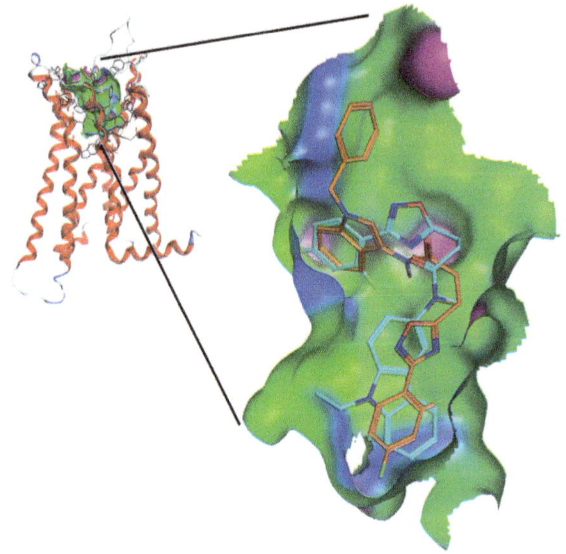

Figure 7 Comparison of the predicted binding modes of 7h and 6h to the human CB2 model. 6h (cyan) binds with the carbazole moiety in the binding pocket. For **7h** (orange), the preferred binding is with ring A pointing outside of the cavity. This figure was created using MOE (Chemical Computing Group Inc., Montreal, Canada).

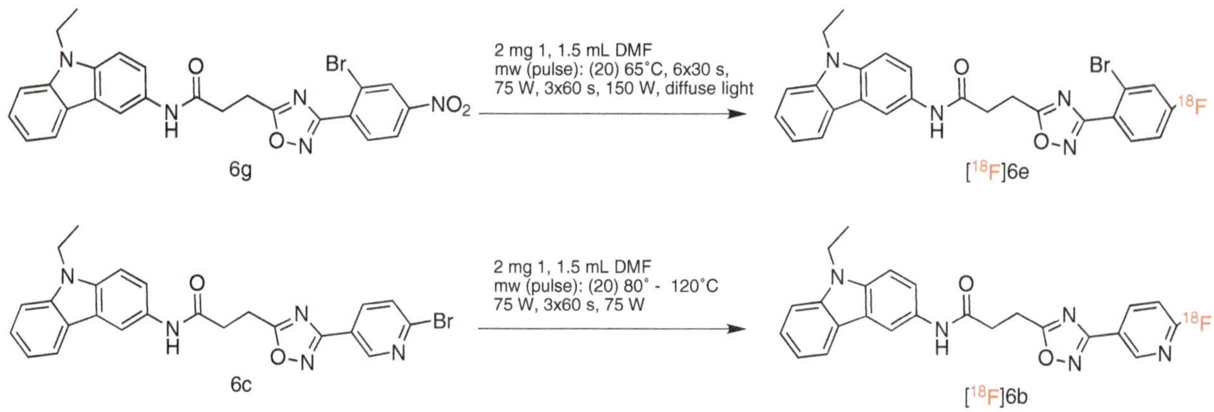

Scheme 4 Radiochemistry.

silica gel (VWR, 60 Å, 40 to 63 µm, VWR GmbH, Darmstadt, Germany) and analytical thin-layer chromatography (TLC) on pre-coated silica gel plates (Roth, 60 Å, F254, 0.25 mm, Carl Roth GmbH & Co. KG, Karlsruhe, Germany). HPLC was performed on silica gel (ReproSil-Pur 120 ODS3, C18, end-capped (endc.)) from JASCO (Jasco Labor- & Datentechnik GmbH, Groß-Umstadt, Germany) with a HPLC from Nordantec GmbH (Bremerhaven, Germany). All compounds were obtained with 95% purity.

3-(3-(2-Bromo-4-fluorophenyl)-1,2,4-oxadiazol-5-yl) propanoic acid (8) and 2-bromo-4-fluorobenzamide (9)

To a mixture of deoxygenated hydroxylamine hydrochloride (517 mg, 7.4 mmol, 1.0 eq.) and sodium carbonate (394 mg, 3.7 mmol, 0.5 eq.), methanol/water (4:1, 35 mL) was added via a cannula, and the reaction mixture was stirred for 10 min. 2-Bromo-4-fluorobenzonitrile (1,487 mg, 7.4 mmol, 1.0 eq.) was added, and the reaction mixture was stirred under diffuse light for 18 h at 80°C. The reaction mixture was diluted with dichloromethane (DCM), washed with water and evaporated to dryness after concentration of the solvent *in vacuo*. To the deoxygenated crude intermediate succinic acid anhydride (638 mg, 6.4 mmol, 0.9 eq.) was added, and the reaction mixture was stirred under diffuse light for 30 min at 140°C. The crude material was purified by column chromatography on silica gel (eluting with petrol spirit or petrol ether/ethyl acetate/acetic acid 1:1:0.01) and by crystallization at room temperature (DCM/methanol/water) to give **8** (566 mg, 1.8 mmol, 24% yield) and **9** (559 mg, 2.6 mmol, 35% yield). **8**: ^{1}H NMR (400 MHz, $CDCl_3$): δ (ppm) = 7.84 (dd, J = 6 Hz, J = 9 Hz, 1H, CH), 7.47 (dd, J = 3 Hz, J = 8 Hz, 1H, CH), 7.14 (ddd, J = 3 Hz, J = 9 Hz, 1H, CH), 3.29 (t, J = 7 Hz, 2H, CH_2), 3.01 (t, J = 7 Hz, 2H, CH_2). ^{19}F NMR (376 MHz, $CDCl_3$): δ (ppm) = −107.89 (dd, J = 8 Hz, J = 14 Hz). ^{13}C NMR (100 MHz, $CDCl_3$): δ (ppm) = 177.7, 176.6, 167.2, 163.4 (d, J = 256 Hz), 133.3 (d, J = 9 Hz), 124.3 (d, J = 4 Hz), 122.8 (d, J = 10 Hz), 121.7 (d, J = 25 Hz), 114.9 (d, J = 22 Hz), 30.1, 21.7. High-resolution mass spectrometry (HRMS) (ESI, negative ion) m/z: 312.9, 314.9 $[M\text{-}H]^-$. **9**: ^{1}H NMR (400 MHz, CD_3OD): δ (ppm) = 7.51 (dd, J = 6 Hz, J = 8 Hz, 1H, CH), 7.47 (dd, J = 3 Hz, J = 9 Hz, 1H, CH), 7.19 (pt, J = 2 Hz, J = 8 Hz, 1H, CH). ^{19}F NMR (376 MHz, CD_3OD): δ (ppm) = −111.64 (dd, J = 8 Hz, J = 15 Hz). ^{13}C NMR (101 MHz, CD_3OD): δ (ppm) = 172.4, 164.2 (d, J = 252 Hz), 136.2 (d, J = 4 Hz), 131.5 (d, J = 9 Hz), 121.5 (d, J = 25 Hz), 121.0 (d, J = 10 Hz), 115.7 (d, J = 22 Hz). HRMS (ESI, positive ion) m/z: 217.96086 $[M+H]^+$.

3-(3-(2-Bromo-4-nitrophenyl)-1,2,4-oxadiazol-5-yl) propanoic acid (10) and 2-bromo-4-nitrobenzamide (11)

The propanoic acid **10** was synthesized similar to the synthesis of **8** but with 2-bromo-4-nitrobenzonitrile as the reacting agent. The mixture was diluted with ethyl acetate, and potassium fluoride (2 mg, 34 µmol, 0.1 eq.) was added during the reaction with succinic acid anhydride. The reaction mixture was stirred under diffuse light for 30 min at 130°C. For the purification, petrol spirit or petrol ether/ethyl acetate/acetic acid (1:1:0.005) was used, resulting in **10** (24 mg, 70 µmol, 16% yield) and **11** (22 mg, 90 µmol, 20% yield). **10**: ^{1}H NMR (300 MHz, $CDCl_3/CD_3OD$ 1:1): δ (ppm) = 8.56 (d, J = 2 Hz, 1H, *CH*), 8.29 (dd, J = 2 Hz, J = 9 Hz, 1H, *CH*), 7.89 (d, J = 9 Hz, 1H, *CH*). ^{13}C NMR (75 MHz, $CDCl_3/CD_3OD$ 1:1): δ (ppm) = 1,178.9, 173.0, 166.0, 148.5, 133.5, 132.2, 128.5, 122.0, 121.7, 29.4, 21.3. HRMS (ESI, negative ion) m/z: 339.95731 $[M\text{-}H^+]^-$, 680.92128 $[2M\text{-}H^+]^-$. **11**: ^{1}H NMR (300 MHz, $CDCl_3/CD_3OD$): δ (ppm) = 8.50 (d, J = 2 Hz, 1H, *CH*), 8.28 (dd, J = 2 Hz, J = 8 Hz, 1H, *CH*), 7.68 (d, J = 8 Hz, 1H, *CH*). ^{13}C NMR (100 MHz, $CDCl_3/CD_3OD$): δ (ppm) = 171.4, 150.0, 145.7, 130.6, 129.1, 123.7, 120.7. HRMS (ESI, positive ion) m/z: 244.95569 $[M+H]^+$.

3-(3-(2-Fluoro-4-nitrophenyl)-1,2,4-oxadiazol-5-yl) propanoic acid (12) and 2-fluoro-4-nitrobenzamide (13)

Compounds **12** and **13** were prepared using 2-fluoro-4-nitrobenzonitrile (prepared as in the synthesis for **10**): **12**: 807 mg, 2.9 mmol, 10% yield; **13**: 93 mg, 0.5 mmol, 2% yield. **12**: ^{1}H NMR (300 MHz, $CDCl_3$): δ (ppm) = 8.26 (dd, J = 7 Hz, J = 8 Hz, 1H, CH), 8.06 to 8.18 (m, 2H, 2xCH), 3.32 (t, J = 7 Hz, 2H, CH_2), 3.03 (t, J = 7 Hz, 2H, CH_2). ^{19}F NMR (282 MHz, $CDCl_3$): δ (ppm) = −103.63 (dd, J = 7 Hz, J = 10 Hz). ^{13}C NMR (75 MHz, $CDCl_3$): δ (ppm) = 178.8, 176.0, 164.1 (d, J = 6 Hz), 160.5 (d, J = 263 Hz), 150.4 (d, J = 8 Hz), 131.8 (d, J = 3 Hz), 121.4 (d, J = 13 Hz), 119.5 (d, J = 4 Hz), 112.8 (d, J = 26 Hz), 30.7, 22.5. HRMS (ESI, negative ion) m/z: 280.03753 $[M\text{-}H^+]^-$, 316.01425 $[M\text{+}Cl^-]^-$, 561.08202 $[2M\text{-}H^+]^-$. **13**: ^{1}H NMR (400 MHz, CD_3OD): δ (ppm) = 8.18 to 8.07 (m, 2H, 2xCH), 7.97 (dd, J = 7 Hz, J = 8 Hz, 2H, CH_2). ^{19}F NMR (376 MHz, CD_3OD): δ (ppm) = −112.07 (t, J = 8 Hz). ^{13}C NMR (101 MHz, CD_3OD): δ (ppm) = 166.9, 160.8 (d, J = 254 Hz), 151.5 (d, J = 9 Hz), 132.8 (d, J = 3 Hz), 130.1 (d, J = 15 Hz), 120.5 (d, J = 4 Hz), 113.1 (d, J = 29 Hz). HRMS (ESI, positive ion) m/z: 185.03583 $[M\text{+}H]^+$, 207.01776 $[M\text{+}Na]^+$, 391.04643 $[2M\text{+}Na]^+$.

3-(3-(2-Bromo-4-methoxyphenyl)-1,2,4-oxadiazol-5-yl) propanoic acid (14) and 2-bromo-4-methoxybenzamide (15)

Compounds **14** and **15** were prepared using 2-bromo-4-methoxybenzonitrile (prepared as in the synthesis of **10**): **14**: 2539 mg, 7.8 mmol, 33% yield; **15**: impure. **14**: ^{1}H NMR (300 MHz, CD_3OD): δ (ppm) = 7.74 (d, J = 9 Hz, 1H, CH), 7.31 (d, J = 2 Hz, 1H, CH), 7.04 (dd, J = 3 Hz, J = 9 Hz, 1H, CH), 3.86 (s, 3H, CH_3), 3.24 (t, J = 7 Hz, 2H, CH_2), 2.92 (t, J = 7 Hz, 2H, CH_2). Impurity: δ (ppm) = 2.56 (s, 1.0H). ^{13}C NMR (76 MHz, CD_3OD): δ (ppm) = 180.2, 175.1, 168.8, 163.2, 133.9, 123.6, 121.5, 120.6, 114.4, 56.3, 31.1, 22.9. Impurity: δ (ppm) = 176.2, 29.9. HRMS (ESI, negative ion) m/z: 324.98282 $[M\text{-}H^+]^-$, 650.97272 $[2M\text{-}H^+]^-$. **15**: ^{1}H NMR (300 MHz, CD_3OD): δ (ppm) = 7.44 (d, J = 9 Hz, 1H, CH), 7.19 (d, J = 3 Hz, 1H, CH), 7.00 (dd, J = 3 Hz, J = 9 Hz, 1H, CH), 3.83 (s, 3H, CH_3). Impurity: δ (ppm) = 3.67 (s, 14.4H), 2.59 (s, 16H), 2.57 (s, 10H). HRMS (ESI, positive ion) m/z: 324.98282 $[M\text{-}H^+]^-$, 229.98094 $[M\text{+}H]^+$.

3-(3-(2,4-Difluorophenyl)-1,2,4-oxadiazol-5-yl)propanoic acid (16)

Carboxylic acid **16** was prepared using 2,4-difluorobenzonitrile (prepared as in the synthesis for **10**): 5684 mg, 22.4 mmol, 64% yield. **16**: ^{1}H NMR (300 MHz, $CDCl_3$/CD_3OD 1:1): δ (ppm) = 8.04 (dd, J = 8 Hz, J = 16 Hz, 1H, CH), 7.14 to 6.96 (m, 2H, 2xCH), 3.24 (t, J = 7 Hz, 2H, CH_2), 2.92 (t, J = 7 Hz, 2H, CH_2). ^{19}F NMR (282 MHz, $CDCl_3$/CD_3OD 1:1): δ (ppm) = −104.91 to −105.25 (m, 1xF), −105.85 to −106.23 (m, 1xF). ^{13}C NMR (75 MHz, $CDCl_3$/CD_3OD 1:1): δ (ppm) = 179.5, 174.2, 165.4 (d, J = 12 Hz, J = 254 Hz), 165.0 (d, J = 6 Hz), 161.9 (d, J = 12 Hz, J = 260 Hz), 132.8 (dd, J = 4 Hz, J = 10 Hz), 112.6 (dd, J = 4 Hz, J = 22 Hz), 112.1 (dd, J = 4 Hz, J = 13 Hz), 105.6 (pt, J = 26 Hz), 30.7, 22.5. HRMS (ESI, positive ion) m/z: 255.05735 $[M\text{+}H]^+$, 277.03917 $[M\text{+}Na]^+$, 531.09038 $[2M\text{+}Na]^+$.

3-(3-(2-Cyano-4-fluorophenyl)-1,2,4-oxadiazol-5-yl) propanoic acid (17)

Lithium hydroxide monohydrate (50 mg, 1.200 mmol, 5.0 eq.) in water (1.2 mL) was added to **24** (66 mg, 241 µmol, 1.0 eq.) in methanol (9.5 mL) and stirred for 2.5 h at room temperature. Ethyl acetate (38 mL) and HCl solution (13 mL, 6 mol/L) were added, and the phases were mixed and separated. The aqueous HCl layer was washed with ethyl acetate, and the solvent was concentrated *in vacuo*. This material was used without further purification; **17**: 58 mg, 221 µmol, 92% yield. **17**: ^{1}H NMR (300 MHz, $CDCl_3$, 50°C): δ (ppm) = 8.51 (s broad, 1H, COOH), 8.15 (dd, J = 5 Hz, J = 9 Hz, 1H, CH), 7.53 (dd, J = 3 Hz, J = 8 Hz, 1H, CH), 7.42 (ddd, J = 3 Hz, J = 9 Hz, 1H, CH), 3.30 (t, J = 7 Hz, 2H, CH_2), 3.01 (t, J = 7 Hz, 2H, CH_2). ^{19}F NMR (282 MHz, $CDCl_3$, 50°C): δ (ppm) = −106.90 (dd, J = 8 Hz, J = 13 Hz). ^{13}C NMR (75 MHz, $CDCl_3$, 50°C): δ (ppm) = 178.9, 175.8, 165.6, 163.3 (d, J = 256 Hz), 132.3 (d, J = 9 Hz), 125.7 (d, J = 4 Hz), 121.8 (d, J = 25 Hz), 120.6 (d, J = 22 Hz), 116.0 (m), 113.3 (d, J = 9 Hz), 52.2, 30.0, 21.9. MS (ESI, positive ion) m/z: 284 $[M\text{+}Na]^+$. MS (ESI, negative ion) m/z: 260 $[M\text{-}H^+]^-$.

3-(3-(2-Cyano-4-nitrophenyl)-1,2,4-oxadiazol-5-yl) propanoic acid (18)

The propanoic acid **18** was prepared using **26** (prepared as for the synthesis of **17**): 119 mg, 412 µmol, 99% yield. **18**: ^{1}H NMR (300 MHz, $CDCl_3$): δ (ppm) = 8.74 (d, J = 2 Hz, 1H, CH), 8.58 (dd, J = 2 Hz, J = 9 Hz, 1H, CH), 8.38 (d, J = 9 Hz, 1H, CH), 3.27 (t, J = 7 Hz, hidden by solvent, CH_2), 2.93 (t, J = 7 Hz, 2H, CH_2). ^{13}C NMR (76 MHz, $CDCl_3$): δ (ppm) = 182.1, 174.9, 166.5, 150.4, 135.4, 132.7, 131.1, 129.1, 116.8, 113.4, 30.9, 23.0. MS (ESI, negative ion) m/z: 287 $[M\text{-}H^+]^-$, 575$[2M\text{-}H^+]^-$.

3-(3-(4-Fluoro-2-hydroxyphenyl)-1,2,4-oxadiazol-5-yl) propanoic acid (19)

To a mixture of deoxygenated tribromoborane (7,528 mg, 30.1 mmol, 8.0 eq.) in dry DCM (130 mL), a mixture of **20** (1,000 mg, 3.8 mmol, 1.0 eq.) in dry DCM (60 mL) was added via a cannula at −70°C. The reaction mixture was stirred for 1 h at −70°C and overnight at room temperature. The reaction mixture was neutralized with saturated aqueous $NaHCO_3$ solution at 1°C, washed with ethyl acetate, and evaporated to dryness after concentration of the solvent *in vacuo*. The crude material was purified by column chromatography on silica gel (eluting with DCM/MeOH = 9:1 and DCM/MeOH = 1:1). Water was added and the product was additionally purified by washing with DCM to give **19** (188 mg, 746 μmol, 20%). **19**: ^{1}H NMR (400 MHz, CD_3OD): δ_H (ppm) = 7.97 (pdd, *J* = 7 Hz, *J* = 9 Hz, 1H, C*H*), 6.79 to 6.71 (m, 2 H, 2xC*H*), 3.27 (t, *J* = 7 Hz, 2H, CH_2), 2.94 (t, *J* = 7 Hz, 2H, CH_2). ^{19}F NMR (376 MHz, CD_3OD): δ_F (ppm) = −109.06 to −109.20 (m). ^{13}C NMR (101 MHz, CD_3OD): δ_C (ppm) = 180.3, 175.1, 167.5, 166.9 (d, *J* = 250 Hz), 160.0 (d, *J* = 13 Hz), 131.6 (d, *J* = 11 Hz), 109.3 (d, *J* = 3 Hz), 108.5 (d, *J* = 23 Hz), 105.1 (d, *J* = 25 Hz), 31.0, 22.9. HR ESI -MS: $C_{11}H_9FN_2O_4$, *m*/*z* = 251.04731 $[M\text{-}H^+]^-$, 503.10122 $[2M\text{-}H^+]^-$.

3-(3-(4-Fluoro-2-methoxyphenyl)-1,2,4-oxadiazol-5-yl) propanoic acid (20)

Carboxylic acid **20** was prepared using 4-fluoro-2-methoxybenzonitrile (prepared as in the synthesis for **8**): 1,250 mg, 4.7 mmol, 15% yield. **20**: ^{1}H NMR (400 MHz, CD_3OD): δ (ppm) = 7.99 (dd, *J* = 7 Hz, *J* = 9 Hz, 1H, C*H*), 6.97 (dd, *J* = 2 Hz, *J* = 11 Hz, 1H, C*H*), 6.82 (ddd, *J* = 2 Hz, *J* = 8 Hz, *J* = 11 Hz, 1H, C*H*), 3.93 (s, 3H, CH_3), 3.21 (t, *J* = 7 Hz, 2H, CH_2), 2.82 (t, *J* = 7 Hz, 2H, CH_2). Impurity: δ (ppm) = 3.16 (q, *J* = 7 Hz, 6.5H), 2.96 (s, 4.6H), 1.28 (t, *J* = 7 Hz, 10.2H). ^{19}F NMR (376 MHz, CD_3OD): δ (ppm) = −108.48 (td, *J* = 7 Hz, *J* = 11 Hz, *J* = 15 Hz). ^{13}C NMR (101 MHz, CD_3OD): δ (ppm) = 180.3, 177.0 (broad), 167.1, 166.9 (d, *J* = 250 Hz), 161.3 (d, *J* = 11 Hz), 133.8 (d, *J* = 11 Hz), 113.2 (d, *J* = 3 Hz), 108.3 (d, *J* = 22 Hz), 101.1 (d, *J* = 27 Hz), 56.7, 33.4 (broad), 22.1 (broad). Impurity: δ (ppm) = 177.6 (broad), 47.5, 23.8, 9.1. HRMS (ESI, negative ion) *m*/*z*: 265.06292 $[M\text{-}H^+]^-$, 531.13261 $[2M\text{-}H^+]^-$.

3-(3-(6-Bromopyridin-3-yl)-1,2,4-oxadiazol-5-yl)propanoic acid (21)

Compound **21** was prepared using 6-bromonicotinonitrile (prepared as in the synthesis for **8**): 164 mg, 550 μmol, 10% yield. **21**: ^{1}H NMR (300 MHz, $CDCl_3/CD_3OD$ 1:1, 30°C): δ (ppm) = 8.95 (dd, *J* = 1 Hz, *J* = 2 Hz, C*H*), 8.22 (dd, *J* = 2 Hz, *J* = 8 Hz, 1H, C*H*), 7.68 (dd, *J* = 1 Hz, *J* = 8 Hz, 1H, C*H*), 3.24 (t, *J* = 7 Hz, 2H, CH_2), 2.92 (t, *J* = 7 Hz, 2H, CH_2). ^{13}C NMR (76 MHz, $CDCl_3/CD_3OD$ 1:1, 30°C): δ (ppm) = 180.6, 174.1, 166.1, 149.2, 145.0, 137.9, 129.3, 123.3, 30.6, 22.5. HRMS (ESI, positive ion) *m*/*z*: 297.98160 $[M+H]^+$, 319.96382 $[M+Na]^+$, 616.93871 $[2M+Na]^+$.

3-(3-(6-Fluoropyridin-3-yl)-1,2,4-oxadiazol-5-yl)propanoic acid (22)

Compound **22** was prepared using 6-fluoronicotinonitrile (prepared as in synthesis for **10**): 197 mg, 830 μmol, 5% yield. **22**: ^{1}H NMR (400 MHz, $CDCl_3/CD_3OD$ 1:1): δ (ppm) = 8.87 to 8.83 (m, 1 H, C*H*), 8.48 (ddd, *J* = 2 Hz, *J* = 7 Hz, *J* = 8 Hz, 1H, C*H*), 7.15 (ddd, *J* = 0.4 Hz, *J* = 3 Hz, *J* = 9 Hz, 1H, C*H*), 3.24 (t, *J* = 7 Hz, 2H, CH_2), 2.93 (t, *J* = 7 Hz, 2H, CH_2). ^{19}F NMR (376 MHz, $CDCl_3/CD_3OD$ 1:1): δ (ppm) = −65.88 (d, *J* = 6 Hz). ^{13}C NMR (101 MHz, $CDCl_3/CD_3OD$ 1:1): δ (ppm) = 180.5, 174.2, 166.0, 165.6 (d, *J* = 244 Hz), 147.4 (d, *J* = 15 Hz), 141.2 (d, *J* = 9 Hz), 122.2 (d, *J* = 5 Hz), 110.9 (d, *J* = 37 Hz), 30.6, 22.5. HRMS (ESI, negative ion) *m*/*z*: 236.04779 $[M\text{-}H^+]^-$, 272.02442 $[M\text{-}Cl^-]^-$, 473.10191 $[2M\text{-}H^+]^-$.

Methyl 3-(3-(2-bromo-4-fluorophenyl)-1,2,4-oxadiazol-5-yl) propanoate (23)

(Diazomethyl)trimethylsilane (2 M in hexane, 1.3 mL, 2.6 mmol, 1.5 eq.) was added dropwise to deoxygenated **8** (547 mg, 1.7 mmol, 1.0 eq.) in dry toluene/methanol (9:1, 20 mL) at 0°C, and the reaction mixture was stirred for 30 min at room temperature. The crude product was purified by column chromatography on silica gel (eluting with petrol spirit or petrol ether/ethyl acetate 2:1) after concentration of the solvent *in vacuo* to give **23** (560 mg, 1.7 mmol, 98% yield). **23**: ^{1}H NMR (400 MHz, $CDCl_3$): δ (ppm) = 7.84 (dd, *J* = 6 Hz, *J* = 9 Hz, 1H, C*H*), 7.47 (dd, *J* = 3 Hz, *J* = 8 Hz, 1H, C*H*), 7.14 (ddd, *J* = 3 Hz, *J* = 9 Hz, 1H, C*H*), 3.73 (s, 3H, CH_3), 3.29 (t, *J* = 7 Hz, 2H, CH_2), 2.94 (t, *J* = 7 Hz, 2H, CH_2). ^{19}F NMR (376 MHz, $CDCl_3$): δ (ppm) = −108.04 (dd, *J* = 8 Hz, *J* = 14 Hz). ^{13}C NMR (101 MHz, $CDCl_3$): δ (ppm) = 178.0, 171.6, 167.2, 163.3 (d, *J* = 256 Hz), 133.3 (d, *J* = 9 Hz), 124.5 (d, *J* = 4 Hz), 122.7 (d, *J* = 10 Hz), 121.6 (d, *J* = 25 Hz), 114.8 (d, *J* = 21 Hz), 52.1, 30.2, 22.0. MS (ESI, positive ion) *m*/*z*: 351 $[M+Na]^+$.

Methyl 3-(3-(2-cyano-4-fluorophenyl)-1,2,4-oxadiazol-5-yl) propanoate (24)

Copper(I) chloride (12 mg, 122 μmol, 0.4 eq.) was added to deoxygenated **10** (100 mg, 304 μmol, 1.0 eq.) in dry dimethylacetamide (2.2 mL). Potassium cyanide (79 mg, 1.215 mmol, 4.0 eq.) was added after 15 min, and the reaction mixture was stirred for 14 h at 130°C. Saturated ammonium chloride (2.2 mL), ethyl acetate (8.7 mL) and water (7.6 mL) were added, and the phases were mixed and separated. The aqueous layer was washed with ethyl acetate. The crude product was purified by column chromatography on silica gel (eluting with petrol spirit or petrol ether/ethyl acetate 2:1) after concentration of the solvent *in vacuo* to give **24** (23 mg, 83 μmol, 27% yield). **24**: ^{1}H NMR (300 MHz, $CDCl_3$): δ (ppm) = 8.15 (dd, *J* = 5 Hz, *J* = 9 Hz, 1H, C*H*), 7.53 (dd, *J* = 3 Hz, *J* =

8 Hz, 1H, *CH*), 7.42 (ddd, *J* = 3 Hz, *J* = 9 Hz, 1H, *CH*), 3.73 (s, 3H, CH_3), 3.03 (t, *J* = 7 Hz, 2H, CH_2), 2.96 (t, *J* = 7 Hz, 2H, CH_2). ^{19}F NMR (282 MHz, $CDCl_3$): δ (ppm) = −106.85 (ddd, *J* = 5 Hz, *J* = 8 Hz). ^{13}C NMR (100 MHz, $CDCl_3$): δ (ppm) = 179.1, 171.6, 165.5, 163.2 (d, *J* = 256 Hz), 132.3 (d, *J* = 9 Hz), 125.6 (d, *J* = 4 Hz), 121.8 (d, *J* = 25 Hz), 120.6 (d, *J* = 21 Hz), 116.2 (d, *J* = 3 Hz), 113.0 (d, *J* = 10 Hz), 52.2, 30.1, 22.0. MS (ESI, positive ion) *m/z*: 276 $[M+H]^+$, 298 $[M+Na]^+$.

Methyl 3-(3-(2-bromo-4-nitrophenyl)-1,2,4-oxadiazol-5-yl) propanoate (25)

Compound **25** was prepared using **10** (prepared as in the synthesis of **23**): 230 mg, 646 µmol, 98% yield. **25**: ^{1}H NMR (400 MHz, $CDCl_3$): δ (ppm) = 8.58 (d, *J* = 2 Hz, 1H, *CH*), 8.25 (dd, *J* = 2 Hz, *J* = 9 Hz, 1H, *CH*), 8.06 (d, *J* = 9 Hz, 1H, *CH*), 3.73 (s, 3H, CH_3), 3.32 (t, *J* = 7 Hz, 2H, CH_2), 2.96 (t, *J* = 7 Hz, 2H, CH_2). ^{13}C NMR (101 MHz, $CDCl_3$): δ (ppm) = 178.7, 171.5, 166.5, 148.9, 133.9, 132.7, 129.2, 122.7, 122.1, 52.2, 30.1, 22.0. MS (ESI, positive ion) *m/z*: 378 $[M+Na]^+$.

Methyl 3-(3-(2-cyano-4-nitrophenyl)-1,2,4-oxadiazol-5-yl) propanoate (26)

The carboxylic acid **26** was prepared using **10** (prepared as for the synthesis of **24**): 83 mg, 275 µmol, 43% yield. **26**: ^{1}H NMR (300 MHz, $CDCl_3$): δ (ppm) = 8.68 (d, *J* = 2 Hz, 1H, *CH*), 8.54 (dd, *J* = 2 Hz, *J* = 9 Hz, 1H, *CH*), 8.39 (d, *J* = 9 Hz, 1H, *CH*), 3.73 (s, 3H, CH_3), 3.34 (t, *J* = 7 Hz, 2H, CH_2), 2.98 (t, *J* = 7 Hz, 2H, CH_2). ^{13}C NMR (75 MHz, $CDCl_3$): δ (ppm) = 179.9, 171.5, 164.9, 148.7, 134.3, 131.3, 129.7, 127.4, 115.4, 112.7, 52.2, 30.0, 22.0. MS (ESI, positive ion) *m/z*: 303 $[M+H]^+$, 325 $[M+Na]^+$.

General amide coupling method A

The coupling reaction was initiated by dropwise addition of *N*-ethyl-*N'*-(3-dimethylaminopropyl)carbodiimide (EDAC; 50 mg, 322 µmol, 1.1 eq.) in dry DCM (2.5 mL) to a mixture of 1.0 eq. of the deoxygenated propanoic acid derivate and 1.1 eq. amine in dry DCM (2.5 mL) at 0°C. The reaction mixture was stirred for 1 h at 0°C followed by stirring for 1 h at room temperature. A tip of spatula of 4-DMAP was added at 0°C, and the reaction mixture was stirred for 1 h at room temperature. EDAC (1.1 eq.) in dry DCM (2.5 mL) was added at 0°C, and the reaction mixture was again stirred for 14 h at room temperature followed by evaporation to dryness after concentration of the solvent *in vacuo*.

3-(3-(6-Bromopyridin-3-yl)-1,2,4-oxadiazol-5-yl)-*N*-(5-*tert*-butylisoxazol-3-yl)propanamide (1a)

Compound **1a** was prepared using **14** and 5-*tert*-butylisoxazol-3-amine according to method A. The crude material was purified by column chromatography on silica gel (elution with petrol spirit/ethyl acetate 2:1) and by HPLC (RP18, ReproSil-Pur 120 ODS3, endc., methanol/water = 85:15) and by crystallization at room temperature (methanol), giving **1a** (19 mg, 44 µmol, 27% yield). **1a**: ^{1}H NMR (400 MHz, $CDCl_3$): δ (ppm) = 10.20 (s broad, 1H, *NH*), 9.01 (d, *J* = 2 Hz, 1H, *CH*), 8.16 (dd, *J* = 2 Hz, *J* = 8 Hz, 1H, *CH*), 7.59 (d, *J* = 8 Hz, 1H, *CH*), 6.69 (s, 1H, *CH*), 3.39 (t, *J* = 7 Hz, 2H, CH_2), 3.11 (t, *J* = 7 Hz, 2H, CH_2), 1.31 (s, 9H, 3×CH_3). ^{13}C NMR (76 MHz, $CDCl_3$): δ (ppm) = 182.2, 179.5, 168.9, 165.8, 158.0, 149.1, 145.0, 137.0, 128.5, 122.5, 93.6, 33.2, 32.5, 28.7, 22.1. HRMS (ESI, positive ion): $C_{17}H_{18}BrN_5O_3$, *m/z* = 420.06635 $[M+H]^+$, 839.12559 $[2M+H]^+$.

3-(3-(6-Fluoropyridin-3-yl)-1,2,4-oxadiazol-5-yl)-*N*-(5-*tert*-butylisoxazol-3-yl)propanamide (1b)

Compound **1b** was synthesized similar to **1a** with **22** (30 mg, 127 µmol, 1.0 eq.) as carboxylic acid component. Before evaporating, water (5.0 mL) was added, and the reaction mixture was washed with ethyl acetate. The crude material was purified as described for **1a**, giving **1b** (14 mg, 38 µmol, 30% yield). **1b**: ^{1}H NMR (300 MHz, CD_3OD): δ_H (ppm) = 8.85 (d, 1H, *CH*), 8.52 (ddd, *J* = 2 Hz, *J* = 8 Hz, *J* = 9 Hz, 1H, *CH*), 7.26 to 7.19 (m, 1H, *CH*), 6.54 (s, 1H, *CH*), 3.34 (t, *J* = 7 Hz, 2H, CH_2), 3.06 (t, *J* = 7 Hz, 2H, CH_2), 1.32 (s, 9H, 3×CH_3). ^{19}F NMR (282 MHz, CD_3OD): δ_F (ppm) = −67.33 (d, *J* = 7 Hz). HR ESI +MS: $C_{17}H_{18}FN_5O_2$, *m/z* = 360.14680 $[M+H]^+$, 382.12896 $[M+Na]^+$, 719.28664 $[2M+H]^+$, 741.26859 $[2M+Na]^+$.

3-(3-(2-Cyano-4-fluorophenyl)-1,2,4-oxadiazol-5-yl)-*N*-(quinolin-3-yl)propanamide (2a)

Compound **2a** was prepared following general amide coupling method A with **17** and quinoline-3-amine. The crude material was purified by column chromatography on silica gel (elution with petrol spirit/ethyl acetate 1:1, ethyl acetate and DCM/methanol 1:1) and by crystallization at room temperature (acetonitrile), giving pure **2a** (25 mg, 64 µmol, 51% yield). **2a**: ^{1}H NMR (300 MHz, $CDCl_3/CD_3OD$ = 1:1, 50°C): δ_H (ppm) = 8.83 (d, *J* = 3 Hz, 1H, *CH*), 8.65 (d, *J* = 2 Hz, 1H, *CH*), 8.14 (dd, *J* = 5 Hz, *J* = 9 Hz, 1H, *CH*), 7.94 (pd, *J* = 8 Hz, 1H, *CH*), 7.77 (d, *J* = 1 Hz, *J* = 8 Hz, 1H, *CH*), 7.64 to 7.42 (m, 4H, *CH*), 3.41 (t, *J* = 7 Hz, 2H, CH_2), 3.11 (t, *J* = 7 Hz, 2H, CH_2). ^{19}F NMR (282 MHz, $CDCl_3$, 50°C): δ_F (ppm) = −107.89 (td, *J* = 5 Hz, *J* = 8 Hz, *J* = 16 Hz). APT NMR (75 MHz, $CDCl_3/CD_3OD$ = 1:1, 50°C): δ_C (ppm) = 180.6, 171.2, 166.3, 164.1, (d, *J* = 255 Hz), 145.1, 144.9, 133.1, 133.0 (d, *J* = 9 Hz), 129.12, 129.08, 128.6, 128.3, 127.9, 127.6, 126.3 (*J* = 4 Hz), 125.2, 122.4 (d, *J* = 26 Hz), 121.5 (d, *J* = 22 Hz), 116.8 (d, *J* = 3 Hz), 113.4 (d, *J* = 9 Hz), 32.9, 22.5. HR ESI +MS: $C_{21}H_{14}FN_5O_2$, *m/z* = 388.12051 $[M+H]^+$, 410.10243 $[M+Na]^+$, 775.23385 $[2M+H]^+$, 797.21557 $[2M+Na]^+$.

3-(3-(6-Fluoropyridin-3-yl)-1,2,4-oxadiazol-5-yl)-*N*-(quinolin-3-yl)propanamide (2b)

The synthesis of **2b** followed the procedure described for **2a** with **21** as reactant. The crude material was purified under the same conditions as **2a**, resulting in 20 mg of **2b** (55 μmol, 44% yield). **2b**: ^{1}H NMR (400 MHz, $CDCl_3/CD_3OD$ = 1:1): δ_H (ppm) = 8.86 to 8.79 (m, 2H, 2x*CH*), 8.68 (d, *J* = 2 Hz, 1H, *CH*), 8.46 (ddd, *J* = 2 Hz, *J* = 8 Hz, *J* = 8 Hz, 1H, *CH*), 7.93 (d, *J* = 8 Hz, 1H, *CH*), 7.77 (dd, *J* = 2 Hz, *J* = 8 Hz, 1H, *CH*), 7.65 to 7.58 (m, 1H, *CH*), 7.55 to 7.48 (m, 1H, *CH*), 7.12 (dd, *J* = 3 Hz, *J* = 9 Hz, 1H, *CH*), 3.34 (t, *J* = 7 Hz, 2H, CH_2), 3.11 (t, *J* = 7 Hz, 2H, CH_2). ^{19}F NMR (376 MHz, $CDCl_3/CD_3OD$ = 1:1): δ_F (ppm) = −66.00 (d, *J* = 7 Hz). ^{13}C NMR (101 MHz, $CDCl_3/CD_3OD$ = 1:1): δ_C (ppm) = 180.7, 171.3, 166.1, 165.6 (d, *J* = 244 Hz), 147.5 (d, *J* = 15 Hz), 145.0, 144.6, 141.2 (d, *J* = 9 Hz), 133.2, 129.19, 129.16, 128.44, 128.41, 128.1, 125.1, 122.3 (d, *J* = 5 Hz), 110.9 (d, *J* = 37 Hz), 32.9, 22.5. HR ESI +MS: $C_{19}H_{14}FN_5O_2$, *m/z* = 364.12066 $[M+H]^+$, 386.10258 $[M+Na]^+$, 727.23464 $[2M+H]^+$, 749.21527 $[2M+Na]^+$.

3-(3-(6-Bromopyridin-3-yl)-1,2,4-oxadiazol-5-yl)-*N*-(quinolin-3-yl)propanamide (2c)

Compound **2c** was synthesized by method A, by coupling **21** (50 mg, 168 μmol, 1.0 eq.) to quinolin-3-amine. Before evaporating to dryness, water (5.0 mL) was added to the reaction mixture and subsequently washed with ethyl acetate. The crude material was purified as described for **2a**, giving **2c** (33 mg, 77 μmol, 46% yield). **2c**: ^{1}H NMR (400 MHz, $CDCl_3/CD_3OD$ = 1:1): δ_H (ppm) = 8.94 (dd, *J* = 1 Hz, *J* = 2 Hz, 1H, *CH*), 8.78 (d, *J* = 2 Hz, 1H, *CH*), 8.70 (d, *J* = 2 Hz, 1H, *CH*), 8.18 (dd, *J* = 2 Hz, *J* = 8 Hz, 1H, *CH*), 7.93 (d, *J* = 8 Hz, 1H, *CH*), 7.76 (d, *J* = 1 Hz, *J* = 8 Hz, 1H, *CH*), 7.63 (dd, *J* = 1 Hz, *J* = 8 Hz, 1H, *CH*), 7.63 to 7.56 (m, 1H, *CH*), 7.53 to 7.47 (m, 1H, *CH*), 3.38 (t, *J* = 7 Hz, 2H, CH_2), 3.10 (t, *J* = 7 Hz, 2H, CH_2). ^{13}C NMR (101 MHz, $CDCl_3/CD_3OD$ = 1:1): δ_C (ppm) = 180.5, 170.8, 166.0, 149.1, 144.9, 144.7, 144.3, 137.7, 132.9, 129.1, 129.0, 128.9, 128.3, 128.2, 127.8, 124.8, 123.1, 32.6, 22.4. HR ESI +MS: $C_{19}H_{14}BrN_5O_2$, *m/z* = 424.04075 $[M+H]^+$, 446.02267 $[M+Na]^+$, 847.07404 $[2M+H]^+$, 869.05547 $[2M+Na]^+$.

3-(3-(6-Fluoropyridin-3-yl)-1,2,4-oxadiazol-5-yl)-*N*-(1-ethyl-1*H*-indol-5-yl)-propanamide (3b)

Compound **3b** was synthesized by coupling deoxygenated **21** (50 mg, 211 μmol, 1.0 eq.) to 1-ethyl-1*H*-indol-5-amine (37 mg, 232 μmol, 1.1 eq.) via method A. The crude material was purified by column chromatography on silica gel (elution with petrol spirit/ethyl acetate 1:1) and by crystallization at room temperature (DCM/petrol spirit), giving **3b** (61 mg, 162 μmol, 77% yield). **3b**: ^{1}H NMR (300 MHz, $CDCl_3$): δ_H (ppm) = 8.91 (d, *J* = 2 Hz, 1H, *CH*), 8.41 (dt, *J* = 2 Hz, *J* = 8 Hz, 1H, *CH*), 7.76 (s, 1H, *CH*), 7.61 (s broad, 1H, N*H*), 7.24 (d, *J* = 10 Hz, 1H, *CH*), 7.21 (d, *J* = 2 Hz, 1H, *CH*), 7.10 (d, *J* = 3 Hz, 1H, *CH*), 7.02 (dd, *J* = 3 Hz, *J* = 9 Hz, 1H, *CH*), 6.41 (d, *J* = 3 Hz, 1H, *CH*), 4.12 (q, *J* = 7 Hz, 2H, CH_2), 3.38 (t, *J* = 7 Hz, 2H, CH_2), 2.97 (t, *J* = 7 Hz, 2H, CH_2), 1.43 (t, *J* = 7 Hz, 3H, CH_3). ^{19}F NMR (282 MHz, $CDCl_3$): δ_F (ppm) = −64.21 (d, *J* = 5 Hz). ^{13}C NMR (76 MHz, $CDCl_3$): δ_C (ppm) = 179.8, 168.4, 165.6, 165.0 (d, *J* = 244 Hz), 147.4 (d, *J* = 16 Hz), 140.2 (d, *J* = 9 Hz), 133.5, 129.7, 128.8, 128.1, 121.5 (d, *J* = 5 Hz), 115.9, 113.2, 110.1 (d, *J* = 38 Hz), 109.5, 41.2, 33.0, 22.5, 15.6. HR ESI +MS: $C_{20}H_{18}FN_5O_2$, *m/z* = 380.15202 $[M+H]^+$, 402.13403 $[M+Na]^+$, 759.29638 $[2M+H]^+$, 781.27720 $[2M+Na]^+$.

3-(3-(2-Bromo-4-fluorophenyl)-1,2,4-oxadiazol-5-yl)-*N*-(9*H*-carbazol-3-yl)propanamide (4e)

Compound **4e** was prepared using **8** and 9*H*-carbazol-3-amine via coupling method A. The crude product was purified by column chromatography on silica gel (elution with petrol spirit/ethyl acetate 1:1, ethyl acetate and DCM/methanol 1:1) and by HPLC (RP18, ReproSil-Pur 120 ODS3, endc., methanol/water = 85:15) and by crystallization at room temperature (chloroform), giving 60 mg of **4e** (125 μmol, 64% yield). **4e**: ^{1}H NMR (300 MHz, CD_3OD): δ (ppm) = 8.26 (d, *J* = 2 Hz, 1H, *CH*), 7.96 (d, *J* = 8 Hz, 1H, *CH*), 7.82 (dd, *J* = 6 Hz, *J* = 9 Hz, 1H, *CH*), 7.55 (dd, *J* = 3 Hz, *J* = 9 Hz, 1H, *CH*), 7.49 to 7.29 (m, 4H, 4×*CH*), 7.21 (td, *J* = 2 Hz, *J* = 8 Hz, 1H, *CH*), 7.11 (t, *J* = 7 Hz, 1H, *CH*), 3.38 (t, *J* = 7 Hz, 2H, CH_2), 3.04 (t, *J* = 7 Hz, 2H, CH_2). ^{19}F NMR (282 MHz, CD_3OD): δ (ppm) = −110.02 (td, *J* = 6 Hz, *J* = 8 Hz). ^{13}C NMR (76 MHz, CD_3OD): δ (ppm) = 180.8, 171.4, 168.5, 164.8 (d, *J* = 254 Hz), 142.1, 138.7, 134.6 (d, *J* = 9 Hz), 131.1, 126.8, 126.1 (d, *J* = 4 Hz), 124.3, 124.2, 123.8 (d, *J* = 10 Hz), 122.4 (d, *J* = 25 Hz), 121.0, 120.7, 119.7, 116.0 (d, *J* = 22 Hz), 113.6, 111.8, 111.6, 33.4, 23.2. HR ESI +MS: $C_{23}H_{16}BrFN_4O_2$, *m/z* = 501.03343 $[M+Na]^+$, 979.07777 $[2M+Na]^+$.

3-(3-(2-Bromo-4-fluorophenyl)-1,2,4-oxadiazol-5-yl)-*N*-(9-methyl-9*H*-carbazol-3-yl)propanamide (5e)

Compound **5e** was synthesized by adding iodomethane (8 mg, 56 μmol, 1.3 eq.) in dry dimethylformamide (0.5 mL) dropwise to deoxygenated **4e** (21 mg, 43 μmol, 1.0 eq.) and potassium carbonate (59 mg, 430 μmol, 10.0 eq.). The reaction mixture was stirred for 20 h at room temperature followed by evaporation to dryness after concentration of the solvent *in vacuo*. The crude product was purified by hot filtration in methanol and by HPLC (RP18, ReproSil-Pur 120 ODS3, endc., acetonitrile/water = 85:15) with subsequent crystallization in the fridge (methanol) to give **5e** (8 mg, 17 μmol, 39% yield). **5e**: ^{1}H NMR (300 MHz, $CDCl_3/CD_3OD$ 1:1): δ

(ppm) = 8.30 (d, J = 2 Hz, 1H, CH), 8.00 (d, J = 8 Hz, 1H, CH), 7.81 (d, J = 9 Hz, 1H, CH), 7.57 to 7.35 (m, hidden by solvent, 4×CH), 7.33 (d, J = 9 Hz, 1H, CH), 7.20 to 7.11 (m, 2 H, 2×CH), 3.81 (s, 3H, CH_3), 3.40 (t, J = 7 Hz, 2H, CH_2), 3.03 (t, J = 7 Hz, 2H, CH_2). ^{19}F NMR (282 MHz, $CDCl_3/CD_3OD$ 1:1): δ (ppm) = −108.76 (td, J = 6 Hz, J = 8 Hz). HR ESI +MS: $C_{23}H_{16}BrFN_4O_2$, m/z = 515.04893 [M+Na]$^+$, 1,007.10847 [2M+Na]$^+$.

3-(3-(2-Cyano-4-nitrophenyl)-1,2,4-oxadiazol-5-yl)-*N*-(9-ethyl-9*H*-carbazol-3-yl)propanamide (6a)

For the synthesis of **6a**, **17** was coupled to 9-ethyl-9*H*-carbazol-3-amine as described in method A. After synthesis, water (5.0 mL) was added, and the reaction mixture was washed with ethyl acetate and evaporated to dryness after concentration of the solvent *in vacuo*. The crude product was purified by column chromatography on silica gel (elution with petrol spirit/ethyl acetate (2:1) + five drops of triethylamine and DCM/methanol (1:1) + five drops of triethylamine) and by crystallization at room temperature (DCM/methanol), giving pure **6a** (27 mg, 60 μmol, 50% yield). **6a**: ^{1}H NMR (300 MHz, $CDCl_3/CD_3OD$ = 1:1, 50°C): δ_H (ppm) = 8.28 (d, J = 2 Hz, 1H, CH), 8.13 (dd, J = 5 Hz, J = 9 Hz, 1H, CH), 7.99 (d, J = 8 Hz, 1H, CH), 7.54 (dd, J = 2 Hz, J = 8 Hz, 1H, CH), 7.52 to 7.37 (m, 3H, 3×CH), 7.35 (d, J = 8 Hz, 1H, CH), 7.31 (d, J = 9 Hz, 1H, CH), 7.13 (pt, J = 7 Hz, 1H, CH), 4.31 (q, J = 7 Hz, 2H, CH_2), 3.40 (t, J = 7 Hz, 2H, CH_2), 3.04 (t, J = 7 Hz, 2H, CH_2), 1.36 (t, J = 7 Hz, 3H, CH_3). ^{19}F NMR (282 MHz, $CDCl_3/CD_3OD$ = 1:1, 50° C): δ_F (ppm) = −107.74 (ps). ^{13}C NMR (75 MHz, $CDCl_3/CD_3OD$ = 1:1, 50°C): δ_C (ppm) = 179.6, 169.2, 165.1, 162.9 (d, J = 255 Hz), 140.1, 136.9, 131.9 (d, J = 9 Hz), 129.5, 125.32, 125.26 (d, J = 4 Hz), 122.5, 122.4, 121.3 (d, J = 26 Hz), 120.3 (d, J = 22 Hz), 119.9, 119.2, 118.2, 115.8, 112.4, 112.2, 108.1, 107.9, 37.0, 32.0, 21.9, 12.9. HR ESI +MS: $C_{26}H_{20}FN_5O_2$, m/z = 496.13901 [M+Na]$^+$, 969.28932 [2M+Na]$^+$.

3-(3-(6-Fluoropyridin-3-yl)-1,2,4-oxadiazol-5-yl)-*N*-(9-ethyl-9*H*-carbazol-3-yl)propanamide (6b)

Compound **6b** was synthesized as **6a** by coupling deoxygenated **22** with 9-ethyl-9*H*-carbazol-3-amine following method A. The crude material was purified by column chromatography on silica gel (elution with petrol spirit/ethyl acetate 1:1 and DCM/methanol 1:1) and by crystallization at room temperature (DCM/methanol), giving **6b** (42 mg, 98 μmol, 47% yield). **6b**: ^{1}H NMR (400 MHz, $CDCl_3/CD_3OD$ = 1:1): δ_H (ppm) = 8.83 (d, J = 2 Hz, 1H, CH), 8.47 to 8.38 (m, 1H, CH), 8.28 (d, J = 2 Hz, 1H, CH), 7.98 (d, J = 8 Hz, 1H, CH), 7.47 (dd, J = 2 Hz, J = 9 Hz, 1H, CH), 7.44 to 7.33 (m, 2H, 2×CH), 7.30 (d, J = 9 Hz, 1H, CH), 7.13 (t, J = 7 Hz, 1H, CH), 7.07 (dd, J = 2 Hz, J = 8 Hz, 1H, CH), 4.30 (q, J = 7 Hz, 2H, CH_2), 3.36 (t, J = 7 Hz, 2 H, CH_2), 3.03 (t, J = 7 Hz, 2H, CH_2), 1.34 (t, J = 7 Hz, 3H, CH_3). ^{19}F NMR (282 MHz, $CDCl_3/CD_3OD$ = 1:1): δ_F (ppm) = −65.79 (d, J = 7 Hz). ^{13}C NMR (101 MHz, $CDCl_3/CD_3OD$ = 1:1): δ_C (ppm) = 180.7, 170.3, 165.9, 165.5 (d, J = 244 Hz), 147.4 (d, J = 15 Hz), 141.1 (d, J = 9 Hz), 141.0, 137.8, 130.5, 126.4, 123.5, 123.3, 122.2 (d, J = 5 Hz), 120.9, 120.1, 119.2, 113.3, 110.8 (J = 37 Hz), 109.1, 109.0, 38.0, 32.8, 22.8, 14.0. HR ESI +MS: $C_{24}H_{20}FN_5O_2$, m/z = 452.14902 [M+Na]$^+$, 859.32705 [2M+H]$^+$, 881.30861 [2M+Na]$^+$.

3-(3-(6-Bromopyridin-3-yl)-1,2,4-oxadiazol-5-yl)-*N*-(9-ethyl-9*H*-carbazol-3-yl)propanamide (6c)

Compound **6c** was prepared as described for **6b** with **21** as carboxylic acid reactant. The crude material was purified as described for **6b**, giving **6c** (42 mg, 86 μmol, 51% yield). **6c**: ^{1}H NMR (300 MHz, $CDCl_3/CD_3OD$ = 1:1): δ_H (ppm) = 8.93 (dd, J = 1 Hz, J = 2 Hz, 1H, CH), 8.28 (d, J = 2 Hz, 1H, CH), 8.16 (dd, J = 2 Hz, J = 8 Hz, 1H, CH), 7.97 (d, J = 8 Hz, 1H, CH), 7.60 (dd, J = 1 Hz, J = 8 Hz, 1H, CH), 7.47 (dd, J = 2 Hz, J = 9 Hz, 1H, CH), 7.44 to 7.33 (m, 2H, 2×CH), 7.30 (d, J = 9 Hz, 1H, CH), 7.17 to 7.09 (m, 1H, CH), 4.30 (q, J = 7 Hz, 2H, CH_2), 3.36 (t, J = 7 Hz, 2H, CH_2), 3.03 (t, J = 7 Hz, 2H, CH_2), 1.35 (t, J = 7 Hz, 3H, CH_3). ^{13}C NMR (76 MHz, $CDCl_3/CD_3OD$ = 1:1): δ_C (ppm) = 180.8, 170.2, 166.0, 149.1, 144.9, 141.0 137.77, 137.75, 130.5, 129.2, 126.4, 123.4, 123.3, 120.9, 120.0, 119.2, 113.3, 109.1, 109.0, 38.0, 32.8, 22.8, 14.0. HR ESI +MS: $C_{24}H_{20}BrN_5O_2$, m/z = 490.08770 [M+H]$^+$, 512.06951 [M+Na]$^+$, 979.16767 [2M+H]$^+$, 1,001.14935 [2M+Na]$^+$.

3-(3-(2-Fluoro-4-nitrophenyl)-1,2,4-oxadiazol-5-yl)-*N*-(9-ethyl-9*H*-carbazol-3-yl)propanamide (6d)

Compound **6d** was synthesized as **6a** using **12**. The crude product was purified by crystallization in the fridge (DCM), resulting in 69 mg of pure compound (145 μmol, 81% yield). **6d**: ^{1}H NMR (400 MHz, CD_3CN, 70°C): δ (ppm) = 8.39 (s broad, 1H, NH), 8.34 to 8.24 (m, 2H, 2×CH), 8.18 to 8.10 (m, 2H, 2xCH), 8.07 (d, J = 8 Hz, 1H, CH), 7.57 to 7.43 (m, 4H, 4×CH), 7.20 (t, J = 7 Hz, 1H, CH), 4.41 (q, J = 7 Hz, 2H, CH_2), 3.40 (t, J = 7 Hz, 2H, CH_2), 3.02 (t, J = 7 Hz, 2H, CH_2), 1.39 (t, J = 7 Hz, 3H, CH_3). ^{19}F NMR (376 MHz, CD_3CN, 90°C): δ (ppm) = −106.52 (s, broad). HR ESI +MS: $C_{25}H_{20}FN_5O_4$, m/z = 496.13901 [M+Na]$^+$, 969.28932 [2M+Na]$^+$.

3-(3-(2-Bromo-4-fluorophenyl)-1,2,4-oxadiazol-5-yl)-*N*-(9-ethyl-9*H*-carbazol-3-yl)propanamide (6e)

Compound **6e** was prepared as described for **6a** using **8** as carboxylic acid. The crude product was purified by column chromatography on silica gel (elution with DCM/methanol 100:1) and by crystallization at room temperature (DCM/

methanol) to give **6e** (112 mg, 221 μmol, 76% yield) **6e**: ^{1}H NMR (300 MHz, $CDCl_3$): δ (ppm) = 8.26 (d, J = 2 Hz, 1H, CH), 8.02 (d, J = 8 Hz, 1H, CH), 7.83 (dd, J = 6 Hz, J = 9 Hz, 1H, CH), 7.69 (s broad, 1H, NH), 7.54 to 7.42 (m, 3H, 3xCH), 7.38 (d, J = 8 Hz, 1H, CH), 7.31 (d, J = 9 Hz, 1H, CH), 7.20 (pt, J = 8 Hz, 1H, CH), 7.12 (ddd, J = 2 Hz, J = 9 Hz, 1H, CH), 4.32 (q, J = 7 Hz, 2H, CH_2), 3.45 (t, J = 7 Hz, 2H, CH_2), 3.02 (t, J = 7 Hz, 2H, CH_2), 1.40 (t, J = 7 Hz, 3H, CH_3). ^{19}F NMR (282 MHz, $CDCl_3$): δ (ppm) = −107.95 (dd, J = 8 Hz, J = 14 Hz). ^{13}C NMR (101 MHz, $CDCl_3$): δ (ppm) = 178.6, 168.4, 167.2, 163.3 (d, J = 255 Hz), 140.4, 137.3, 133.3 (d, J = 9 Hz), 129.2, 125.9, 124.5 (d, J = 4 Hz), 123.0, 122.8 (d, J = 10 Hz), 122.7, 121.6 (d, J = 25 Hz), 120.6, 119.5, 118.8, 114.9 (d, J = 21 Hz), 113.0, 108.6, 108.5, 37.6, 33.1, 22.4, 13.78. HR ESI +MS: $C_{25}H_{20}BrFN_4O_2$, m/z = 507.08249 $[M+H]^+$, 529.06444 $[M+Na]^+$, 1013.15637 $[2M+H]^+$, 1035.13966 $[2M+Na]^+$.

3-(3-(2-Cyano-4-nitrophenyl)-1,2,4-oxadiazol-5-yl)-*N*-(9-ethyl-9*H*-carbazol-3-yl)propanamide (6f)

Compound **6f** was synthesized as **6a** using **18**. The crude product was purified by column chromato- graphy on silica gel (elution with petrol spirit/ethyl acetate (2:1) + five drops of triethylamine and DCM/methanol (1:1) + five drops of triethylamine) and by crystallization at room temperature (DCM/methanol and acetonitrile), resulting in **6f** (25 mg, 51 μmol, 25%). **6f**: ^{1}H NMR (300 MHz, CD_3CN, 70°C): δH (ppm) = 8.71 (d, J = 2 Hz, 1H, CH), 8.54 (dd, J = 2 Hz, J = 9 Hz, 1H, CH), 8.38 (d, J = 9 Hz, 1H, CH), 8.32 (ps, 1H, CH), 8.07 (pd, J = 8 Hz, 1H, CH), 7.54 (dd, J = 2 Hz, J = 9 Hz, 1H), 7.51 to 7.43 (m, 3H, 3×CH), 7.20 (pt, J = 7 Hz, 1H, CH), 4.41 (q, J = 7 Hz, 2H, CH_2), 3.43 (t, J = 7 Hz, 2H, CH_2), 3.04 (t, J = 7 Hz, 2H, CH_2), 1.39 (t, J = 7 Hz, 3H CH_3). HR ESI +MS: $C_{26}H_{20}N_6O_4$, m/z = 503.14351 $[M+Na]^+$, 983.29765 $[2M+Na]^+$.

3-(3-(2-Bromo-4-nitrophenyl)-1,2,4-oxadiazol-5-yl)-*N*-(9-ethyl-9*H*-carbazol-3-yl)propanamide (6g)

Compound **6g** was prepared as **6a** but with **10** as the reactant. The crude product was purified as described for **6e**, yielding **6g** (106 mg, 198 μmol, 68%). **6g**: ^{1}H NMR (300 MHz, $CDCl_3$, 50°C): δ_H (ppm) = 8.57 (d, J = 2 Hz, 1H, CH), 8.36 to 8.14 (m, 2H, 2×CH), 8.03 (pd, J = 8 Hz, 2H, 2×CH), 7.62 to 7.13 (m, hidden by solvent), 4.35 (q, J = 7 Hz, 2H, CH_2), 3.49 (ps broad, 2H, CH_2), 3.04 (ps broad, 2H, CH_2), 1.43 (t, J = 7 Hz, 3H, CH_3). HR ESI +MS: $C_{25}H_{20}BrN_5O_4$, m/z = 556.05940 $[M+Na]^+$, 1,067.14721 $[2M+H]^+$, 1,089.12816 $[2M+Na]^+$.

3-(3-(2,4-Difluorophenyl)-1,2,4-oxadiazol-5-yl)-*N*-(9-ethyl-9*H*-carbazol-3-yl)propanamide (6h)

Compound **6h** was synthesized similar to the procedure described for **6a** using **16** as carboxylic acid. The crude product was purified by column chromatography on silica gel (elution with petrol spirit/ethyl acetate 2:1, petrol spirit/ethyl acetate 2:1 and DCM/methanol 1:1) and by crystallization at room temperature (DCM/methanol 1:1), yielding **6h** (39 mg, 88 μmol, 49%). **6h**: ^{1}H NMR (400 MHz, $CDCl_3/CD_3OD$ = 1:1): δ_H (ppm) = 8.29 (d, J = 2 Hz, 1H, CH), 8.04 (pdd, J = 8 Hz, J = 16 Hz, 1H, CH), 8.00 (d, J = 8 Hz, 1H, CH), 7.49 (dd, J = 2 Hz, J = 9 Hz, 1H, CH), 7.46 to 7.36 (m, 2H, 2xCH), 7.33 (d, J = 8 Hz, 1H, CH), 7.14 (pt, J = 6 Hz, 1H, CH), 7.06 to 6.97 (m, 2H, 2xCH), 4.33 (q, J = 7 Hz, 2H, CH_2), 3.38 (t, J = 7 Hz, 2H, CH_2), 3.03 (t, J = 7 Hz, 2H, CH_2), 1.37 (t, J = 7 Hz, 3H, CH_3). ^{19}F NMR (376 MHz, $CDCl_3/CD_3OD$ = 1:1): δ_F (ppm) = −105.08 (pdd, J = 7 Hz, J = 14 Hz, 1xF), −105.89 to −106.04 (m, 1×F). ^{13}C NMR (101 MHz, $CDCl_3/CD_3OD$ = 1:1): δ_C (ppm) = 179.8, 170.4, 165.4 (dd, J = 12 Hz, J = 254 Hz), 165.0 (d, J = 6 Hz), 161.9 (dd, J = 12 Hz, J = 260 Hz), 141.1, 137.9, 132.7 (dd, J = 4 Hz, J = 10 Hz), 130.5, 126.4, 123.5, 123.4, 120.9, 120.2, 119.2, 113.4, 112.6 (dd, J = 4 Hz, J = 22 Hz), 112.1 (dd, J = 4 Hz, J = 13 Hz), 109.2, 109.0, 105.6 (t, J = 26 Hz), 38.0, 32.9, 22.8, 14.0. HR ESI +MS: $C_{25}H_{20}F_2N_4O_2$, m/z = 447.16279 $[M+H]^+$, 469.14455 $[M+Na]^+$, 893.31771 $[2M+H]^+$, 915.29946 $[M+Na]^+$.

3-(3-(4-Amino-2-fluorophenyl)-1,2,4-oxadiazol-5-yl)-*N*-(9-ethyl-9*H*-carbazol-3-yl)propanamide (6i)

Tin(II) chloride (40 mg, 211 μmol, 5.0 eq.) was added to deoxygenated **6d** (20 mg, 42 μmol, 1.0 eq.) in ethanol (1.0 mL), and the reaction mixture was stirred for 30 min at reflux. Saturated sodium carbonate solution (2.0 mL) was added at 0°C. The precipitate was filtered up, washed with water, diluted in chloroform/methanol (1:1), filtered and evaporated to dryness after concentration of the solvent *in vacuo*. The crude material was purified by column chromatography on silica gel (elution with chloroform/methanol 100:1) and by crystallization in the fridge (acetonitrile) to give **6i** (12 mg, 26 μmol, 62% yield) **6i**: ^{1}H NMR (300 MHz, CD_3CN, 65°C): δ (ppm) = 8.38 (s broad, 1H, NH), 8.32 (s, 1H, CH), 8.07 (d, J = 8 Hz, 1H, CH), 7.74 (t, J = 8 Hz, 1H, CH), 7.60 to 7.36 (m, 4H, 4×CH), 7.19 (t, J = 7 Hz, 1H, CH), 6.61 to 6.41 (m, 2H, 2×CH), 4.71 (s broad, 2 H, $NH2$), 4.39 (q, J = 7 Hz, 2H, CH_2), 3.31 (t, J = 7 Hz, 2H, CH_2), 2.96 (t, J = 7 Hz, 2H, CH_2), 1.38 (t, J = 7 Hz, 3H, CH_3). ^{19} F NMR (282 MHz, CD_3CN, 65°C): δ (ppm) = −110.20 (dd, J = 9 Hz, J = 13 Hz). HRMS (ESI, positive ion) m/z: 466.16522 $[M+Na]^+$, 909.34029 $[2M+Na]^+$.

3-(3-(4-Fluoro-2-hydroxyphenyl)-1,2,4-oxadiazol-5-yl)-*N*-(9-ethyl-9*H*-carbazol-3-yl)propanamide (6j)

Compound **6j** was prepared using **19** as described in the synthesis of **6a**. The crude material was purified as described for **6h**, giving 38 mg of **6j** (85 µmol, 23% yield). **6j**: ^{1}H NMR (300 MHz, CD_3CN): δ (ppm) = 8.55 (s, broad, 1H, N*H*), 8.35 (d, *J* = 1 Hz, 1H, C*H*), 8.06 (pd, *J* = 6 Hz, 1H, C*H*), 8.00 (dd, *J* = 5 Hz, *J* = 7 Hz, 1H, C*H*), 7.55 to 7.42 (m, 4H, 4xC*H*), 7.18 (td, *J* = 1 Hz, *J* = 5 Hz, 1H, C*H*), 6.84 to 6.74 (m, 2H, 2xC*H*), 4.38 (q, *J* = 5 Hz, 2H, CH_2), 3.37 (t, *J* = 5 Hz, 2H, CH_2), 3.02 (t, *J* = 5 Hz, 2H, CH_2), 1.35 (t, *J* = 5 Hz, 3H, CH_3). ^{19}F NMR (282 MHz, CD_3CN): δ (ppm) = −108.31 to −108.44 (m). HR ESI +MS: $C_{25}H_{21}FN_4O_3$, *m/z* = 445.16724 $[M+H]^+$, 467.14897 $[M+Na]^+$, 889.32803 $[2M+H]^+$, 911.30937 $[2M+Na]^+$.

3-(3-(4-Fluoro-2-(2-fluoroethoxy)phenyl)-1,2,4-oxadiazol-5-yl)-*N*-(9-ethyl-9*H*-carbazol-3-yl)-propanamide (6k)

Potassium carbonate (14 mg, 101 µmol, 2.0 eq.) was added to deoxygenated **6j** (22 mg, 50 µmol, 1.0 eq.) in dry dimethylformamide (0.5 mL), and the reaction mixture was stirred for 5 min. To the reaction mixture, 1-fluoro-2-iodoethane (18 mg, 101 µmol, 2.0 eq.) was added, and the reaction mixture was stirred for 20 h at 50°C. The reaction mixture was added to ice water, washed with ethyl acetate and evaporated to dryness after concentration of the solvent *in vacuo*. The crude material was purified by column chromatography on silica gel (elution with petrol spirit or petrol ether/ethyl acetate 1:1) and by crystallization at room temperature (DCM/methanol) to give **6k** (11 mg, 22 µmol, 43% yield). **6k**: ^{1}H NMR (300 MHz, $CDCl_3/CD_3OD$ 1:1): δ (ppm) = 8.52 (s, broad, 1H, N*H*), 8.36 (d, *J* = 2 Hz, 1H, C*H*), 8.06 (pd, *J* = 8 Hz, 1H, C*H*), 7.94 (dd, *J* = 7 Hz, *J* = 9 Hz, 1H, C*H*), 7.58 to 7.39 (m, 4H, 4×C*H*), 7.18 (pt, *J* = 7 Hz, 1H, C*H*), 6.93 (dd, *J* = 2 Hz, *J* = 11 Hz, 1H, C*H*), 6.86 (dt, *J* = 2 Hz, *J* = 8 Hz, 1H, C*H*), 4.88 to 4.78/4.71 to 4.61 (dm, *J* = 48 Hz, 1 H/1H, CH_2), (m, 1H, CH_2), 4.47 to 4.32/4.31 to 4.22 (m, 2H, 1H/1H, 2×CH_2), 3.31 (t, *J* = 7 Hz, 2H, CH_2), 2.98 (t, *J* = 7 Hz, 2H, CH_2), 1.35 (t, *J* = 7 Hz, 3H, CH_3). ^{19}F NMR (282 MHz, $CDCl_3/CD_3OD$ 1:1): δ (ppm) = −108.79 to −108.96 (m, 1F), −223.78 to −224.42 (m, 1F). HR ESI +MS: $C_{27}H_{24}F_2N_4O_3$, *m/z* = 513.17095 $[M+Na]^+$, 1,003.35233 $[2M+Na]^+$.

3-(3-(4-Fluoro-2-methoxyphenyl)-1,2,4-oxadiazol-5-yl)-*N*-(9-ethyl-9*H*-carbazol-3-yl)-propanamide (6 l)

Compound **6l** was synthesized via coupling method A as described for **6a** with **20** as carboxylic acid. The crude material was purified following the procedure for **6e**, yielding **6l** (76 mg, 166 µmol, 57%). **6l**: ^{1}H NMR (400 MHz, $CDCl_3/CD_3OD$ = 1:1): δ_H (ppm) = 8.29 (d, *J* = 2 Hz, 1H, C*H*), 8.02 to 7.91 (m, 2H, 2×C*H*), 7.48 (dd, *J* = 2 Hz, *J* = 8 Hz, 1H, C*H*), 7.43 to 7.33 (m, 2H, 2×C*H*), 7.30 (d, *J* = 9 Hz, 1H, C*H*), 7.13 (pt, *J* = 7 Hz, 1H, C*H*), 6.79 (dd, *J* = 2 Hz, *J* = 11 Hz, 1H, C*H*), 6.72 (dd, *J* = 2 Hz, *J* = 8 Hz, 1H, C*H*), 4.29 (q, *J* = 7 Hz, 2 H, CH_2), 3.88 (s, 3H, CH_3), 3.35 (t, *J* = 7 Hz, 2H, CH_2), 3.01 (t, *J* = 7 Hz, 2H, CH_2), 1.34 (t, *J* = 7 Hz, 3H, CH_3). ^{13}C NMR (101 MHz, $CDCl_3/CD_3OD$ = 1:1): δ_C (ppm) = 178.7, 170.5, 166.6, 166.2 (d, *J* = 251 Hz), 160.4 (d, *J* = 11 Hz), 141.1 137.8, 133.3 (d, *J* = 11 Hz), 130.5, 126.4, 123.5, 123.4, 120.9, 120.1, 119.2, 113.4, 112.3 (d, *J* = 3 Hz), 109.2, 109.0, 108.0 (d, *J* = 22 Hz), 100.5 (d, *J* = 26 Hz), 56.4, 38.0, 33.0, 22.8, 14.0. HR ESI +MS: $C_{26}H_{23}FN_4O_3$, *m/z* = 459.18247 $[M+H]^+$, 917.35797 $[2M+H]^+$.

3-(3-(2-Bromo-4-methoxyphenyl)-1,2,4-oxadiazol-5-yl)-*N*-(9-ethyl-9*H*-carbazol-3-yl)propanamide (6m)

Compound **6m** was synthesized as **6a** with **14** as carboxylic acid reactant. The crude material was purified by column chromatography on silica gel (elution with DCM/methanol 100:1 and DCM/methanol 100:2) and by crystallization at room temperature (DCM/methanol), yielding **6m** (83 mg, 159 µmol, 54%). **6m**: ^{1}H NMR (400 MHz, $CDCl_3/CD_3OD$ = 1:1): δ_H (ppm) = 8.29 (s, 1H, C*H*), 8.00 (d, *J* = 8 Hz, 1H, C*H*), 7.72 (d, *J* = 8 Hz, 1H, C*H*), 7.55 to 7.27 (m, hidden by solvent, 4×C*H*), 7.22 (d, *J* = 2 Hz, 1H, C*H*), 7.15 (t, *J* = 7 Hz, 1H, C*H*), 6.92 (dd, *J* = 2 Hz, *J* = 9 Hz, 1H, C*H*), 4.32 (q, *J* = 7 Hz, 2H, CH_2), 3.80 (s, 3H, CH_3), 3.38 (t, *J* = 7 Hz, 2H, CH_2), 3.02 (t, *J* = 7 Hz, 2H, CH_2), 1.36 (t, *J* = 7 Hz, 3H, CH_3). ^{13}C NMR (101 MHz, $CDCl_3/CD_3OD$ = 1:1): δ_C (ppm) = 179.4, 170.4, 168.2, 162.4, 141.0, 137.8, 133.3, 130.5, 126.4, 123.4, 123.3, 123.2, 120.9, 120.7, 120.13, 120.09, 119.2, 113.9, 113.4, 109.1, 109.0, 56.0, 38.0, 32.9, 22.8, 14.0. HR ESI +MS: $C_{26}H_{23}BrN_4O_3$, *m/z* = 519.10249 $[M+H]^+$, 541.08500 $[M+Na]^+$, 1,037.19973 $[2M+H]^+$, 1,059.18045 $[2M+Na]^+$.

3-(3-(2,4-Difluorophenyl)-1,2,4-oxadiazol-5-yl)-*N*-(1-benzyl-1*H*-indol-3-yl)-propanamide (7h)

Compound **7h** was prepared by coupling of **16** with 1-benzyl-1*H*-indol-3-amine hydrochloride according to coupling method A. The crude product was purified by column chromatography on silica gel (elution with petrol spirit/ethyl acetate 2:1 and ethyl acetate), yielding **7h** (71 mg, 155 µmol, 87%). For affinity data, the product (20 mg) was further purified by HPLC (RP18, ReproSil-Pur 120 ODS3, endc., acetonitrile/0.057 M triethylammonium acetate = 65:35) and by crystallization at room temperature (ethanol/water) to an aspic. The aspic was dried in a speed vacuum to give 14.7 mg of pure solid product. **7h**: ^{1}H NMR (400 MHz, $CDCl_3$): δ_H (ppm) = 8.07 to 7.98 (m, 1H, C*H*), 7.92 (s broad, 1H, N*H*), 7.78 (s, 1H, C*H*), 7.51 (d, *J* = 8 Hz, 1H, C*H*), 7.36 to 7.22 (m, hidden by solvent, 4×C*H*), 7.19 (pt, *J* = 7 Hz, 1H, C*H*), 7.16 to 7.10 (m, 2H, 2×C*H*), 7.07 (pt, *J* = 7 Hz, 1H, C*H*), 7.02 to 6.92 (m, 2H, 2×C*H*), 5.24 (s, 2H, CH_2),

3.42 (t, J = 7 Hz, 2H, CH_2), 3.06 (t, J = 7 Hz, 2H, CH_2). ^{19}F NMR (376 MHz, $CDCl_3$): δ_F (ppm) = −104.01 to −104.26 (m, 1xF), −104.97 to −105.20 (m, 1xF). ^{13}C NMR (101 MHz, $CDCl_3$): δ_C (ppm) = 178.8, 167.7, 164.7 (dd, J = 12 Hz, J = 254 Hz), 164.6 (d, J = 6 Hz), 161.3 (dd, J = 12 Hz, J = 260 Hz), 137.4, 134.1, 132.1 (dd, J = 4 Hz, J = 10 Hz), 128.9, 127.8, 127.0, 122.6, 121.1, 119.9, 119.3, 116.8, 114.1, 112.1 (dd, J = 4 Hz, J = 22 Hz), 111.6 (dd, J = 4 Hz, J = 13 Hz), 110.1, 105.3 (t, J = 25 Hz), 50.3, 32.6, 22.6. HR ESI +MS: $C_{26}H_{20}F_2N_4O_2$, m/z = 481.14447 $[M+Na]^+$, 939.29960 $[2M+Na]^+$.

X-ray structural analysis

The single-crystal X-ray diffraction data of compound **6f** were collected on a diffractometer IPDS-2T (Stoe & Cie GmbH, Darmstadt, Germany) at 180 K using Mo-K_α radiation (l = 71.073 pm). The data reduction was performed using the STOE X-AREA software package (2006, Stoe & Cie, Darmstadt, Germany). The structure was solved by direct methods using the program SHELXS-97 and refined using SHELXL-97 [46]. All non-H atoms were refined anisotropically, and hydrogen (H) atoms were added geometrically using a riding model. Graphical visualization of the structure was performed using the program Diamond 3.2e (DIAMOND 3.2e, K. Brandenburg, 2010, Crystal Impact GbR, Bonn, Germany). The crystal structure has been deposited at the Cambridge Crystallographic Data Centre and allocated the deposition number CCDC 841516.

Cell culture

CHO cell lines stably transfected with human CB1 (hCB1-CHO; obtained from Euroscreen, Gosselies, Belgium) or human CB2 (hCB2-CHO; obtained from Paul L. Prather, Department of Pharmacology and Toxicology, College of Medicine, University of Arkansas for Medical Sciences, USA) were cultured in Ham's F12 medium or Dulbecco's modified Eagle's medium (DMEM) with 10% fetal calf serum, 100 IU/mL penicillin, 100 μg/mL streptomycin and 250 or 400 μg/mL of the selection antibiotic Geneticin (G418), respectively. The cells were cultured in a humidified atmosphere with 5% CO_2 at 37°C. Confluent cell layers of 175-cm^2 flasks were scraped; cells were harvested by centrifugation (800 rpm, 3 min), counted by trypan blue staining, suspended in 200 μL of 50 mM tris(hydroxymethyl)aminomethane (TRIS; pH 7.4) at 4°C and stored at −32°C until the binding experiment.

Determination of CB receptor affinity

Competitive binding experiments were performed with crude membrane homogenates obtained from hCB1-CHO or hCB2-CHO cells as described above. Increasing concentrations of test compounds (0.01 nM to 10 μM) diluted from 10 mM stock solutions in DMSO were incubated with 30 to 50 μg of membrane protein (equivalent to 0.5 to 1 × 10^6 hCB1-CHO or hCB2-CHO cells) and 0.5 nM [^{3}H]CP55,940 (6,438 GBq/mmol; PerkinElmer Life and Analytical Sciences, Rodgau, Germany) in a final volume of 1 mL in a binding buffer (50 mM TRIS (pH 7.4) at 21°C, 0.1% bovine serum albumin (BSA), 5 mM $MgCl_2$, 1 mM EDTA) for 90 min at room temperature. Non-specific binding of [^{3}H] CP55,940 was determined in the presence of 10 μM CP55,940. Incubations were terminated by rapid filtration through a GF-B glass fibre filter pre-incubated for 90 min at room temperature in freshly prepared 0.5% polyvinylpyrrolidone + 0.1% Tween 20 solution using a 48-well cell harvester (Brandel, Gaithersburg, MD, USA).

Saturation binding of CP55,940 towards hCB1-CHO or hCB2-CHO cell membranes was analysed in homologous competition experiments performed with increasing concentrations of CP55,940 (0.01 nM to 10 μM) and one concentration of [^{3}H]CP55,940 (0.5 nM). Kinetic analysis of the binding of CP55,940 towards hCB2-CHO cell membranes was performed in one association experiment using three concentrations of [^{3}H]CP55,940 (0.207, 0.458 and 0.873 nM) and incubation times of up to 120 min.

Binding data were analysed using GraphPad Prism version 2.01 (GraphPad Software, Inc., San Diego, CA, USA) by non-linear regression to provide estimates of the half maximal inhibitory concentration (IC_{50}) values and the rate of association. K_D values of [^{3}H]CP55,940 from homologous radioligand displacement experiments were estimated according to Jeffries et al. [47] by K_D = IC_{50} − [radioligand] and from kinetic experiments according to Hulme and Trevethick [48]. The corresponding inhibition constants (K_i) of test compounds were derived from the IC_{50} values using the Cheng-Prusoff equation [49]. All binding experiments were performed in triplicates, and data are given as mean values from independent experiments.

Animals

Animal experiments were performed under procedures approved by the State of Saxony Animal Care and Use Committee and conducted in accordance with the German Law for the Protection of Animals. Female CD-1 mice (10 to 12 weeks old, 20 to 25 g), obtained from the Medizinisch-Experimentelles Zentrum der Universität Leipzig (Leipzig, Germany), were used for the experiments.

Autoradiographic binding study

The animals were anesthetized and sacrificed, and their spleens were rapidly removed and frozen in isopentane at −35°C. The spleens were brought to −15°C in a cryostat (Microm International GmbH, Walldorf, Germany), and a series of 12-μm-thick coronal sections obtained from the spleens of three animals were collected in parallel on microscopic glass slides. The sections were dried at room temperature and stored at −35°C until they were processed for receptor binding autoradiography.

For autoradiographic experiments, the slides were brought to room temperature, dried in a stream of cold air, pre-incubated in a binding buffer (50 mM TRIS (pH 7.4) at 21°C, 5% BSA) for 15 min at room temperature and dried again in a stream of cold air. To account for total binding, samples were incubated for 2 h at room temperature with 6 nM [^{3}H]CP55,940 (5,328 GBq/mmol, PerkinElmer Life and Analytical Sciences, Rodgau, Germany). Sections were incubated in the presence of 1 μM CP55,940 (non-specific binding), SR144528 (CB2-selective inverse agonist), SR141716A (CB1-selective antagonist), or a test compound in binding buffer. Samples were washed twice for 30 min at 4°C in 50 mM TRIS (pH 7.4) at 4°C, containing 1% BSA, dipped briefly in ice-cold deionized water (5 s), dried in a stream of cold air and exposed along with [^{3}H] standards (Amersham/GE Healthcare, Piscataway, NJ, USA) for 14 days to [^{3}H]-sensitive screen plates (Fuji Photo Film, Co. Ltd., Tokyo, Japan).

The image plates were analysed using a BAS-1800II system bioimaging analyser (Fuji Photo Film, Co. Ltd., Tokyo, Japan). Scan data were visualized and processed by computer-assisted microdensitometry (Aida version 2.31, Raytest Isotopenmessgeräte GmbH, Straubenhardt, Germany). Irregular regions of interest (ROIs) were drawn on selected areas of the spleen labelled as red pulp (low-density binding) and white pulp (high-density binding) according to Lynn and Herkenham [18] and Massi et al. [39]. The intensity of the radioligand binding was assessed by measuring the background-corrected optical density in each ROI expressed as photostimulated luminescence per square millimetre The theoretical fractional occupancy (f) of [^{3}H]CP55,940 and the reference and test compounds at CB2 was calculated using the Gaddum equation: $fA = [A] / ([A] + K_{D,A}(1 + [B]/K_{D,B}))$ [50].

Receptor modelling

The receptor model was created employing the 'Homology Modeling' module of the program Molecular Operation Environment (MOE, version 2010.11, Chemical Computing Group Inc. Montreal, Canada). For this purpose, the sequence of the human CB2 [Swiss-Prot: P34972] [4] was subjected to a PDB search on the protein structure database implemented in MOE 2010.11 with the Z cut-off set to 2.0 while leaving the other parameters at their default values. The search suggested the human adenosine receptor A2a (hAA2R) as the template for the comparative modelling procedure. Since the recently published structure of the agonist-bound hAA2 receptor [43] is not included in the MOE protein database, the hAA2R structure [PDB:3EML] [51] was chosen as reference for the sequence alignment. The alignment of the human CB2 sequence with that of hAA2R is given as Additional files 1, 2, and 3. After downloading the 3D structure of [PDB:3QAK] [43] from the RCSB database, the structure was superimposed on the crystal structure 3eml. After removal of all lipid molecules, ions and water molecules, the residues between 209 and 222, which belong to lysozyme T4, were removed from the structure. In order to improve the modelling accuracy, the co-crystalized agonist UK-432097 of [PDB:3QAK] remained in the system during the modelling procedure. Out of ten independently generated models employing the default parameters of the Homology Modeling module, a consensus model was computed. To remove clashes and optimize the overall geometry of the protein, the system was subjected to an energy minimization employing the implemented AMBER89 force field using the default values. The quality of the model was verified by running the Protein Report module of MOE. After removal of the template ligand UK-432097, the apo receptor was energy-minimized to convergence, giving the final hCB2 model structure.

Docking studies

The small compounds were built in MOE with subsequent geometry optimization based on the MMFF force field as incorporated in the program package with a distance-dependent dielectric constant. The residues of the proposed binding pocket were defined based on the Site Finder module of MOE. The docking site included residue Y190$^{5.39}$ (numbering scheme according to Ballesteros and Weinstein [52]), which is known to be involved in ligand binding (*cf.* [53] and references cited therein). For the molecular docking studies, the program GOLD [54] (version 5) with parameters set to their default values was employed. All single bonds of the small ligands were allowed to rotate freely during the docking simulation. The side chains of the residues composing the binding pocket were treated as flexible, and the atoms of the protein backbone were kept at fixed positions. This approach is considered to represent the main characteristics of an induced fit [55]. The predicted poses were clustered by the GOLD software with a cut-off of 1.0 Å (heavy atoms only), giving representative geometries of the small molecules. For each of the compounds, all final poses were subjected to a further analysis with the program PostDock [45].

Radiochemistry

The radiolabelling procedure was initiated by addition of K[^{18}F]/K2.2.2 and K_2CO_3 to 2 mg of precursor in dry *N*,*N*-dimethylformamide under diffuse light and argon atmosphere (**6g**: 293 MBq [^{18}F]fluoride, K2.2.2 (7.4 μmol/GBq) and K_2CO_3 (3.2 μmol/GBq); **6c**: 303.2 MBq [^{18}F]fluoride, K2.2.2 (7.4 μmol/GBq) and K_2CO_3 (3.2 μmol/GBq)). The reaction mixtures were subjected to microwave radiation in closed vessels employing a Discover microwave synthesizer (CEM GmbH, Kamp-Lintfort, Germany) with the following scheme: heating to 60°C (30 s, 45 to 75 W with subsequent cooling to 20°C followed by three radiation cycles (100°C (60 s, 150 W); 20°C). Subsequently, 5 eq. $SnCl_2$ was added and the reaction mixture was subjected to three heating cycles (120°C (60 s, 150 W); 20°C). The yields of the labelled compounds were determined by radio-TLC (EE/petrol ether = 2:1).

Conclusions

Various *N*-aryl-3-((hetero)aromatic)-oxadiazolyl-propionamides have been synthesized. Among those, 9-ethyl-9*H*-carbazole-substituted compounds showed the highest affinity towards CB2 and good selectivity against CB1 receptors. The study revealed strong relationships between the structure of the CB2 ligands and their CB2 affinity and selectivity. The data of this study indicate that a modification of the compounds at the amide moiety shows a stronger impact on binding and specificity of the compounds toward CB2 than variation at the (hetero)aromatic ring located at the 3-position of the oxadiazoles. Thus, introduction of functional groups for subsequent ^{18}F labelling at this moiety is a promising strategy for the creation of CB2-selective radioligands suitable for (neuro)imaging by PET. Such imaging studies are currently in process at our laboratory.

Endnotes

[a]Vendors of chemicals (details can be obtained from the authors upon request): ABCR GmbH (Karlsruhe, Germany), Activate Scientific GmbH (Prien, Germany), Alfa Aesar Johnson Matthey Forschungschemikalien GmbH (Karlsruhe, Germany), Apollo Scientific LTD (Cheshire, UK), AppliChem GmbH (Darmstadt, Germany), Carl Roth GmbH & Co. KG (Karlsruhe, Germany), Fisher Scientific GmbH (Schwerte, Germany), Green Chempharm, Inc. (Bardonia, NY, USA), Hande Sciences (Suzhou, China), Oakwood Products Inc. (West Columbia, SC, USA), Princeton BioMolecular Research (Munich, Germany), Sigma-Aldrich Chemie GmbH (Munich, Germany), VWR International GmbH (Darmstadt, Germany).

Additional files

Additional file 1: Contains crystal data and structure refinement for compound X-ray structural data of 6f. Crystal data: $C_{26}H_{20}N_6O_4$, M_m = 480.48 g mol^{-1}, triclinic, space group $P\bar{1}$ (no. 2), a = 766.4(1) pm, b = 1236.3(1) pm, c = 1278.1(2) pm, α = 109.04(1)°, β = 100.34(1)°, γ = 91.31 (1)°, V = 1,121.8(2)·× 10^6 pm^3, Z = 2, r_{calc} = 1.423 g cm^{-3}, μ(Mo-K$_\alpha$) = 0.10 mm^{-1}, crystal size 0.32 × 0.08 × 0.07 mm^3, Q_{max} = 50°, 6,766 reflections collected, 3,761 unique, R_{int} = 0.046, 2,382 observed reflections, 330 parameters, $R1$ = 0.043 [$I > 2s(I)$], $wR2$ = 0.082 (all data), maximum and minimum residual electron density 0.18 and −0.14 × 10^{-6} Å^{-3}, respectively.

Additional file 2: Contains the alignment of the sequence of hCB2 with hAA2R.

Additional file 3: Contains the 3D coordinates of the modelled human cannabinoid receptor 2.

Competing interests

The authors declare that they have no competing interests.

Acknowledgements

This work has been supported by the DFG (project BR 1360/12-1). The authors wish to thank Bernhard Wünsch from Westfälische Wilhelms-Universität Münster for the fruitful discussions. The authors are grateful to Claudia Birkenmeyer, Ramona Oehme and Aniko Kretschmar from Universität Leipzig for the mass spectrometry and the HRMS data.

Disclaimer

Some of the syntheses described here have partially been disclosed in the patent DE 10 2010 063 974 A1.

Author details

[1]Department of Neuroradiopharmaceuticals, Institute of Radiopharmacy, Research Site Leipzig, Helmholtz-Zentrum Dresden-Rossendorf e.V., Permoserstr. 15, Leipzig 04318, Germany. [2]Institute of Organic Chemistry, Faculty of Chemistry and Mineralogy, Universität Leipzig, Johannisallee 29, Leipzig 04103, Germany. [3]Institute of Inorganic Chemistry, Faculty of Chemistry and Mineralogy, Universität Leipzig, Johannisallee 29, Leipzig 04103, Germany.

References

1. Fowler CJ, Rojo ML, Rodriguez-Gaztelumendi A (2010) Modulation of the endocannabinoid system: neuroprotection or neurotoxicity? Exp Neurol 224(1):37–47
2. Matsuda LA, Lolait SJ, Brownstein MJ, Young AC, Bonner TI (1990) Structure of a cannabinoid receptor and functional expression of the cloned cDNA. Nature 346(6284):561–564
3. Alger B (2002) Retrograde signaling in the regulation of synaptic transmission: focus on endocannabinoids. Prog Neurobiol 68(4):247–286
4. Munro S, Thomas KL, Abu-Shaar M (1993) Molecular characterization of a peripheral receptor for cannabinoids. Nature 365(6441):61–65
5. Stella N (2004) Cannabinoid signaling in glial cells. Glia 48(4):267–277
6. Howlett AC, Barth F, Bonner TI, Cabral G, Casellas P, Devane WA, Felder CC, Herkenham M, Mackie K, Martin BR, Mechoulam R, Pertwee RG (2002) International Union of Pharmacology. XXVII Classification of cannabinoid receptors Pharmacol Rev 54(2):161–202
7. Wilson RI, Nicoll RA (2002) Endocannabinoid signaling in the brain. Science 296(5568):678–682
8. Guzmán M, Sánchez C, Galve-Roperh I (2002) Cannabinoids and cell fate. Pharmacol Ther 95(2):175–184
9. Witkin JM, Tzavara ET, Davis RJ, Li X, Nomikos GG (2005) A therapeutic role for cannabinoid CB1 receptor antagonists in major depressive disorders. Trends Pharmacol Sci 26(12):609–617
10. Shohami E, Novikov M, Bass R (1995) Long-term effect of HU-211, a novel non-competitive NMDA antagonist, on motor and memory functions after closed head injury in the rat. Brain Res 674(1):55–62

11. Maas A, Murray G, Henney H, Kassem N, Legrand V, Mangelus M, Muizelaar J, Stocchetti N, Knoller N (2006) Efficacy and safety of dexanabinol in severe traumatic brain injury: results of a phase III randomised, placebo-controlled, clinical trial. Lancet Neurol 5(1):38–45
12. Alexander A, Smith PF, Rosengren RJ (2009) Cannabinoids in the treatment of cancer. Cancer Lett 285(1):6–12
13. Oesch S, Gertsch J (2009) Cannabinoid receptor ligands as potential anticancer agents - high hopes for new therapies? J Pharm Pharmacol 61 (7):839–853
14. Pertwee RG, Thomas A (2010) Therapeutic applications for agents that act at CB1 and CB2 receptors. In: Reggio PH (ed) The cannabinoid receptors. Humana, New York, pp 361–392
15. Mackie K (2006) Cannabinoid receptors as therapeutic targets. Annu Rev Pharmacol Toxicol 46:101–122
16. Turu G, Hunyady L (2010) Signal transduction of the CB1 cannabinoid receptor. J Mol Endocrinol 44(2):75–85
17. Ludányi A, Hu SS-J, Yamazaki M, Tanimura A, Piomelli D, Watanabe M, Kano M, Sakimura K, Maglóczky Z, Mackie K, Freund TF, Katona I (2011) Complementary synaptic distribution of enzymes responsible for synthesis and inactivation of the endocannabinoid 2-arachidonoylglycerol in the human hippocampus. Neuroscience 174:50–63
18. Lynn AB, Herkenham M (1994) Localization of cannabinoid receptors and nonsaturable high-density cannabinoid binding-sites in peripheral-tissues of the rat - implications for receptor-mediated immune modulation by cannabinoids. J Pharmacol Exp Ther 268(3):1612–1623
19. Palazuelos J, Aguado T, Egia A, Mechoulam R, Guzmán M, Galve-Roperh I (2006) Non-psychoactive CB2 cannabinoid agonists stimulate neural progenitor proliferation. FASEB J 20(13):2405–2407
20. Skaper S, Buriani A, DalToso R, Petrelli L, Romanello S, Facci L, Leon A (1996) The ALIAmide palmitoylethanolamide and cannabinoids, but not anandamide, are protective in a delayed postglutamate paradigm of excitotoxic death in cerebellar granule neurons. P Natl Acad Sci USA 93(9):3984–3989
21. Van Sickle MD, Duncan M, Kingsley PJ, Mouihate A, Urbani P, Mackie K, Stella N, Makriyannis A, Piomelli D, Davison JS, Marnett LJ, Di Marzo V, Pittman QJ, Patel KD, Sharkey KA (2005) Identification and functional characterization of brainstem cannabinoid CB2 receptors. Science 310 (5746):329–332
22. Gong J-P, Onaivi ES, Ishiguro H, Liu Q-R, Tagliaferro PA, Brusco A, Uhl GR (2006) Cannabinoid CB2 receptors: immunohistochemical localization in rat brain. Brain Res 1071(1):10–23
23. Onaivi ES, Ishiguro H, Gong J-P, Patel S, Meozzi PA, Myers L, Perchuk A, Mora Z, Tagliaferro PA, Gardner E, Brusco A, Akinshola BE, Hope B, Lujilde J, Inada T, Iwasaki S, Macharia D, Teasenfitz L, Arinami T, Uhl GR (2008) Brain neuronal CB2 cannabinoid receptors in drug abuse and depression: from mice to human subjects. PLoS One 3(2):e1640
24. Suárez J, Bermúdez-Silva FJ, Mackie K, Ledent C, Zimmer A, Cravatt BF, de Fonseca FR (2008) Immunohistochemical description of the endogenous cannabinoid system in the rat cerebellum and functionally related nuclei. J Comp Neurol 509(4):400–421
25. Atwood BK, Mackie K (2010) CB2: a cannabinoid receptor with an identity crisis. Br J Pharmacol 160(3):467–479
26. Ashton JC, Wright JL, McPartland JM, Tyndall JDA (2008) Cannabinoid CB1 and CB2 receptor ligand specificity and the development of CB2-selective agonists. Curr Med Chem 15(14):1428–1443
27. Halleskog C, Mulder J, Dahlström J, Mackie K, Hortobágyi T, Tanila H, Kumar Puli L, Färber K, Harkany T, Schulte G (2011) WNT signaling in activated microglia is proinflammatory. Glia 59(1):119–131
28. Scotter EL, Abood ME, Glass M (2010) The endocannabinoid system as a target for the treatment of neurodegenerative disease. Br J Pharmacol 160 (3):480–498
29. Graham ES, Ashton JC, Glass M (2009) Cannabinoid receptors: a brief history and "what's hot". Front Biosci 14:944–957
30. Evens N, Vandeputte C, Coolen C, Janssen P, Sciot R, Baekelandt V, Verbruggen AM, Debyser Z, Van Laere K, Bormans GM (2011) Preclinical evaluation of [^{11}C]NE40, a type 2 cannabinoid receptor PET tracer. Nuclear Med Biol 39(3):389–399
31. Roche M, Finn DP (2010) Brain CB2 receptors: implications for neuropsychiatric disorders. Pharmaceuticals 3(8):2517–2553
32. Lavey BJ, Kozlowski JA, Hipkin RW, Gonsiorek W, Lundell DJ, Piwinski JJ, Narula S, Lunn CA (2005) Triaryl bis-sulfones as a new class of cannabinoid CB2 receptor inhibitors: identification of a lead and initial SAR studies. Bioorg Med Chem Lett 15(3):783–786
33. Evens N, Muccioli GG, Houbrechts N, Lambert DM, Verbruggen AM, Van Laere K, Bormans GM (2009) Synthesis and biological evaluation of carbon-11- and fluorine-18-labeled 2-oxoquinoline derivatives for type 2 cannabinoid receptor positron emission tomography imaging. Nucl Med Biol 36(4):455–465
34. Gao M, Wang M, Miller KD, Hutchins GD, Zheng Q-H (2010) Synthesis and in vitro biological evaluation of carbon-11-labeled quinoline derivatives as new candidate PET radioligands for cannabinoid CB2 receptor imaging. Bioorg Med Chem 18(6):2099–2106
35. Evens N, Bormans GM (2010) Non-invasive imaging of the type 2 cannabinoid receptor, focus on positron emission tomography. Curr Top Med Chem 10(15):1527–1543
36. Cheng Y, Albrecht BK, Brown J, Buchanan JL, Buckner WH, DiMauro EF, Emkey R, Fremeau RT, Harmange J-C, Hoffman BJ, Huang L, Huang M, Lee JH, Lin F-F, Martin MW, Nguyen HQ, Patel VF, Tomlinson SA, White RD, Xia X, Hitchcock SA (2008) Discovery and optimization of a novel series of N-arylamide oxadiazoles as potent, highly selective and orally bioavailable cannabinoid receptor 2 (CB2) agonists. J Med Chem 51(16):5019–5034
37. Shoemaker JL, Joseph BK, Ruckle MB, Mayeux PR, Prather PL (2005) The endocannabinoid noladin ether acts as a full agonist at human CB2 cannabinoid receptors. J Pharmacol Exp Ther 314(2):868–875
38. Gullapalli S, Amrutkar D, Gupta S, Kandadi MR, Kumar H, Gandhi M, Karande V, Narayanan S (2010) Characterization of active and inactive states of CB1 receptor and the differential binding state modulation by cannabinoid agonists, antagonists and inverse agonists. Neuropharmacology 58(8):1215–1219
39. Massi P, Patrini G, Rubino T, Fuzio D, Parolaro D (1997) Changes in rat spleen cannabinoid receptors after chronic CP-55,940: an autoradiographic study. Pharmacol Biochem Behav 58(1):73–78
40. McPartland JM, Glass M, Pertwee RG (2007) Meta-analysis of cannabinoid ligand binding affinity and receptor distribution: interspecies differences. Br J Pharmacol 152(5):583–593
41. Shire D, Calandra B, Rinaldi-Carmona M, Oustric D, Pessegue B, Bonnin-Cabanne O, LeFur G, Caput D, Ferrara P (1996) Molecular cloning, expression and function of the murine CB2 peripheral cannabinoid receptor. Biochim Biophys Acta 1307(2):132–136
42. Warne T, Moukhametzianov R, Baker JG, Nehmé R, Edwards PC, Leslie AGW, Schertler GFX, Tate CG (2011) The structural basis for agonist and partial agonist action on a β(1)-adrenergic receptor. Nature 469(7329):241–244
43. Xu F, Wu H, Katritch V, Han GW, Jacobson KA, Gao Z-G, Cherezov V, Stevens RC (2011) Structure of an agonist-bound human A2A adenosine receptor. Science 332(6027):322–327
44. Poso A, Huffman JW (2008) Targeting the cannabinoid CB2 receptor: modelling and structural determinants of CB2 selective ligands. Br J Pharmacol 153(2):335–346
45. Wiley EA, Deslongchamps G (2006) PostDock: a novel visualization tool for the analysis of molecular docking. Comput Visual Sci 12(1):1–7
46. Sheldrick GM (2008) A short history of SHELX. Acta Crystallogr, A, Found Crystallogr 64(Pt 1):112–122
47. Jeffries WB, Waugh D, Abel PW (1997) Analysis of data from "cold saturation" radioligand binding experiments. Methods Mol Biol 73:331–342
48. Hulme EC, Trevethick MA (2010) Ligand binding assays at equilibrium: validation and interpretation. Br J Pharmacol 161(6):1219–1237
49. Cheng Y, Prusoff WH (1973) Relationship between the inhibition constant (K_i) and the concentration of inhibitor which causes 50 per cent inhibition (IC_{50}) of an enzymatic reaction. Biochem Pharmacol 22(23):3099–3108
50. Foreman JC, Johansen T (2003) Textbook of receptor pharmacology, 2nd edn. CRC, Boca Raton
51. Jaakola V-P, Griffith MT, Hanson MA, Cherezov V, Chien EYT, Lane JR, Ijzerman AP, Stevens RC (2008) The 2.6 Ångström crystal structure of a human A_{2A} adenosine receptor bound to an antagonist. Science 322:1211–1217
52. Ballesteros JA, Weinstein H (1995) Integrated methods for the construction of three-dimensional models and computational probing of structure-function relations in G protein-coupled receptors. In: Sealfon SC (ed) Receptor molecular biology. Methods in neurosciences, vol 25. Elsevier, San Diego, pp 366–428
53. Abood ME (2005) Molecular biology of cannabinoid receptors. Handb Exp Pharmacol 168:81–115

54. Verdonk ML, Cole JC, Hartshorn MJ, Murray CW, Taylor RD (2003) Improved protein–ligand docking using GOLD. Proteins 52(4):609–623
55. Gunasekaran K, Nussinov R (2007) How different are structurally flexible and rigid binding sites? Sequence and structural features discriminating proteins that do and do not undergo conformational change upon ligand binding. J Mol Biol 365(1):257–273

Increase of leishmanicidal and tubercular activities using steroids linked to aminoquinoline

Luciana MR Antinarelli[1†], Arturene ML Carmo[2†], Fernando R Pavan[3], Clarice Queico F Leite[3], Adilson D Da Silva[2*], Elaine S Coimbra[1] and Deepak B Salunke[4]

Abstract

Background: Aminoquinoline/steroid conjugates were synthesized based on the fact that steroid transporters have been shown to accept and carry a variety of drugs. So, in continuing our research of antileishmanial and antitubercular drugs, aminoquinoline/steroid conjugates (**12**, **13**, and **14**) were regioselectively synthesized via 1, 3-dipolar cycloaddition of alkynes **3**, **5**, and **7** with azide **12**. The aminoquinoline/steroids conjugates were evaluated *in vitro* against *Leishmania major* and *Mycobacterium tuberculosis*.

Results: Regioselective synthesis of the novel aminoquinoline/steroid conjugates was achieved in very high yield. All aminoquinoline/steroid conjugates (**12**, **13**, and **14**) exhibited best results against *Leishmania* and *M. tuberculosis* than the respective alkyne intermediate structures (**3**, **5**, and **7**, respectively). Among them, the compound **12** exhibited the best activity for *M. tuberculosis* (MIC = 8.8 μM). This result is comparable to drugs commonly used in tuberculosis treatment. Also, for antileishmanial assay, the aminoquinoline/steroid conjugates demonstrated a significant activity against promastigote and amastigote forms of *L. major*.

Conclusions: Addition of a steroid group to aminoquinoline molecules enhanced the leishmanicidal and antitubercular activities. These results highlight the importance of steroids as carrier.

Keywords: Antileishmanial drugs, Antituberculosis drugs, Click chemistry, Quinoline, Steroid

Background

Quinolines are among the most important antimalarial drugs ever used [1,2]. In addition, quinoline derivatives have also demonstrated a variety of biological properties that includes antiviral, anti-inflammatory, antitubercular, and antileishmanial activities [2-5]. Leishmaniasis is a disease caused by parasitic protozoans of the genus *Leishmania*. Over 20 different *Leishmania* species can infect humans and cause a wide spectrum of symptoms. It has an estimated prevalence of 12 million cases worldwide, which is continuing to increase, with 1.5–2 million new cases each year [6]. With no available vaccine, the chemotherapy is a major control for the disease. However, the treatment options are severely limited and first line treatment is based on pentavalent antimonials that have been used in therapeutics for more than half a century [7]. Tuberculosis (TB) is another important neglected disease. TB is more prevalent in the world today than at any other time in human history. *Mycobacterium tuberculosis* (MTB), the pathogen responsible for TB, uses diverse strategies to survive in a variety of host lesions and to evade immune surveillance [7,8]. The last 20 years have seen the worldwide appearance of multidrug-resistant TB, followed by extensively drug-resistant TB, and most recently, strains that are resistant to all antituberculosis drugs [9]. Since the discovery of rifampicin (1960), no new drugs have been developed specifically against mycobacteria [10]. Also, only within the last few years some promising drug candidates have emerged [11]. Considering the inefficacy and the high toxicity of the currently used drugs for the treatment of these infectious diseases, as well as the emergence of drug-resistant strains of the causative organisms, the development of new leishmanicidal and antitubercular agents is extremely important.

Bioconjugation has emerged as a fast growing technology and aims at the ligation of two or more molecules to form new complexes with the combined properties of their individual components [12]. To make this linkage,

* Correspondence: david.silva@ufjf.edu.br
[†]Equal contributors
[2]Departamento de Química, I.C.E., Universidade Federal de Juiz de Fora, Campus Universitário, Juiz de Fora, MG 36036-900, Brazil
Full list of author information is available at the end of the article

the 1,2,3-triazole moieties are attractive as connecting units, since they are stable to metabolic degradation and capable of hydrogen bonding, which can be favorable in binding to biomolecular targets and also improves solubility [13]. Although the 1,2,3-triazole structural moiety does not occur in nature, the synthetic molecules containing the 1,2,3-triazole unit show diverse biological activities including antibacterial, herbicidal, fungicidal, anti-allergic, and anti-HIV [14]. Aminoquinoline/cholic acid conjugates were synthesized based on the fact that steroid transporters have been shown to accept and carry a variety of drugs [15]. Cholic acid is the most common form of the steroid and its derivatives are known to exhibit antimicrobial activities [16]. Bile acids are amphiphilic molecules which may represent alternatives for chemotherapeutic agents by acting synergistically with antibiotics as membrane permeabilizers [17-21]. Moreover, several bile acid/drug conjugates are shown to possess better activity than the precursor [22,23].

In a previous study, we demonstrate that 4-amino-7-chloroquinoline derivatives showed an interesting antileishmanial and anti-MTB activities [24]. In continuation of this study were synthesized aminoquinoline conjugate with steroids in the expectation of improving its biological activity.

Methods

General experimental techniques and apparatus

TLC was performed on precoated silica gel F254 plates (0.25 mm; E. Merck). Infrared spectra were recorded on Schimadzu 8400 series FTIR instrument. ^{1}H NMR spectra were recorded on a Bruker AC-300 and 500 spectrometers at 300.13 and 500.13 MHz and ^{13}C NMR spectra were recorded on a Bruker AC-300 at 75 MHz. The chemical shifts are given in parts per million relative to tetramethylsilane. Mass spectra were recorded on LC–MS/MS-TOF API QSTAR PULSAR spectrometer, and samples were introduced by infusion method using Electro spray Ionization Technique. Standard work up: after extraction of all the reactions, the organic extracts were washed with water and brine and dried over anhydrous Na_2SO_4 and concentrated in vacuum.

Synthesis of terminal acetylenes

General synthetic procedure for N-(7-chloroquinolin-4-yl) alkyl-diamine) (2, 4, and 6)

A mixture of 4,7-dichloroquinoline (2.0 g, 10.1 mmol) and the corresponding diamines (50.0 mmol), ethane-1,2-diamine, propane-1,3-diamine, or buthane-1,4-diamine, was heated at 80°C for 1 h without stirring for 1 h and then at 110°C for 4–6 h with continued stirring to drive the reaction to completion. The reaction mixture was cooled to room temperature and diluted with dichloromethane. The organic layer was successively washed with 5% NaOH (30 mL) followed by water wash and then finally with brine. The organic layer was dried over anhydrous Na_2SO_4 and solvent was removed under reduced pressure to afford the compounds **2**, **4**, and **6**, at 80–90% yield.

N-(7-chloroquinolin-4-yl)ethane-1,2-diamine (2) [25]: Yellow solid, yield: 90%; mp = 141°C (145-147°C).
N-(7-chloroquinolin-4-yl)propane-1,3-diamine (4) [25]: Yellow solid, yield: 90%; mp = 97°C (96–98°C) [25].
N-(7-chloroquinolin-4-yl)buthane-1,4-diamine (6) [25]: Yellow solid, yield: 80%; mp = 123°C (122–124°C).

General synthetic procedure for 7-chloro-N-(3-(prop-2-ynylamino)alquil)quinolin-4-amine (3, 5, and 7)

The compounds **2**, **4**, and **6** (6.8 mmol) and propargyl bromide (13.6 mmol), in presence of K_2CO_3 (13.6 mmol), were dissolved in EtOH (5.0 mL). The reaction mixture was stirred at 0°C for 2 h and then at 25°C for 48 h. Solvent was removed in vacuum until dry. The crude reaction product was purified by flash chromatography (eluent: $MeOH/CH_2Cl_2$ 5:95) producing the compounds **3**, **5**, and **7**, respectively (2.5 mmol) in 60% yield as yellow solid.

7-chloro-N-(2-(prop-2-ynylamino)ethyl)quinolin-4-amine (3) [24]: Yield: 60%, mp = 99°C.
7-chloro-N-(3-(prop-2-ynylamino)propyl)quinolin-4-amine (5) [24]: Yield: 60%, mp = 75°C.
7-chloro-N-(4-(prop-2-ynylamino)butyl)quinolin-4-amine (7) [24]: Yield: 62%, mp = 72°C.

Synthesis of terminal azide

Synthesis of methyl 3α,7α,12α-trihydroxy-5β-cholane-24-oate (9)

Compound **9** was synthesized in overall good yield starting from bile acid **8** using the literature procedure [24]. White solid, m.p. 158°C.

*Methyl-3α-mesyloxy-7α-12α-dihydroxy-5β-cholane-24-oate (**10**)* [23]: To a solution of **9** (2.0 g, 4.92 mmol) in CH_2Cl_2 (20 mL) was added triethylamine (6.4 mL, 49.2 mmol) at 0°C. Methane sulfonyl chloride (0.5 mL, 4.92 mmol) was added dropwise for 10 min at 0°C. The reaction mixture was extracted with CH_2Cl_2/H_2O. Organic layer was washed with $NaHCO_3$, water, and brine. The solvent was evaporated under reduced pressure. The crude product was purified by column chromatography (AcOEt/Hex 2:8) to obtain pure product 7 (1.9 g).

Synthesis of methyl-3β-azido-7α,12α-dihydroxy-5β-cholane-24-oate (11)

The compound **10** was reacted with NaN_3 (5 equiv) in DMF for 24 h at 120°C to give product **11** [23]. White solid, m.p. 175°C.

General procedure for cycloaddition (12–14)

The alkyne **3**, **5**, or **7** (1 equiv) and the azide **11** (1.3 equiv) were dissolved in DMSO/H_2O 4:1 (5 mL). To this solution, $CuSO_4.5H_2O$ (0.05 equiv) and sodium ascorbate (0.40 equiv) were added. The reaction mixture was stirred for 48 h at room temperature and it was then extracted with CH_2Cl_2/H_2O. Organic layer was washed with $NaHCO_3$, water, and brine. The solvent was evaporated under reduced pressure and crude product was purified by column chromatography on silica gel using 30% $MeOH/CH_2Cl_2$ system to obtain aminoquinoline/bile acid conjugates **12**, **13**, or **14**, respectively, linked with 1,4-disubstituted 1,2,3-triazole in 60% yield.

*Methyl 3β-(N-[(7-chloroquinolin-4-yl)amino]ethylaminomethyl)-1 H-1,2,3-triazol-1-yl)]7α-12α-dihydroxy-5β-cholane-24-oate (**12**)*: Yellow crystalline solid; m.p. 128°C, υ_{max} (KBr): 3340 (NH), 2930 (CH); ^1H NMR (300 MHz, CD_3OD): 8.31 (d, 1 H, $J_{2,3}=4$ Hz, H-2'); 8.08 (d, 1 H, $J_{5,6}=6$ Hz, H-5'); 7.88 (s, 1 H, H-4" triazole); 7.73 (s, 1 H, H-8'); 7.37 (dd, 1 H, $J_{6,5}=6$ Hz, $J=2$ Hz, H-6'); 6.51 (d, 1 H, $J_{3,2}=4$ Hz, H-3'); 4.53 (s, 1 H, H-12); 3.60 (s, 1 H, H-7); 3.89 (s, 2 H, H-3"); 3.49 (s, 3 H, H-25); 3.45 (m, 2 H, H-1"); 2.93 (m, 2 H, H-2"); 0.97 (d, 3 H, $J=6$ Hz, H-21); 0.76 (s, 3 H, H-18); 0.65 (s, 3 H, H-19); ^{13}C NMR (75 MHz, CD_3OD): 176.4 (C-24); 152,6 (C-4'); 152.0 (C-2'); 149.3 (C-9'); 146.3 (C-3" triazole); 136.3 (C-7'); 127.3 (C-8'); 125.9 (C-6'); 124.3 (C-4" triazole); 123.3 (C-5'); 118.6 (C-10'); 99.5 (C-3'); 73.7 (C-12); 68.7 (C-7); 58.2 (C-3); 51.8 (C-13); 48.8 (C-25); 47.1 (C-2); 23.3 (C-21); 17.4 (C-19); 12.8 (C-18); HRMS ESI $[M+H]^+$: m/z: Calc for $C_{39}H_{56}N_6O_4Cl$ 707.4052 $[M+H]^+$, found 707.4059 $[M+H]^+$.

*Methyl 3β-(N-[(7-chloroquinolin-4-yl)amino]propylaminomethyl)-1 H-1,2,3-triazol-1-yl)]7α-12α-dihydroxy-5β-cholane-24-oate (**13**)*: Yellow oil; υ_{max} (KBr): 3345 (NH), 2928 (CH); ^1H NMR (300 MHz, $CDCl_3$): 8.38 (d, 1 H, $J_{2,3}=4$ Hz, H-2'); 7.87 (s, 1 H, H-8'); 7.74 (d, 1 H, $J_{5,6}=6$ Hz, H-5'); 7.52 (s, 1 H, H-5" triazole); 7.20 (dd, 1 H, $J_{6,5}=6$ Hz, $J=2$ Hz, H-6'); 6.27 (d, 1 H, $J_{3,2}=4$ Hz, H-3'); 4.53 (s, 2 H, H-4"); 3.87 (s, 1 H, H-7); 3.65 (s, 3 H, H-25); 3.45 (m, 2 H, H-1"); 0.97 (d, 3 H, $J=6$ Hz, H-21); 0.81 (s, 3 H, H-18); 0.68 (s, 3 H, H-19); ^{13}C NMR (75 MHz, $CDCl_3$): 174.9 (C-24); 151.4 (C-4'); 150.2 (C-2'); 144.6 (C-9'); 144.6 (C-4" triazole); 135.5 (C-7'); 126.8 (C-8'); 125.4 (C-6'); 123.0 (C-5" triazole); 122.9 (C-5'); 121.4 (C-10'), 114.0 (C-3'), 73.0 (C-12), 68.2 (C-7), 57.0 (C-3), 51.7 (C-13), 48.4 (C-25), 47.4 (C-2), 38.3 (C-14); 22.9 (C-21); 17.5 (C-19); 12.7 (C-18); HRMS ESI $[M+H]^+$: m/z: Calc for $C_{40}H_{58}N_6O_4Cl$ 721.4108 $[M+H]^+$, found 721.4210 $[M+H]^+$.

*Methyl 3β-(N-[(7-chloroquinolin-4-yl)amino]buthylaminomethyl)-1 H-1,2,3-triazol-1-yl)]7α-12α-dihydroxy-5β-cholane-24-oate (**14**).*

Yellow oil; υ_{max} (KBr): 3347 (NH), 2931 (CH); ^1H NMR (300 MHz, $CDCl_3$): 8.44 (d, 1 H, $J_{2,3}=2$ Hz, H-2'); 7.88 (s, 1 H, H-8'); 7.77 (d, 1 H, $J_{5,6}=6$ Hz, H-5'); 7.51 (s, 1 H, H-7" triazol); 7.23 (dd, 1 H, $J_{6,5}=6$ Hz, $J=2$ Hz, H-6'); 6.32 (d, 1 H, $J_{3,2}=2$ Hz, H-3'); 3.92 (s, 2 H, H-4"); 3.88 (s, 1 H, H-7); 3.66 (s, 3 H, H-25); 3.28 (m, 2 H, H-1"); 0.99 (d, 3 H, $J=6$ Hz, H-21); 0.82 (s, 3 H, H-18); 0.68 (s, 3 H, H-19); ^{13}C NMR (75 MHz, $CDCl_3$): 174.9 (C-24); 151.6 (C-4'); 150.5 (C-2'); 148.7 (C-9'); 145.3 (C-6" triazole); 134.8 (C-7'); 127.8 (C-8'); 124.9 (C-6'); 122.3 (C-7" triazole); 121.2 (C-5'); 117.4 (C-10'); 98.8 (C-3'); 72.9.0 (C-12); 68.0 (C-7); 56.9 (C-3); 51.6 (C-13); 48.7 (C-25); 47.3 (C-2); 22.9 (C-21); 17.5 (C-19); 12.7 (C-18); HRMS ESI $[M+H]^+$: m/z: Calc for $C_{41}H_{60}N_6O_4Cl$ 735.4365 $[M+H]^+$, found 735.4362 $[M+H]^+$.

Biological evaluation

Anti-MTB activity

The anti-MTB activity of the compounds was determined by the *Resazurin Microtiter Assay* (REMA) [26]. Stock solutions of the test compounds were prepared in dimethyl sulfoxide (DMSO) and diluted in Middlebrook 7 H9 broth (Difco), supplemented with oleic acid, albumin, dextrose and catalase (OADC enrichment—BBL/Becton Dickinson, Sparks, MD, USA), to obtain final drug concentration ranges from 0.15 to 250 μM. The serial dilutions were realized in a Precision XS Microplate Sample Processor (Biotek™). The isoniazid was dissolved in distilled water, as recommended by the manufacturer (Difco laboratories, Detroit, MI, USA), and used as a standard drug. MTB $H_{37}Rv$ ATCC 27294 was grown for 7 to 10 days in Middlebrook 7 H9 broth supplemented with OADC, plus 0.05% Tween 80 to avoid clumps. Cultures were centrifuged for 15 min at 3,150 *g*, washed twice, and resuspended in phosphate-buffered saline and aliquots were frozen at −80°C. After 2 days, an aliquot was thawed to determine the viability and the CFU after freezing. MTB $H_{37}Rv$ (ATCC 27294) was thawed and added to the test compounds, yielding a final testing volume of 200 μL with 2×10^4 CFU/mL. Microplates with serial dilutions of each compound were incubated for 7 days at 37°C, after resazurin was added to test viability. Wells that turned from blue to pink, with the development of fluorescence, indicated growth of bacterial cells, while maintenance of the blue color indicated bacterial inhibition [26]. The fluorescence was read (530 nm excitation filter and 590 nm emission filter) in a SPECTRAfluor Plus (Tecan®) microfluorimeter. The MIC was defined as the lowest concentration resulting in 90% inhibition of growth of MTB. As a standard test, the MIC of isoniazid was determined on each microplate. The acceptable range of isoniazid MIC is from 0.11 to 0.44 μM [10,33]. Each test was set up in triplicate.

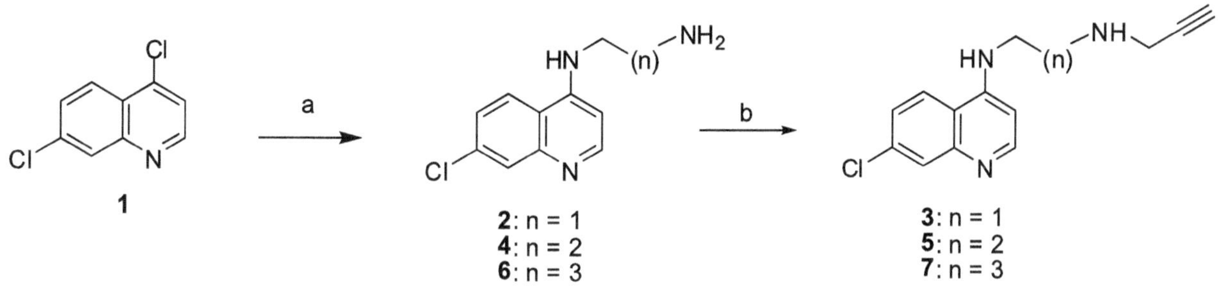

Figure 1 Reagents and conditions: (a) ethane-1,2-diamine, propane-1,3-diamine, or butane-1,4-diamine, 80°C for 1 h, 110°C for 4 h, 90%; (b) propargyl bromide, K_2CO_3, EtOH, 25°C, 48 h, 60%.

In vitro antileishmanial activity

Parasites and cell culture

Promastigote forms of *L. major* (MRHO/SU/59/P) were maintained in Medium BHI supplemented with 10% fetal bovine serum (FBS) at 24°C. FBS was purchased from Cultilab (Campinas, São Paulo, Brazil) and brain heart infusion (BHI) from Himédia (Mumbai, India).

Promastigote forms

The viability of parasites was determined by the colorimetric 3-(4,5-dimethylthiazol-2-yl)-2,5-diphenyl-tetrazolium bromide (purchased by Sigma Chemical Co., St. Louis, MO, USA) or MTT method, based on tetrazolium salt reduction by mitochondrial dehydrogenases [27]. Briefly, promastigotes of *L. major* from a logarithmic phase culture were suspended to yield 2 million cells/mL after Neubauer chamber counting. The screening was performed in 96-well microtiter plates maintained at 24°C. Controls with DMSO and without drugs were performed. Absorbance was measured at 570 nm (Multiskan MS microplate reader, LabSystems Oy, Helsink, Finland). The results are expressed as the concentrations inhibiting parasite growth by 50% (IC_{50}) after a 3-day incubation period. Amphotericin B (supplied by Cristália, São Paulo, Brazil) was used as the reference standard. For data analysis: IC_{50} values were carried out at 5% significance level ($p < 0.05$, CI 95%), calculated using a non-linear regression curve, by using *GraFit* Version 5 software (Erithacus Software Ltd., Horley, UK).

Amastigote forms

Concerning the amastigotes *in vitro* model, inflammatory macrophages were obtained from BALB/c mice previously inoculated with 3% thioglycollate medium (Sigma Chemical Co.). Briefly, peritoneal macrophages were plated at 2×10^6 cells/mL on coverslips (13-mm diameter) previously arranged in a 24-well plate in RPMI 1640 medium supplemented with 10% inactivated FBS, and allowed to adhere for 24 h at 37°C in 5% CO_2. Adherent macrophages were infected with *L. major* (MRHO/SU/59/P) promastigotes in the stationary growth phase using a ratio of 1:10 at 37°C for 3 h. Non-internalized promastigotes were eliminated and

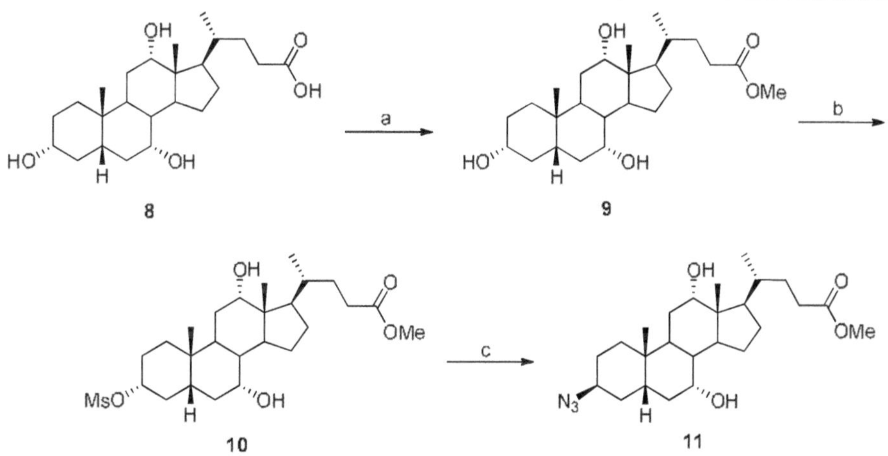

Figure 2 Reagents and conditions: (a) HCl/MeOH, 25°C, 24 h, 98%; (b) MsCl, Et_3N, CH_2Cl_2, 0°C, 2 h, 80%; (c) NaN_3, DMF, 120°C, 24 h, 70%.

solutions of tested compounds were added and maintained at 37°C in 5% CO_2 for 72 h. Slides were fixed and stained with Giemsa for parasite counting (optical microscopy, 1000× magnification). Amphotericin B was used as a standard drug and the reduction of the number of amastigotes was evaluated after only 24-h post-infection (0.1 μM = 35% and 1.0 μM = 48% of reduction of intracellular amastigotes). The data were analyzed using GraphPad Prism 5.0 (GraphPad Software, San Diego, CA, USA), which considered the mean of two assays performed in duplicate. One-way ANOVA was applied to compare all the groups. Differences were regarded as significant when $p < 0.0001$ (***) and $p < 0.001$ (**).

Results and discussion

Chemistry

The aminoquinoline/steroids conjugates **12**, **13**, **and 14** were synthesized via 1,3-dipolar cycloaddition of alkyne **3**, **5**, or **7**, respectively, with an azide group of the bile acid **11**. 4,7-dichloroquinoline **1** on treatment with ethylenediamine, propanediamine, or butanediamine at 80–110°C for 4 h furnished the intermediates *N*-(2-aminoethyl)-7-chloroquinolin-4-amine (**2**), *N*-(3-aminopropyl)-7-chloroquinolin-4-amine (**4**), and *N*-(4-aminobutyl)-7-chloroquinolin-4-amine (**6**) in 90% yield [25]. These intermediates **2**, **4**, or **6** on further treatment with propargyl bromide and K_2CO_3 in EtOH at 25°C for 48 h yielded compounds **3**, **5**, and **7**, respectively, in 60% yield (see Figure 1) [28].

The C-3-azido steroid (bile acid) derivative **11** was synthesized according to the literature procedures [29,30] with small modifications (see Figure 2). Finally, the

Table 1 Effect of the compounds on promastigote forms of *L. major*, murine peritoneal macrophages and *M. tuberculosis*

Compounds	Biological tests (μM)	
	M. tuberculosis (MIC)[a]	*L. major*(IC_{50})[b]
3	60.1[c]	20.6[c]
5	60.1[c]	45.0[c]
7	54.2[c]	>87.0[c]
12	8.8	10.6
13	17.3	21.2
14	17.0	25.6
AmB*	–	0.3
Isoniazid*	0.11–0.44	–

Values represent the mean of triplicate samples.*AmB (amphotericin B) and isoniazid were used as reference drug for antileishmanial and anti-MTB assays, respectively. [a]IC_{50} values (concentrations inhibiting parasite growth by 50%). [b]MIC: lowest concentration resulting in 90% inhibition of growth of MTB. [c]Data have been reported previously [24].

3 + 11 →

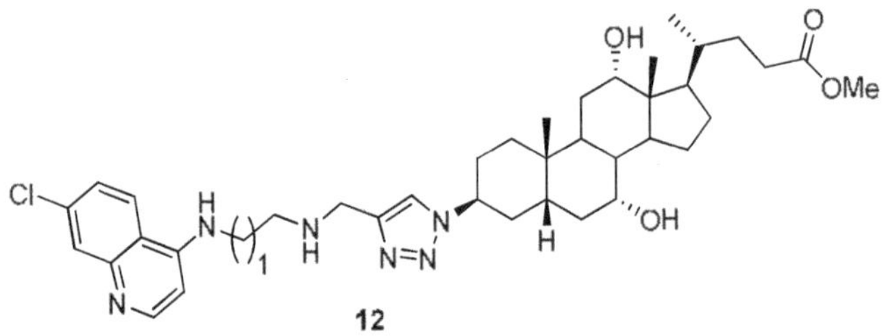

12

5 + 11 →

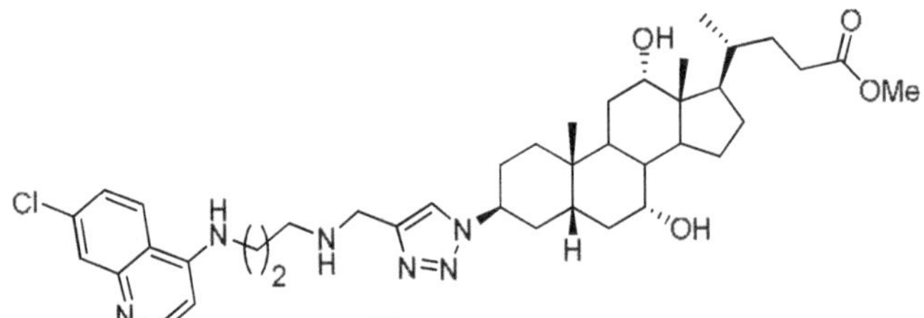

13

7 + 11 →

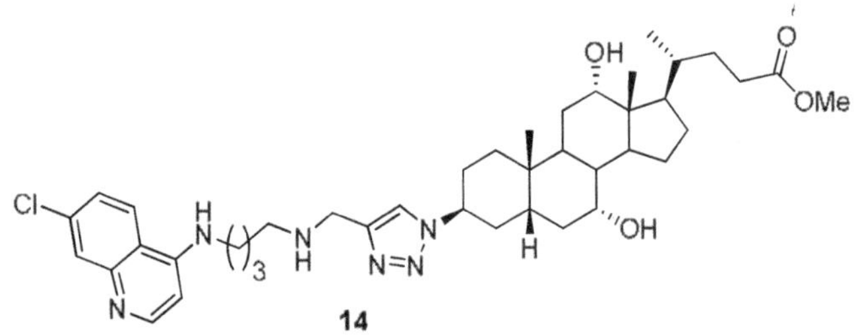

14

Figure 3 Reagents and conditions: (a) $CuSO_4.5H_2O$, sodium ascorbate, DMSO/H_2O (1:1), 25°C, 96 h, 60%.

aminoquinoline/steroid (bile acid) conjugates **12**, **13**, and **14** were synthesized in very high yield via 1,3-dipolar cycloaddition of alkyne **3**, **5**, or **7** with an azide group of the bile acid **11**, respectively, using $CuSO_4 \cdot 5H_2O$, sodium ascorbate, DMSO/H_2O (1:1) at 25°C for 96 h, in 60% yield (see Figure 3). All the compounds were well characterized by ^1H NMR, ^{13}C NMR, and HRMS.

Biological evaluation

Previous study demonstrated that 4-amino-7-chloroquinoline derivatives (**2–7**) showed an interesting antileishmanial and anti-MTB activities [24]. In continuation of this study, novel steroid linked aminoquinolines were synthesized in an anticipation to improve its biological activity. Table 1 shows the biological results comparing

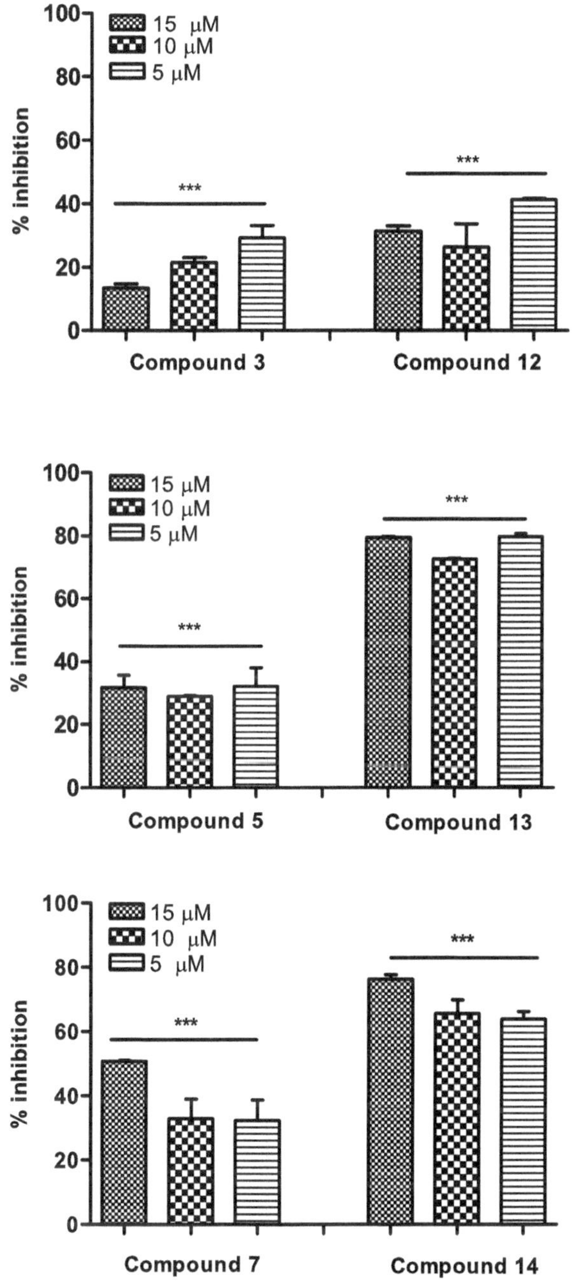

Figure 4 Effect of alkyne intermediate structures (3, 5 and 7) and aminoquinoline/steroid conjugates (12, 13 and 14) on intracellular amastigotes. Peritoneal macrophages previously infected with *L. major* promastigotes in the stationary growth phase were exposed to the compounds for 72 h. Results from two assays in duplicate are shown as percentage of growth inhibition in relation to untreated control. All results were significant (***$p < 0.0001$).

the alkyne intermediate structures (**3**, **5**, and **7**) and their corresponding aminoquinoline/steroid conjugate products (**12**, **13**, and **14**).

Anti-MTB activity of the compounds increased in the following order: alkyne intermediate structures (**3**, **5**, and **7**) < aminoquinoline/steroid conjugates (**12–14**). The aminoquinoline/steroid conjugates (**12–14**) showed excellent results with MICs ranging from 8.8 to 17.3 μM. Within these conjugates, the compound **12** was the most active against MTB bacilli (8.8 μM) and the presence of the shortest ethylenodiamine linker was enough to demonstrate the improved activity. The minimum inhibitory concentration (MIC) value found for the compound **12** is comparable or better than the MIC of some "second-line" drugs currently used in TB therapy such as cycloserine (122.4–489.7 μM), kanamycin (2.1–8.6 μM), tobramycin (8.6–17.1 μM), and clarithromycin (10.7–21.4 μM) [31].

For antileishmanial test, the assay was performed in both promastigote and amastigote forms of *Leishmania* since both stages of parasite are used for drug screening research [32-34]. Table 1 shows IC_{50} values of synthesized compounds on promastigote forms of *L. major*. Aminoquinoline/steroid conjugates (**12–14**) were more active than the respective alkyne intermediate structures (**3**, **5**, and **7**, respectively). Among them, the compound **12** was the most active in promastigotes of *L. major*, inhibiting two times more the viability of the parasite than the alkyne intermediate **3**.

Although the promastigotes of the *Leishmania* genus are used for screening of compounds, this assay must be considered as preliminary because: this stage of parasite is significantly more susceptible to drug-induced effects than amastigote, the amastigote are responsible for all clinical manifestations in humans and the intracellular amastigote model has been cited as the golden standard for *in vitro Leishmania* drug discovery research [33,34]. *L. major*-macrophage treated with the aminoquinoline/steroid compounds (**12–14**) showed a significant inhibitory effect against the intracellular amastigotes, as evidenced in Figure 4. Addition of a steroid group to aminoquinoline molecules again enhanced the biological activity of the compounds. Results showed that the compounds **13** and **14** showed the best antiproliferative effects on intracellular amastigotes, inhibiting between 64 and 80% of the parasite burden. These assays were performed in concentrations above those toxic for murine macrophages.

Antileishmanial and anti-MTB results confirm the importance of steroid groups such cholic acid acting as carriers. The cholic acid-derived carriers can possibly increase the solubility in physiological conditions and it could lead to increased cell permeability due to the amphiphilic character of the molecule and could function as an ionophore [22]. Further *in vivo* mouse model studies could better elucidate the role of bile acid derivatives as carriers.

Conclusions

Regioselective synthesis of the novel aminoquinoline/steroid conjugates was achieved in very high yield. Addition of a steroid group to aminoquinoline molecules enhanced the anti-MTB activity, having lower MICs than some drugs commonly used to treat TB. For antileishmanial assay, the aminoquinoline/steroid conjugates demonstrated a significant activity against promastigote and amastigote forms of *L. major*.

Abbreviations

BHI: Brain heart infusion; FBS: Fetal bovine serum; IC_{50}: Concentrations inhibiting parasite growth by 50%; MIC: Minimum inhibitory concentration; MTB: *Mycobacterium* tuberculosis; TB: Tuberculosis.

Competing interests

The authors declare that they have no competing interests.

Acknowledgments

This study was supported by the FAPEMIG, FAPESP, CAPES, CNPq and BIC/UFJF.

Author details

[1]Departamento de Parasitologia, Microbiologia e Imunologia, I.C.B, Universidade Federal de Juiz de Fora, Campus Universitário, Juiz de Fora, MG 36036-900, Brazil. [2]Departamento de Química, I.C.E., Universidade Federal de Juiz de Fora, Campus Universitário, Juiz de Fora, MG 36036-900, Brazil. [3]Departamento de Ciências Biológicas, F.C. F., Universidade Estadual Paulista "Júlio de Mesquita Filho", Rod. Araraquara-Jaú Km.01 s/n, Campus, 14801-902, Araraquara, SP, Brazil. [4]Centre National de la Recherche Scientifique, Institut de Chimie des Substances Naturelles, UPR 2301 CNRS, Avenue de la Terrasse, 91198, Gif-sur-Yvette, France.

References

1. Kaur K, Jain M, Reddy RP, Jain R: **Quinolines and structurally related heterocycles as antimalarials.** *Eur J Med Chem* 2010, **45**:3245.
2. Kaur K, Jain M, Khan SI, Jacob MR, Tekwani BL, Singh S, Singh PP, Jain R: **Synthesis, antiprotozoal, antimicrobial, β-hematin inhibition, cytotoxicity and methemoglobin (MetHb) formation activities of bis(8-aminoquinolines).** *Bioorg Med Chem* 2011, **19**:197.
3. Vieira NC, Herrenknecht C, Vacus J, Fournet A, Bories C, Figadère B, Espindola LS, Loiseau PM: **Selection of the most promising 2-substituted quinoline as antileishmanial candidate for clinical trials.** *Biomed Pharmacother* 2008, **62**:684.
4. Tekwani BL, Walker LA: **8-Aminoquinolines: future role as antiprotozoal drugs.** *Curr Opin Infect Dis* 2006, **19**:623.
5. Kaur K, Patel SR, Patil P, Jain M, Khan SI, Jacob MR, Ganesan S, Tekwani BL, Jain R: **Synthesis, antimalarial, antileishmanial, antimicrobial, cytotoxicity, and methemoglobin (MetHB) formation activities of new 8-quinolinamines.** *Bioorg Med Chem* 2007, **15**:915.
6. World Health Organization: *Leishmaniasis*; http://www.who.int/leishmaniasis/en/. Accessed May 16, 2011.
7. Baiocco P, Colotti G, Franceschini S, Ilari A: **Molecular basis of antimony treatment in leishmaniasis.** *J Med Chem* 2009, **23**:2603.
8. Koul A, Arnoult E, Lounis N, Guillemont J, Andries K: **The challenge of new drug discovery for tuberculosis.** *Nature* 2011, **469**:483.
9. Gandhi NR, Nunn P, Dheda K, Schaaf HS, Zignol M, van Soolingen D, Jensen P, Bayona J: **Multidrug-resistant and extensively drug-resistant tuberculosis: a threat to global control of tuberculosis.** *Lancet* 2010, **22**:1830.

10. Pavan FR, Poelhsitz GV, Do Nascimento FB, Leite SR, Batista AA, Deflon VM, Sato DN, Franzblau SG, Leite CQ: **Ruthenium (II) phosphine/picolinate complexes as antimycobacterial agents.** *Eur J Med Chem* 2010, **45:**598.
11. Barry CE 3rd, Slayden RA, Sampson AE, Lee RE: **Use of genomics and combinatorial chemistry in the development of new antimycobacterial drugs.** *Biochem Pharmacol* 2000, **59:**221.
12. Hermanson GT: *Bioconjugate techniques.* San Diego: Academic; 1996.
13. Breinbauer R, Kohn M: **Azide-alkyne coupling: a powerful reaction for bioconjugate chemistry.** *Chembiochem* 2003, **4:**1147.
14. Kharb R, Sharma PC, Yar MS: **Pharmacological significance of triazole scaffold.** *J Enz Inhib Med Chem* 2011, **26:**1.
15. Bhat L, Jandeleit B, Dias TM, Moors TL, Gallop MA: **Synthesis and biological evaluation of novel steroidal pyrazoles as substrates for bile acid transporters.** *Bioorg Med Chem Lett* 2005, **15:**85.
16. Savage PB, Li C: **Cholic acid derivatives: novel antimicrobials.** *Exp Opin Investig Drugs* 2000, **9:**263.
17. Bavikar SN, Salunke DB, Hazra BG, Pore VS, Dodd RH, Thierry J, Shirazi F, Deshpande MV, Kadreppa S, Chattopadhyay S: **Synthesis of chimeric tetrapeptide-linked cholic acid derivatives: impending synergistic agents.** *Bioorg Med Chem Lett* 2008, **18:**5512.
18. Pore VS, Aher NG, Kumar M, Shukla PK: **Design and synthesis of fluconazole/bile acid conjugate using click reaction.** *Tetrahedron* 2006, **62:**11178.
19. Enhsen A, Kramer W, Wess G: **Bile acids in drug discovery.** *Drug Discov Today* 1998, **3:**409.
20. Kannan A, De Clercq E, Pannecouque C, Witvrouw M, Hartman TL, Turpin JA, Buckheit RW Jr, Cushman M: **Synthesis and anti-HIV activity of a bile acid analog of cosalane.** *Tetrahedron* 2001, **57:**9385.
21. Anelli PL, Lattuada L, Lorusso V, Lux G, Morisetti A, Morosini P, Serleti M, Uggeri FJJ: **Conjugates of gadolinium complexes to bile acids as hepatocyte-directed contrast agents for magnetic resonance imaging.** *J Med Chem* 2004, **47:**3629.
22. Solaia BA, Terzic N, Pocsfalvi G, Gerena L, Tinant B, Opsenica D, Milhous WKJ: **Mixed steroidal 1,2,4,5-tetraoxanes: antimalarial and antimycobacterial activity.** *Med Chem* 2002, **45:**3331.
23. Salunke DB, Hazra BG, Pore VS: **Steroidal conjugates and their pharmacological applications.** *Curr Med Chem* 2006, **13:**813.
24. Carmo AML, Silva FMC, Machado PA, Fontes AP, Pavan FR, Leite CQ, Leite SR, Coimbra ES, Da Silva AD: **Synthesis of 4-aminoquinoline analogues and their platinum(II) complexes as new antileishmanial and antitubercular agents.** *Biomed Pharmacother* 2011, **65:**204.
25. De Souza NB, Carmo AML, Lagatta DC, Alves MJM, Fontes APS, Coimbra ES, Da Silva AD, Abramo C: **4-aminoquinoline analogues and its platinum (II) complexes as antimalarial agents.** *Biomed Pharmacother* 2011, **65:**313.
26. Palomino JC, Martin A, Camacho M, Guerra H, Swings J, Portaela F: **Resazurin microtiter assay plate: simple and inexpensive method for detection of drug resistance in Mycobacterium tuberculosis.** *Antimicrob Agents Chemother* 2002, **46:**2720.
27. Mossman T: **Rapid colorimetric assay for cellular growth and survival: application to proliferation and cytotoxicity assays.** *J Immunol Meth* 1983, **65:**55.
28. Musonda CC, Gut J, Rosenthal PJ, Yardley V, de Souza RCC, Chibale K: **Application of multicomponent reactions to antimalarial drug discovery. Part 2. New antiplasmodial and antitrypanosomal 4-aminoquinoline gamma- and delta-lactams via a 'catch and release protocol.** *Bioorg Med Chem* 2006, **14:**5605.
29. Aher NG, Pore VS: **Synthesis of Bile Acid Dimers Linked with 1,2,3-Triazole Ring at C-3, C-11, and C-24 Positions.** *Synlett* 2005, **14:**2155.
30. Salunke DB, Hazra BG, Pore VS, Bhat MK, Nahar PB, Deshpande MV: **New steroidal dimers with antifungal and antiproliferative activity.** *J Med Chem* 2004, **47:**1591.
31. Collins L, Franzblau SG: **Microplate alamar blue assay versus BACTEC 460 system for high-throughput screening of compounds against *Mycobacterium tuberculosis* and *Mycobacterium avium*.** *Antimicrob Agents Chemother* 1997, **41:**1004.
32. Sereno D, Cordeiro da Silva A, Mathieu-Daude F, Ouassi A: **Advances and perspectives in *Leishmania* cell based drug-screening procedures.** *Parasitol Int* 2007, **56:**3.
33. Vermeersch M, da Luz RI, Tote K, Timmermans JP, Cos P, Maes L: **In vitro susceptibilities of *Leishmania donovani* promastigote and amastigote stages to antileishmanial reference drugs: practical relevance of stage-specific differences.** *Antimicrob Agents Chemother* 2009, **53:**3855.
34. Tempone AG, Martins de Oliveira C, Berlinck RG: **Current approaches to discover marine antileishmanial natural products.** *Planta Med* 2011, **77:**572.

Synthesis and characterization of Schiff's bases of sulfamethoxazole

Zainab Hussain[1], Emad Yousif[2*], Ahmed Ahmed[2] and Ali Altaie[1]

Abstract

Background: Schiff's bases are excellent ligands which are synthesized from the condensation of primary amines with carbonyl groups.

Findings: The classical reaction for the synthesis of Schiff's bases in an ethanolic solution and glacial acetic acid as a catalyst was followed in the synthesis of substituted sulfamethoxazole compounds.

Conclusions: Some Schiff's bases containing sulfamethoxazole nucleus have been synthesized and characterized. The present compounds are hoped to be applied in the photostability of PVC.

Keywords: Schiff bases; Sulfamethoxazole; Synthesis

Findings

Background

Schiff's bases are an important class of organic compounds [1]. They were first reported by Hugo Schiff in 1864 [2]. Schiff's bases are condensation products of primary amines with carbonyl compounds. The common structural feature of these compounds is the azomethine group with the general formula RHC = N-R_1, where R and R_1 are alkyl, aryl, cycloalkyl, or heterocyclic groups [1]. Structurally, a Schiff's base (also known as imine or azomethine) is a nitrogen analogue of an aldehyde or ketone in which the carbonyl group (>C = O) is replaced by an imine or azomethine group. Schiff's bases have also been shown to exhibit a broad range of biological activities, including antifungal, antibacterial, antimalarial, antiproliferative, anti-inflammatory, antiviral, and antipyretic properties [3,4]. Imine or azomethine groups are present in various natural, naturally derived, and nonnatural compounds. The imine group present in such compounds has been shown to be critical to their biological activities [5-7]. Schiff's bases are important compounds owing to their wide range of industrial applications [8]. Schiff's bases are used in the photostabilization of poly (vinyl chloride) polymers against photodegradation by ultraviolet radiation [9-11] and are also used to improve poly(methyl methacrylate) from degradation [12] and to prevent polystyrene from photodegradation by their addition to polymer films [13,14].

* Correspondence: emad_yousif@hotmail.com
[2]Department of Chemistry, College of Science, Al-Nahrain University, Baghdad, Iraq
Full list of author information is available at the end of the article

Methods

Fourier transform infrared (FTIR) spectra were registered on a SHIMADZU (8300, Kyoto, Japan) infrared spectrophotometer, using KBr discs. Proton nuclear magnetic resonance (^{1}H-NMR; 600 MHz) spectra were obtained at room temperature with Bruker equipment (Madison, WI, USA) using TMS as an internal standard in dimethyl sulfoxide (DMSO). Melting points were recorded using hot-stage Gallenkamp melting point apparatus (Loughborough, UK) and were uncorrected. Analytical grade chemicals (BDH, G.C.C., Hopkin & William Corporation, Poole, UK) were used throughout the project.

Results and discussion

The synthesis of Schiff's bases with different specific aldehydes in ethanol as a solvent and catalyst (glacial acetic acid) resulted in five new series of Schiff's bases with the general formula RHC = N-R_1. Here R_1 = sulfamethoxazole and R = benzaldehyde, 4-bromobenzaldehyde, 2-hydroxybenzaldehyde (salicylaldehyde), 4-*N,N*-dimethylbenzaldehyde, and 3-nitrobenzaldehyde were synthesized by the reaction of sulfamethoxazole and substituted aldehydes in ethanol (Scheme 1). Such compounds were characterized by different physicochemical techniques like melting point, elemental analysis, FTIR spectroscopy, and multinuclear NMR (^{1}H).

Physical properties of the prepared Schiff's bases

The physical properties of sulfamethoxazole and its derivatives including melting point, color, and elemental analysis are tabulated in Table 1.

The structure of the prepared Schiff's bases was confirmed by infrared spectroscopy. The FTIR spectra of sulfamethoxazole and its prepared compounds, as shown in Table 2, showed that the band of NH_2 was found in sulfamethoxazole in the location 3,298 cm^{-1} and then vanished. After that, the band of NH appeared in the prepared Schiff's bases with different shifting from 3,250 to 3,287 cm^{-1}. The band of C = N for imine stretching vibration was also not found in sulfamethoxazole, and it

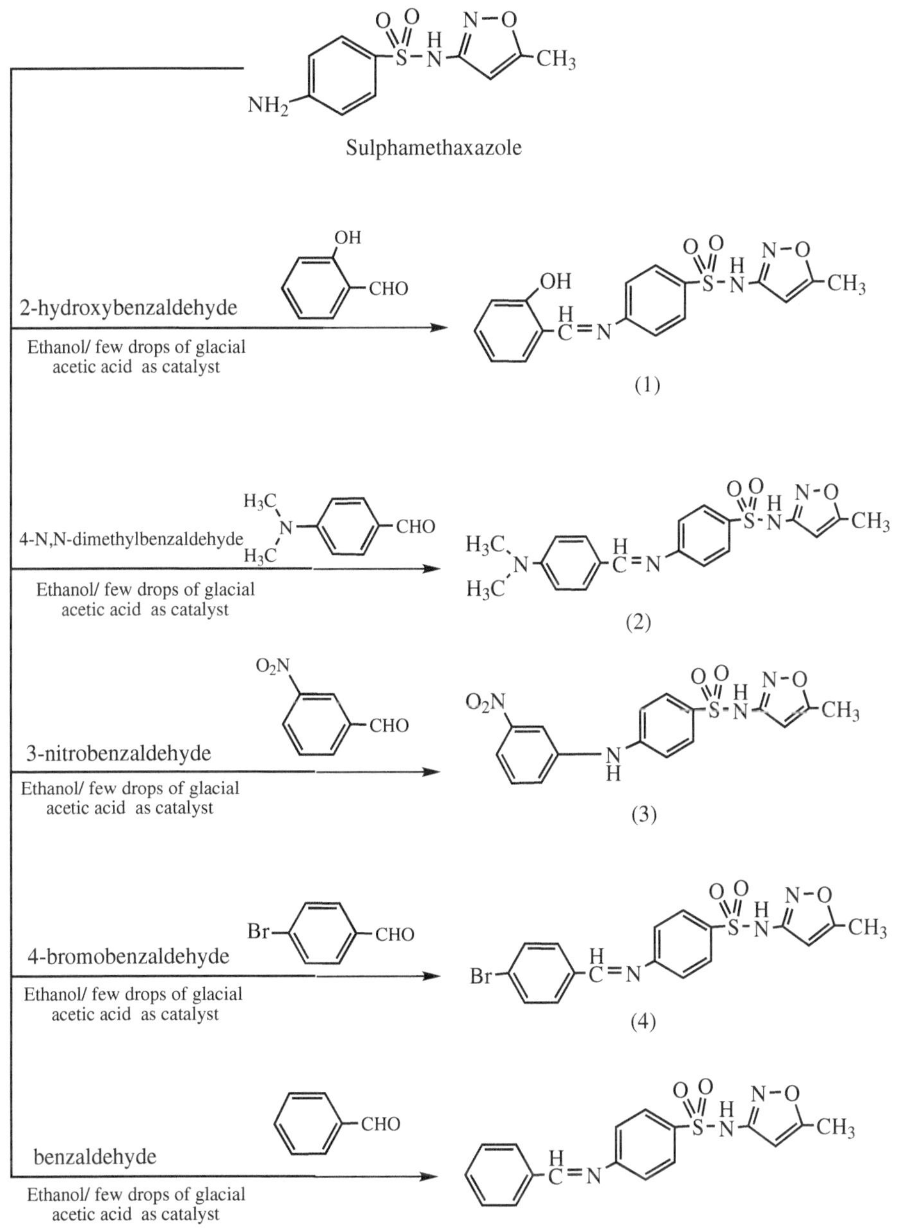

Scheme 1 Scheme of the preparation of Schiff's bases from sulfamethoxazole. (1) 4-[(2-Hydroxy-benzylidene)-amino]-*N*-(5-methyl-isoxazol-3-yl)-benzene sulfonamide. (2) *N*-(5-Methyl-isoxazol-3-yl)-4-[(4-nitroox-benzylidene)-amino]-benzene sulfonamide. (3) 4-[(4-Dimethylamino-benzylidene)-amino]-*N*-(5-methyl-isoxazol-3-yl)-benzene sulfonamide. (4) 4-[(4-Bromo-benzylidene)-amino]-*N*-(5-methyl-isoxazol-3-yl)-benzene sulfonamide. (5) (*N*-(5-Methyl-isoxazol-3-yl)-4-[(3-nitro-benzylidene)-amino]-benzene sulfonamide.

Table 1 Physical data of the prepared compounds

Compounds	Color	MP (°C)	Elemental analysis, theoretical (actual)				
			% C	% H	% N	% O	% S
(1)	Yellow	190 to 192	57.13 (57.23)	4.23 (4.88)	11.76 (10.39)	17.91 (16.88)	8.97 (9.11)
(2)	Brown	148 to 150	60.85 (59.82)	6.23 (6.43)	13.52 (13.63)	11.58 (12.09)	7.74 (8.10)
(3)	Orange	122 to 124	52.84 (53.88)	3.65 (3.22)	14.50 (13.91)	20.70 (19.33)	8.30 (8.21)
(4)	Light yellow	142 to 143	48.58 (49.59)	3.36 (3.51)	10.00 (9.33)	11.42 (10.21)	7.63 (8.33)
(5)	Orange	110 to 112	59.81 (69.88)	4.43 (3.89)	12.31 (12.49)	14.06 (14.63)	9.39 (10.21)

appeared in the prepared Schiff's bases with shifting from 1,603 to 1,650 cm^{-1}. Also, the band of C = N for ring stretching vibration shifted from 1,620 cm^{-1} in sulfamethoxazole to 1,615 to 1,630 cm^{-1} in the prepared compounds.

The ultraviolet-visible spectrophotometry technique is used to characterize sulfamethoxazole and its derivatives in DMSO as a solvent. The ultraviolet-visible electronic spectra of the prepared Schiff's bases showed absorption bands that could be attributed to $\pi \to \pi^*$ electronic transitions; these transitions are assigned in relevance to the structures of the compounds. The electronic spectrum of sulfamethoxazole shows a band at the wavelength 280 nm; this may be attributed to the $\pi \to \pi^*$ electronic transition. In the prepared Schiff's bases, the bands shifted to wavelengths different from that of the corresponding band in sulfamethoxazole, as shown in Table 3, which appear in the wavelength range between 270 and 360 nm. These transitions may be attributed to $\pi \to \pi^*$ and $n \to \pi^*$ electronic transitions.

The ^{1}H-NMR spectrum of compound (1) showed the following characteristic chemical shifts (DMSO as a solvent): the singlet signal at $\delta = 2.212$ ppm suggested the attribution of the protons of the CH_3 group, the singlet signal at $\delta = 6.029$ ppm suggested the attribution of the proton of CH of the isoxazole ring, the multiplet signal at $\delta = 6.743$ to 7.768 ppm suggested the attribution of the protons of two aromatic benzene rings, the singlet signal at $\delta = 8.764$ ppm suggested the attribution of the proton of the CH = N group, the singlet signal at $\delta = 9.352$ ppm suggested the attribution of the proton of the NH group, and the singlet signal at $\delta = 10.525$ ppm suggested the attribution of the proton of the OH group.

Also, the ^{1}H-NMR spectrum of compound (5) showed the following characteristic chemical shifts (DMSO as a solvent): the singlet signal at $\delta = 2.200$ ppm suggested the attribution of the protons of the CH_3 group, the singlet signal at $\delta = 5.833$ ppm suggested the attribution of the proton of CH of the isoxazole ring, the multiplet signal at $\delta = 6.789$ to 7.749 ppm suggested the attribution of the protons of two aromatic benzene rings, the singlet signal at $\delta = 8.698$ ppm suggested the attribution of the proton of the CH = N group, and the singlet signal at $\delta = 9.602$ ppm suggested the attribution of the proton of the NH group [15], as shown in Table 4.

Table 2 FTIR spectroscopy for sulfamethoxazole and its derivatives

Compounds	υ (NH_2) (cm^{-1})	υ (N-H) (cm^{-1})	υ (C = N) imine (cm^{-1})	υ (C = N) ring (cm^{-1})
Sulfamethoxazole	3,298	-	-	1,620
(1)	-	3,250	1,650	1,616
(2)	-	3,266	1,603	1,620
(3)	-	3,290	1,650	1,600
(4)	-	3,270	1,650	1,630
(5)	-	3,287	1,633	1,615

Table 3 UV spectroscopy for sulfamethoxazole and its derivatives

Compounds	Absorption bands (nm)	Assigned transition
Sulfamethoxazole	280	$\pi \to \pi^*$
(1)	282, 310	$\pi \to \pi^*$, $n \to \pi^*$
(2)	250, 360	$\pi \to \pi^*$, $n \to \pi^*$
(3)	270	$\pi \to \pi^*$
(4)	271	$\pi \to \pi^*$
(5)	270	$\pi \to \pi^*$

Experimental

A solution of sulfamethoxazole (0.001 mol) in absolute ethanol (30 ml) was slowly added to a solution of aldehyde (0.001 mol) in absolute ethanol (20 ml). The stirred reaction mixture was refluxed for 12 h. After cooling, a precipitate was formed which was collected by filtration, then washed with cold ethanol, and recrystallized from ethanol.

Table 4 ^{1}H-NMR data of sulfamethoxazole and its derivatives

Compounds	CH_3	C-H isoxazole ring	Aromatic benzene rings	Imine	N-H	OH
(1)	2.212	6.029	6.743 to 7.768	8.764	9.352	10.525
(5)	2.200	5.833	6.789 to 7.749	8.698	9.602	-

Conclusion

Five Schiff's bases: (1), (2), (3), (4), and (5), were synthesized as derivatives of sulfamethoxazole and characterized by UV, FTIR, and ^{1}H-NMR spectroscopies and elemental analysis (CHNS).

Competing interests

The authors declare that they have no competing interests.

Acknowledgements

The authors acknowledge the Department of Chemistry, College of Science, Al-Nahrain University for their encouragement.

Author details

[1]Department of Chemistry, College of Science for Women, Baghdad University, Baghdad, Iraq. [2]Department of Chemistry, College of Science, Al-Nahrain University, Baghdad, Iraq.

References

1. Arulmurugan S, Kavitha PH, Venkatraman RP (2010) Biological activities of Schiff base and its complexes: a review. Rasayan J Chem 3(3):385–410
2. Schiff H (1864) Mitteilungen aus dem universitats laboratorium in Pisa: Eineneue reihe organischer basen. Justus Liebigs Ann Chem 131:118–119
3. Dhar DN, Taploo CL (1982) Schiff bases and their applications. J Sci Ind Res 41:501–506
4. Przybylski P, Huczyński A, Pyta K, Brzezinski B, Bartl F (2009) Biological properties of Schiff bases and azo derivatives of phenols. Curr Org Chem 13:124–148
5. Bringmann G, Dreyer M, Faber JH, Dalsgaard PW, Staerk D, Jaroszewski JW (2004) Ancistrotanzanine C and related 5,1'- and 7,3'-coupled naphthylisoquinoline alkaloids from *Ancistrocladus tanzaniensis*. J Nat Prod 67(5):743–748
6. Salimon J, Salih N, Ibraheem H, Yousif E (2010) Synthesis of 2-N-salicylidene-5-(substituted)-1,3,4-thiadiazole as potential antimicrobial agents. Asian J Chem 22(7):5289–5296
7. Guo Z, Xing R, Liu S, Zhong Z, Ji X, Wang L (2007) Antifungal properties of Schiff bases of chitosan, N-substituted chitosan and quaternized chitosan. Carbohydr Res 342(10):1329–1332
8. Li Y, Yang ZS, Zhang H, Cao BJ, Wang FD (2003) Artemisinin derivatives bearing Mannich base group: synthesis and antimalarial activity. Bioorg Med Chem 11:4363–4368
9. Yousif E, Salih N, Salimon J (2011) Improvement of the photostabilization of PVC films in the presence of 2 N-salicylidene-5-(substituted)-1,3,4-thiadiazole. J Appl Polym Sci 120:2207–2214
10. Yousif E, Ahmed A, Mahmoud M (2012) New organic photostabilizers for rigid PVC against photodegradation. Lambert Academic, Saarbrücken
11. Yousif E (2012) Photostabilization of PVC: principles and applications. Lambert Academic, Saarbrücken
12. Yousif E, Salimon J, Salih N, Ahmed A (2012) Improvement of the photostabilization of PMMA films in the presence 2 N-salicylidene-5-(substituted)-1,3,4-thiadiazole. J King Saud University Sci 24:131–137
13. Yousif E, Salimon J, Salih N (2012) New stabilizers for polystyrene based on 2-N-salicylidene-5-(substituted)-1,3,4-thiadiazole compounds. J Saudi Chem Soc 16:299–306
14. Yousif E, Haddad R, Ahmed A (2013) Photodegradation and photostabilization of polystyrene. Lambert Academic, Saarbrücken
15. Haddad R, Yousif E, Ahmed A (2013) Synthesis and characterization of transition metal complexes of 4-amino-5-pyridyl-4H-1,2,4-triazole-3-thiol. Springerplus 2:510

Assessing the pharmacokinetic profile of the CamMedNP natural products database: an *in silico* approach

Fidele Ntie-Kang[1,2,3*], James A Mbah[4], Lydia L Lifongo[2], Luc C Owono Owono[1,5], Eugene Megnassan[6], Luc Meva'a Mbaze[7], Philip N Judson[8], Wolfgang Sippl[3] and Simon MN Efange[4]

Abstract

Background: Drug metabolism and pharmacokinetic (DMPK) assessment has come to occupy a place of interest during the early stages of drug discovery today. Computer-based methods are slowly gaining ground in this area and are often used as initial tools to eliminate compounds likely to present uninteresting pharmacokinetic profiles and unacceptable levels of toxicity from the list of potential drug candidates, hence cutting down the cost of the discovery of a drug.

Results: In the present study, we present an *in silico* assessment of the DMPK profile of our recently published natural products database of 1,859 unique compounds derived from 224 species of medicinal plants from the Cameroonian forest. In this analysis, we have used 46 computed physico-chemical properties or molecular descriptors to predict the absorption, distribution, metabolism and elimination (ADME) of the compounds. This survey demonstrated that about 50% of the compounds within the Cameroonian medicinal plant and natural products (CamMedNP) database are compliant, having properties which fall within the range of ADME properties of >95% of currently known drugs, while >73% of the compounds have ≤2 violations. Moreover, about 72% of the compounds within the corresponding 'drug-like' subset showed compliance.

Conclusions: In addition to the previously verified levels of 'drug-likeness' and the diversity and the wide range of measured biological activities, the compounds in the CamMedNP database show interesting DMPK profiles and, hence, could represent an important starting point for hit/lead discovery from medicinal plants in Africa.

Keywords: ADMET; Database collection; Descriptors; *In silico*; Medicinal plants; Natural products

Background

Natural products (NPs) play an increasingly important role in drug discovery today [1-5], both serving as drugs and as templates for the design of nature-inspired medicines [3,6]. In fact, it has been reported that a significant proportion of drugs that undergo clinical trials are either naturally occurring or are derived from NPs [7]. What characterises NPs are their richness in stereogenic centres and coverage of segments of chemical space which are typically not occupied by a majority of synthetic molecules and drugs [8,9]. In addition, they generally contain more oxygen atoms and less aromatic atoms on average, when compared with 'drug-like' molecules [8-11]. It is needless to say that NPs sometimes fail the famous 'drug-likeness' test due to the often bulky nature of naturally occurring metabolites [11].

It is also worth mentioning that designing drug-like molecules having interesting pharmacokinetic properties is an important paradigm in drug discovery programs [12,13]. This entails the search for lead compounds which can be easily orally absorbed, easily transported to their desired site of action, not easily attacked by metabolising enzymes so as to form toxic metabolic products before reaching the targeted site of action and easily eliminated from the body before accumulating in sufficient amounts

* Correspondence: ntiekfidele@gmail.com
[1]CEPAMOQ, Faculty of Science, University of Douala, P.O. Box 8580, Douala, Cameroon
[2]Chemical and Bioactivity Information Centre, Department of Chemistry, Faculty of Science, University of Buea, P.O. Box 63, Buea, Cameroon
Full list of author information is available at the end of the article

that may produce adverse side effects. The ensemble of the above properties is often referred to as absorption, distribution, metabolism and elimination (ADME) properties, or better still ADMET or ADME/T or ADMETox (i.e. if toxicity criteria are also taken into consideration).

Computer-based *in silico* approaches for the prediction of ADMET profiles of drug leads at early stages of drug discovery are increasingly gaining ground [14-16]. This could be explained by the relative cost advantage added to the time factor, when compared to standard experimental approaches for ADMET profiling [17,18]. On these grounds, several theoretical methods for the determination of ADMET parameters have been developed and implemented in a number of currently available software for drug discovery protocols [19-22], even though the predictions are sometimes disappointing [23]. Such software often make use of quantitative structure-activity relationships [22-24] or knowledge-base methods [25-27]. The goal has been to considerably cut down on the currently very high cost of discovery of a drug [17]. A promising lead is often defined as a compound which combines potency with an admirable ADMET profile. As such, compounds with unfavourably predicted pharmacokinetic profiles are either completely dismissed from the list of potential drug candidates (even if they prove to be highly potent) or the drug metabolism and pharmacokinetics (DMPK) properties are 'fine tuned' in order to improve their chances of making it to clinical trials [28]. This explains why the 'graveyard' of very highly potent compounds which do not make it to clinical trials keeps filling up, to the extent that the process of drug discovery often presents the challenge of either resorting to new leads or 'resurrecting' some buried leads with the view of fine-tuning their ADMET profiles.

In a recent paper, we have presented a database of 1,859 compounds derived from the Cameroonian flora, Cameroonian medicinal plant and natural products (CamMedNP), the compounds being predicted to be sufficiently orally available and diverse to be employed in lead discovery programs [29]. Additional arguments in favour of the use of this database are the wide range of the previously observed biological activities of the compounds and the wide range of ailments being treated by traditional medicine with the help of the herbs from which the compounds have been derived [29,30].

Numerous drugs at a late stage of pharmaceutical development and many more lead compounds fail due to adverse pharmacokinetic properties [18]. It is, therefore, important to incorporate the prediction of the ADME properties into the lead compound selection, by means of molecular descriptors. A molecular descriptor is often defined as a structural or physico-chemical property of a molecule or part of a molecule, for example the logarithm of the *n*-octanol/water partition coefficient (log *P*), molar weight (MW) and total polar surface area. A number of relevant molecular properties (descriptors) are often used to help predict the pharmacokinetic behaviour of potential drug leads. In the present study, we have carried out an *in silico* assessment of the ADMET profile of the CamMedNP database by the use of computed molecular descriptors currently implemented in a wide range of software tools as indicators of the pharmacokinetic properties of a large proportion of currently known drugs.

Methods

Data sources and generation of 3D structures

The plant sources, geographical collection sites, chemical structures of pure compounds and their measured biological activities were retrieved from literature sources and have been previously described [29]. The three-dimensional (3D) structures were generated using the builder module of MOE [31], and energy minimization was subsequently carried out using the MMFF94 [32] until a gradient of 0.01 kcal/mol was reached.

Initial treatment of chemical structures and calculation of ADMET-related descriptors

The 1,859 low-energy 3D chemical structures in the CamMedNP library were saved in mol2 format and initially treated with LigPrep [33], distributed by Schrodinger, Inc. (New York, USA). This implementation was carried out with the graphical user interface of the Maestro software package (New York, USA) [34], using the OPLS force field [35-37]. Protonation states at biologically relevant pH were correctly assigned (group I metals in simple salts were disconnected, strong acids were deprotonated and strong bases protonated, while topological duplicates and explicit hydrogens were added). All molecular modelling was carried out on a Linux workstation (San Francisco, USA) with a 3.5 GHz Intel Core2 Duo processor (Santa Clara, USA). A set of the ADMET-related properties (a total of 46 molecular descriptors) were calculated using the QikProp program (New York, USA) [21] running in normal mode. QikProp generates physically relevant descriptors and uses them to perform ADMET predictions. An overall ADME-compliance score, drug-likeness parameter (indicated by #stars), was used to assess the pharmacokinetic profiles of the compounds within the CamMedNP library. The #stars parameter indicates the number of property descriptors computed by QikProp, which falls outside the optimum range of values for 95% of known drugs. The methods implemented were developed by Jorgensen et al. [38-40]. Among the calculated descriptors are the total solvent-accessible molecular surface, S_{mol} in Å^2 (probe radius 1.4 Å; range for 95% of drugs is 300 to 1,000 Å^2); the hydrophobic portion of the solvent-accessible molecular surface, $S_{mol,hfob}$ in Å^2 (probe radius 1.4 Å; range for 95% of drugs is 0 to 750 Å^2); the total volume of molecule enclosed by solvent-accessible molecular surface, V_{mol} in Å^3 (probe radius 1.4 Å; range for 95% of drugs is 500 to 2,000 Å^3); the logarithm of aqueous solubility, logS_{wat} (range for 95% of drugs is −6.0 to 0.5) [36,38]; the logarithm of predicted binding constant to human serum albumin, logK_{HSA} (range for 95% of drugs is −1.5 to 1.2) [41]; the logarithm of predicted blood/brain barrier partition coefficient, log *B/B* (range for 95% of drugs is −3.0 to 1.0) [42-44]; the predicted apparent Caco-2 cell membrane permeability ($BIP_{Caco\text{-}2}$) in Boehringer-Ingelheim scale, in nm/s (range for 95% of drugs is <5 low, >100 high) [45-47]; the predicted apparent Madin-Darby canine kidney (MDCK) cell permeability in nm s^{-1} (<25 poor, >500 great) [46]; the index of cohesion interaction in solids, Ind_{coh}, calculated from the number of hydrogen bond acceptors (HBA), hydrogen bond donors (HBD) and the surface area accessible to the solvent (S_{mol}) by the relation $Ind_{coh} = HBA \times \sqrt{HBD}/S_{mol}$ (0.0 to 0.05 for 95% of drugs) [40]; the globularity descriptor, Glob = $(4\pi r^2)/S_{mol}$, where *r* is the radius of the sphere whose volume is equal to the molecular volume (0.75 to 0.95 for 95% of drugs); the predicted polarizability, QP_{polrz} (13.0 to 70.0 for 95% of drugs); the predicted IC_{50} value for blockage of HERG K^+ channels, logHERG (concern <−5) [48,49]; the predicted skin permeability, logK_p (−8.0 to −1.0 for 95% of drugs) [50,51]; and the number of likely metabolic reactions, #metab (range for 95% of drugs is 0 to 15).

Results and discussion

Overall DMPK compliance of the CamMedNP library

The 24 most relevant molecular descriptors calculated by QikProp are used to determine the #star parameter [52]. A plot of the #stars parameter (on the *x*-axis) against the corresponding counts (on the *y*-axis) in the CamMedNP is shown within the same set of axes with those of the 'drug-like', 'lead-like' and 'fragment-like' standard subsets, Figure 1. The criteria for the respective standard subsets were defined as MW < 500, log *P* < 5, HBD ≤ 5, HBA ≤ 10 [14]; 150 ≤ MW ≤ 350, log *P* ≤ 4, HBD ≤ 3, HBA ≤ 6 [53-55] and MW ≤ 250, −2 ≤ log *P* ≤ 3, HBD < 3, HBA < 6, NRB < 3 [56]. QikProp was unable to compute the ADMET descriptors for 25 compounds out of the total library due to limitations that were not clear to us. Of the remaining 1,834 compounds, 48.04% showed #star = 0, while 74.21% had #star ≤ 2. Among the 1,122 compounds of the drug-like subset, 79.12% had pharmacokinetic descriptors within the acceptable range for 95% of known drugs, while 97.33% showed #stars ≤ 2. The lead-like and fragment-like subsets were, respectively, 81.15% and 55.56% compliant for all of the 24 most relevant computed descriptors. The mean values for 19 selected computed descriptors have been shown in Table 1 for all four compound libraries, while the percentage compliances for 14 selected ADMET-related descriptors are shown in

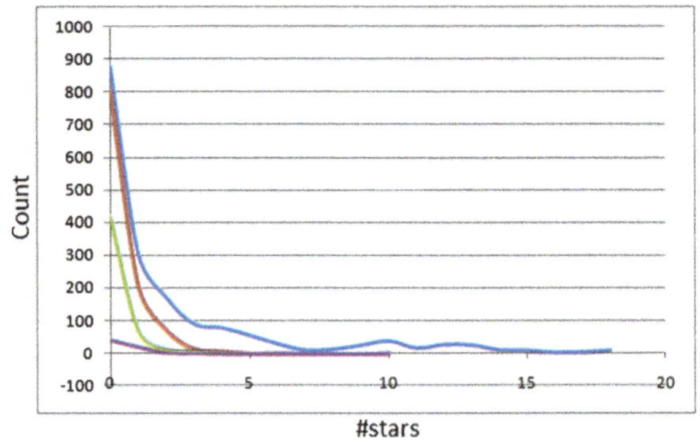

Figure 1 Distribution curves for #stars within the CamMedNP library and subsets. Blue = CamMedNP library, red = drug-like subset, green = lead-like subset and violet = fragment-like subset.

Table 2. The mean values and percentage compliances indicate a high probability of finding drug leads within the CamMedNP compound library.

Bioavailability prediction

The bioavailability of a compound depends on the processes of absorption and liver first-pass metabolism [57]. The absorption, in turn, depends on the solubility and permeability of the compound, as well as on the interactions with transporters and metabolizing enzymes in the gut wall. The computed parameters used to assess oral absorption are the predicted aqueous solubility, logS_{wat}, the conformation-independent predicted aqueous solubility, CI logS_{wat}, the predicted qualitative human oral absorption, the predicted % human oral absorption and compliance to Jorgensen's famous 'Rule of Three' (ro3). The solubility calculation procedure implemented depends on the similarity property space between the given molecule and its most similar analogue within the experimental training set used to develop the model implemented in QikProp, i.e. if the similarity is <0.9, then the QikProp predicted value is taken; otherwise, the predicted property, P_{pred}, is adjusted such that

$$P_{pred} = SP_{exp} + (1 - S)P_{QP} \quad (1)$$

where *S* is the similarity and P_{exp} and P_{QP} are, respectively, the experimental and QikProp predictions for the most similar molecule within the training set. In Equation 1, if *S* = 1, then the predicted property is equal to the measured experimental property of the training set compound. According to Jorgensen's ro3, if a compound complies to all or some of the rules (logS_{wat} > −5.7, $BIP_{Caco\text{-}2}$ > 22 nm/s and number of primary metabolites < seven), then it is more likely to be orally available. The distribution curves for two of the three determinants for the ro3 (logS_{wat} and $BIP_{Caco\text{-}2}$) are shown in Figure 2A,B. In general, 47.22% of the CamMedNP library was compliant

Table 1 Average pharmacokinetic property distributions of total CamMedNP library in comparison with various subsets

	Library name	Subset		
	CamMedNP	Drug-like	Lead-like	Fragment-like
Lib. size[a]	1,859	1,122	520	81
No. compl.[b]	881	807	422	45
MW (Da)[c]	426.70	330.33	276.46	195.75
Log *P*[d]	4.18	2.82	2.24	1.42
HBA[e]	5.85	5.18	4.39	3.53
HBD[f]	2.39	1.40	1.29	0.81
NRB[g]	5.31	4.51	3.39	2.06
Log *B/B*[h]	−1.30	−0.77	−0.64	−0.36
BIP_{Caco-2} (nm s^{-1})[i]	1,199.37	1,216.27	1,207.91	1,577.16
S_{mol} (Å^2)[j]	696.28	569.69	501.44	393.20
$S_{mol,hfob}$ (Å^2)[k]	409.24	280.66	200.91	131.61
V_{mol} (Å^3)[l]	1,304.41	1,024.64	870.65	645.16
LogS_{wat} (*S* in mol L^{-1})[m]	−5.11	−3.87	−3.13	−1.77
LogK_{HSA}[n]	0.46	0.15	−0.05	−0.44
MDCK[o]	661.25	671.02	663.83	907.31
Ind$_{coh}$[p]	0.013	0.009	0.009	0.006
Glob[q]	0.84	0.86	0.88	0.92
QP_{polrz} (Å^3)[r]	42.47	33.56	28.23	19.86
LogHERG[s]	−4.64	−4.41	−4.22	−3.40
LogK_p[t]	−2.96	−2.86	−2.89	−2.63
#metab[u]	5.56	4.62	3.57	2.07

[a]Size or number of compounds in library; [b]number of compounds with #star = 0; [c]molar weight (range for 95% of drugs is 130 to 725 Da); [d]logarithm of partitioning coefficient between *n*-octanol and water phases (range for 95% of drugs is −2 to 6); [e]number of hydrogen bonds accepted by the molecule (range for 95% of drugs is 2 to 20); [f]number of hydrogen bonds donated by the molecule (range for 95% of drugs is 0 to 6); [g]number of rotatable bonds (range for 95% of drugs is 0 to 15); [h]logarithm of predicted blood/brain barrier partition coefficient (range for 95% of drugs is −3.0 to 1.0); [i]predicted apparent Caco-2 cell membrane permeability in Boehringer-Ingelheim scale, in nm/s (range for 95% of drugs is <5 low, >100 high); [j]total solvent-accessible molecular surface, in Å^2 (probe radius 1.4 Å; range for 95% of drugs is 300 to 1,000 Å^2); [k]hydrophobic portion of the solvent-accessible molecular surface, in Å^2 (probe radius 1.4 Å; range for 95% of drugs is 0 to 750 Å^2); [l]total volume of molecule enclosed by solvent-accessible molecular surface, in Å^3 (probe radius 1.4 Å; range for 95% of drugs is 500 to 2,000 Å^3); [m]logarithm of aqueous solubility in g/dm^3 (range for 95% of drugs is −6.0 to 0.5); [n]logarithm of predicted binding constant to human serum albumin (range for 95% of drugs is −1.5 to 1.2); [o]predicted apparent MDCK cell permeability in nm/sec (<25 poor, >500 great); [p]index of cohesion interaction in solids (0.0 to 0.05 for 95% of drugs); [q]globularity descriptor (0.75 to 0.95 for 95% of drugs); [r]predicted polarizability (13.0 to 70.0 for 95% of drugs); [s]predicted IC_{50} value for blockage of HERG K^+ channels (concern <−5); [t]predicted skin permeability (−8.0 to −1.0 for 95% of drugs); [u]number of likely metabolic reactions (range for 95% of drugs is 0 to 15).

to the ro3, while the respective percentage compliances for the various subsets were 72.28%, 92.11% and 100% for the drug-like, lead-like and fragment-like libraries. Among the individual computed parameters, the most remarkable was logS_{wat}, which was met by 75.74% of the compounds within the CamMedNP library, while this property shows a Gaussian distribution for the drug-like and lead-like subsets. Only 37.94% of the compounds fell within the respected range for the BIP_{Caco-2} criterion. The predicted apparent Caco-2 cell permeability, BIP_{Caco-2} (in nm s^{-1}), models the permeability of the gut-blood barrier (for non-active transport), even though this parameter is not often correctly predicted computationally [58]. The histograms of the predicted qualitative human oral absorption parameter (in the scale 1 = low, 2 = medium and 3 = high) are shown in Figure 3. It was observed that 52.45% of the compounds in CamMedNP were predicted to have high human oral absorption. The predicted % human oral absorption (on 0 to 100% scale) shows a similar trend, with 41.06% of the compounds being predicted to be absorbed at 100%, and 57.96% of the compounds predicted to be absorbed at >90%.

The size of a molecule, as well as its capacity to make hydrogen bonds, its overall lipophilicity, its shape and flexibility are important properties to consider when determining permeability. Molecular flexibility has been seen as a parameter which is dependent on the number of rotatable bonds (NRB), a property which influences the bioavailability in rats [58]. The distribution of the NRB for this dataset has been previously discussed [29] and revealed that the compounds within the CamMedNP library show some degree of conformational flexibility, the peak

Table 2 Percentage compliances of selected ADMET-related descriptors of total CamMedNP library in comparison with various subsets

	Library name	Subset		
	Total library	Drug-like	Lead-like	Fragment-like
Log *B/B*	88.22	99.55	100.00	100.00
BIP_{Caco-2} (nm s^{-1})	43.95	41.80	39.04	25.93
S_{mol} (Å^2)	89.69	99.55	100.00	95.06
$S_{mol,hfob}$ (Å^2)	90.89	100.00	100.00	100.00
V_{mol} (Å^3)	90.95	99.47	99.81	95.06
$LogS_{wat}$ (*S* in mol L^{-1})	69.08	89.57	100.00	97.53
$LogK_{HSA}$	85.77	99.82	100.00	100.00
MDCK	49.94	58.02	56.73	49.38
Ind_{coh}	95.20	98.75	99.62	100.00
Glob	87.90	96.97	96.73	83.95
ro3[a]	47.22	72.28	91.92	100.00
LogHERG	55.02	61.94	73.27	100.00
$LogK_p$	91.44	95.99	97.50	97.53
#metab	79.61	89.30	97.31	93.83

The descriptors of the entries in the first column are defined in Table 1; [a]percentage compliance to Jorgensen's Rule of Three.

value for the NRB being between 1 and 2, while the average value is 5.31 (Table 1).

Prediction of blood-brain barrier penetration

Too polar drugs do not cross the BBB. The blood/brain partition coefficients (log *B/B*) were computed and used as a predictor for access to the central nervous system (CNS). The predicted CNS activity was computed on a −2 (inactive) to +2 (active) scale and showed that only 1.85% of the compounds in the CamMedNP could be active in the CNS (predicted CNS activity >1). A distribution of the log *B/B* (Figure 4) shows a right-slanted Gaussian-shaped curve with a peak at −0.5 log *B/B* units (the same for all the standard subsets), with >88% of the compounds in the CamMedNP falling within the recommended range for the predicted brain/blood partition coefficient (−3.0 to 1.2). The MDCK monolayers are widely used to make oral absorption estimates, the reason being that these cells also express transporter proteins, but only express very low levels of metabolizing enzymes [58]. They are also used as an additional criterion to predict BBB penetration. Thus, our calculated apparent MDCK cell permeability could be considered to be a good mimic for the BBB (for non-active transport). It was estimated that only about 50% of the compounds had apparent MDCK cell permeabilities falling within the recommended range of 25 to 500 nm s^{-1} for 95% of known drugs. This situation was not greatly improved in the drug-like and lead-like subsets (58% and 57%, respectively).

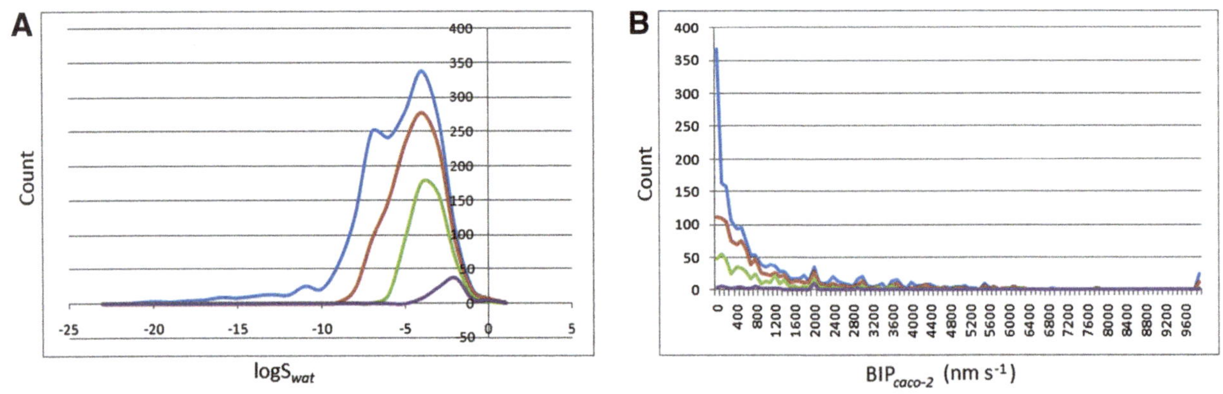

Figure 2 Distribution curves for compliance to Jorgensen's 'Rule of Three'. (A) calculated $logS_{wat}$ against count. **(B)** Predicted BIP_{Caco-2} against count. Blue = CamMedNP library, red = drug-like subset, green = lead-like subset and violet = fragment-like subset.

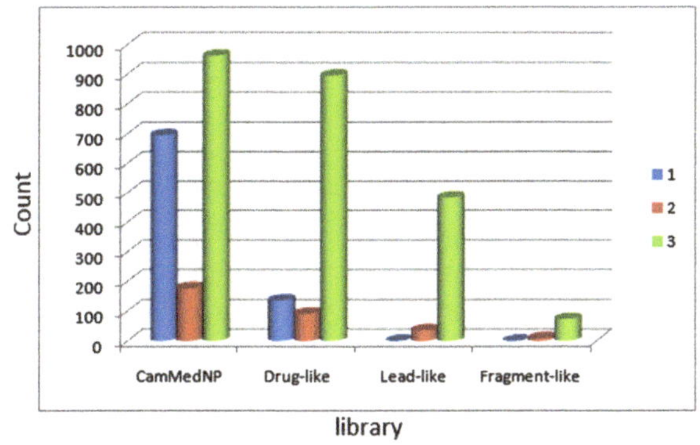

Figure 3 Histograms showing the distribution of human oral absorption predictions.

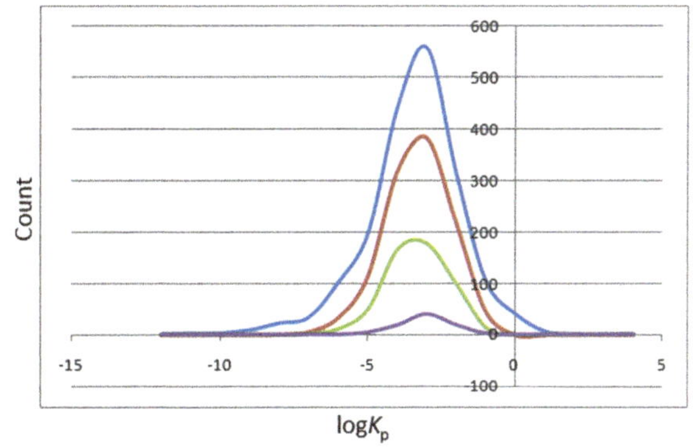

Figure 5 Distribution curves for the predicted skin penetration parameter. Blue = CamMedNP library, red = drug-like subset, green = lead-like subset and violet = fragment-like subset.

Prediction of dermal penetration

This factor is important for drugs administered through the skin. The distribution of computed skin permeability parameter, logK_p, showed smooth Gaussian-shaped graphs centred at −2.5 logK_p units for all the four datasets (Figure 5), with approximately 91% of the compounds in the CamMedNP database falling within the recommended range for >95% of known drugs. The predicted maximum transdermal transport rates, J_m (in μ cm^{-2} h^{-1}), were computed from the aqueous solubility (S_{wat}), the MW and skin permeability (K_p) using the relation (2):

$$J_m = K_p \times \mathrm{MW} \times S_{wat} \quad (2)$$

This parameter showed variations from 0 to 1,603 μ cm^{-2} h^{-1}, with only about 1.39% of the compounds in CamMedNP having the predicted value of J_m > 100 μ cm^{-2} h^{-1}.

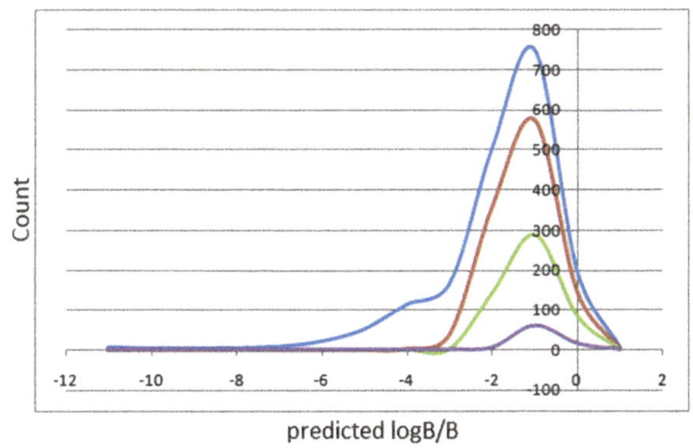

Figure 4 Plot of the physico-chemical descriptor used to predict BBB penetration. Predicted log *B/B* against count. The *x*-axis label is the lower limit of the binned data, e.g. 0 is equivalent to 0.0 to 1.0. Blue = CamMedNP library, red = drug-like subset, green = lead-like subset and violet = fragment-like subset.

Prediction of plasma-protein binding

The efficiency of a drug may be affected by the degree to which it binds to the proteins within the blood plasma. It is noteworthy that the binding of drugs to the plasma proteins (like human serum albumin, lipoprotein, glycoprotein, α, β and γ globulins) greatly reduces the quantity of the drug in the general blood circulation, and hence, the less bound a drug is, the more efficiently it can traverse cell membranes or diffuse. The predicted plasma-protein binding has been estimated by the prediction of binding to human serum albumin; the logK_{HSA} parameter recommended range is −1.5 to 1.5 for 95% of known drugs. Figure 6 shows the variation of this calculated parameter within the CamMedNP dataset, as well as for the standard subsets. This equally gave smooth Gaussian-shaped curves centred on −0.5 logK_{HSA} units for all the four datasets. In addition, our calculations revealed that >85% of the compounds within the CamMedNP library are compliant to this parameter, indicating that a majority of the compounds are likely to circulate freely within the blood stream and, hence, have access to the target site.

Metabolism prediction

An estimated number of possible metabolic reactions has also been predicted by QikProp and used to determine whether the molecules can easily gain access to the target site after entering the blood stream. The average estimated number of possible metabolic reactions for the CamMedNP library was between five and six, while those of the standard subsets drop sequentially by one step in a progressive manner (Table 1). Even though some of the compounds are likely to undergo as many as up to 26 metabolic reactions due to the complexity of some of the plant secondary metabolites within the database (Figure 7), about 80% of the compounds are predicted to undergo the recommended number of metabolic steps (one to eight reactions), with the situation improving to around 90% and approximately

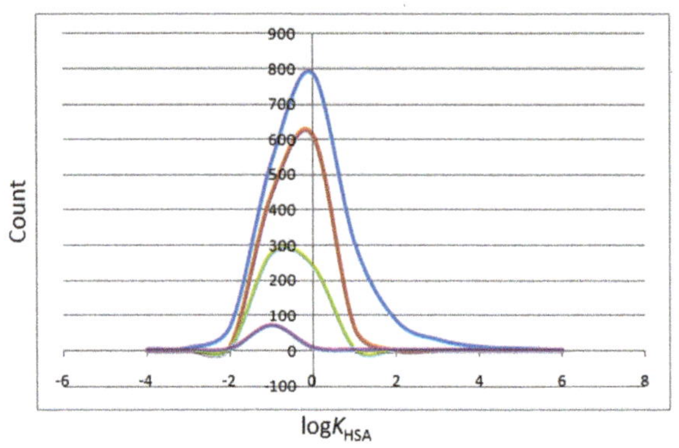

Figure 6 Distribution curves for predicted plasma-protein binding. Blue = CamMedNP library, red = drug-like subset, green = lead-like subset and violet = fragment-like subset.

97% in the drug-like and lead-like subsets, respectively. From Figure 7, it can be observed that, except for the fragment-like subsets which peaks at two predicted metabolic reactions, the peak values for the number of predicted metabolic reactions were at three for all of the datasets.

Prediction of blockage of human ether-a-go-go-related gene potassium channel

Human ether-a-go-go-related gene (HERG) encodes a potassium ion (K^+) channel that is implicated in the fatal arrhythmia known as *torsade de pointes* or the long QT syndrome [59]. The HERG K^+ channel, which is best known for its contribution to the electrical activity of the heart which coordinates the heart's beating, appears to be the molecular target responsible for the cardiac toxicity of a wide range of therapeutic drugs [60]. HERG has also been associated with modulating the functions of some cells of the nervous system and with establishing and maintaining cancer-like features in leukemic cells [61]. Thus, HERG K^+ channel blockers are potentially toxic, and the predicted IC_{50} values often provide reasonable predictions for cardiac toxicity of drugs in the early stages of drug discovery [62]. In this work, the estimated or predicted IC_{50} values for blockage of this channel have been used to model the process *in silico*. The recommended range for the predicted log IC_{50} values for blockage of the HERG K^+ channels (logHERG) is >–5. A distribution curve for the variation of the predicted logHERG is shown in Figure 8, which is left-slanted Gaussian-shaped curve with a peak at –5.5 logHERG units for both the total library and the drug-like subset, meanwhile the lead-like library rather peaks at –4.5 units. It was observed that, in general, this parameter is predicted to fall within the recommended range for about 55% of the compounds within the CamMedNP database, approximately 62% for the drug-like subset and around 73% for the lead-like subset.

Usefulness of the CamMedNP library

The usefulness of the CamMedNP database in lead generation has been exemplified with the docking and pharmacophore-based screening for potential inhibitors of a validated anti-malarial drug target in our laboratory, and the results will be published in a subsequent paper. It is important to mention that virtual screening results could provide insight and direct natural products chemists to search for theoretically active principles with attractive ADMET profiles, which have been previously isolated, but not tested for activity against specified drug targets (if samples are absent). This 'resurrection' process could prove to be a better procedure for lead search than the random screening, which is a common practice in our Cameroonian laboratories. CamMedNP is constantly being updated; meanwhile, a MySQL platform (Cupertino, USA) to facilitate the searching of this database and ordering of compound samples is under development within our group and will also be published subsequently. However, 3D structures of the compounds, as well as their physico-chemical properties that were used to evaluate the DMPK profile, can be

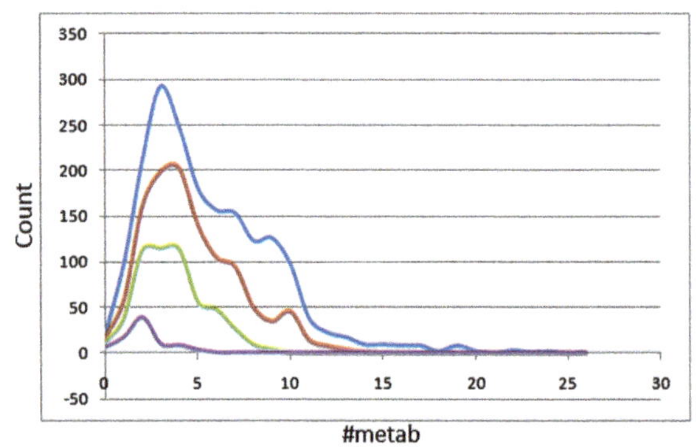

Figure 7 Distribution of the predicted number of metabolic reactions for compounds in the CamMedNP. Blue = CamMedNP library, red = drug-like subset, green = lead-like subset and violet = fragment-like subset.

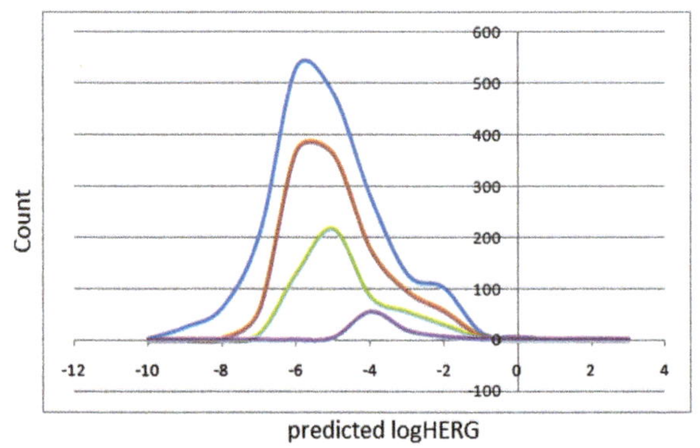

Figure 8 A plot of the predicted logHERG values for the CamMedNP and standard subsets. Blue = CamMedNP library, red = drug-like subset, green = lead-like subset and violet = fragment-like subset.

freely downloaded as additional files accompanying this publication (see Additional file 1, Additional file 2, Additional file 3, Additional file 4). In addition, information about compound sample availability can be obtained on request from the authors of this paper or from the pan-African Natural Products Library (p-ANAPL) project [63,64].

Conclusion

Modern drug discovery programs usually involve the search for small molecule leads with attractive pharmacokinetic profiles. The presence of such within the CamMedNP library is of major importance and, therefore, renders the database attractive, in addition to the already-known properties (drug-like, lead-like fragment-like and diverse). This is an indication that the 3D structures of naturally occurring compounds within the CamMedNP could be a good starting point for docking, neural networking and pharmacophore-based virtual screening campaigns, thus rendering the CamMedNP as a useful asset for the drug discovery community. 3D structures of the compounds, as well as their physico-chemical properties that were used to evaluate the DMPK profile of the CamMedNP library, can be freely downloaded (for non-commercial use) as additional files which accompany this publication (see Additional file 1, Additional file 2, Additional file 3, Additional file 4). The physical samples for testing are available at the various research laboratories in Cameroon in varying quantities. Questions regarding the availability of the compound samples could be addressed directly to the authors of this paper. Otherwise, the samples could be obtainable from the p-ANAPL consortium, which has a mandate to collect samples of NPs from the entire continent of Africa and make them available for biological screening. This network is being set up under the auspices of the Network for Analytical and Bioassay Services in Africa [63,64].

Additional files

Additional file 1: Compounds currently included in CamMedNP. 1 3D structures of compounds currently included in CamMedNP with calculated pharmacokinetic descriptors.

Additional file 2: Drug-like subset. 3D structures of the drug-like subset with calculated pharmacokinetic descriptors.

Additional file 3: Lead-like subset. 3D structures of the lead-like subset with calculated pharmacokinetic descriptors.

Additional file 4: Fragment-like subset. 3D structures of the fragment-like subset with calculated pharmacokinetic descriptors.

Abbreviations

3D: Three dimensional; ADME/T: Absorption distribution, metabolism, excretion and toxicity; CamMedNP: Cameroonian medicinal plant and natural products database; DMPK: Drug metabolism and pharmacokinetics; log *P*: logarithm of the octan-1-ol/water partition coefficient; MDCK: Madin-Darby canine kidney; MW: Molar weight; NP: Natural product; NRB: Number of rotatable bonds; p-ANAPL: pan-African natural products library.

Competing interests

The authors declare that they have no competing interests.

Authors' contributions

WS, EM, LCOO and SMNE conceived the project. All authors participated in the data generation and analysis, discussion of results and the conception of the paper. FNK wrote the first draft of the paper. This work is part of the PhD project of FNK. All authors read and approved the final manuscript.

Authors' information

WS and SMNE are professors of Medicinal Chemistry with an interest in CADD, while SMNE also focuses on organic synthesis and on natural product leads from the Cameroonian medicinal plants. LMM and JAM are natural products chemists actively involved in the isolation and characterization of secondary metabolites from the Cameroonian medicinal plants. LLL holds a PhD in Environmental Science and manages the Chemical and Bioactivity Information Centre (CBIC) with a focus on developing databases for information from medicinal herbs in Africa. PNJ is a retired research officer of Lhasa Ltd., who currently leads the CBIC branch in Leeds, UK. FNK is a PhD student working on CADD under the joint supervision of LCOO and EM.

Acknowledgements

Financial support is acknowledged from the German Academic Exchange Service (DAAD) to FNK for his stay in Halle, Germany for part of his PhD and from the International Centre for Theoretical Physics (ICTP), Trieste, Italy, via the OEA-AC71 Program. The authors also acknowledge the academic licence generously offered by Schrodinger Inc., for this work. The assistance of Mr. Vincent de Paul Nzuwah Nziko (graduate student, Chemistry and Biochemistry, Utah State University, USA) is also acknowledged for proofreading the manuscript.

Author details

[1]CEPAMOQ, Faculty of Science, University of Douala, P.O. Box 8580, Douala, Cameroon. [2]Chemical and Bioactivity Information Centre, Department of Chemistry, Faculty of Science, University of Buea, P.O. Box 63, Buea, Cameroon. [3]Department of Pharmaceutical Sciences, Martin Luther University of Halle-Wittenberg, Wolfgang-Langenbeck Str. 4, Halle (Saale) 06120, Germany. [4]Department of Chemistry, Faculty of Science, University of Buea, P.O. Box 63, Buea, Cameroon. [5]Laboratory for Simulations and Biomolecular Physics, Advanced Teachers Training College, University of Yaoundé I, P.O. Box 47, Yaoundé, Cameroon. [6]Laboratory of Fundamental and Applied Physics, University of Abobo-Adjame, Abidjan 02 BP 801, Cote d'Ivoire, Africa. [7]Department of Chemistry, Faculty of Science, University of Douala, P.O. Box 24157, Douala, Cameroon. [8]Chemical and Bioactivity Information Centre, 22-23 Blenheim Terrace, Woodhouse Lane, Leeds LS2 9HD, UK.

References

1. Li JWH, Vederas JC (2009) Drug discovery and natural products: end of an era or an endless frontier? Science 325:161–165
2. Chin YW, Balunas MJ, Chai HB, Kinghorn AD (2006) Drug discovery from natural sources. AAPS J 8(2):E239–E253
3. Newman DJ (2008) Natural products as leads to potential drugs: an old process or the new hope for drug discovery? J Med Chem 51:2589–2599
4. Harvey AL (2008) Natural products in drug discovery. Drug Discov Today 13:894–901
5. Koehn FE, Carter GT (2005) The evolving role of natural products in drug discovery. Nat Rev Drug Discov 4:206–220
6. Efange SMN (2002) Natural products: a continuing source of inspiration for the medicinal chemist. In: Iwu MM, Wootton JC (eds) Advances in phytomedicine. Elsevier, Amsterdam
7. Butler MS (2005) Natural products to drugs: natural product derived compounds in clinical trials. Nat Prod Rep 22:162–195
8. Wetzel S, Schuffenhauer A, Roggo S, Ertl P, Waldmann H (2007) Cheminformatic analysis of natural products and their chemical space. Chimia Int J Chem 61:355–360

9. Grabowski K, Baringhaus K-H, Schneider G (2008) Scaffold diversity of natural products: inspiration for combinatorial library design. Nat Prod Rep 25:892–904
10. Grabowski K, Schneider G (2007) Properties and architecture of drugs and natural products revisited. Curr Chem Biol 1:115–127
11. Quinn RJ, Carroll AR, Pham MB, Baron P, Palframan ME, Suraweera L, Pierens GK, Muresan S (2008) Developing a drug-like natural product library. J Nat Prod 71:464–468
12. Hodgson J (2001) ADMET – turning chemicals into drugs. Nat Biotechnol 19:722–726
13. Navia MA, Chaturvedi PR (1996) Design principles for orally bioavailable drugs. Drug Dev Today 1:179–189
14. Lipinski CA, Lombardo F, Dominy BW, Feeney PJ (1997) Experimental and computational approaches to estimate solubility and permeability in drug discovery and development settings. Adv Drug Delivery Rev 23:3–25
15. Lombardo F, Gifford E, Shalaeva MY (2003) In silico ADME prediction: data, models, facts and myths. Mini Rev Med Chem 3:861–875
16. Gleeson MP, Hersey A, Hannongbua S (2011) In-silico ADME models: a general assessment of their utility in drug discovery applications. Curr Top Med Chem 11(4):358–381
17. DiMasi JA, Hansen RW, Grabowsk HG (2003) The price of innovation: new estimates of drug development costs. J Health Econ 22:151–185
18. Darvas F, Keseru G, Papp A, Dormán G, Urge L, Krajcsi P (2002) *In silico* and *ex silico* ADME approaches for drug discovery. Top Med Chem 2:1287–1304
19. eADMET (2011) OCHEM - our platform for the creation of in silico ADME/tox prediction models http://www.eadmet.com/en/ochem.php. Accessed 21 June 2013
20. Lhasa Ltd (2010) Meteor, version 13.0.0. Lhasa Ltd, Leeds, UK
21. Schrödinger (2011) QikProp, version 3.4. LLC, New York, NY
22. Cruciani C, Crivori P, Carrupt PA, Testa B (2000) Molecular fields in quantitative structure-permeation relationships: the VolSurf approach. J Mol Struc-Theochem 503:17–30
23. Tetko IV, Bruneau P, Mewes H-W, Rohrer DC, Poda GI (2006) Can we estimate the accuracy of ADMET predictions? Drug Discov Today 11:700–707
24. Hansch C, Leo A, Mekapatia SB, Kurup A (2004) QSAR and ADME. Bioorg Med Chem 12:3391–3400
25. Greene N, Judson PN, Langowski JJ (1999) Knowledge-based expert systems for toxicity and metabolism prediction: DEREK, StAR and METEOR. SAR QSAR Environ Res 10:299–314
26. Button WG, Judson PN, Long A, Vessey JD (2003) Using absolute and relative reasoning in the prediction of the potential metabolism of xenobiotics. J Chem Inf Comput Sci 43:1371–1377
27. Cronin MTD (2003) Computer-assisted prediction of drug toxicity and metabolism in modern methods of drug discovery. In: Hilgenfeld R, Hillisch A (eds) Modern methods of drug discovery. Birkhäuser, Basel
28. Hou T, Wang J (2008) Structure-ADME relationship: still a long way to go? Expert Opin Drug Metab Toxicol 4(6):759–770
29. Ntie-Kang F, Mbah JA, Mbaze LM, Lifongo LL, Scharfe M, Ngo Hanna J, Cho-Ngwa F, Amoa Onguéné P, Owono Owono LC, Megnassan E, Sippl W, Efange SMN (2013) CamMedNP: building the Cameroonian 3D structural natural products database for virtual screening. BMC Complement Altern Med 13:88
30. Ntie-Kang F, Lifongo LL, Mbaze LM, Ekwelle N, Owono Owono LC, Megnassan E, Judson PN, Sippl W, Efange SMN (2013) Cameroonian medicinal plants: a bioactivity versus ethnobotanical survey and chemotaxonomic classification. BMC Complement Altern Med 13:147
31. Chemical Computing Group, Inc (2010) Molecular operating environment software. CCG, Montreal
32. Halgren TA (1996) Merck molecular force field. J Comput Chem 17:490–641
33. Schrödinger (2011) LigPrep software, version 2.5. LLC, New York, NY
34. Schrödinger (2011) Maestro, version 9.2. LLC, New York, NY
35. Shivakumar D, Williams J, Wu Y, Damm W, Shelley J, Sherman W (2010) Prediction of absolute solvation free energies using molecular dynamics free energy perturbation and the OPLS force field. J Chem Theory Comput 6:1509–1519
36. Jorgensen WL, Maxwell DS, Tirado-Rives J (1996) Development and testing of the OPLS all-atom force field on conformational energetics and properties of organic liquids. J Am Chem Soc 118(45):11225–11236
37. Jorgensen WL, Tirado-Rives J (1988) The OPLS (optimized potentials for liquid simulations) potential functions for proteins, energy minimizations for crystals of cyclic peptides and crambin. J Am Chem Soc 110(6):1657–1666
38. Jorgensen WL, Duffy EM (2002) Prediction of drug solubility from structure. Adv Drug Deliv Rev 54:355–366
39. Duffy EM, Jorgensen WL (2000) Prediction of properties from simulations: free energies of solvation in hexadecane, octanol, and water. J Am Chem Soc 122:2878–2888
40. Jorgensen WL, Duffy EM (2000) Prediction of drug solubility from Monte Carlo simulations. Bioorg Med Chem Lett 10:1155–1158
41. Colmenarejo G, Alvarez-Pedraglio A, Lavandera J-L (2001) Cheminformatic models to predict binding affinities to human serum albumin. J Med Chem 44:4370–4378
42. Luco JM (1999) Prediction of brain–blood distribution of a large set of drugs from structurally derived descriptors using partial least squares (PLS) modelling. J Chem Inf Comput Sci 39:396–404
43. Kelder J, Grootenhuis PD, Bayada DM, Delbresine LP, Ploemen JP (1999) Polar molecular surface as a dominating determinant for oral absorption and brain penetration of drugs. Pharm Res 16:1514–1519
44. Ajay BGW, Murkco MA (1999) Designing libraries with CNS activity. J Med Chem 42:4942–4951
45. Yazdanian M, Glynn SL, Wright JL, Hawi A (1998) Correlating partitioning and Caco-2 cell permeability of structurally diverse small molecular weight compounds. Pharm Res 15:1490–1494
46. Irvine JD, Takahashi L, Lockhart K, Cheong J, Tolan JW, Selick HE, Grove JR (1999) MDCK (Madin-Darby canine kidney) cells: a tool for membrane permeability screening. J Pharm Sci 88:28–33
47. Stenberg P, Norinder U, Luthman K, Artursson P (2001) Experimental and computational screening models for the prediction of intestinal drug absorption. J Med Chem 44:1927–1937
48. Cavalli A, Poluzzi E, De Ponti F, Recanatini M (2002) Toward a pharmacophore for drugs inducing the long QT syndrome: insights from a CoMFA Study of HERG K^+ channel blockers. J Med Chem 45:3844–3853
49. De Ponti F, Poluzzi E, Montanaro N (2001) Organising evidence on QT prolongation and occurrence of *Torsades de Pointes* with non-antiarrhythmic drugs: a call for consensus. Eur J Clin Pharmacol 57:185–209
50. Potts RO, Guy RH (1992) Skin permeability. Pharm Res 9:663–669
51. Potts RO, Guy RH (1995) A predictive algorithm for skin permeability: the effects of molecular size and hydrogen bond activity. Pharm Res 12:1628–1633
52. Schrödinger Press (2011) QikProp 3.4 user manual. LLC, New York, NY
53. Teague SJ, Davis AM, Leeson PD, Opea TI (1999) The design of leadlike combinatorial libraries. Angew Chem Int Ed 38:3743–3748
54. Oprea TI (2002) Current trends in lead discovery: are we looking for the appropriate properties? J Comput-Aided Mol Des 16:325–334
55. Schneider G (2002) Trends in virtual computational library design. Curr Med Chem 9:2095–2102
56. Verdonk ML, Cole JC, Hartshorn ML, Murray CW, Taylor RD (2003) Improved protein-ligand docking using GOLD. Proteins 52:609–623
57. Van de Waterbeemd H, Gifford E (2003) ADMET *in silico* modelling: towards prediction paradise? Nat Rev Drug Discov 2:192–204
58. Veber DF, Johnson SR, Cheng HY, Smith BR, Ward KW, Kopple KD (2002) Molecular properties that influence the oral bioavailability of drug candidates. J Med Chem 45:2615–2623
59. Hedley PL, Jørgensen P, Schlamowitz S, Wangari R, Moolman-Smook J, Brink PA, Kanters JK, Corfield VA, Christiansen M (2009) The genetic basis of long QT and short QT syndromes: a mutation update. Hum Mutat 30:1486–1511
60. Vandenberg JI, Walker BD, Campbell TJ (2001) HERG K^+ channels: friend or foe. Trends Pharmacol Sci 22:240–246
61. Chiesa N, Rosati B, Arcangeli A, Olivotto M, Wanke E (1997) A novel role for HERG K^+ channels: spike-frequency adaptation. J Physiol 501:313–318
62. Aronov AM (2005) Predictive *in silico* modeling for hERG channel blockers. Drug Discov Today 10:149–155
63. Chibale K, Davies-Coleman M, Masimirembwa C (2012) Drug discovery in Africa: impacts of genomics, natural products, traditional medicines, insights into medicinal chemistry, and technology platforms in pursuit of new drugs. Springer, Berlin
64. pan-ANAPL pan-African Natural Products Library [http://www.linkedin.com/groups/pANPL-4098579/about] Accessed 21 June 2013

Facile synthesis of symmetrical bis(benzhydryl) ethers using *p*-toluenesulfonyl chloride under solvent-free conditions

Goutam Brahmachari* and Bubun Banerjee

Abstract

Background: The benzhydryl ether moiety is widely distributed in nature and constitutes a key structural motif in numerous molecules of significant biological potential and of prospective clinical uses. Solvent-free and cost-effective facile synthesis of symmetrical bis(benzhydryl)ethers is, thus, much desirable.

Results: A simple and efficient method for the facile synthesis of symmetrical bis(benzhydryl)ethers directly from the corresponding benzhydrols has been developed using a catalytic amount of *p*-toluenesulfonyl chloride (5 mol%) at an oil bath temperature of 110°C under solvent-free conditions.

Conclusions: Operational simplicity, low reagent loading, high product yields, short reaction time, and solvent-free conditions are the notable advantages of the present method.

Keywords: Bis(benzhydryl)ethers, Benzhydrols, *p*-Toluenesulfonyl chloride, Solvent-free

Background

The benzhydryl ether moiety is abundant in a number of naturally occurring and biologically active compounds as well as molecules of potential clinical uses [1-8]; this motif was also found as a partial structure in a few new chemical entities showing therapeutic activity as well [9]. A number of reports are available describing the synthesis of molecules bearing this structural motif, which were shown to exhibit various pharmacological potentials such as non-nucleoside reverse transcriptase inhibition [10], anti-plasmodial and anti-trypanosomal action [11], monoamine uptake inhibition, anti-depressant and anti-parkinsonian activity [12,13], and anti-histaminic [14] and anti-spasmodic [15] action. Naturally occurring symmetrical bis(benzhydryl)ethers are also known to show promising therapeutic potentials including significant anti-platelet aggregation efficacy [16]. Very recently, application of such ether substructures in the total syntheses of a number of natural products has nicely been reviewed by Pitsinos et al. [17]. Although there are a good number of reports on the synthetic methodology of diaryl ethers, there are only two such reports so far on bis (benzhydryl)ethers in the literature [18-20]; symmetrical bis(benzhydryl)ethers were conventionally synthesized from corresponding benzhydrols using 100% sulfuric acid in large excess [18-20] and *p*-toluenesulfonic acid in equivalent amount [21]. Both of these earlier methods require the use of strong acids in relatively large excess. Under this purview, we have been motivated to undertake systematic planning to develop a convenient and efficient protocol for the conversion of benzhydrols into their bis (benzhydryl)ether derivatives.

In continuation of our effort to develop green and solvent-free synthetic methodologies for organic transformations [22-28], we wish to report in this communication a convenient and straightforward protocol for the efficient synthesis of symmetrical bis(benzhydryl)ethers in excellent yields using a catalytic amount of *p*-toluenesulfonyl chloride under solvent-free conditions (Scheme 1). The process is very simple, cost-effective, and environmentally benign.

Methods

Infrared spectra were recorded using a Shimadzu (FT-IR 8400S) Fourier transform infrared (FT-IR) spectrophotometer (Shimadzu, Kyoto, Japan) using KBr disc. ^{1}H and ^{13}C nuclear magnetic resonance (NMR) spectra were

* Correspondence: brahmg2001@yahoo.co.in
Laboratory of Natural Products and Organic Synthesis, Department of Chemistry, Visva-Bharati University, Santiniketan, West Bengal 731 235, India

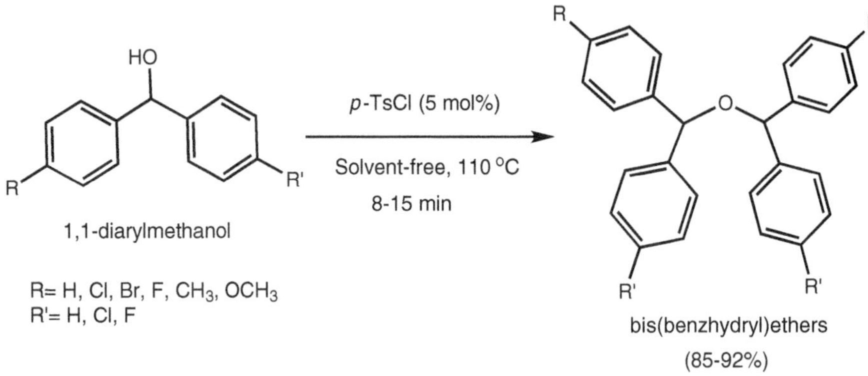

Scheme 1 Synthesis of symmetrical bis(benzhydryl)ethers.

obtained at 400 and 100 MHz, respectively, using a Bruker DRX400 spectrometer (Bruker Instruments, Billerica, MA, USA) and $CDCl_3$ as the solvent. Mass spectra (time-of-flight mass spectrometry (TOF-MS)) were measured on a Q-Tof Micro™ mass spectrometer (Waters MS Technologies, Manchester, UK). Elemental analyses were performed with an Elementar Vario EL III Carlo Erba 1108 micro-analyzer instrument (Carlo Erba Reagenti SpA, Rodano, Italy). Melting point was recorded on a Sunvic melting point apparatus (Sunvic, Glasgow, UK) and is uncorrected. Column chromatography was carried out over silica gel (60 to 120 mesh, Merck & Co., Inc., Whitehouse Station, NJ, USA), and thin layer chromatography (TLC) was performed using silica gel 60 F_{254} (Merck) plates.

Results and discussion

Firstly, we carried out the synthesis of bis(benzhydryl) ether **1** from benzhydrol as our model reaction in order to optimize the best suited reaction conditions (Figure 1); it was observed (Table 1) that the alcohol in the presence of *p*-TsCl (5 mol%) afforded the best result with 86% isolated yield at 110°C within a short period of time (15 min) under solvent-free conditions.

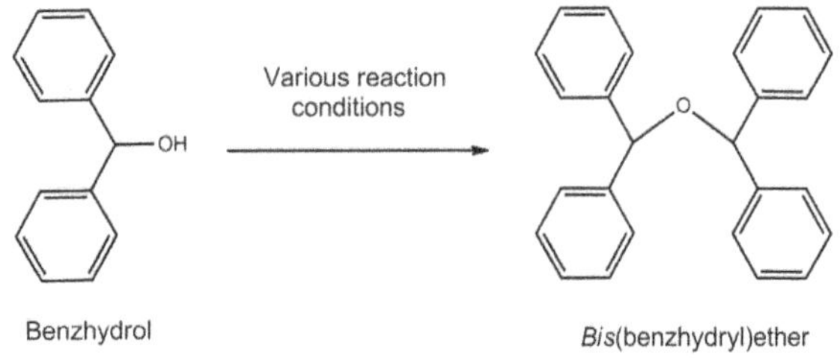

Figure 1 Optimization of the reaction conditions.

A number of benzhydrol derivatives containing mono- and di-chloro, mono-bromo, di-fluoro, mono-methoxy, and mono-methyl phenyl groups were then screened for studying the generality as well as the efficacy of this present procedure (Figure 2; Table 2). All the entries find an easy and efficient route to their symmetrical bis (benzhydryl)ether derivatives in the presence of *p*-TsCl under solvent-free conditions (Figure 2) within 8 to 15 min affording excellent yields (85% to 92%). The workup of the reaction mixtures is simple and highly convenient. Each product has been characterized by detailed spectral analyses including FT-IR, ^{1}H NMR, ^{13}C NMR, and TOF-MS. In addition, the molecular structure of bis(bis-

Table 1 Optimization of the reaction conditions following Figure 1

Entry	*p*-TsCl (mol%)	Solvent	Temperature (°C)	Time (min)	Yield (%)[a]
1	0	-	110	120	No reaction
2	10	-	90	25	82
3	10	-	110	15	87
4	5	-	90	35	80
5	*5*	-	*110*	*15*	*86*
6	5	-	Rt	240	Trace
7	3	-	110	75	28
8	10	CH_2Cl_2	Rt	1,050	19
9	5	CH_2Cl_2	Rt	1,050	Trace
10	10	THF	Rt	600	Trace
11	10	CH_3CN	Rt	720	17
12	10	CH_2Cl_2	Reflux	300	36
13	50	-	110	5	43 (tosylate: 47)
14	100	-	110	5	7 (tosylate: 91)

[a]Isolated yield; RT, room temperature; *p*-TsCl, *p*-toluenesulfonyl chloride; Tosylate, benzhydryl *p*-toluenesulfonate.

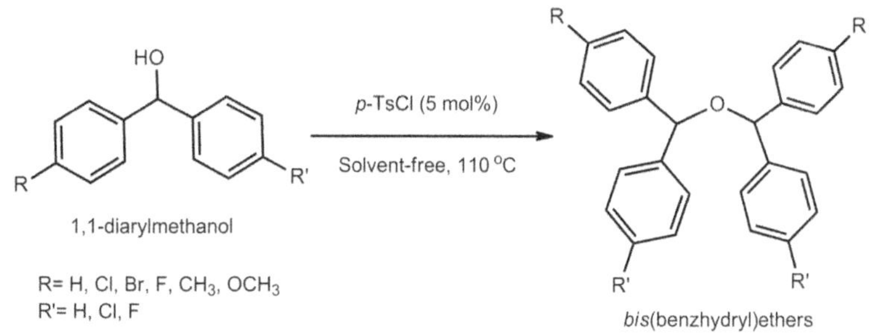

Figure 2 Synthesis of symmetrical bis(benzhydryl)ethers using *p*-TsCl as reagent under solvent-free conditions.

phenylmethyl)ether (Table 2, entry 1) has unambiguously been confirmed from X-ray crystallographic analysis [29-33] (Figure 3).[a]

We propose the following mechanistic pathway for the reaction (Scheme 2). *p*-TsCl reacts rapidly with an equivalent amount of diarylmethanol to generate HCl (and a tosylate derivative as side product) *in situ* that eventually catalyzes the etherification following a catalytic cycle. The corresponding tosylate derivative remains intact as side product. To ensure the fact, we have checked the reaction with 50 and 100 mol% *p*-TsCl in two separate entries (entries 13 and 14; Table 1) where benzhydryl *p*-toluenesulfonate was isolated as 47% and 91% yields, respectively. In addition, we have carried out the reaction with benzhydrol separately using dry HCl gas (passed for a while into the reaction vessel) and concentrated hydrochloric acid; it has been found that dry HCl could also act as an efficient catalyst producing the corresponding ether derivative **1** with 82% yield in 30 min at 110°C, while concentrated HCl (45 mg added to 1 mmol of benzhydrol) required much more time (45 min) producing less amount of yield (62%) at the same reaction temperature. These experimental observations support our proposed mechanistic pathway as well.

Experimental

General procedure for the synthesis of symmetrical bis (benzhydryl)ethers (entries 1 to 7)

An oven-dried screw cap test tube was charged with a magnetic stir bar, benzhydrol (1 mmol), and *p*-toluenesulfonyl chloride (5 mol%). The tube was then evacuated and back-filled with nitrogen. The evacuation/backfill sequence was repeated two additional times. The tube was placed in a preheated oil bath at 110°C, and the reaction mixture was stirred vigorously. The progress of the reaction was monitored by TLC, and on completion, the reaction mixture was cooled to room temperature. The reaction mixture was extracted with dried ethyl acetate (10 ml), and the extract was then concentrated under reduced pressure; the residue was purified via column chromatography using silica gel (60 to 120 mesh) and petrol ether-ethyl acetate mixture. The structure of each purified symmetrical bis(benzhydryl) ethers was confirmed by analytical as well as spectral studies including FT-IR, ^{1}H NMR, ^{13}C NMR, and TOF-MS. Respective physical and spectral properties of bis (diarylmethyl)ethers are described below.

The spectral and analytical data of all the compounds including all new entries are given below (see also Additional file 1):

- *Bis(bis-phenylmethyl)ether (1)*: white solid, 86% yield, m.p. 106°C to 107°C (Lit. 105°C to 107°C [34]. 107°C [18]). IR (ν_{max}, KBr) cm^{-1}: 3,057, 3,028, 2,953, 1,595, 1,489, 1,445, 1,250, 1,163, 1,098, 1,072, 1,029, 6,98. ^{1}H NMR ($CDCl_3$, 200 MHz, δ): 7.40 to 7.23 (m, 20H, Ar H), 5.41 (s, 2H, CH). ^{13}C NMR ($CDCl_3$, 100 MHz, δ): 142.28, 128.45, 127.51, 127.33, 80.05. TOF-MS: 373.44 ([M + Na]$^{+}$). Anal. found: C, 89.13; H, 6.28. $C_{26}H_{22}O$ requires C, 89.11; H, 6.33%
- *Bis[[1-(4-methylphenyl)-1-phenyl]methyl]ether (2)*: yellowish white, semi solid, 89% yield. IR (ν_{max}, KBr) cm^{-1}: 3,060, 3,025, 2,923, 2,852, 1,655, 1,460, 1,277, 1,124, 1,071, 824, 810, 699. ^{1}H NMR ($CDCl_3$, 400 MHz, *δ*): 7.6 (d, 4H, Ar H, *J* = 7.6 Hz), 7.53 to 7.45 (m, 8H, Ar H), 7.43 to 7.41 (m, 2H, Ar H), 7.34 (d, 4H, Ar H, *J* = 7.6 Hz), 5.63 (s, 2H, CH), 2.53 (s, 6H, CH_3). ^{13}C NMR ($CDCl_3$, 100 MHz, δ): 142.82, 142.70, 139.59, 139.48, 137.26, 137.22, 129.33, 129.30, 128.57, 128.54, 127.53, 127.49, 127.46, 127.41, 127.34, 79.96, 21.37. TOF-MS: 401.05 ([M + Na]$^{+}$). Anal. found: C, 89.89; H, 6.90. $C_{28}H_{26}O$ requires C, 89.85; H, 6.92%
- *Bis[[1-(4-chlorophenyl)-1-phenyl]methyl]ether (3)*: white semi solid, 85% yield. IR (ν_{max}, KBr) cm^{-1}: 3,063, 3,029, 2,925, 2,854, 1,595, 1,490, 1,449, 1,259, 1,185, 1,086, 1,057, 843, 811, 700. ^{1}H NMR ($CDCl_3$, 400 MHz, *δ*): 7.31 to 7.30 (m, 8H, Ar H), 7.28 to 7.25 (m, 10H, Ar H), 5.33 (s, 2H, CH). ^{13}C NMR ($CDCl_3$, 100 MHz, *δ*): 141.49, 141.39, 140.65, 140.54, 133.37, 133.30, 128.69, 128.63, 128.60, 128.56, 128.48, 127.87, 127.81, 127.22, 127.13, 79.53. TOF-

Table 2 Synthesis of symmetrical bis(benzhydryl)ethers using *p*-TsCl as reagent under solvent-free conditions following Figure 2

Entry	Alcohol	Product	Time (min)	Yield (%)[a]	Melting point (°C)	
					Found	Reported
1	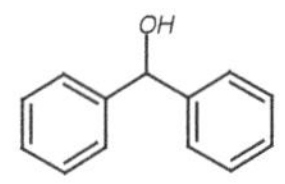	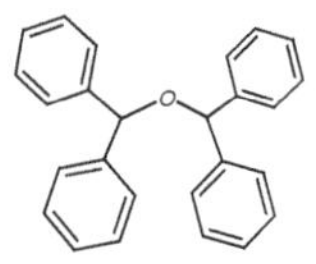 1	15	86	106 to 107	105 to 107 [34]
2	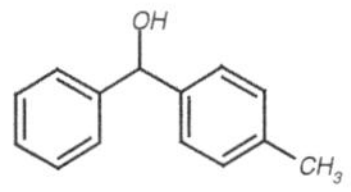	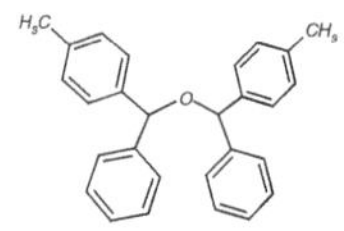 2	15	89	Semisolid	Present work
3	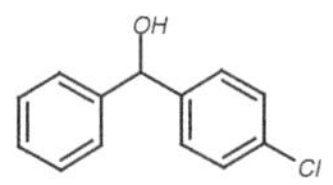	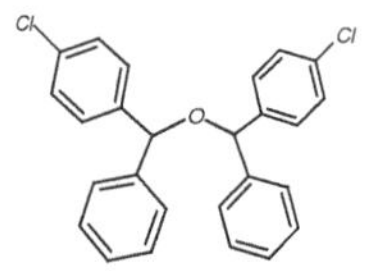 3	10	85	Semisolid	Present work
4	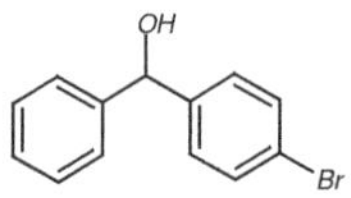	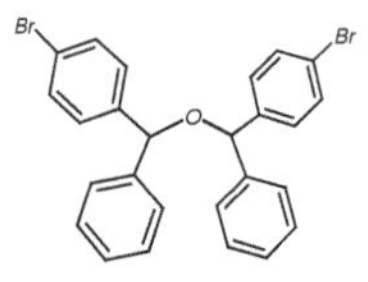 4	10	92	Semisolid	Present work
5	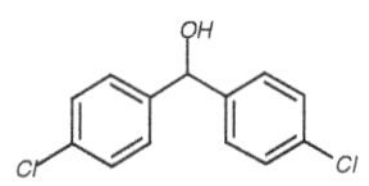	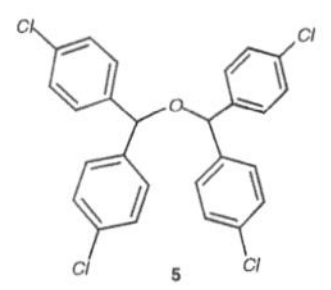 5	10	88	125 to 127	126 to 127 [34,35]
6	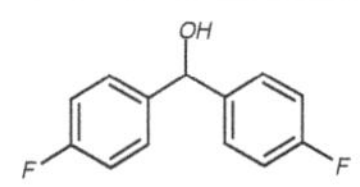	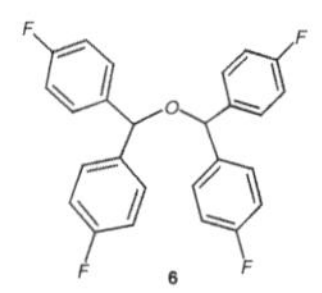 6	8	91	88 to 90	Present work
7	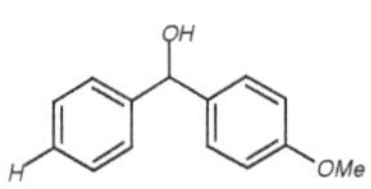	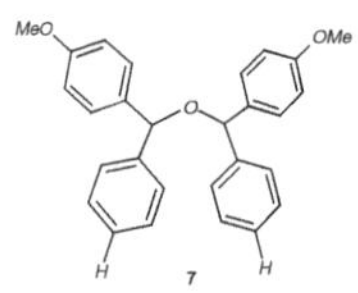 7	12	90	Semisolid	Present work

[a]Isolated yield.

MS: 441.94 ([M + Na]$^+$). Anal. found: C, 74.45; H, 4.83. $C_{26}H_{20}Cl_2O$ requires C, 74.47; H, 4.81%

- *Bis[[1-(4-bromophenyl)-1-phenyl]methyl]ether (4)*: white semi solid, 92% yield. IR (ν_{max}, KBr) cm^{-1}: 3,085, 3,062, 3,028, 2,924, 2,854, 1,602, 1,590, 1,486, 1,454, 1,290, 1,185, 1,107, 1,070, 1,028, 847, 793, 700. ^{1}H NMR ($CDCl_3$, 400 MHz, δ): 7.33 (dd, 4H, Ar H, J = 8.4, 5.2 Hz), 7.21 to 7.15 (m, 10H, Ar H), 7.12 (dd, 4H, Ar H, J = 8.4, 3.2 Hz), 5.23 (s, 2H, CH). ^{13}C NMR ($CDCl_3$, 100 MHz, δ): 141.43, 141.33, 141.20, 141.08, 131.68, 131.62, 128.94, 128.86, 128.70, 128.65, 127.94, 127.87, 127.26, 127.17, 121.60, 121.52, 79.61. TOF-MS: 528.74 ([M + Na]$^+$). Anal. found: C, 61.49; H, 3.93. $C_{26}H_{18}Br_2O$ requires C, 61.44; H, 3.97%
- *Bis[bis(4-chlorophenyl)methyl]ether (5)*: white solid, 88% yield, m.p. 125°C to 127°C (Lit. 126°C to 127°C) [35,36]. IR (ν_{max}, KBr) cm^{-1}: 3,031, 2,924, 1,594, 1,491, 1,410, 1,290, 1,188, 1,089, 1,013, 854, 824, 735, 726. ^{1}H NMR ($CDCl_3$, 200 MHz, δ): 7.31 (d, 8H, Ar H, J = 8.6 Hz), 7.23 (d, 8H, Ar H, J = 8.6 Hz), 5.29 (s, 2H, CH). ^{13}C NMR ($CDCl_3$, 75 MHz,

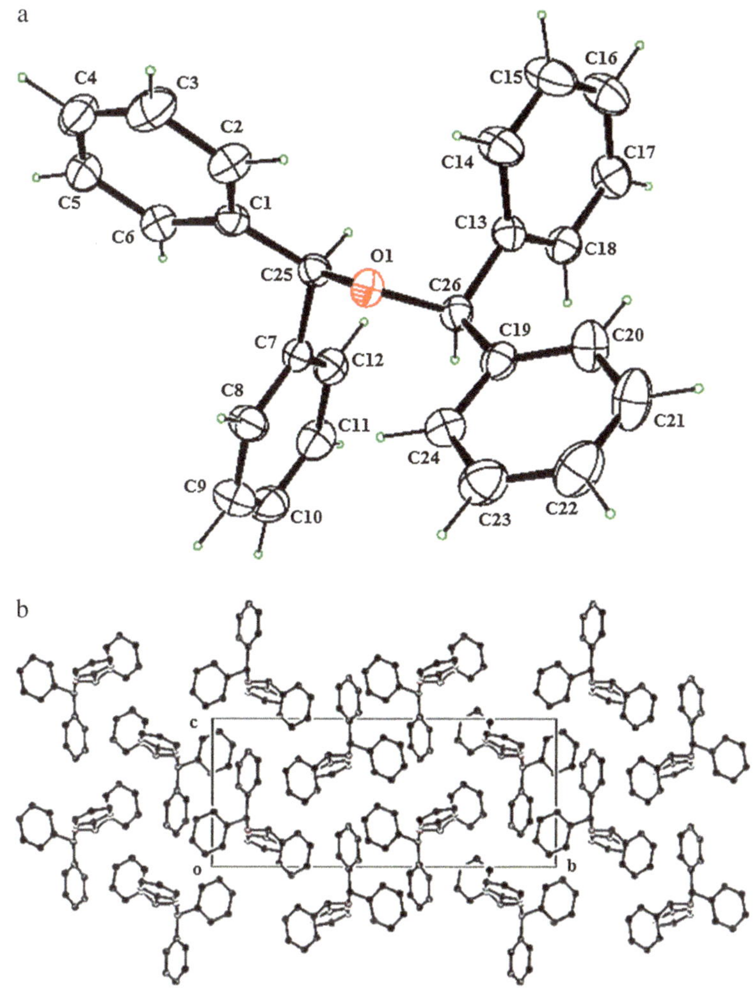

Figure 3 Diagram and packing arrangement. (**a**) ORTEP diagram of compound **1** (CCDC 840259). (**b**) The packing arrangement of molecules viewed down the a-axis.

δ): 139.72, 133.71, 128.82, 128.36, 78.97. TOF-MS: 509.12 ([M + Na]$^+$). Anal. found: C, 63.94; H, 3.69; $C_{26}H_{18}Cl_4O$ requires C, 63.96; H, 3.72%

- *Bis[bis[4-fluorophenyl]methyl]ether (6)*: white solid, 91% yield, m.p. 88°C to 90°C. IR (ν_{max}, KBr) cm^{-1}: 3,069, 3,057, 2,925, 1,603, 1,507, 1,422, 1,408, 1,298, 1,225, 1,178, 1,155, 1,101, 1,029, 859, 837, 818. ^{1}H NMR ($CDCl_3$, 400 MHz, δ): 7.19 to 7.16 (m, 8H, Ar H), 6.94 to 6.88 (m, 8H, Ar H), 5.22 (s, 2H, CH). ^{13}C NMR ($CDCl_3$, 100 MHz, δ): 163.52, 161.07, 137.51, 137.48, 128.82, 128.74, 115.59, 115.38, 78.91. TOF-MS: 445.98 ([M + Na]$^+$). Anal. found: C, 73.89; H, 4.28. $C_{26}H_{18}F_4O$ requires C, 73.93; H, 4.30%
- *Bis[[1-(4-methoxyphenyl)-1-phenyl]methyl]ether (7)*: colorless liquid, 90% yield. IR (ν_{max}, KBr) cm^{-1}: 3,062, 3,029, 2,953, 2,932, 2,906, 2,835, 1,510, 1,494, 1,451, 1,249, 1,171, 1,111, 1,080, 849, 819, 698. ^{1}H NMR ($CDCl_3$, 400 MHz, δ): 7.35 (d, 4H, Ar H, J = 7.6 Hz), 7.32 to 7.28 (m, 4H, Ar H), 7.27 to 7.24 (m, 6H, Ar H), 6.84 (d, 4H, Ar H, J = 8.4 Hz), 5.34 (s, 2H, CH), 3.77 (s, 6H, OCH_3). ^{13}C NMR ($CDCl_3$, 100 MHz, δ): 158.97, 158.93, 142.72, 142.52, 134.53, 134.32, 128.67, 128.60, 128.35, 128.32, 127.30, 127.24, 127.17, 127.09, 113.80, 113.77, 79.43, 79.40, 55.26. TOF-MS: 432.99 ([M + Na]$^+$). Anal. found: C, 81.95; H, 6.37. $C_{28}H_{26}O_3$ requires C, 81.92; H, 6.38%

Conclusions

In conclusion, we have developed a very simple and highly efficient solvent-free protocol for the synthesis of symmetrical bis(benzhydryl)ethers using inexpensive *p*-toluenesulfonyl chloride as reagent. The significant features of this environmentally benign and cost-effective straightforward protocol for direct conversion of benzhydrols into symmetrical bis(benzhydryl)ethers include operational simplicity, low reagent loading, high

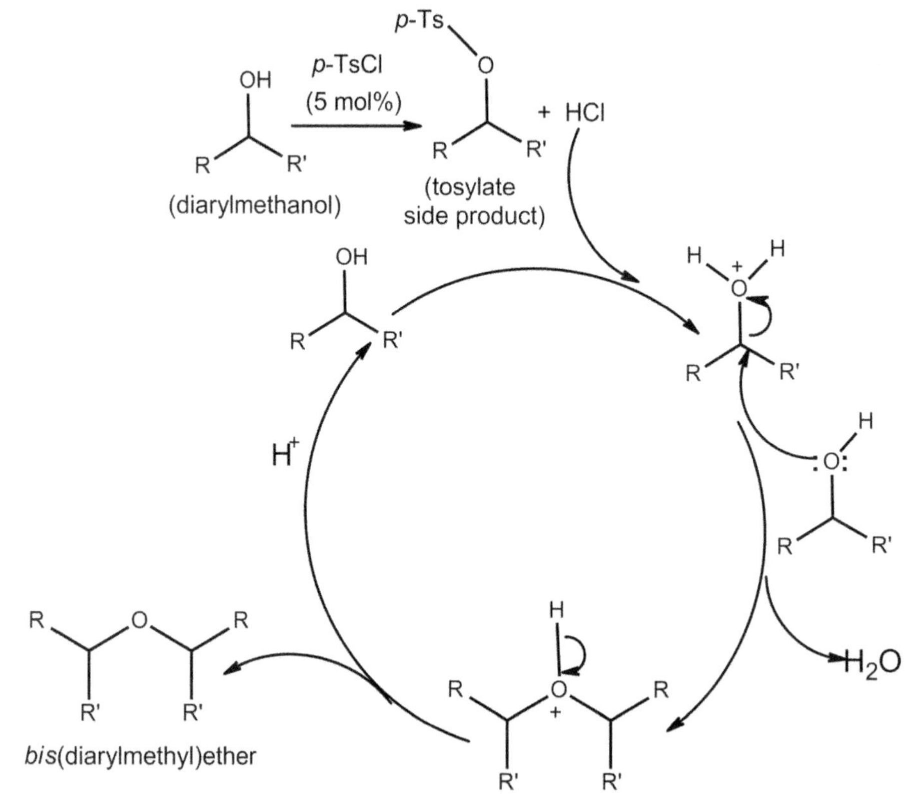

Scheme 2 Proposed mechanistic pathway for etherification.

product yields, short reaction time, and solvent-free conditions.

Endnote

[a]The molecular structure of the product, bis(bis-phenylmethyl)ether (**1**), was determined by means of X-ray crystallographic studies. CCDC 840259 (**1**) contains the supplementary crystallographic data for this article. These data can be obtained free of charge from The Cambridge Crystallographic Data Centre via http://www.ccdc.cam.ac.uk/data_request/cif.

Competing interests

The authors declare that they have no competing interests.

Acknowledgments

The authors are thankful to I.I.C.B., Kolkata and Chemistry Department, Kalyani University, India for the spectral measurements. B.B. is grateful to the UGC, New Delhi for awarding him a Senior Research Fellowship. G.B. is thankful to the CSIR, New Delhi for financial support (No. 02(0110)/12/EMR-II dated 01.11.2012). The authors are grateful to Dr. Vivek K. Gupta, Post-Graduate Department of Physics, University of Jammu, Jammu Tawi 180 006, India for collecting the X-ray data.

This study was conducted in memory of Santosh Kr. Brahmachari.

References

1. Brahmachari G (2010) Handbook of pharmaceutical natural products, 1st edn. Wiley-VCH, Weinheim
2. Li X, Upton TG, Gibb CLD, Gibb BC (2003) Resorcinarenes as templates: a general strategy for the synthesis of large macrocycles. J Am Chem Soc 125:650–651
3. Ley SV, Thomas AW (2003) Modern synthetic methods for copper-mediated C(aryl)-O, C(aryl)-N, and C(aryl)-S bond formation. Angew Chem Int Ed 42:5400–5449
4. Tlili A, Monnier F, Taillefer M (2010) Selective one-pot access to symmetrical or unsymmetrical diaryl ethers by copper-catalyzed double arylation of a simple oxygen source. Chem Eur J 16:12299–12302
5. Tan ES, Miyakawa M, Bunzow JR, Grandy DK, Scanlan TS (2007) Exploring the structure-activity relationship of the ethylamine portion of 3-iodothyronamine for rat and mouse trace amine-associated receptor 1. J Med Chem 50:2787–2798
6. Nicolaou KC, Boddy CNC, Brase S, Winssinger N (1999) Chemistry, biology and medicine of the glycopeptide antibiotics. Angew Chem Int Ed 38:2097–2152
7. Harris CM, Kopecka H, Harris TM (1983) Vancomycin: structure and transformation to CDP-I. J Am Chem Soc 105:6915–6922
8. Barna JCJ, Williams DH, Stone DJM, Leung TWC, Doddrell DM (1984) Structure elucidation of the teicoplanin antibiotics. J Am Chem Soc 106:4895–4902
9. Hayashi M (1997) Drug Data Report 704 (JP 97077745). J. R. Prous Science, Barcelona

10. Su D, Lim JJ, Tinney E, Wan B, Young MB, Anderson KD, Rudd D, Munshi V, Bahnck C, Felock PJ, Lu M, Lai M, Touch S, Moyer G, DiStefano DJ, Flynn JA, Liang Y, Sanchez R, Perlow-Poehnelt R, Miller M, Vacca JP, Williams TM, Anthony NJ (2009) Biaryl ethers as novel non-nucleoside reverse transcriptase inhibitors with improved potency against key mutant viruses. J Med Chem 52:7163–7169
11. Weis R, Schlapper C, Brun CR, Kaiser M, Seebacher W (2006) Antiplasmodial and antitrypanosomal activity of new esters and ethers of 4-dialkylaminobicyclo[2.2.2]octan-2-ols. Eur J Pharm Sci 28:361–368
12. Van Der Zee P, Hespe W (1978) A comparison of the inhibitory effects of aromatic substituted benzhydryl ethers on the uptake of catecholamines and serotonin into synaptosomal preparations of the rat brain. Neuropharmacol 17:483–490
13. Nilsson JL, Wågermark J, Dahlbom R (1969) Potential antiparkinsonism agents. Quinuclidinyl benzhydryl ethers. J Med Chem 12:1103–1105
14. McGavack TH, Schulman PM, Boyd LJ (1948) A clinical investigation of beta-morpholino-ethyl benzhydryl ether hydrochloride (linadryl) as an antihistamine agent. J Allergy 19:141–145
15. Loew ER, Kaiser ME (1945) Alleviation of anaphylactic shock in guinea pigs with synthetic benzhydryl alkamine ethers. Exp Biol Med 58:235–237
16. Pyo MK, Jin JL, Koo YK, Yun-Choi S (2004) Phenolic and furan type compounds isolated from *Gastrodia elata* and their anti-platelet effects. Arch Pharm Res 27:381–385
17. Pitsinos EN, Vidali VP, Couladouros EA (2011) Diaryl ether formation in the synthesis of natural products. Eur J Org Chem 7:1207–1222
18. Pratt EF, Draper JD (1949) Reaction rates by distillation. I. The etherification of phenylcarbinols and the transetherification of their ethers1. J Am Chem Soc 71:2846–2849
19. Welch CM, Smith HA (1950) The properties of benzhydrol in sulfuric acid solution. J Am Chem Soc 72:4748–4750
20. Smith HA, Thompson RG (1955) Preparation and properties of substituted benzhydryl carbonium ions. J Am Chem Soc 77:1778–1783
21. Toda F, Takumi H, Akehi M (1990) Efficient solid-state reactions of alcohols: dehydration, rearrangement, and substitution. J Chem Soc Chem Commun 1270–1271
22. Brahmachari G, Laskar S (2010) A very simple and highly efficient procedure for *N*-formylation of primary and secondary amines at room temperature under solvent-free conditions. Tetrahedron Lett 51:2319–2322
23. Brahmachari G, Laskar S, Sarkar S (2010) Metal acetate/metal oxide in acetic acid: an efficient reagent for the chemoselective *N*-acetylation of amines. J Chem Res 34:288–295
24. Brahmachari G, Laskar S, Sarkar S (2010) A green approach to chemoselective *N*-acetylation of amines using catalytic amount of zinc acetate in acetic acid under microwave irradiation. Indian J Chem 49B:1274–1281
25. Brahmachari G, Das S (2012) Bismuth nitrate-catalyzed multicomponent reaction for efficient and one-pot synthesis of densely functionalized piperidine scaffolds at room temperature. Tetrahedron Lett 53:1479–1484
26. Brahmachari G, Banerjee B (2012) A comparison between catalyst-free and $ZrOCl_2{\cdot}8H_2O$-catalyzed Strecker reactions for the rapid and solvent-free one-pot synthesis of racemic α-aminonitrile derivatives. Asian J Org Chem 1:251–258
27. Brahmachari G, Das S (2013) One-pot synthesis of 3-[(*N*-alkylanilino)(aryl) methyl] indoles via a transition metal assisted three-component condensation at room temperature. J Het Chem, in press
28. Brahmachari G, Das S (2013) A simple and straightforward method for one-pot synthesis of 2,4,5-triarylimidazoles using titanium dioxide as an eco-friendly and recyclable catalyst under solvent-free conditions. Indian J Chem Sec B, 52B:387–393
29. Sheldrick GM (1997) SHELXS97, Program for the solution of crystal structures. University of Gottingen, Gottingen
30. Farrugia LJ (1997) ORTEP-3 for windows—a version of ORTEP-III with a graphical user interface (GUI). J Appl Cryst 30:565–566
31. Farrugia LJ (1999) WinGX suite for small-molecule single-crystal crystallography. J Appl Cryst 32:837–838
32. Nardelli M (1995) PARST95-An update to PARST. A system of Fortran routines for calculating molecular structure parameters from the results of the crystal structure analysis. J Appl Cryst 28:659
33. Spek AL (2009) Structure validation in chemical crystallography. Acta Cryst D65:148–155
34. Koloves M, Froussios C (1984) *O*-diphenylmethylation of alcohols and carboxylic acids using diphenylmethyl diphenyl phosphate as alkylating agent. Tetrahedron Lett 25:3909–3912
35. Grummitt O, Buck AC (1945) Di-(p, p/-dichlorobenzohydryl) ether. J Am Chem Soc 67:693
36. Welch CM, Smith HA (1953) Reactions of carboxylic acids in sulfuric acid. J Am Chem Soc 75:1412–1415

Free radical scavenging properties of pyrimidine derivatives

Tabassum Bano[1*], Nitin Kumar[2] and Rupesh Dudhe[2]

Abstract

Free radicals are well known for playing a dual role in our body- deleterious as well as beneficial. It includes a metabolic pathway for its generation. Oxidative stress in our body occurs due to excessive generation of free radicals and reduced level of antioxidants, but at low concentrations, these radicals help to perform normal physiological functions of the body. Scientific evidence suggests that antioxidants reduce the risk for chronic diseases including cancer and heart disease. This review shows current tendency in the pyrimidine synthesis and reveals the pyrimidine core to be a very potent moiety which can be a rich source for the synthesis of new compounds having desirable antioxidant activity.

Keywords: Free radical, Antioxidant, Pyrimidine, Oxidative stress

Review

Introduction

Free radicals can be defined as the atoms, molecules, or ions with unpaired electrons in an open shell configuration. Sometimes, these free radicals may bear some charge, either positive, negative, or zero. They also play a significant role in combustion, atmospheric chemistry, polymerization, plasma chemistry, and many other chemical processes. Free radicals may generate different kinds of chemical and biological reactions in the body. Development of free radicals in the body is believed to involve in the development of various degenerative diseases; huge generation of free radicals particularly reactive oxygen species and their high activity may lead to progression of a number of pathological disturbances such as inflammation, atherosclerosis, cancer, Parkinson's disease, and Alzheimer's disease. This phenomenon of excessive production of free radicals is termed as oxidative stress. This oxidative stress has also been found to be implicated in many ailments such as heart disease and some age-related diseases. Thus, in a concise way, it can be said that excessive production of free radicals is harmful for the body.

Many heterocyclic compounds have been synthesized because of their wide range of biological activity [1]. Pyrimidine is a six-member heterocyclic compound that contains two nitrogen atoms at positions 1 and 3 (Figure 1). Pyrimidine derivatives have showed various biological activities such as antimicrobial, antitumor, antifungal, and antileishmanial activities and are also useful for the treatment of thyroid and leukemia [2]. In this article, the authors give an emphasis on antioxidant activity by pyrimidine-containing nucleus.

Types of free radical reaction

There are three main types of free radical reactions:

1. Initiation reaction
2. Propagation reaction
3. Termination reaction [3]

Sources of free radical generation

Various sources lead to the generation of free radicals:

- UV radiations, X-rays, gamma rays, and microwave radiation
- Reaction catalyzed by metals
- Oxygen free radicals in the atmosphere considered as pollutants
- Inflammation that initiates neutrophils and macrophages to produce reactive oxygen species and reactive nitrogen species

* Correspondence: tabassumald@gmail.com
[1]Department of Pharmaceutical Technology, Meerut Institute of Engineering and Technology, Baghpat Bypass Crossing, NH-58, Delhi-Roorkee Highway, Meerut, Uttar Pradesh 250005, India
Full list of author information is available at the end of the article

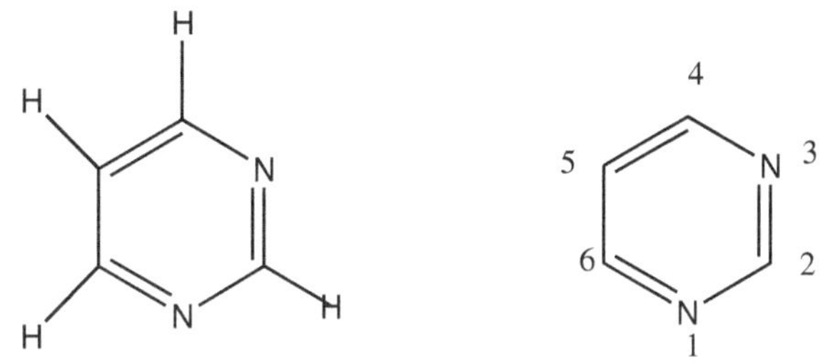

Figure 1 Basic structure of a pyrimidine ring.

- In mitochondria-catalyzed electron transport reactions, oxygen free radicals produced as by-product
- Reactive oxygen species (ROS) generated by the metabolism of arachidonic acid, platelets, macrophages and smooth muscle cells
- Interaction with chemicals, automobile exhaust fumes, smoking of cigarettes and cigars
- Burning of organic matter during cooking, forest fires, volcanic activities
- Industrial effluents, excess chemicals, alcoholic intake, certain drugs, asbestos, certain pesticides and herbicides, some metal ions, fungal toxins, and xenobiotics

Generation of free radical by metabolic pathway

Free radicals are mainly generated by various metabolic pathways such as lipid and peroxidation, gluconeogenesis, and glucuronidation. Generation of free radicals is first converted to hydrogen peroxide which is further reduced to water. This detoxification occurs during oxidative stress, where in the oxygen generates inside the body. The superoxide released by the oxidative phosphorylation pathway is the result of multiple enzymes; superoxide dismutase catalyzes the first step, and then various peroxides help in removing the hydrogen peroxide.

Role of free radicals in our body

Free radicals are naturally produced within the body (Figure 2), and their various effects are exhibited. The immune system is the main site for their attack. Generation of these free radicals decreases the effectiveness of the immune system. Free radicals also attack the cell membrane, resulting in the damage of a cell at such point that it must be discarded by the immune system. If the formation of free radicals and attacks are not controlled within the muscle during exercise, a large quantity of muscle could easily be damaged. Damaged muscles could in turn inhibit performance by the induction of fatigue [4,5].

Diseases caused by the free radical generation in the human body

Oxygen is an element that is essential to life. Living systems have evolved to survive in the presence of molecular oxygen, which is also applicable to most biological systems. Oxidative properties of oxygen play a vital role in diverse biological systems. It includes the following:

- Neurodegenerative disorders such as Alzheimer's disease, Parkinson's disease, multiple sclerosis, amyotrophic lateral sclerosis, memory loss, and depression
- Cardiovascular diseases such as atherosclerosis, ischemic heart disease, cardiac hypertrophy, hypertension, shock, and trauma

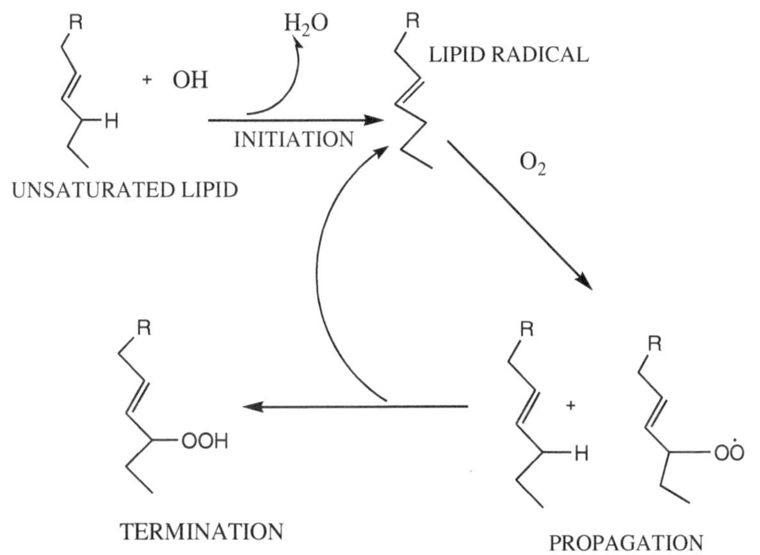

Figure 2 Biological pathway for the generation of free radical in living organisms.

- Pulmonary disorders such as inflammatory lung diseases such as asthma and chronic obstructive pulmonary disease
- Diseases associated with premature infants, including bronchopulmonary, dysplasia, periventricular leukomalacia, and intraventricular hemorrhage, retinopathy of prematurity, and necrotizing enterocolitis
- Autoimmune disease such as rheumatoid arthritis
- Renal disorders such as glomerulonephritis and tubulointerstitial nephritis, chronic renal failure, proteinuria, and uremia
- Gastrointestinal diseases such as peptic ulcer, inflammatory bowel disease, and colitis
- Tumors and cancer such as lung cancer, leukemia, and breast, ovary, and rectum cancers
- Eye diseases such as cataract and age-related retinal maculopathy. Aging process, diabetes, skin lesions, immunodepression, liver disease, pancreatitis, AIDS, infertility [6]

General properties of antioxidants

The main characteristic of an antioxidant is its ability to trap free radicals. Scientific evidence suggests that antioxidants reduce the risk of chronic diseases including cancer and heart disease. Antioxidant activity was performed by DPPH free radical scavenging method using ascorbic acid as a standard drug.

Classification of antioxidants

Natural antioxidants

Antioxidants obtained from the natural source are known as natural antioxidants. They can be divided into following categories:

1. *Enzymes.* Enzyme such as superoxide dismutase, catalase, and glutathione peroxidase (GPx) attenuate the generation of reactive oxygen species by removing potential oxidants or by transferring ROS/RNS into relatively stable compounds (Figure 3). GPx reduces lipid peroxides (ROOH), formed by the oxidation of polyunsaturated fatty acids, to a stable nontoxic molecule - hydroxyl fatty acid (ROH).
2. *Lipid-soluble antioxidants.* This group of antioxidants is supposed to act as highly efficient scavengers, against lipid peroxyl radical, which is formed within the lipoprotein as a consequence of free radical chain reaction of lipid peroxidation.
3. *Water-soluble antioxidants.* These antioxidants cannot enter the lipid moiety of low density lipoprotein (LDL); these will be less efficient as these are principally unable to encounter most of these lyophilic radicals.
4. *Low molecular weight antioxidants.* These are subdivided into lipid-soluble antioxidants (tocopherol, carotenoids, quinones, bilirubin, and some polyphenols) and water-soluble antioxidants (ascorbic acid, uric acid, and polyphenols). These delay or inhibit cellular damage mainly through their free radical scavenging property.

Table 1 Various ROS and corresponding neutralizing antioxidants

ROS	Neutralizing antioxidants
Lipid peroxides	Beta-carotene, flavonoids, vitamin E, ubiquinone, glutathione1 peroxidase
Superoxide radical	Flavonoids, vitamin C, glutathione
Hydrogen peroxide	Vitamin E, vitamin C, glutathione, lipoic acid beta-carotene, flavonoids
Hydroxyl radical	Lipoic acid, vitamin C, glutathione, flavonoids

Synthetic antioxidants

These are the compounds which are synthesized inside the laboratory. It includes butylated hydroxyl anisole, butylated hydroxy toluene, and tertiary butylated hydroxy quinone. These are most effective antioxidants and also come under the category of synthetic chemicals. ROS is a term which encompasses all highly reactive, oxygen-containing molecules, including free radicals. Some of the ROS along with their neutralizing antioxidants are given in Table 1 [7-10].

Chemistry of the pyrimidine ring

The structure of the pyrimidine ring (Figure 4) is similar to benzene and pyridine. In a pyrimidine ring, as the number of nitrogen atoms increases the ring π electrons become less energetic; electrophilic aromatic substitution gets more difficult, while nucleophilic aromatic substitution resonance stabilization properties of pyrimidine may lead to the addition and ring cleavage reactions rather than substitutions.

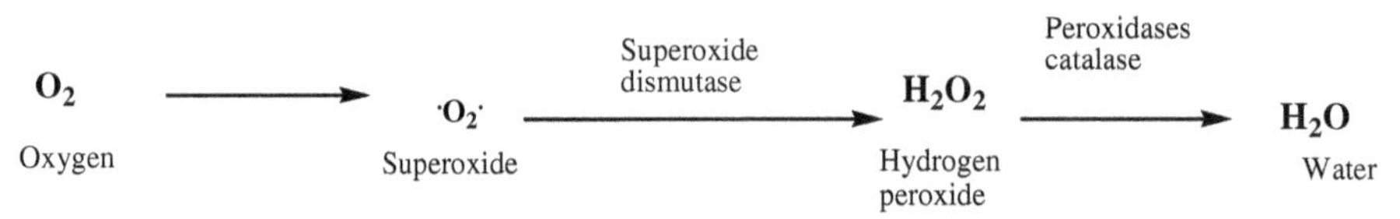

Figure 3 Enzymatic pathway for the detoxification of reactive oxygen species.

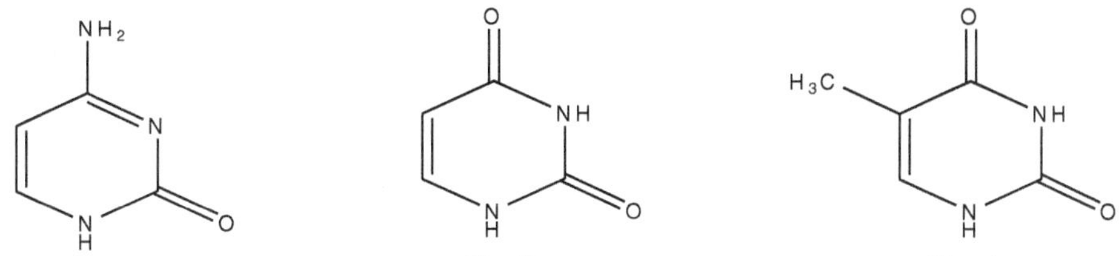

Cytosine (I) Uracil (II) Thymine (III)

Figure 4 Basic unit of body building material.

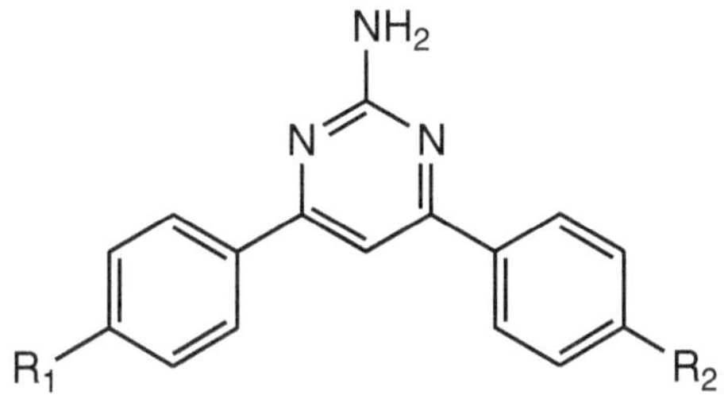

	5d	5e
R_1	Cl	Cl
R_2	Cl	Br

Figure 5 Compounds 5d and 5e.

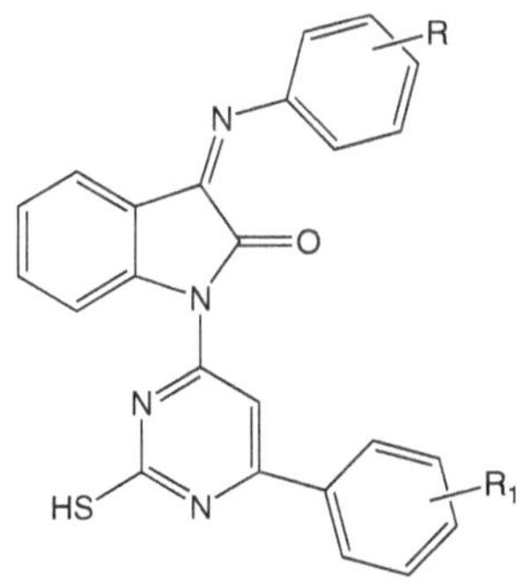

($7a_1$- $7a_3$) - ($7b_1$-$7b_3$)

R= Cl , NO_2
$R_1 = NO_2$, OH, OCH_3

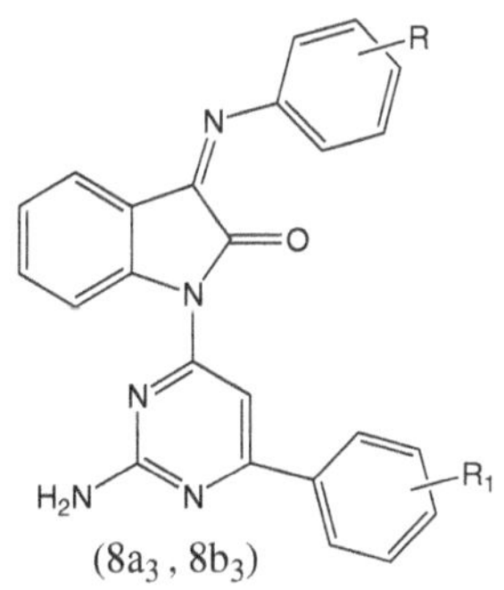

($8a_3$, $8b_3$)

Figure 6 Substituted (Z)-3-(phenylimino)-1-(6-phenylpyrimidin-4-yl)indolin-2-one.

a

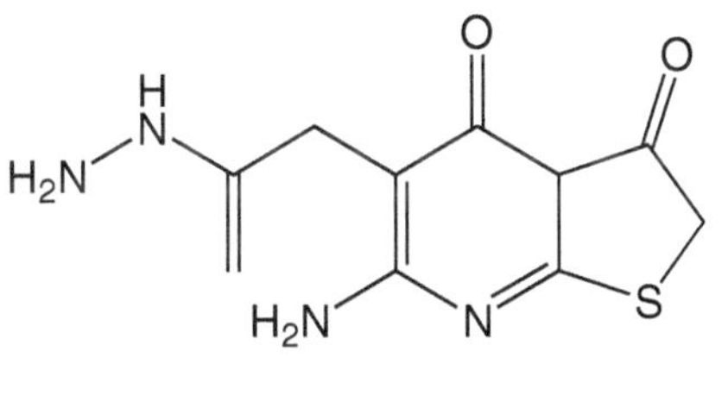

b

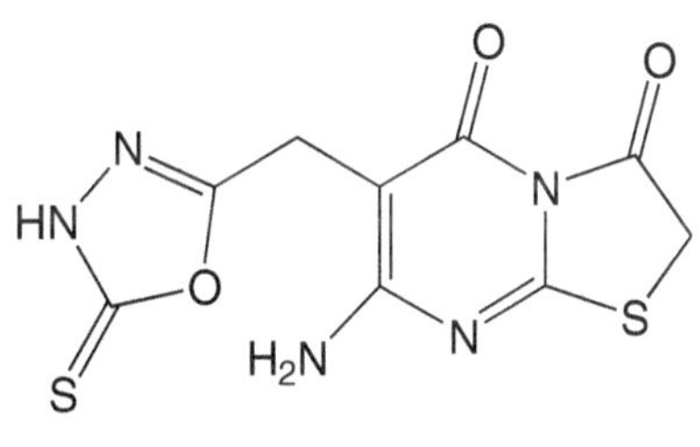

Figure 7 Thiazole and oxadiazole containing pyrimidine derivatives.

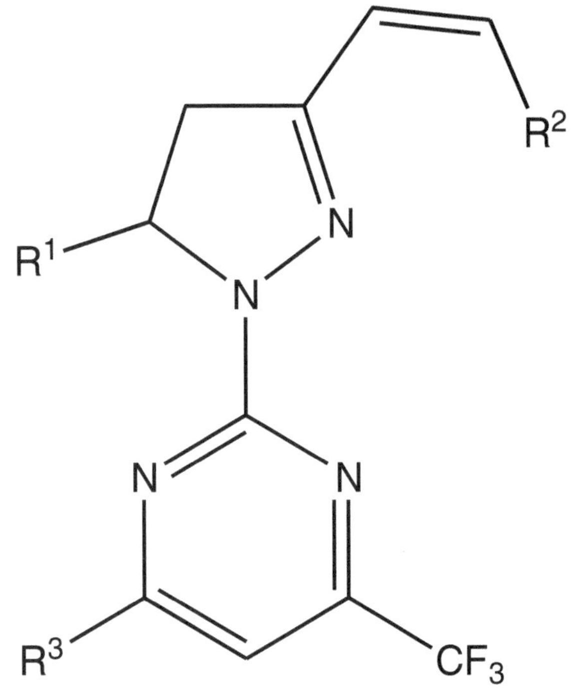

Figure 8 2-(4,5-Dihydro-1 *H*-pyrazol-1-yl)-pyrimidine.

Leading compound as antioxidant templates

Kumar et al. synthesized a novel series of 4,6-bisaryl-pyrimidin-2-amine derivative. All the synthesized compounds were evaluated for their antioxidant activity by nitric oxide and hydrogen peroxide free radical scavenging method using ascorbic acid as a standard drug. Among these synthesized derivatives, compound 5d by nitric oxide free radical scavenging method and compound 5e (Figure 5) by hydrogen peroxide free radical scavenging method show potent antioxidant activity as compare with the standard drug due to the presence of -Cl and -Br as the electron withdrawing group at positions $R_1$and R_2. IC_{50} values of the compounds are 0.019 and 0.020 mol/lit, respectively [11].

Mondal et al. synthesized a series of 1-(2-mercapto-6-

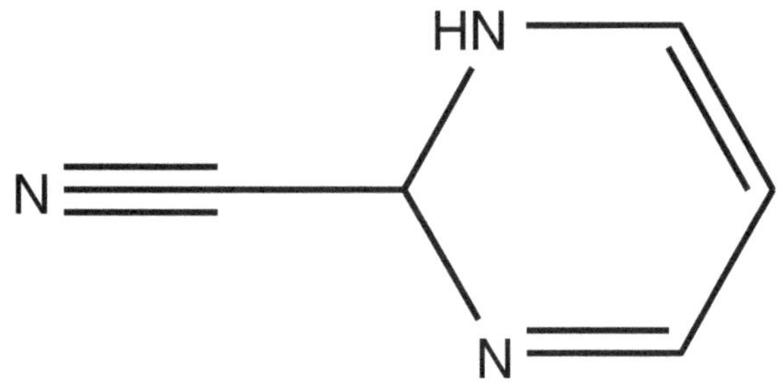

Figure 10 Structure of dihydropyrimidine carbonitrile.

indoline-2-one and 1-(2-amino-6-(substituted phenyl)pyrimidine-4-yl)-3-(2-subsitutedphenylimino) indolin-2-one from different substituted chalconised indole-2,3-dione. Compounds $7a_2$, $7a_3$, $7b_2$, $7b_3$, $8a_3$, and $8b_3$ show more promising antioxidant activity due to the substitution of the SH and NH_2 groups at the second position of the pyrimidine ring. (Figure 6) [12].

Abu-Hashem et al. synthesized a series of pyrimidine derivatives 6-amino-2-thiouracil with ethyl bromoacetate yielded ethyl 2-(7-amino-2,5-dioxo-3,5-dihydro-2 *H*-thiazolo[3,2-*a*]pyrimidin-6-yl)acetate and 7-amino-6-[(5-thioxo-4,5-dihydro-1,3,4-oxadiazol-2-yl)-methyl]-5 *H*-thiazolo[3,2-*a*]pyrimidine-3,5(2 *H*)-dione. The newly prepared compounds were subjected for their antioxidant activity; out of the synthesized compounds, compounds 7a and 7b (Figure 7) manifested potent antioxidative activity by lipid peroxidation assay. Novel thiazolopyrimidine derivatives incorporated with carbohydrazide, amino, oxadiazol, and other moieties which possess potential antioxidant activities [13].

Gressler et al. synthesized a series of 4-trifluoromethyl-2-(5-aryl-3-styryl-1 *H*-pyrazol-1yl)-pyrimidine derivatives and were screened for their *in vitro* antioxidant activity. The antioxidant activity was evaluated using the DPPH and HRP/luminol/H_2O_2chemiluminescence assay method. The DPPH antioxidant assay measures the hydrogen-donating capacity of the molecules

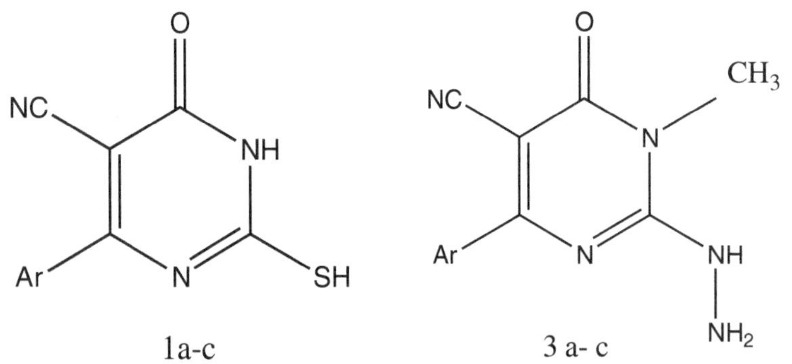

Figure 9 Structures of novel dihydropyrimidine carbonitrile and hydrazine derivative.

in the sample. On the other hand, the chemiluminescence method is based on the light emission produced by a chemical reaction. For the series 8a to 8e (Figure 8), resonance stabilization is not possible because the molecules do not have chain flexibility. Compound 8c shows potent antioxidant activity because of the presence of the SH group at R^3 position [14].

Bhalgat et al. synthesized a series of novel dihydropyrimidine carbonitrile (compounds 1a to 1c), its dimethylated adduct (compounds 2a to 2c), and hydrazine derivative (compounds 3a to 3c); from compounds 2a to 2c, they also prepared its triazole fused derivatives (compounds 4a to 4c, 5a to 5c, and 6a to 6c). The tested compounds1a to 1c and 3a to 3c revealed potent antioxidant activity and showed the most promising results. This may be due to the presence of -NH and -SH groups in compounds1a to 1c and the presence of $-NH-NH_2$ group in compounds 3a to 3c. The investigation of antioxidant screening revealed that some of the tested compounds particularly 1a, 1c, 3b, and 3c have shown more promising antioxidant activity as compare with the standard drug ascorbic acid, while other derivatives showed moderate activity (Figures 9 and 10) [15].

Conclusions

The present review is concentrating on the synthesis and antioxidant activity of the pyrimidine nucleus. Pyrimidine is a unique molecule that is associated with several other biological activities. Among the antioxidants, it has the ability to trap the free radicals which are responsible for the generation of different diseases such as inflammation, skin lesions, immune depression, liver disease, pancreatitis, AIDS, infertility. Mainly antioxidants having pyrimidine nucleus are not able to enter in the lipid moiety of low density lipoprotein, so the penetration power of these types of compounds is very low, and they are least effective. To rectify this problem, the substitution on pyrimidine nucleus was made by different substitutions of Cl, Br, CF_3, and NO_2, which increased the penetration of molecules into the lipid membrane so that they increase the antioxidant activity by combining with the reactive oxygen species, which is generated by the different disease conditions. By making these changes on the pyrimidine nucleus, we are able to find out the most potent pyrimidine-substituted antioxidant compounds.

Competing interests

The authors declare that they have no competing interests.

Acknowledgments

The authors are highly thankful to NISCARE and NML, India for providing the necessary library and internet facilities to complete this article.

Author details

[1]Department of Pharmaceutical Technology, Meerut Institute of Engineering and Technology, Baghpat Bypass Crossing, NH-58, Delhi-Roorkee Highway, Meerut, Uttar Pradesh 250005, India. [2]Department of Pharmacy, Galgotias University, Yamuna Expressway, Greater Noida, Uttar Pradesh 201306, India.

References

1. Kumar SM, Pavani M, Bhalgat CM, Deepthi R, Mounika A, Mudshinge SR, Reas IJ, Ghomi JS, Ghasemzadeh MA (2011) Novel pyrimidine and its triazole fused derivatives: synthesis and investigation of antioxidant and anti-inflammatory activity. J Serb Chem Soc 76:679–684
2. Gayathri G, Nair BR, Babu V (2011) Analysis of proximate and nutritional composition in the leaves of *Azima tetracantha* Lam. Pharma Bio Sci 2:1568–1570
3. March J (1985) Advanced organic chemistry reactions mechanism and structure, 3rd edn. Wiley, New York, pp 165–179
4. Morrison RT, Boyd RN, Boyd RK (1992) Organic Chemistry, 6th edn. Prentice Hall, Upper Saddle River, pp 218–232
5. Acworth IN, Bailey B (1997) Reactive oxygen species. In: (ed) The handbook of oxidative metabolism. ESA Inc, Chelmsford, pp 89–95
6. Alessio HM, Blasi ER (1997) Physical activity as a natural antioxidant booster and its effect on a healthy lifestyle. Res Q Exerc Sport 68(4):292–302
7. Saikat S, Chakraborty R, Sridhar C, Reddy YS, Biplab D (2010) Free radicals, antioxidants, diseases and phytomedicines: current status and future prospect. Int J Ph Sci R 3(1):91–100
8. Butkovica VL, Bors KWJ (2004) Kinetic study of flavonoid reactions with stable radicals. Agric Food Chem 52:2816–2820
9. Singh RP, Sharad S, Kapur S (2004) Free radicals and oxidative stress in neurodegenerative diseases, relevance of dietary antioxidants. JIACM 5 (3):218–225
10. Lonita P (2005) Plasma polymerisation: study and application. Chem Pap 59:11–16
11. Kumar SM, Pavani M, Bhalgat CM, Deepthi R, Mounika A, Mudshinge SR (2009) In-vitro antioxidant studies of 4,6-bis aryl-pyrimidin- 2-amine derivatives. Inter JR Ph Bio Sci 2:1568–1570
12. Mondal P, Jana S, Kanthal LK (2010) Synthesis of novel mercapto-pyrimidine and amino-pyrimidine derivatives of indoline-2-one as potential antioxidant & antibacterial agent. T Ph Res 3:17–26
13. Abu-Hashem AA, Youssef MM, Hoda AR (2011) Synthesis, antioxidant, antituomer activities of some new thiazolopyrimidines, pyrrolothiazolopyrimidines and triazolopyrrolothiazolopyrimidines derivatives. J Chi Chem Soc 58:41–48
14. Gressler V, Moura S, Flores AFC, Flores DC, Colepicolo P, Pinto E (2010) Antioxidant and antimicrobial properties of 2-(4,5-dihydro-1H-pyrazol-1-yl)-pyrimidine and 1-carboxamidino-1H-pyrazole derivatives. J Braz Chem Soc 21:1–7
15. Bhalgat CM, Ali MI, Arsab GR (2011) In-vitro antioxidant studies of 4,6-bis aryl-pyrimidin- 2-amine derivatives. J Chem (in press)

Synthesis of phenylazonaphtol-β-D-O-glycosides, evaluation as substrates for beta-glycosidase activity and molecular studies

Marco Brito-Arias[1*], Carlos Aguilar-Lemus[1], Pamela B Hurtado-Ponce[1], Guadalupe Martínez-Barrón[2] and Miguel Ibañez-Hernandez[2]

Abstract

Background: Phenylazonaphtol-β-D-*O*-glycosides are alternative substrates for the detection of enzymatic activity of β-glycosidases which are involved in various important processes. These azoic compounds are currently exploited as prodrugs for colonic disease due the presence of β-glycosidase activity in the gut flora and therefore allowing the release of the drug at the specific site.

Results: Phenylazonaphtol-β-D-*O*-glucoside **3a** and galactoside **3b** were prepared via diazonium salt conditions under weak acidic conditions which do not compromise the *O*-glycosidic bond stability, by coupling reaction between 2-naphtol sodium salt with aminoglycosides **1a** and **1b**. The resulting phenylazonaphtol glycosides **2a** and **2b** were deprotected affording the phenylazonaphtol glycosides **3a** and **3b** in quantitative yield. The galactoside glycoside **3b** was assayed as substrate for *in vitro* β-galactosidase enzymatic activity showing strong absorbance after releasing of the azoic chromophore. Also, docking studies were performed to determine the best pose as well as the interactions between the ligand and the residues located at the active site.

Conclusions: The methodology developed for synthesizing the phenylazonaphtol glycosides described proved to be convenient for generating azoic functionalities in the presence of glycosidic bonds and the glycosides suitable as alternative substrates and potentially useful prodrugs in the treatment of colonic diseases.

Keywords: β-galactosidase; Synthesis; Phenylazonaphtol glycoside; Substrate; Docking

Background

β-glycosidases are hydrolytic enzymes involved in a number of important processes such as defense mechanism, growth regulation [1], gene markers in transgenic plants [2], and prodrugs [3]. The most commonly used substrates for the histochemical localization of β-glycosidases contain the 5-bromo-4-chloro-3-indolyl chromophore attached to most of the known monosaccharides through an *O*-glycosidic bond [4]. After enzymatic hydrolysis, the water soluble indoxyl intermediate must undergo an oxidative dimerization to produce a blue precipitate. However, in some cases before dimerization occurs to produce the indigo dye, some diffusion takes place, producing false positives at some regions in cells lacking enzymatic activity [5]. In addition, phenylazonaphtol glucosides have been synthetically prepared and tested in transgenic plants containing the β-glucuronidase activity which is a widely used gene marker. A comparative test between the commercially available glycosidic indoxyl substrates with the alternative phenylazonaphtol glucuronides resulted in partial diffusion for the indigo dye and no detectable diffusion for the phenylazonaphtol chromophore [6,7].

On the other hand, glycosides when attached to pharmacologically active substances can be used as prodrugs for improving availability, stability, and particularly for specific delivery of the active compound at the target organ. For instance, steroids, antitumor, and anti-inflammatory compounds have been attached to glycosides and evaluated as specific delivery prodrugs [8]. Also, azoic β-glycosides provided to be useful as prodrugs particularly against colitis,

* Correspondence: mbrito@ipn.mx
[1]Unidad Profesional Interdisciplinaria de Biotecnología del Instituto Politécnico Nacional, Avenida Acueducto s/n La Laguna Ticomán DF cp 07340, Mexico
Full list of author information is available at the end of the article

Crohn's disease, and colorectal cancer since the delivery at colon level might be achieved by the action of azoreductase or glycosidase present at the colonic microflora [9].

Due the potential usefulness of phenylazonaphtol glycosides in processes mentioned above, we developed a methodology for preparing phenylazonaphtol glycosides under weak acidic conditions and the resulting azoic glycosides evaluated as β-galactosidase substrates with potential application as prodrugs for colon diseases.

Methods

The preparation of the phenylazonaphtol glycosides **3a** and **3b** was achieved according to Scheme 1 consisting in the coupling reaction between 2-naphtol in the sodium salt form with 4-aminophenyl tetracetyl glycopyranoside [10-12] **1a** and **1b** under modified diazonium salt condition, which is mainly the use of acetic acid instead of stronger acids, with sodium nitrite at 0°C to produce the diazonium salts which was condensed *in situ* with 2-naphtol sodium salt providing the corresponding phenylazonaphtol tetracetyl glucopyranoside **2a** and **2b**. Final removal of the acetate protecting groups under Zemplen conditions provided the target phenylazonaphtol glycosides **3a** and **3b** as a reddish solid in 60% yield.

Scheme

The beta galactosidase assay. β-galactosidase (2 mg; 2.1 U/mg) was suspended in 0.8 mL of buffer containing 0.06 M Na_2HPO_4, 0.04 M NaH_2PO_4, 0.01 M KCl, 0.001 M $MgSO_4$, and 1 mM DTT, pH 7.0, and then incubated with glycoside **3b** (4 mg; 9.3×10^{-3} mM) in a mixture of 50 mM acetate buffer with pH 5.0 (0.5 mL) and methanol (0.5 mL) at 37°C for 3 h. The reaction was stopped by adding 0.5 mL 1 M Na_2CO_3. The amount of the released phenylazonaphtol chromophore was measured spectrophotometrically at 410 and 455 nm [13].

Results and discussion

The deprotected glycoside **3b** was tested as substrate for the detection of glycosidase activity using commercial *Escherichia coli* β-galactosidase. Thus, the hydrolytic activity resulted in the cleavage of the glycosidic linkage, releasing the phenylazonaphtol chromophore which is observed as an intense reddish color with absorption at 410 and 455 nm, as it is observed in the absorption graphic (Figure 1) and as observed in the vials (Figure 2).

Docking studies

The active site architecture showing the interactions between the phenylazonaphtol galactoside **3b** and *E. coli* β-galactosidase pocket was performed using AutoDock 4.2 [14] and Chimera [15] software packages as visualization system. The protein assigned for the docking analysis was *E. coli* β-galactosidase (PDB IDs: 1JYN), and the residues chosen were Asn102, Asp201, Asn460, His418, Glu461, Glu537, His540, Phe 601, and Trp999 which have been described to participate in the interactions with its natural substrate lactose [16]. β-galactosidase is a retaining glycosidase with a double displacement mechanism, and

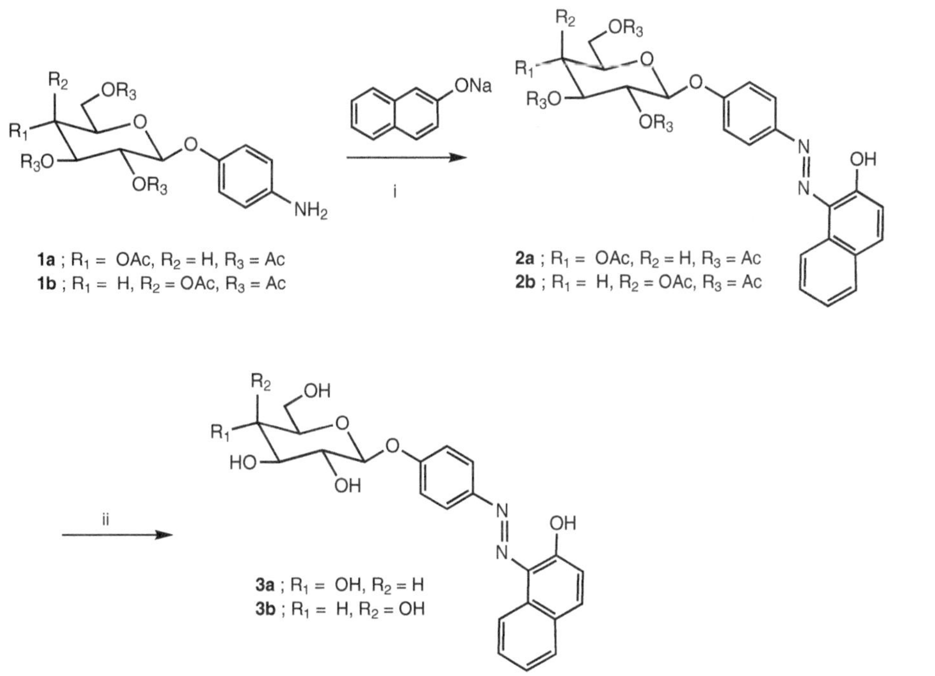

Scheme 1 The preparation of the phenylazonaphtol glycosides 3a and 3b.

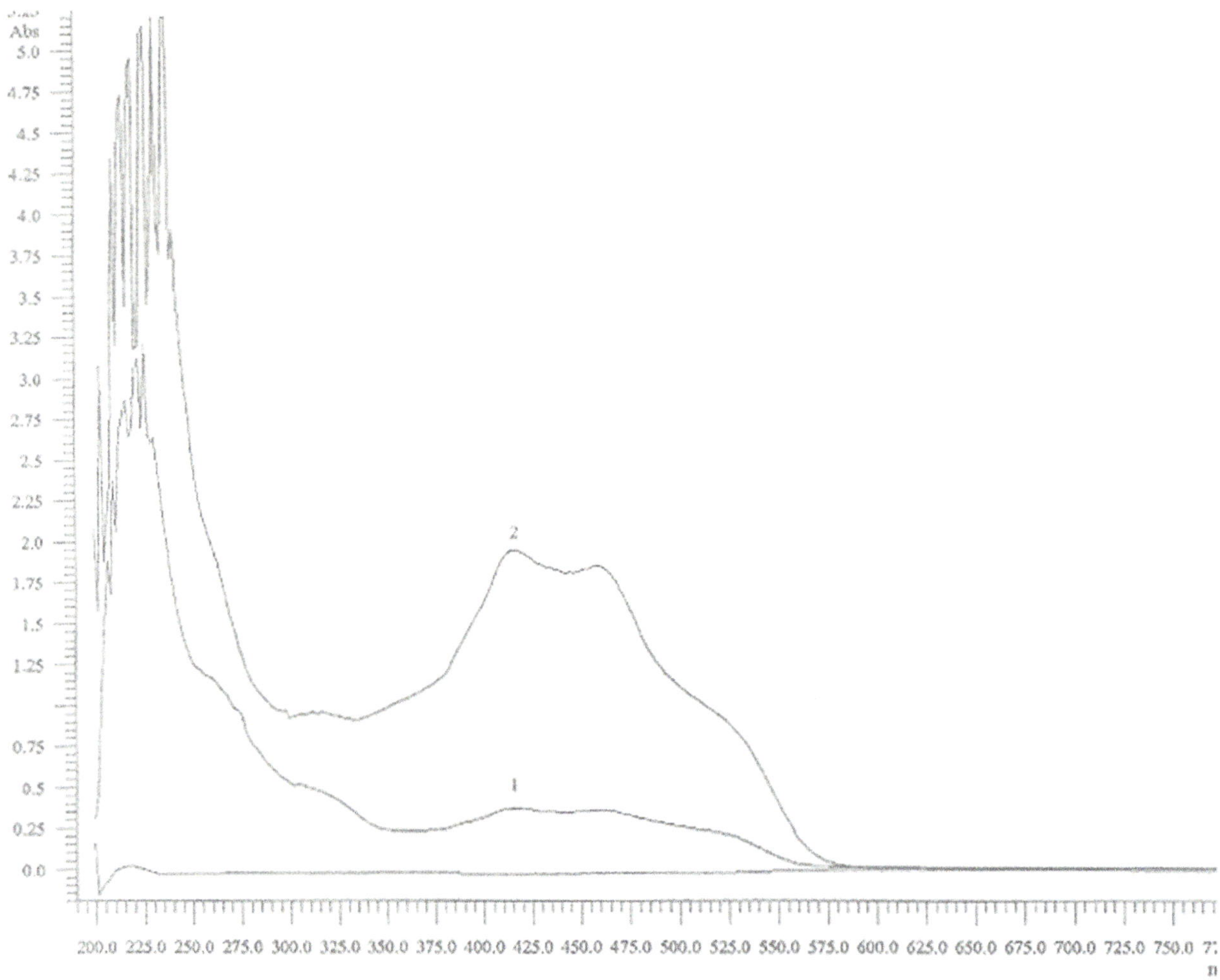

Figure 1 Adsorption of 3b without β-galactosidase (1) and with β-galactosidase (2).

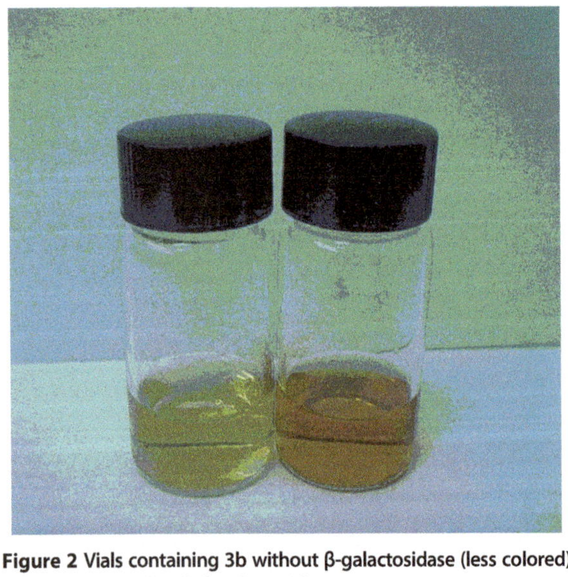

Figure 2 Vials containing 3b without β-galactosidase (less colored) and 3b incubated with β-galactosidase.

its interactions with the ligand proceed with participation of water and the ions Mg^{2+} and Na^{1+} within the catalytic cavity [17]. The docking analysis was performed to find the minimized conformations according to the docking protocols which use the Lamarckian Genetic Algorithm for searching the most favorable ligand-protein complex interactions. Thus, as a result of the docking analysis, we found the minimized conformer with the galactose moiety positioned toward the active site having a binding energy of −11.62, showing hydrogen bond interactions of C-3 and C-4 hydroxyl groups of galactoside moiety with Glu461 residue, in agreement with those reported for the natural substrate lactose [16] (Figure 3).

The ribbon representation was also analyzed by using the chimera visualizing system to show the region of the cavity and the residues involved in the interaction with the substrate **3b** (Figure 4).

In addition, the surface representation shows that the galactopyranoside moiety is embedded into the pocket interacting with the residues while the azoic chromophore

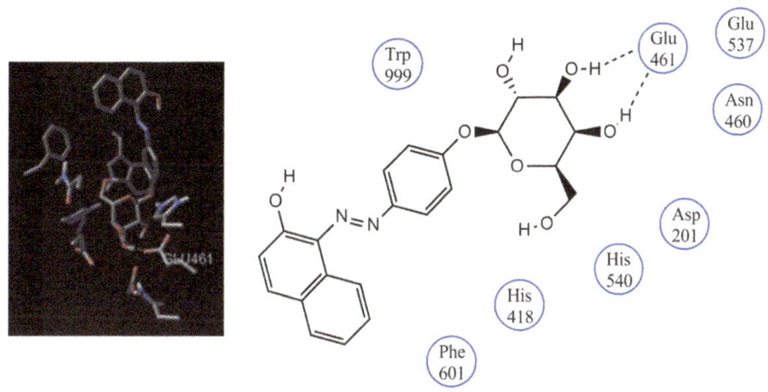

Figure 3 The first scored conformation assumed by 3b presenting hydrogen bond interactions with Glu461 residue.

is pointed out toward the pocket exit as shown in Figure 5.

Experimental

All the reagents were purchased from Aldrich Chemical Co. (St. Louis, MO, USA) except HBr/acetic acid which was purchased from Fluka Chemical Co. (Buchs, Switzerland). Column chromatography was performed on silica gel with a 70-230 mesh, and thin-layer chromatography on Kieselgel, both from Merck Co. (Darmstadt, Germany), which was used as a detection system. A cerium sulfate solution followed by heating on hot plate. Infrared (IR) spectra were obtained on Perkin-Elmer spectrometer (Waltham, MA, USA); nuclear magnetic resonance (NMR) spectra were recorded on Varian 300-MHz spectrometer (Palo Alto, CA, USA) and Bruker 500 MHz (Karlsruhe, Germany). Mass spectrum (MS) spectra were obtained using a Hewlett-Packard 5989A (Palo Alto, CA, USA). Optical rotations were measured with a Perkin-Elmer 341 polarimeter at 23°C. Enzyme galactosidase was purchased from Sigma Chemical Company (St. Louis, MO, USA).

1-[(4-tetra-*O*-acetyl-β-D-glucopyranosyloxy phenyl)azo]-2-naphtol (2a)

Compound **1a** (0.543 g, 1.23 mmol) was dissolved in 8 mL of THF, and the flask was cooled to 0°C. After the addition of sodium nitrite (85 mg, 1.23 mmol) and 0.5 mL of acetic acid/H_2O (1:1, *v*/*v*), the reaction was kept under ice-bath temperature with stirring for 15 min. 2-naphtol sodium salt dissolved in 5 mL of THF/H_2O (1:1, *v*/*v*) was added dropwise in another flask, and the reaction was kept at 0°C with stirring for 30 min, allowing the reaction to reach room temperature and stirred for another 60 min. The solvent was removed under *vacuo*, diluted with CH_2Cl_2 (30 mL) and washed with cold 2 N NaOH solution (3 × 15 mL) and water (20 mL). The organic phase was dried over anhydrous sodium sulfate and evaporated on

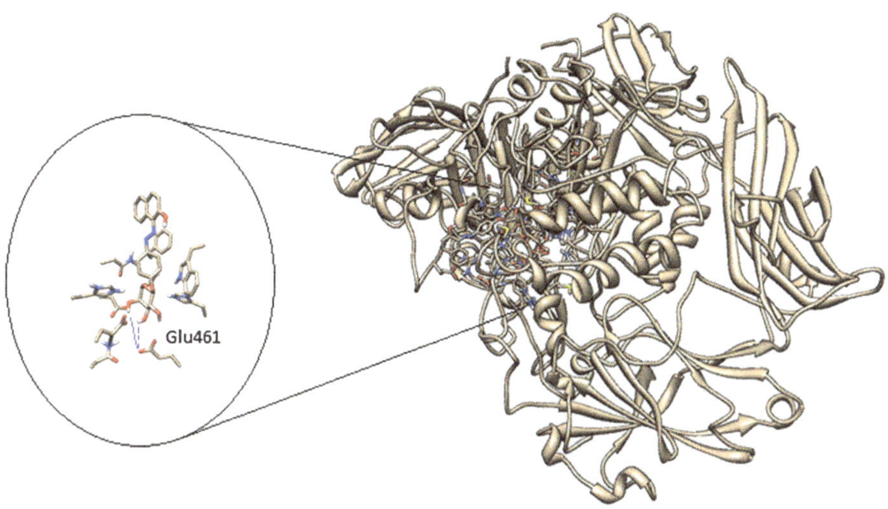

Figure 4 Ribbon representation. This shows the region of the active site among the protein and residues involved in the interaction with the ligand.

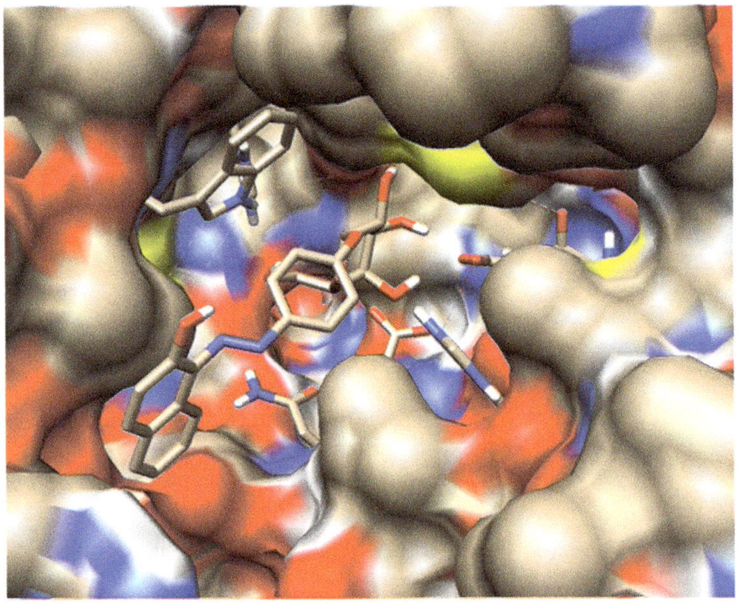

Figure 5 Surface representation showing the pose of ligand 3b at the active.

rotavapor. The crude was purified by column chromatography with AcOEt/hexane (1:3) to give an orange-red solid (325 mg, 60%). m.p. 81°C to 83°C, [α]D −13.1 (c 0.6, $CHCl_3$), IR (thin film) 1,738 cm^{-1}, ^1H NMR ($CDCl_3$) δ 2.05 to 2.14 (4 s, 12 H), 3.92 (m, H-5), 4.20 (dd, H-6, *J* = 12.3 Hz, 2.1 Hz), 4.33 (dd, H-6′, *J* = 12.3 Hz, 5.1 Hz), 5.17 (d, H-1, *J* = 7.5 Hz), 5.20 (t, H-4, *J* = 9.6 Hz), 5.31 (t, H-2, *J* = 9.6 Hz), 5.34 (t, H-3, *J* = 9.6 Hz), 6.97 (d, H-13, *J* = 9.3), 7.15 (d, H-8, 8′, *J* = 5.1 Hz), 7.41 (t, H-16, *J* = 7.5 Hz, 7.2 Hz), 7.58 (t, H-17, *J* = 7.5 Hz, 7.2 Hz), 7.66 (d, H-15, *J* = 8.1 Hz), 7.75 (d, H-14, *J* = 9.6 Hz), 7.76 (d, H-9,9′, *J* = 9.0 Hz), 8.62 (d, H-18, *J* = 7.8 Hz). ^{13}C NMR ($CDCl_3$) δ 20.5, 20.6 (4 CH_3-), 61.8 (C-6), 68.1 (C-4), 71.1 (C-3), 72.1 (C-2), 72.6 (C-5), 98.9 (C-1), 117.8 (C-8), 121.0 (C-9), 121.5 (C-18), 123.0 (C-13), 125.2 (C-16), 127.7 (C-14a), 128.1 (C-11), 128.4 (C-17), 129.7 (C-15), 133.3 (C-18a), 138.2 (C-10), 142.6 (C-14), 156.8 (C-7), 165.1 (C-12), 169.2, 169.3, 170.1, 170.4 (4 C = O). HRMS calculated for $C_{30}H_{30}N_2O_{11}$ (M+) 594.1850, found 594.1845 (Figure 6).

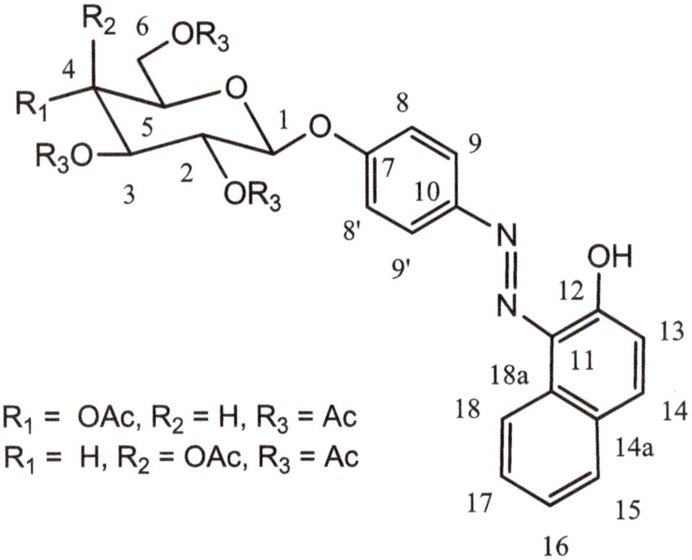

2a ; R_1 = OAc, R_2 = H, R_3 = Ac
2b ; R_1 = H, R_2 = OAc, R_3 = Ac

Figure 6 Structure of 1-[(4-tetra-*O*-acetyl-β-D-glucopyranosyloxy phenyl)azo]-2-naphtol (2a).

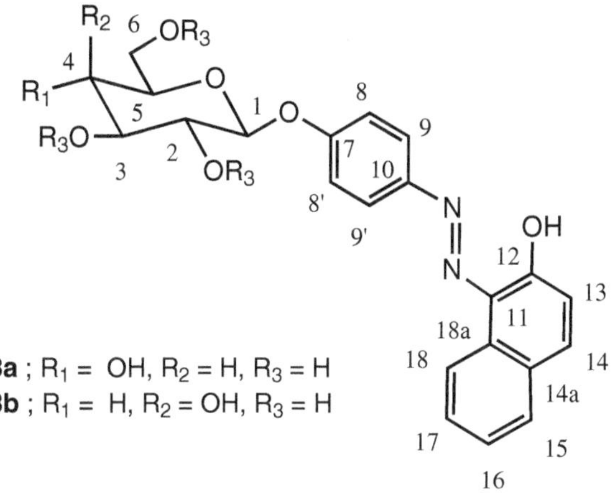

3a ; R_1 = OH, R_2 = H, R_3 = H
3b ; R_1 = H, R_2 = OH, R_3 = H

Figure 7 Structure of 1-[(4-β-D-glucopyranosyloxy phenyl)azo]-2-naphtol (3a).

1-[(4-tetra-*O*-acetyl-β-D-galactopyranosyloxy phenyl azo]-2-naphtol (2b)

Same reaction conditions as for **2a** except that compound **1b** is used instead of **1a**.

^{1}H NMR ($CDCl_3$) δ 2.09 to 2.12 (4 s, 12 H), 4.12 (1H, m, H-5), 4.22 (1H, dd, H-6), 4.26 (1-H, dd, H6′), 5.11 (1H, d, H-1), 5.13 (1H, dd, H-4), 5.48 (1H, t, H-2), 5.54 (1H, dd, H-3), 6.97 (d, H-13, *J* = 9.3), 7.15 (d, H-8, 8′, *J* = 5.1 Hz), 7.41 (t, H-16, *J* = 7.5 Hz, 7.2 Hz), 7.58 (t, H-17, *J* = 7.5 Hz, 7.2 Hz), 7.66 (d, H-15, *J* = 8.1 Hz), 7.75 (d, H-14, *J* = 9.6 Hz), 7.76 (d, H-9,9′, *J* = 9.0 Hz), 8.62 (d, H-18, *J* = 7.8 Hz). ^{13}C NMR ($CDCl_3$) δ 20.8, 20.9 (4 CH_3-), 61.5 (C-6), 67.0 (C-4), 68.7 (C-2), 71.2 (C-3), 71.4 (C-5), 99.7 (C-1), 117.8 (C-8), 121.0 (C-9), 121.5 (C-18), 123.0 (C-13), 125.2 (C-16), 127.7 (C-14a), 128.1 (C-11), 128.4 (C-17), 129.7 (C-15), 133.3 (C-18a), 138.2 (C-10), 142.6 (C-14), 156.8 (C-7), 165.1 (C-12), 169.2, 169.3, 170.1, 170.4 (4 C = O). MS (EI) m/z 594.18 [M^+], 169 (100), 264 (62).

1-[(4-β-D-glucopyranosyloxy phenyl)azo]-2-naphtol (3a)

To protected phenylazonaphtol glycoside **2a** (0.3 g, 0.504 mmol), 5 mL of 10% NaOMe in MeOH was added and stirred in a room temperature for 2 h. Ion exchange resin Dowex 50WX2-100 was added to neutralize and the resin filtered. The solvent was removed under *vacuo* to give 0.193 g, 90% as a red solid (Figure 7).

m.p. 177°C to 178°C, [α]D −23.4 (c 0.9, MeOH), ^{1}H NMR (DMSO d-6) δ 3.13 (H-2), 3.30 (H-4), 3.35 (H-5), 3.37 (H-3), 3.60 (H-6), 3.75 (H-6′), 4.99 (H-1, *J* = 7.8), 6.97 (d, H-13, *J* = 9.3), 7.15 (d, H-8, 8′, *J* = 5.1 Hz), 7.41 (t, H-16, *J* = 7.5 Hz, 7.2 Hz), 7.58 (t, H-17, *J* = 7.5 Hz, 7.2 Hz), 7.66 (d, H-15, *J* = 8.1 Hz), 7.75 (d, H-14, *J* = 9.6 Hz), 7.76 (d, H-9,9′, *J* = 9.0 Hz), 8.62 (d, H-18, *J* = 7.8 Hz). ^{13}C NMR (DMSO d-6) δ 61.7 (C-6), 76.8 (C-5), 71.6 (C-4), 74.1 (C-2), 76.7 (C-3), 96.7 (C-1), 117.8 (C-8), 121.0 (C-9), 121.5 (C-18), 123.0 (C-13), 125.2 (C-16), 127.7 (C-14a), 128.1 (C-11), 128.4 (C-17), 129.7 (C-15), 133.3 (C-18a), 138.2 (C-10), 142.6 (C-14), 156.8 (C-7), 165.1 (C-12), 169.2, 169.3, 170.1, 170.4 (4 C = O). HRMS calculated for $C_{22}H_{22}N_2O_7$ (M + H) 427.1505, found 427.1509.

1-[(4-β-D-galactopyranosyloxy phenyl)azo]-2-naphtol (3b)

Same reaction conditions as for **3a** except that compound **2b** is used instead of **2a**. ^{1}H NMR (DMSO d-6) δ 3.41 (t, H-2), 3.56 (dd, H-3), 3.61 (m, H-5), 3.62 (H-6), 3.70 (H-6′), 3.84 (dd, H-4), 4.98 (d, H-1, *J* = 8.0), 6.97 (d, H-13, *J* = 9.3), 7.15 (d, H-8, 8′, *J* = 5.1 Hz), 7.41 (t, H-16, *J* = 7.5 Hz, 7.2 Hz), 7.58 (t, H-17, *J* = 7.5 Hz, 7.2 Hz), 7.66 (d, H-15, *J* = 8.1 Hz), 7.75 (d, H-14, *J* = 9.6 Hz), 7.76 (d, H-9,9′, *J* = 9.0 Hz), 8.62 (d, H-18, *J* = 7.8 Hz). ^{13}C NMR (DMSO d-6) δ 62.0 (C-6), 69.7 (C-4), 72.9 (C-2), 73.8 (C-3), 76.0 (C-5), 97.3 (C-1), 117.8 (C-8), 121.0 (C-9), 121.5 (C-18), 123.0 (C-13), 125.2 (C-16), 127.7 (C-14a), 128.1 (C-11), 128.4 (C-17), 129.7 (C-15), 133.3 (C-18a), 138.2 (C-10), 142.6 (C-14), 156.8 (C-7), 165.1 (C-12), 169.2, 169.3, 170.1, 170.4 (4 C = O). FABMS (M + 1) 427.1.

The Additional file 1 (as word document) shows the ^{1}H, ^{13}C NMR spectra for the synthesized compounds **2a-b** and **3a-b**, and high-resolution mass spectrometry and elemental analysis are also included.

Conclusions

The methodology developed for synthesizing the phenylazonaphtol glycosides described proved to be convenient for generating azoic functionalities in the presence of glycosidic bonds, and the glycosides are suitable as alternative substrates and potentially useful prodrugs in the treatment of colonic diseases.

Additional file

Additional file 1: Bidimensional NMR spectroscopy for compound 2a. Homonuclear through-bond correlation bidimensional spectroscopy (COSY), heteronuclear single quantum coherence (HSQC), and heteronuclear multiple bond correlation (HMBC) experiments are included to provide further evidence for compound **2a.**

Competing interests

The authors declare that they have no competing interests.

Acknowledgements

We wish to thank COFAA-IPN for the scholarship and SIP-IPN for the financial support. We also want to thank Dr. Carlos Cerda Garcia-Rojas for MS and optical rotation, Mabel Fragoso for mass spectroscopy, and Gerardo Zepeda for NMR bidimensional determinations.

Author details

[1]Unidad Profesional Interdisciplinaria de Biotecnología del Instituto Politécnico Nacional, Avenida Acueducto s/n La Laguna Ticomán DF cp 07340, Mexico. [2]Escuela Nacional de Ciencias Biológicas del Instituto

Politécnico Nacional, Carpio y Plan de Ayala Colonia Santo Tomas DF cp11340, Mexico.

References

1. Esen A (1993) β-glucosidase: Biochemistry and Molecular Biology, ACS Symposium Series 533. Washington DC, pp 2–5
2. Jefferson RA, Kavanagh TA, Bevan MW (1987) GUS fusions: beta-glucuronidase as a sensitive and versatile gene fusion marker in higher plants. EMBO J 6:3901–3907
3. Tietze LF, von Hof JM, Krewer B, Müller M, Major F, Schuster HJ, Schuberth I, Alves F (2008) Asymmetric synthesis and biological evaluation of glycosidic prodrugs for a selective cancer therapy. Chem Med Chem 3(12):1946–1955
4. Manafi M, Kneifel W, Bascomb S (1991) Fluorogenic and chromogenic substrates used in bacterial diagnostics. Microbiol Rev 55:335–348
5. Lodja Z (1970) An improved histochemical method for the demonstration of disaccharidases with natural substrates. Histochemie 22:347–361
6. Terryn N, Brito-Arias M, Engler G, Tiré C, Villaroel R, Van Montagu M, Inzé D (1993) rha1, a gene encoding a small GTP binding protein from *Arabidopsis*, is expressed primarily in developing guard cells. Plant Cell 5:1761–1769
7. Van der Eycken E, Terryn N, Goemans JL, Carlens G, Nerinckx W, Claeyssens M, Van der Eycken J, Van Montagu M, Brito-Arias M, Engler G (2000) Sudan-b-D-glucuronides and their use for the histochemical localization of b-glucuronidase activity in transgenic plants. Plant Cell Rep 19:966–970
8. Friend DR, Chang GW (1985) Drug glycosides: potential prodrugs for colon-specific drug delivery. J Med Chem 28:51–57
9. Friend DR, Chang GW (1984) A colon-specific drug-delivery system based on drug glycosides and the glycosidases of colonic bacteria. J Med Chem 27:261–266
10. Ganjian I, Basile DV (1997) Reductive syntheses of *p*-aminophenyl-β-D-glucoside and its conversion to β-glucosyl Yariv reagent. Anal Biochem 246:152–155
11. Barni E, Barolo C, Quagliotto PL, Valldeperas J, Viscardi G (2000) Novel azobenzene derivatives containing a glucopyranoside moiety. Dyes Pigments 46:29–36
12. Amaike M, Kobayashi H, Sakurai K, Shinkai S (2002) Novel attempts to change the colour of dye molecules utilizing the aggregation mode of saccharides. Supramol Chem 14:245–253
13. Stiborová M, Asfaw B, Frei E, Schmeiser HH, Wiessler M (1994) Identification of 1-(3,4-dihydroxyphenylazo)-2-hydroxynaphthalene as the product of oxidation of 1-phenylazo-2-hydroxynaphthalene (Sudan I, solvent yellow 14) by rat liver microsomes. Collect Czech Chem Commun 59:2727–2733
14. Sanner MF, Huey R, Dallakyan S, Karnati S, Lindstrom W, Morris GM, Norledge B, Omelchenko A, Stoffler D, Vareille G (2007) AutoDockTools, version 1.4.5. The Scripps Research Institute, La Jolla
15. Pettersen EF, Goddard TD, Huang CC, Couch GS, Greenblatt DM, Meng EC, Ferrin TE (2004) UCSF chimera—a visualization system for exploratory research and analysis. J Comput Chem 25(13):1605–1612
16. Juers DH, Tom D, Heightman TD, Vasella A, McCarter JD, Mackenzie L, Withers SG, Matthews BW (2001) A structural view of the action of *Escherichia coli* (lacZ) α-galactosidase. Biochemistry 40:14781–14794
17. Jancewicz LJ, Wheatley RW, Sutendra G, Lee M, Fraser ME, Huber RE (2012) Ser-796 of b-galactosidase (*Escherichia coli*) plays a key role in maintaining a balance between the opened and closed conformations of the catalytically important active site loop. Arch Biochem Biophys 517:111–122

Radiofluorination and biological evaluation of *N*-aryl-oxadiazolyl-propionamides as potential radioligands for PET imaging of cannabinoid CB_2 receptors

Rodrigo Teodoro[1†], Rareş-Petru Moldovan[1†], Corinna Lueg[2†], Robert Günther[1], Cornelius K Donat[1], Friedrich-Alexander Ludwig[1], Steffen Fischer[1], Winnie Deuther-Conrad[1], Bernhard Wünsch[2] and Peter Brust[2*]

Abstract

Background: The level of expression of cannabinoid receptor type 2 (CB_2R) in healthy and diseased brain has not been fully elucidated. Therefore, there is a growing interest to assess the regional expression of CB_2R in the brain. Positron emission tomography (PET) is an imaging technique, which allows quantitative monitoring of very low amounts of radiolabelled compounds in living organisms at high temporal and spatial resolution and, thus, has been widely used as a diagnostic tool in nuclear medicine. Here, we report on the radiofluorination of *N*-aryl-oxadiazolyl-propionamides at two different positions in the lead structure and on the biological evaluation of the potential of the two tracers $[^{18}F]$**1** and $[^{18}F]$**2** as CB_2 receptor PET imaging agents.

Results: High binding affinity and specificity towards CB_2 receptors of the lead structure remained unaffected by the structural changes such as the insertion of the aliphatic and aromatic fluorine in the selected labelling sites of **1** and **2**. Aliphatic and aromatic radiofluorinations were optimized, and $[^{18}F]$**1** and $[^{18}F]$**2** were achieved in radiochemical yields of ≥30% with radiochemical purities of ≥98% and specific activities of 250 to 450 GBq/μmol. Organ distribution studies in female CD1 mice revealed that both radiotracers cross the blood–brain barrier (BBB) but undergo strong peripheral metabolism. At 30 min after injection, unmetabolized $[^{18}F]$**1** and $[^{18}F]$**2** accounted for 60% and 2% as well as 68% and 88% of the total activity in the plasma and brain, respectively. The main radiometabolite of $[^{18}F]$**2** could be identified as the free acid $[^{18}F]$**10**, which has no affinity towards the CB_1 and CB_2 receptors but can cross the BBB.

Conclusions: *N*-aryl-oxadiazolyl-propionamides can successfully be radiolabelled with ^{18}F at different positions. Fluorine substitution at these positions did not affect affinity and specificity towards CB_2R. Despite a promising *in vitro* behavior, a rather rapid peripheral metabolism of $[^{18}F]$**1** and $[^{18}F]$**2** in mice and the generation of brain permeable radiometabolites hamper the application of these radiotracers *in vivo*. However, it is expected that future synthetic modification aiming at a replacement of metabolically susceptible structural elements of $[^{18}F]$**1** and $[^{18}F]$**2** will help to elucidate the potential of this class of compounds for CB_2R PET studies.

Keywords: Blood–brain barrier; Cannabinoid receptors; ^{18}F labelling; Molecular imaging; Positron emission tomography

* Correspondence: p.brust@hzdr.de
†Equal contributors
[2]Department of Pharmaceutical and Medicinal Chemistry
University of Münster, Correnstraße 58-62, 48149 Münster, Germany
Full list of author information is available at the end of the article

Background

Cannabinoid receptors (CBR) belong to the superfamily of G protein-coupled receptors (GPCR) and are involved in various physiological processes. Besides the CBR identified so far, the cannabinoid receptor type 1 (CB$_1$R) [1] and type 2 (CB$_2$R) [2], another GPCR natively interacting with endogenous cannabinoids (GPR55) has been proposed as a third type of CBR [3,4]. While the CB$_1$R is primarily expressed in the central nervous system, the CB$_2$R is predominantly located in the periphery, especially in tissues related to the immune system. In pathological conditions, the up-regulation of CB$_2$R expression is mostly associated with inflammatory processes [5,6], neuropathic pain [7-9], Alzheimer's disease, and amyotrophic lateral sclerosis (ALS) [10-13]. It has also been shown that the activation of CB$_2$R is connected with the induction of apoptosis in several cancer cell lines [14-17]. However, CB$_2$R are also expressed in healthy brain under physiological conditions at very low expression levels [18,19]. Therefore, the non-invasive quantification of CB$_2$R in the brain, possibly in general by application of highly sensitive imaging techniques such as positron emission tomography (PET), requires the availability of radioligands binding with high affinity and high specificity towards CB$_2$R [20]. Apart from the numerous specific pharmacologically relevant ligands of CB$_2$R reported so far (see [21,22]), only a limited number have been applied for the development of PET radiotracers for imaging of CB$_2$R [23-29]. As we reported earlier, the increase of brain uptake and metabolic stability and decrease of non-specific binding remained as a challenge for further development [29]. Even a follow-up study on [^{11}C]AZD1940 in non-human primate with PET confirmed a relatively low CNS exposure of this radioligand [28]. Mu et al. reported on *N*-(1-adamantyl)-8-methoxy-4-oxo-1-phenyl-1, 4-dihydroquinoline-3-carboxamide as a ^{11}C-labelled PET probe for imaging of CB$_2$R [30]. Although the study showed a rather low brain uptake, and two blocking experiments with GW4058233 to demonstrate the specificity of brain uptake were not conclusive, the potential of the compound for PET imaging of amyotrophic lateral sclerosis has been proposed.

Further, a whole-body biodistribution and radiation dosimetry study of the CB$_2$R ligand [^{11}C]NE40 has been performed in healthy subjects [31]. It showed the expected biodistribution being compatible with lymphoid tissue (spleen) uptake and an appropriate uptake and kinetics in the brain. This underscores the potential of this tracer for application in central and peripheral inflammation imaging. Despite this considerable progress in CB$_2$R PET imaging, a suitable ligand [32] radiolabelled with the advantageous longer-lived isotope ^{18}F is still missing.

Recently, we reported on the synthesis, radiofluorination, and first biological investigation of the *N*-aryl-oxadiazolyl-propionamide [^{18}F]**2** as a potential radioligand for the PET imaging of CB$_2$R [29]. Although the initial radiofluorination approach using a nitro precursor proved to be unsatisfactory (yields ≤ 3%), the promising biological findings encouraged us to revise and upgrade the radiosynthesis of [^{18}F]**2** and to perform a more detailed biological evaluation.

Methods

We describe an improved synthesis of [^{18}F]**2** using a trimethylammonium precursor for the radiolabelling at the aromatic site of the lead structure (Figure 1, compound **13**, X^2 = NMe_3^+I). In parallel, we explored the aliphatic radiofluorination at the carbazole *N*-alkyl chain (Figure 1, compound **15**, X^1 = OTs). The labelling of the lead compound at two different sites opens up the possibility to investigate the dependence of affinity, biodistribution and metabolism of these radiotracers on the site of radiolabelling.

Results and discussion

Synthesis of *N*-arylamide oxadiazoles: precursors for radiochemistry and reference compounds

In a previous study, we have described the synthesis of >20 fluorinated *N*-arylamide oxadiazoles including labelling precursors for radiochemistry [29]. Here we describe a modified and improved route to obtain novel derivatives for high-yield radiochemistry. In brief, treatment of the nitriles **3** and **4** with excess of hydroxylamine hydrochloride under alkaline conditions delivered the (Z)-amidoximes **5** and **6** in 55% and 73% yield together with amides **7** and **8** (Scheme 1), which have been separated by column chromatography on silica. The Z configuration of

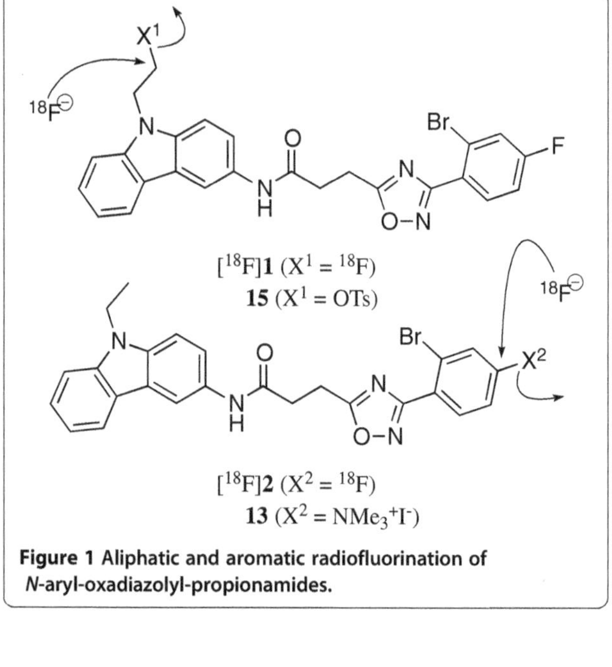

[^{18}F]**1** (X^1 = ^{18}F)
15 (X^1 = OTs)

[^{18}F]**2** (X^2 = ^{18}F)
13 (X^2 = $NMe_3^+I^-$)

Figure 1 Aliphatic and aromatic radiofluorination of *N*-aryl-oxadiazolyl-propionamides.

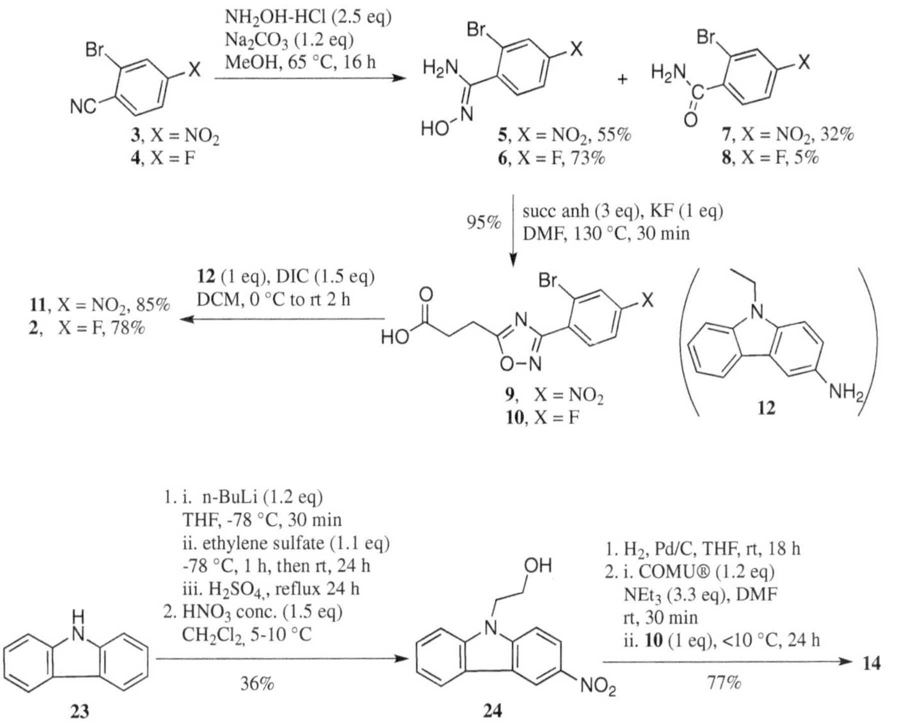

Scheme 1 Synthesis of the *N*-aryl-oxadiazolyl-propionamide derivatives 11, 2, and 14. NH_2OH-HCl, hydroxylamine hydrochloride; succ anh, succinic anhydride; DIC, *N,N'*-diisopropylcarbodiimide; COMU®, (1-Cyano-2-ethoxy-2-oxoethylidenaminooxy) dimethylamino-morpholino-carbenium hexafluorophosphate.

the amidoximes was determined by two-dimensional nuclear magnetic resonance (NMR) spectroscopy. Treatment of the amidoximes **5** and **6** with excess of succinic anhydride delivered the acids **9** and **10** in a nearly quantitative manner. The *N*-aryl-oxadiazolyl-propionamides **11** and **2** were obtained in high yields (85% and 78%) by using *N, N'*-diisopropylcarbodiimide (DIC) as coupling reagent [33].

For the aromatic radiofluorination, trimethylammonium iodide has been used as a leaving group. Although methyl iodide (MeI) has a very high nucleophilicity, the choice of I^- as a counter ion speeds up the displacement of the trimethylammonium salt in an aromatic ring during radiofluorination under mild conditions [34], thus lowering the amount of potential formation of non-radioactive and radioactive by-products. The trimethylammonium salt **13** was synthesized from the nitro derivative **11** by reduction, reductive methylation with paraformaldehyde and $NaBH_4$ [35], and quaternization by employing large excess of MeI (Scheme 2) [36].

The ethanol derivative **14** was synthesized in four steps and 28% overall yield starting from the commercially available carbazole (**23**). The synthesis started with deprotonation of carbazole with *n*-BuLi, reaction of the carbazolyl anion with ethylene sulfate, and subsequent hydrolysis with dilute H_2SO_4 to afford the hydroxyethyl derivative **25** (see 'Experimental' section). The crystalline cyclic ethylene sulfate represents a non-toxic but reactive alternative to the gaseous and toxic oxirane. However, there are only few examples for the introduction of a 2-hydroxyethyl group using ethylene sulfate. Nitration of the hydroxyethylcarbazole **25** was performed with concentrated nitric acid at 5°C to 10°C to give the 3-nitro carbazole derivative [37] **24** in 54% yield (Scheme 1). Reduction of the nitrocarbazole **24** with H_2 in the presence of Pd/C provided the primary aromatic amine **26**, which was precipitated as HCl salt. The final coupling of the carbazolamine **26** with the propionic acid **10** was induced by COMU® providing the amide **14** (Scheme 1).

The fluoroethyl reference compound **1** was prepared by treatment of **14** with the fluorinating agent diethylaminodifluorosulfonium tetrafluoroborate (XtalFluor-E®) (Scheme 2). In order to obtain the precursor for the radiosynthesis, the alcohol **14** was transformed into the tosylate **15** since the tosyloxy moiety represents a good leaving group for the nucleophilic substitution with [^{18}F]fluoride.

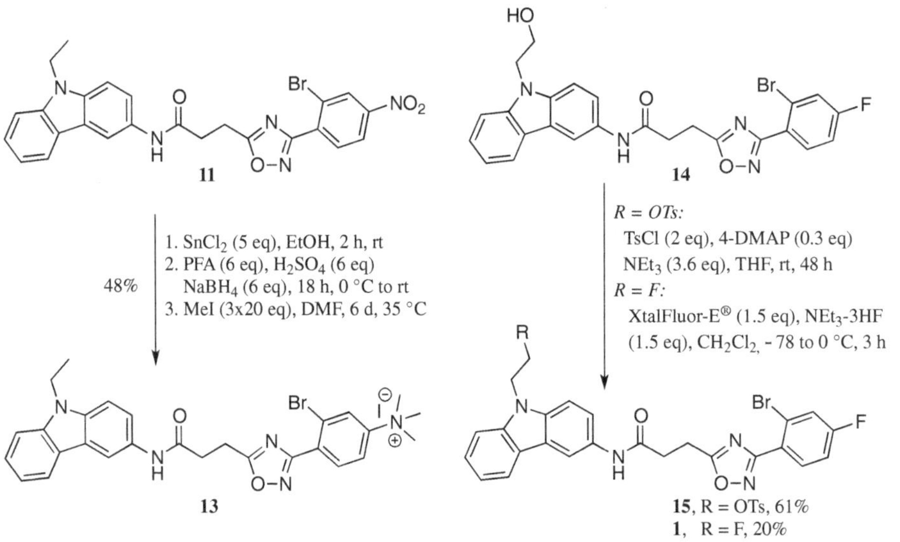

Scheme 2 Synthesis of precursors 13 and 15 and reference compound 1. $SnCl_2$, tin(II) chloride; PFA, paraformaldehyde; MeI, methyl iodide; 4-DMAP, 4-dimethylaminopyridine; XtalFluor-E®, diethylaminodifluorosulfonium tetrafluoroborate; NEt_3-3HF, triethylamine trihydrofluoride.

For investigations regarding the main metabolite [^{18}F]**10**, the trimethylammonium salt **18** and reference compound **17** were synthesized. Intermediate **16** was obtained by acid protection followed by reduction from **9**. To synthesize the reference compound **17**, Sandmeyer reaction has been applied [38]. The use of tetrafluoroborate as fluorinating reagent led to the formation of a complex reaction mixture whereas the use of KF delivered **17** in 40% yields. Alternatively, **17** could also be obtained from **10** (not shown in Scheme 3, see 'Experimental' section) in improved yield. The trimethylammonium salt **18** was obtained as described above in 48% over two steps.

Radiochemistry

Reaction conditions, purification, and formulation procedures were optimized to achieve a high radiochemical yield (RCY) and a high radiochemical purity in a short synthesis time. Aliphatic and aromatic radiolabellings were carried out at 82°C in MeCN under no-carrier-added (NCA) conditions (Scheme 4). High labelling yields (Figure 2) were obtained using 2 mg of precursor. For [^{18}F]**1**, the optimal conversion of the tosylate **15** was achieved after 10 min (53 ± 6%, n = 12). For [^{18}F]**2**, a maximum was reached after 10 min (63 ± 5%, n = 7), along with a steady loss of product (51 ± 6%, 15 min)

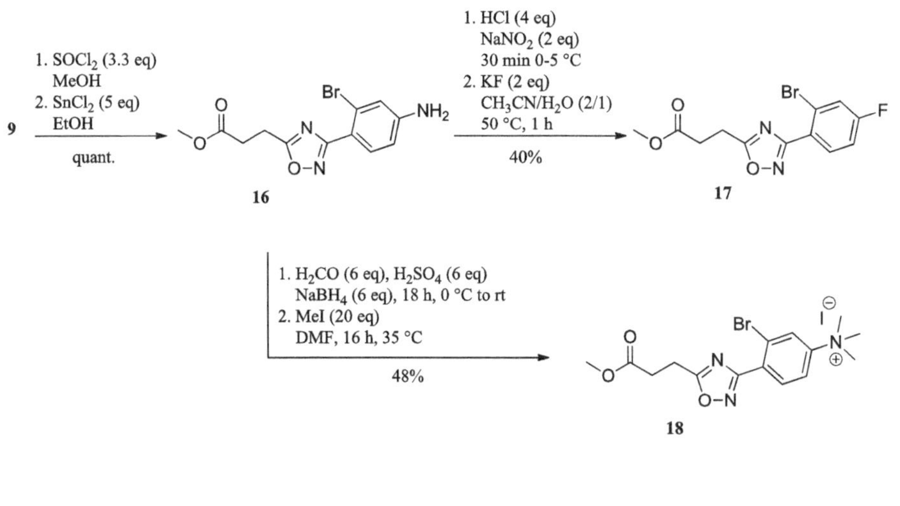

Scheme 3 Synthesis of the trimethylammonium salt 18 and reference compound 17.

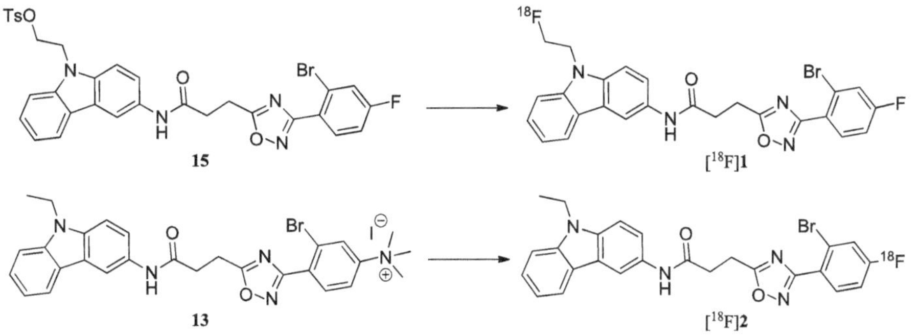

Scheme 4 Radiosynthesis of [^{18}F]1 and [^{18}F]2. K[^{18}F]F-$K_{2.2.2}$-carbonate complex (5.6 mg, 15 μmol), 2 mg (**15** or **13**), MeCN, 82°C, 10 min.

thereafter, probably due to the decomposition of the trimethylammonium salts under prolonged heating [39]. Altogether, evaluating the current results of labelling of [^{18}F]**2**, a great improvement was obtained by using the herein described new trimethylammonium precursor **13** instead of the formerly applied nitro compound **11** (see Scheme 4) where a radiochemical yield of only 3% has been achieved [29].

Reaction mixtures were separated by isocratic semipreparative HPLC, fractions were collected, and the identities confirmed by spiked analytical HPLC samples with the respective reference compounds of [^{18}F]**1** and [^{18}F]**2** (Figure 3). Final purification was performed by solid phase extraction (SPE) using Sep-Pack cartridges, and for biological investigations, the products were formulated in isotonic saline containing 10% EtOH. The radiotracers were produced with 30% to 35% RCY, high radiochemical purities (≥98%), and high specific activities (250 to 450 GBq/μmol, n = 4).

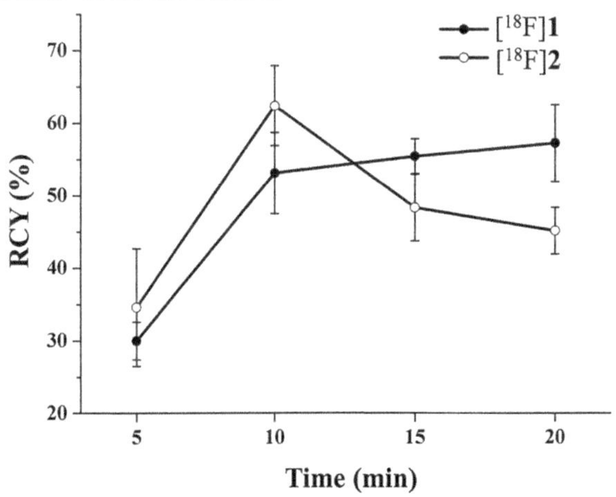

Figure 2 Time-yield curves of the aliphatic ([^{18}F]1) and aromatic ([^{18}F]2) radiolabellings in MeCN up to 20 min.

In vitro stability and logD determination

Investigations on the *in vitro* stability of [^{18}F]**1** and [^{18}F]**2** were performed prior to the experimental determination of logD values. [^{18}F]**1** exhibited a slight tendency to de-fluorinate at 40°C in Tris–HCl, EtOH, 0.9% NaCl, and Dulbecco's phosphate buffer with 89%, 93%, 95%, and 94% of intact tracer after 30 min of incubation and no further decrease up to 90 min. [^{18}F]**2** showed a very high stability with ≥98% of intact tracer at incubation in all selected media up to 90 min. Radio-thin-layer chromatography (TLC) and radio-HPLC analyses were in good agreement, and no further radioactive degradation products were observed.

Regarding the HPLC-based logD determination, differences were noticed between isocratic and gradient elutions using the same column. However, as compiled in Table 1, the logD values using Reprosil-Pur C18 AQ column under gradient conditions are in good agreement with those found with Prodigy 5 μm C8 column.

Receptor affinity

The substitution of the ethyl chain of the carbazole moiety in **2** with a fluorine-ethyl chain in **1** had little effect on target affinity and specificity as reflected by comparable K_i values for the CB_2R (**1**, K_i 2.32 ± 2.12 nM; **2**, K_i 4.27 ± 3.03 nM) [29]. Based on the data published by Cheng et al. [40] (JCPDS 42–44), an agonistic profile of **1** and **2** can be assumed. Both compounds possess no affinity towards the CB_1R (K_i > 1 μM). By contrast, one major brain-penetrating metabolite, compound **10,** shows almost no binding towards the CBRs ($K_{i\ CB1R}$ > 1 μM, $K_{i\ CB2R}$ > 1 μM). In accordance with the *ex vivo* autoradiographic studies on [^{18}F]**2** in spleen tissue slices [29], compound [^{18}F]**1** targets CB_2R *in vivo* too. The autoradiograms are shown in Figure S1 of Additional file 1.

Organ distribution of [^{18}F]1 and [^{18}F]2 in mice

The biodistribution of compounds [^{18}F]**1** and [^{18}F]**2** in percentage of injected dose per gram (% ID/g) at 5, 30,

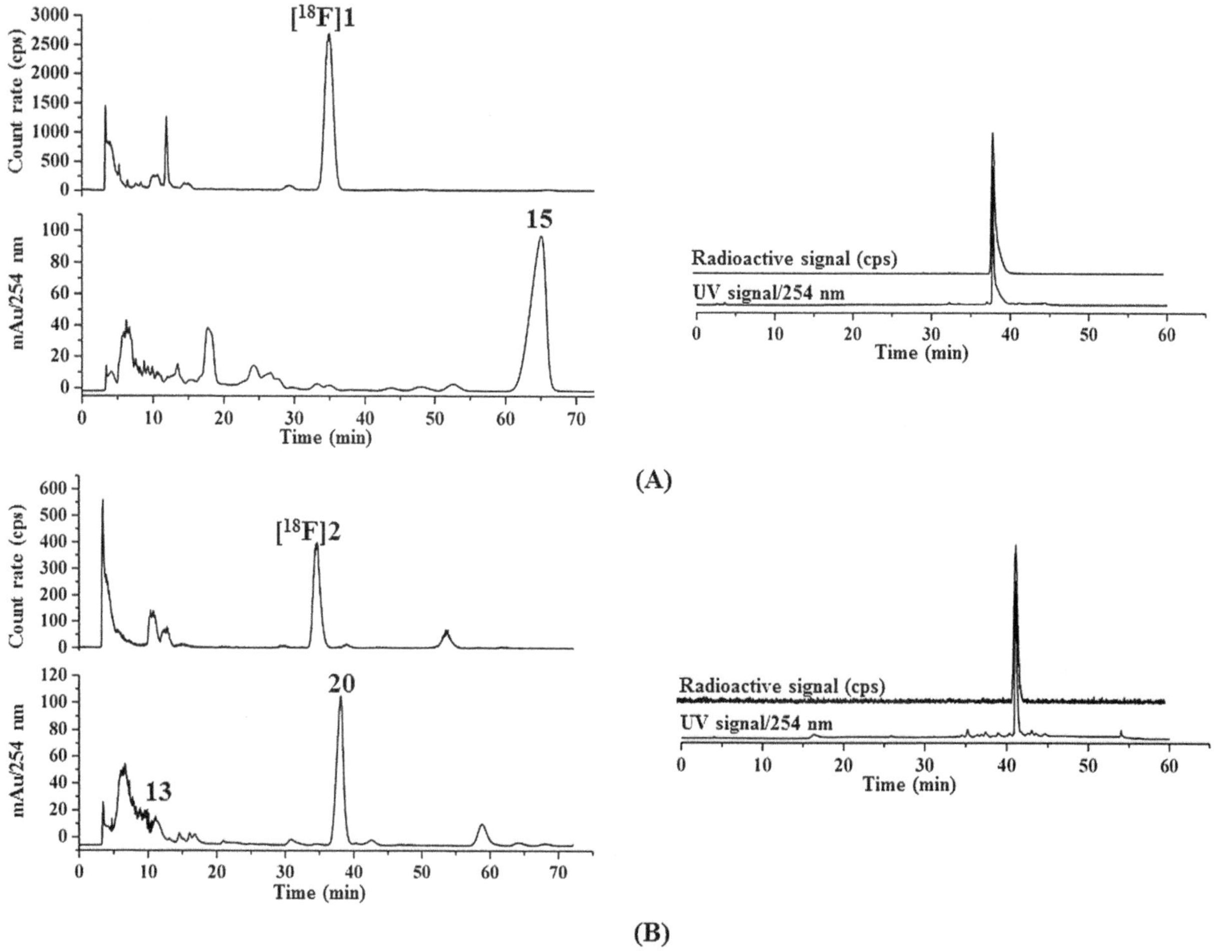

Figure 3 High-performance liquid chromatography. Isocratic semi-preparative RP-HPLC chromatograms (left) and the analytical HPLC chromatograms (right) of the radiotracers spiked with the respective reference compounds. **(A)** [^{18}F]**1** (t_R = 35.3 min), eluent: 58% MeCN/10 mM NH_4OAc aq. on a Reprosil Gold C18, 10 μm, 150 × 4.6 mm; flow rate: 2.5 mL/min. **(B)** [^{18}F]**2** (t_R = 35.6 min), eluent: 60% MeCN/20 mM NH_4OAc aq. on a Multospher 120 RP-18 AQ, 5 μm, 150 × 10 mm; flow rate: 2.0 mL/min. The precursors for radiolabelling (**13** and **15**) and compound **20** (see 'Experimental' section) were also identified by analytical HPLC on a Multospher 120 RP 18 AQ column, 5 μm, 250 × 4.6 mm; solvents: A: 10% MeCN/20 mM NH_4OAc, B: 90% MeCN/20 mM NH_4OAc. Gradient elution(A%): 0 to 10 min, 100%; 10 to 40 min, gradient from 100% to 0%; 40 to 45 min, 0%; 45 to 50 min, 100% at a flow rate of 1 mL/min.

and 60 min post injection (p.i.) is compiled in Tables 2 and 3. For both radiotracers, the highest uptake was detected at 5 min p.i. in the spleen. Comparable kinetics were observed in the brain and most other organs such as the lung, liver, kidney, thymus, and adrenals after administration of [^{18}F]**1** and [^{18}F]**2**, respectively. Both compounds showed a high gastrointestinal excretion as reflected by the constant increase of activity uptake in the small intestine. A constantly low uptake of activity in the femur indicates no confounding defluorination during the experiment.

Table 1 Experimental logD coefficients of compounds 1 and 2

Compound	Reposil-Pur C18-AQ[a]		Prodigy 5 μ C8[a]
	Isocratic	Gradient	Isocratic
1	4.21 ± 0.32	3.82 ± 0.10	3.86 ± 0.33
2	4.87 ± 0.36	4.35 ± 0.11	4.40 ± 0.35

[a]Experiments performed with the respective reference compounds (n = 3 to 6).

The highest accumulation of activity was found in the kidneys and liver for both compounds. While the activity uptake is higher in the kidneys for [^{18}F]**1**, the values for [^{18}F]**2** are higher in the liver, indicating different excretion patterns.

Blocking experiments were performed with pre-administration of the CB_2R-specific inverse agonist SR144528. At 60 min, the animals were sacrificed and the percentage of injected dose per gram of activity uptake was calculated for the various organs. No significant reduction of percentage of injected dose per gram could be observed for both compounds in any of

Table 2 Radioactivity uptake in major organs of female CD1mice after intravenous administration of 300 to 400 kBq [^{18}F]1

Organ	Control (% ID/g)			Blocking (% ID/g)
	5 min[a]	30 min[b]	60 min[b]	60 min[c]
Blood	1.94 ± 0.44	1.44 ± 0.41	1.94 ± 0.69	1.43 ± 0.34
Plasma	2.52 ± 0.58	1.88 ± 0.58	2.50 ± 0.87	1.87 ± 0.41
Brain	1.31 ± 0.24	0.76 ± 0.22	0.92 ± 0.27	0.66 ± 0.11
Heart	3.39 ± 0.45	1.43 ± 0.47	1.66 ± 0.37	1.49 ± 0.29
Lung	3.68 ± 0.62	1.65 ± 0.70	1.77 ± 0.74	1.47 ± 0.29
Stomach	2.05 ± 0.33	1.23 ± 0.36	2.70 ± 1.47	1.84 ± 1.28
Small intestine	4.36 ± 2.09	10.51 ± 8.38	22.03 ± 8.32	19.39 ± 5.53
Large intestine	1.91 ± 2.66	3.24 ± 5.61	1.54 ± 0.42	1.63 ± 0.64
Liver	11.00 ± 1.04	4.38 ± 1.19	5.29 ± 1.22	4.22 ± 0.96
Kidney	13.40 ± 5.66	2.68 ± 0.37	1.65 ± 0.49	1.74 ± 0.48
Bladder	2.23 ± 1.39	1.65 ± 0.43	3.27 ± 1.94	5.07 ± 3.84
Spleen	3.44 ± 0.77	1.46 ± 0.56	1.52 ± 0.62	0.98 ± 0.21
Thymus	3.30 ± 0.58	1.57 ± 0.80	1.90 ± 0.98	1.50 ± 0.35
Pancreas	4.97 ± 0.62	1.50 ± 0.74	1.13 ± 0.11	1.03 ± 0.26
Adrenals	4.16 ± 6.23	3.31 ± 0.99	3.16 ± 1.25	3.00 ± 0.64
Gonads	1.06 ± 0.94	1.02 ± 0.26	1.33 ± 0.50	1.19 ± 0.30
Muscle	2.10 ± 0.33	1.02 ± 0.50	0.89 ± 0.19	0.93 ± 0.23
Femur	2.00 ± 0.38	1.37 ± 0.50	1.84 ± 0.35	1.49 ± 0.45

Blocking was performed with pre-administration of SR144528 (3 mg/kg i.p.). Values are mean ± SD. [a]*n* = 4, [b]*n* = 5, [c]*n* = 6.

the organs investigated including CB_2R-expressing organs (details are compiled in Additional file 1: Table S1). For [^{18}F]**2**, the pre-administration of SR144528 led to an increase of percentage of injected dose per gram in some organs, which might be related to metabolic processes.

Interestingly, major differences between the radioactivity uptakes in various organs were found for [^{18}F]**1** and [^{18}F]**2**. Figure 4 shows all organs (plus the blood and liver) in which significant differences in radioactivity uptake were found at 60 min after injection of the two radiotracers. The measured radioactivity was higher after application of [^{18}F]**1** in those organs expressing CB_2R natively [18] in comparison to the data obtained after injection of [^{18}F]**2**. This relation is reversed in those organs associated to excretion. The cause of this is probably related to the much faster metabolism of [^{18}F]**2** and its radiometabolites compared to that of [^{18}F]**1**, which is in agreement with the observation of significantly lower accumulation of radiolabelled compounds in the plasma and kidney.

The significant differences in the pancreas and femur can be considered as a further indicator of different metabolic processes of [^{18}F]**1** and [^{18}F]**2** leading to different radiometabolites with diverse organ distribution patterns. Thus, the activity measured in the *ex vivo* biodistribution study is largely determined by metabolites bearing the ^{18}F label.

Metabolism of [^{18}F]1 and [^{18}F]2 in mice

Typical HPLC radiochromatograms of brain extracts are shown in Figure 5. In general, radio-TLC analytics of plasma, urine, and brain samples obtained at 30 and 60 min p.i. of [^{18}F]**1** or [^{18}F]**2** are consistent with the data obtained by radio-HPLC. As shown in Table 4, unmetabolized [^{18}F]**1** accounted for 60% of the recovered activity in plasma samples at 30 min p.i., while 36% of the total radioactivity can be addressed to a more hydrophilic metabolite $\mathbf{M1_a}$. The amount of intact radiotracer [^{18}F]**1** is further reduced at 60 min p.i. to 7% with a concomitant increase of $\mathbf{M1_a}$ to 92%.

Radiochromatograms of brain samples at 30 min p.i. shown in Figure 5 revealed that unmetabolized radiotracer corresponded to 68% and 88% of the total activity after administration of [^{18}F]**1** and [^{18}F]**2**, respectively. Paralleled by the constantly increasing accumulation of radiometabolites in the brain, these values decreased to 35% and 43%, respectively, at 60 min p.i. In particular, these radiometabolites account for 13% ($\mathbf{M1_a}$) and 10% ($\mathbf{M2_a}$) as well as 8% ($\mathbf{M1_b}$) and 3% ($\mathbf{M2_b}$) of total activity at 30 min p.i. of [^{18}F]**1** and [^{18}F]**2**, respectively, with the main radiometabolites $\mathbf{M1_a}$ and $\mathbf{M1_b}$ reaching values of 58% and 51% at 60 min p.i., respectively. The radiometabolite $\mathbf{M2_a}$ of [^{18}F]**1** corresponds most likely to the amine, which is formed by enzymatic hydrolysis of the amide bond in the compound.

Table 3 Radioactivity uptake in major organs of female CD1 mice after intravenous administration of 300 to 400 kBq [18F]2

Organ	Control (%ID/g)			Blocking (%ID/g)
	5 min[a]	30 min[b]	60 min[a]	60 min[a]
Blood	2.29 ± 0.48	3.42 ± 0.39	2.50 ± 0.42	3.40 ± 0.21
Plasma	3.87 ± 0.90	6.82 ± 1.19	5.22 ± 0.73	5.78 ± 0.07
Brain	0.62 ± 0.22	0.86 ± 0.34	0.26 ± 0.07	0.28 ± 0.03
Heart	3.42 ± 0.57	2.32 ± 0.24	1.45 ± 0.20	1.53 ± 0.13
Lung	4.62 ± 0.21	3.36 ± 0.02	2.52 ± 0.60	2.31 ± 0.19
Stomach	1.57 ± 1.18	2.09 ± 0.81	2.21 ± 0.43	3.24 ± 2.10
Small intestine	3.86 ± 2.64	20.78 ± 3.28	27.31 ± 2.44	29.64 ± 5.10
Large intestine	0.46 ± 0.06	1.25 ± 0.30	1.86 ± 0.36	1.78 ± 0.23
Liver	31.31 ± 9.91	8.84 ± 0.83	6.27 ± 0.68	10.51 ± 1.10
Kidney	5.86 ± 0.96	5.90 ± 0.15	3.96 ± 1.25	4.91 ± 1.51
Bladder	1.01 ± 0.29	2.02 ± 0.39	1.45 ± 0.57	1.77 ± 0.16
Spleen	10.42 ± 7.67	1.34 ± 0.10	0.68 ± 0.11	0.74 ± 0.10
Thymus	2.30 ± 1.06	1.96 ± 0.22	1.04 ± 0.08	1.77 ± 0.14
Pancreas	2.04 ± 0.59	1.71 ± 0.15	0.82 ± 0.21	1.02 ± 0.11
Adrenals	7.67 ± 2.18	5.38 ± 0.61	2.44 ± 0.72	3.34 ± 0.15
Gonads	1.14 ± 0.32	2.08 ± 0.03	2.29 ± 0.57	1.97 ± 0.39
Muscle	1.00 ± 0.30	0.92 ± 0.15	0.70 ± 0.27	0.70 ± 0.06
Femur	1.63 ± 0.93	1.10 ± 0.03	0.58 ± 0.11	0.61 ± 0.09

Blocking was performed with pre-administration of SR144528 (3 mg/kg i.p.). Values are mean ± SD. [a]$n = 3$, [b]$n = 2$.

The total amount of activity measured in, e.g. the plasma at particular times p.i. also depends on the kinetics of the excretion of radiotracer/radiometabolites. For [^{18}F]**2**, this is more pronounced than for [^{18}F]**1** with unmetabolized [^{18}F]**2** accounting for only 2% of the total radioactivity in the plasma at 30 min p.i. At this time, more than 90% of the recovered activity in plasma samples for [^{18}F]**2** consisted of the single radiometabolite $\mathbf{M1_b}$. As this value decreases only slightly up to 60 min p.i. (88%), $\mathbf{M1_b}$ can be assumed as a rather metabolically stable compound. This radiometabolite of [^{18}F]**2** probably corresponds to the *N*-aryl-oxadiazolyl-propanoic acid resulting from enzymatic hydrolysis of the amide bond of **2** [40]. To prove this assumption, the trimethylammonium salt **18** was synthesized as the precursor of this metabolite. In order introduce ^{18}F into the molecule, the carbon acid moiety was protected as a methyl ester resulting in the labelled compound [^{18}F]**17** (Scheme 5). It was expected that after injection of this compound in mice, the ester will be converted into the free acid [^{18}F]**10**. Those metabolic pathways are common for drug inactivation and excretion [41] as well as for the prodrug concept providing pharmacologically active metabolites *in vivo* from pharmacologically inactive compounds [42]. After intravenous injection of [^{18}F]**17** in CD1 mice, samples of the plasma, brain, and spleen were analyzed at 30 and 60 min p.i. (Table 5).

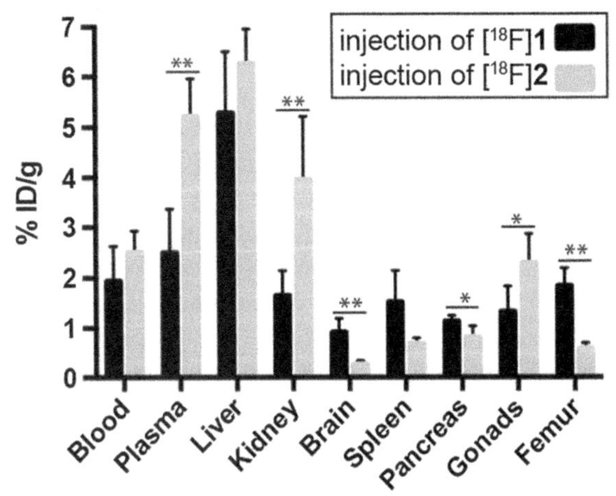

Figure 4 Distribution of radioactivity at 60 min in selected organs after administration of the tracers [^{18}F]1 and [^{18}F]2. Values are mean ± SD. Significant differences are indicated ($^{*}p < 0.05$, $^{**}p < 0.01$). Plasma, $p = 0.0041$; kidney, $p = 0.0086$; brain, $p = 0.0070$; pancreas, $p = 0.0288$; gonads, $p = 0.0445$; femur, $p = 0.0011$.

As expected, the methylester [^{18}F]**17** (t_R = 36 min) is completely converted to free acid [^{18}F]**10** (t_R = 22 min) in the plasma samples already at 30 min p.i. (Scheme 5). Radio-HPLC analysis of brain samples at 60 min p.i., spiked with the reference compounds **2** and **10**, confirmed

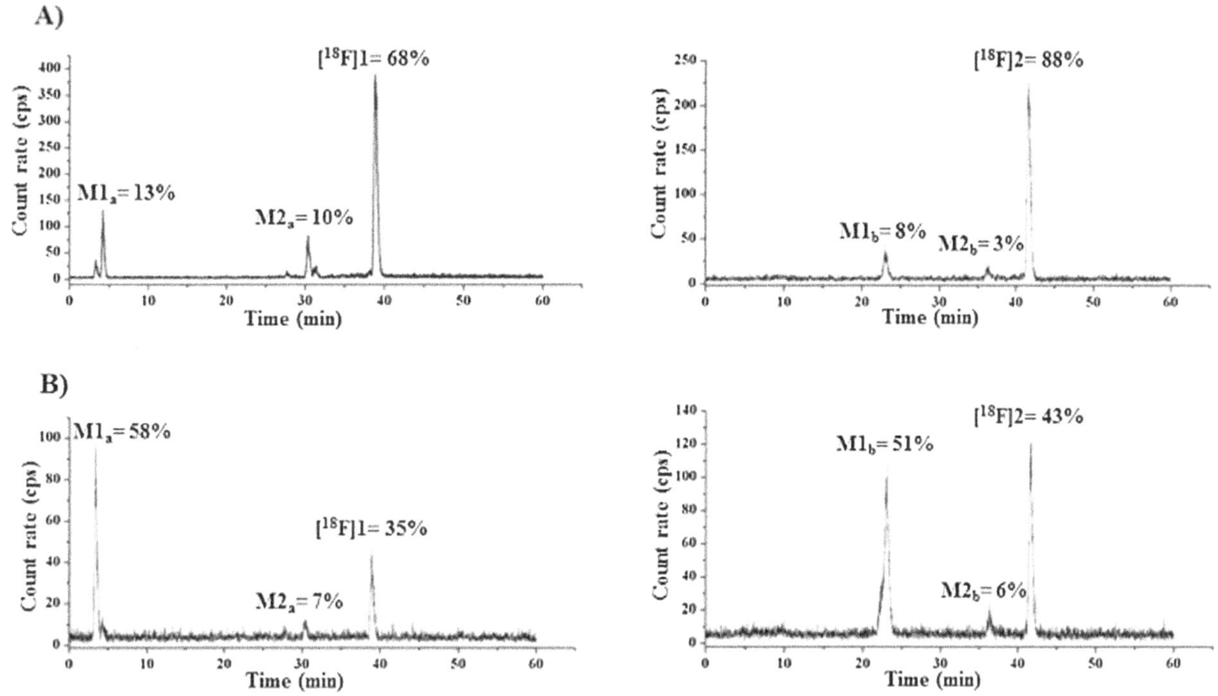

Figure 5 Analytical radio-HPLC profile of acetonitrile extracts of brain homogenates. (A) At 30 min p.i. and **(B)** 60 min p.i. Conditions: Multospher 120 RP 18 AQ, 5 μm, 250 × 4.6 mm. Solvents: A: 10% MeCN/20 mM NH_4OAc, B: 90% MeCN/20 mM NH_4OAc. Gradient elution (A%): 0 to 10 min, 100%; 10 to 40 min, gradient from 100% to 0%; 40 to 45 min, 0%; 45 to 50 min, 100% at a flow rate of 1 mL/min.

that the radiometabolite $\mathbf{M1_b}$ co-elutes with compound **10** (Figure 6).

Furthermore, in combination with the time-activity data presented in Table 5, this result indicates that the main radiometabolite $\mathbf{M1_b}$ of $[^{18}F]$**2** derived from peripheral metabolism ($[^{18}F]$**10**) penetrates the blood–brain barrier (BBB). In addition, analyses of brain and spleen sample data revealed that no further metabolic transformation of $[^{18}F]$**10** could be observed up to 60 min p.i. as shown in Figure 7.

In vitro investigation of the affinity of **10** towards both hCB_2R and hCB_1R revealed no specific binding (K_i > 1 μM). Altogether, these data suggest that non-target binding radiometabolites of $[^{18}F]$**1** and $[^{18}F]$**2** account for the vast majority of *ex vivo* activity measured in the spleen and other organs known to express CB_2R. This corresponds very well with the insignificant displacement of activity after administration of $[^{18}F]$**1** and $[^{18}F]$**2** by the CB_2R-specific SR144528. Hence, radiometabolites generated in the periphery penetrate the BBB leading to a pronounced accumulation of the main radiometabolites in the brain, hampering the application of $[^{18}F]$**1** and $[^{18}F]$**2** for imaging of CB_2R in the brain.

Table 4 Relative percentages of intact tracer and radiometabolites in plasma samples

Compound	t_R (min)[a]	Plasma	
		30 min p.i. (%)	60 min p.i. (%)
$[^{18}F]$**1**	38.8	60	7
$\mathbf{M1_a}$	4.2	36	92
$\mathbf{M2_a}$	30.2	3	1
$[^{18}F]$**2**	41.7	2	2
$\mathbf{M1_b}$	22.9	95	88
$\mathbf{M2_b}$	36.4	≤1	≤1

At 30 and 60 min p.i. of $[^{18}F]$**1** and $[^{18}F]$**2**. [a]Radio-HPLC (separation conditions, see 'Experimental' section).

Experimental

Materials and general procedures

Unless otherwise noted, moisture-sensitive reactions were performed under dry nitrogen or argon. All chemicals and reagents were purchased from commercially available sources and used without further purification unless otherwise specified. Tetrahydrofuran (THF) was dried with sodium/benzophenone and was freshly distilled before use. For the TLC, silica gel 60 F254 plates (Merck KGaA, Darmstadt, Germany) were used. For the flash chromatography (fc), silica gel 60, 40 to 64 μm, (Merck) was used. Room temperature (rt) was 20°C. Melting point was determined using Stuart™ Melting point apparatus SMP3 (Bibby Scientific Ltd, Staffordshire, UK), uncorrected. Mass spectrometry (MS) was done using MAT GCQ (Thermo Finnigan

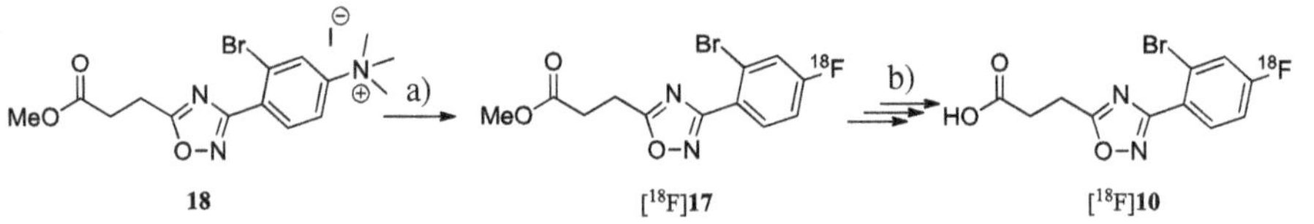

Scheme 5 Radiosynthesis and metabolism of [^{18}F]17. (a) Radiolabelling with K[^{18}F]F-$K_{2.2.2}$-carbonate complex (5.6 mg, 15 μmol), 2 mg of **18**, MeCN, 82°C, 10 min; **(b)** *in vivo* metabolism.

MAT GmbH, Bremen, Germany). ^{1}H, ^{13}C, and ^{19}F NMR spectra were recorded on VARIAN GEMINI 2000 (200 MHz for ^{1}H NMR, 50 MHz for ^{13}C NMR, 188 MHz for ^{19}F NMR), VARIAN MERCURY plus (300 MHz for ^{1}H NMR, 75 MHz for ^{13}C NMR, 228 MHz for ^{19}F NMR), and VARIAN MERCURY plus and BRUKER DRX-400 (400 MHz for ^{1}H NMR, 100 MHz for ^{13}C NMR, 367 MHz for ^{19}F NMR); δ (in ppm)was related to tetramethylsilane and trichloro-fluoro-methane (CF_3Cl), respectively; coupling constants (*J*) were given with 0.1-Hz resolution. Multiplicities of NMR signals are indicated as follows: s (singlet), d (doublet), t (triplet), m (multiplet), dd (doublet of doublets), and dt (doublet of triplets). HPLC method for determination of the product purity was done with Merck Hitachi Equipment; L-7400 UV detector, L-7200 autosampler, L-7100 pump, and L-7614 degasser were used. The following conditions were used in the experiment: column, LiChrospher® 60 RP-select B, 5 μm, 250 × 4.0 mm; flow rate, 1 mL/min; injection volume, 5.0 μL; detection at λ = 210 nm. Solvents: A: water with 0.05% (*v*/*v*) trifluoroacetic acid, B: MeCN with 0.05% (*v*/*v*) trifluoroacetic acid. Gradient elution (A%): 0 to 4 min, 90%; 4 to 29 min, gradient from 90% to 0%; 29 to 31 min, 0%; 31 to 31.5 min, gradient from 0% to 90%; 31.5 to 40 min, 90%.

For radiochemistry, TLC was performed on silica gel pre-coated plates (Polygram, SIL G/UV254) with petroleum ether/ethyl acetate/ammonia (2:1:0.1, *v*/*v*/*v*), and the spots were visualized using UV light at 254 nm. Radio-TLC was recorded using a BAS-1800 II system Bioimaging Analyzer (Fuji Photo Film, Co. Ltd., Tokyo, Japan), and images were evaluated with AIDA 2.31 software (raytest Isotopenmessgeräte GmbH, Straubenhardt, Germany). Purification and isolation of the radiotracers were conducted on a semi-preparative radio-HPLC consisting of a S1021 pump (Sykam GmbH, Eresing, Germany), UV detector (WellChrom Filter-Photometer K-2001; Wissenschaftl. Gerätebau Dr. Ing. Herbert Knauer GmbH, Berlin, Germany), NaI(Tl) counter, and data acquisition by an automated system (Nina, Nuclear Interface, GE Medical Systems, Munich, Germany) on a Reprosil Gold C18, 10 μm, 150 × 4.6 mm, eluent: 58% MeCN/10 mM NH_4OAc aq. at a flow rate of 2.5 mL/min, and Multospher 120 RP-18 AQ, 5 μm, 150 × 10 mm, eluent: 60% MeCN/20 mM NH_4OAc aq. at a flow rate of 2.0 mL/min, respectively for [^{18}F]**1** (t_R = 35.3 min) and [^{18}F]**2** (t_R = 35.6 min). For the *in vivo* pharmacokinetic metabolite evaluation of [^{18}F]**17** (t_R = 19.5 min) semi-preparative isolation was performed on a Multospher 120 RP 18 AQ, 5 μm, 150 × 10 mm, eluent: 56% MeCN/20 mM NH_4OAc aq. at a flow rate of 2.0 mL/min. Analytical chromatographic separations were performed on a JASCO LC-2000 system (JASCO Labor- und Datentechnik GmbH, Gross-Umstadt, Germany), incorporating a PU-2080Plus pump, AS-2055Plus auto injector (100 μL sample loop) and a UV-2070Plus UV detector (monitoring at 254 nm). All analytical radio-HPLC analyses were performed using a gradient mode on a Multospher 120 RP18 AQ, 5 μm, 250 × 4.6 m. Solvents: A: 10% MeCN/20 mM NH_4OAc, B: 90% MeCN/20 mM NH_4OAc.Gradient elution (A%): 0 to10 min, 100%; 10 to 40 min, gradient from 100% to 0%; 40 to 45 min, 0%; 45 to 50 min, 100% at a flow rate of 1 mL/min.

Table 5 [^{18}F]10 uptake in female CD1mice after intravenous administration of 100 to 200 kBq [^{18}F]17

Sample	30 min p.i. (% ID/g)	60 min p.i. (% ID/g)
Plasma	18.21	15.38
Brain	0.28	0.29
Spleen	1.35	1.31

(Z)-2-Bromo-N'-hydroxy-4-nitrobenzimidamide (5) and 2-bromo-4-nitrobenzamide (7)

To a solution of 2-bromo-4-nitrobenzonitrile **3** (100 mg, 0.44 mmol, 1 eq.) in 5 mL MeOH under argon, Na_2CO_3 (56 mg, 0.52 mmol, 1.2 eq.) and NH_2OH-HCl (76 mg, 1.1 mmol, 2.5 eq.) were added at rt, and the reaction mixture was refluxed for 15 h. Upon cooling to rt, 10 mL of H_2O was added and the aqueous phase was washed three times with 10 mL ethyl acetate (EtOAc). The combined organic extracts were dried over sodium sulfate and filtered. Upon evaporation of the solvent, column chromatography was performed (silica, EtOAc/isohexane (IH) 2:8) to give **5** (62 mg, 0.24 mmol, 55%) and **7** (41 mg, 0.17 mmol, 32%) as colorless solids. **5**: ^{1}H NMR (400 MHz, DMSO-d_6): δ

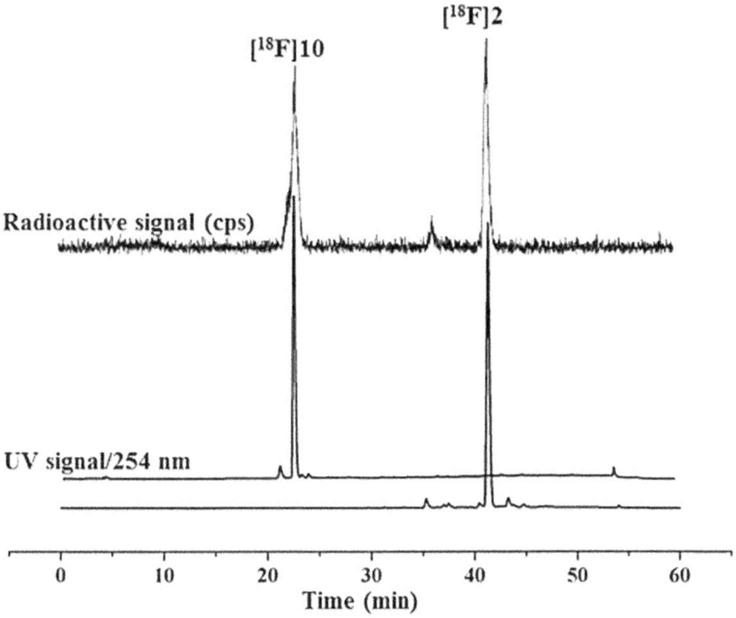

Figure 6 Analytical radio-HPLC profile of [^{18}F]2 at 60 min p.i spiked with the reference 2 and 10 (M1$_b$). Conditions: Multospher 120 RP 18 AQ, 5 µm, 250 × 4.6 mm. Solvents: A: 10% MeCN/20 mM NH_4OAc, B: 90% MeCN/20 mM NH_4OAc.Gradient elution (A%): 0 to 10 min, 100%; 10 to 40 min, gradient from 100% to 0%; 40 to 45 min, 0%; 45 to 50 min, 100% at a flow rate of 1 mL/min.

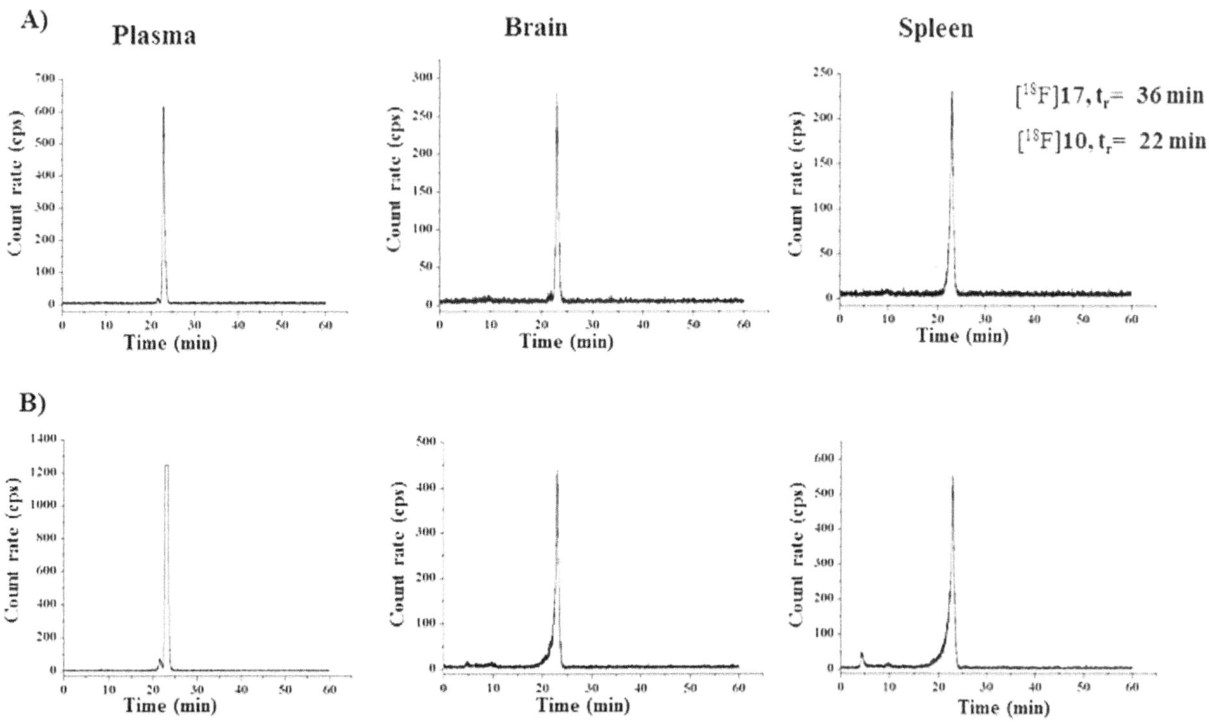

Figure 7 *In vivo* metabolism conversion of [^{18}F]17 to [^{18}F]10. Analytical radio-HPLC profiles of the *in vivo* metabolism conversion of [^{18}F]**17** (t_R = 36 min) to [^{18}F]**10** (t_R = 22 min, Scheme 5b) in plasma, brain, and spleen samples. **(A)** At 30 min p.i. and **(B)** at 60 min p.i. Conditions: Multospher 120 RP 18 AQ, 5 µm, 250 × 4.6 mm. Solvents: A: 10% MeCN/20 mM NH_4OAc, B: 90% MeCN/20 mM NH_4OAc.Gradient elution (A%): 0 to 10 min, 100%; 10 to 40 min, gradient from 100% to 0%; 40 to 45 min, 0%; 45 to 50 min, 100% at a flow rate of 1 mL/min.

(ppm) = 9.70 (s, 1H), 8.41 (d, J = 2.3 Hz, 1H), 8.21 (dd, J = 8.4/2.3 Hz, 1H), 7.64 (d, J = 8.4 Hz, 1H), 5.99 (s, 2H), 5.99 (s, 2H); ^{13}C NMR (100 MHz, DMSO-d_6): δ (ppm) = 150.4, 147.8, 141.7, 132.2, 127.3, 122.5, 122.3; MS (ESI+): m/z (%) = 260/262 (100/100) $[M+H]^+$. 7: ^{1}H NMR (400 MHz, $CDCl_3$): δ (ppm) = 8.49 (d, J = 2.2 Hz, 1H), 8.24 (dd, J = 8.5, 2.2 Hz, 1H), 7.79 (d, J = 8.5 Hz, 1H); ^{13}C NMR (100 MHz, $CDCl_3$): δ (ppm) = 164.0, 130.6, 128.7, 122.7, 120.0; MS (ESI+): m/z (%) = 245/247 (100/100) $[M+H]^+$.

(Z)-2-Bromo-4-fluoro-N'-hydroxybenzimidamide (6) and 2-bromo-4-fluorobenzamide (8)

Compounds **6** and **8** (pale yellow solids) were obtained under the same synthetic procedure described for compounds **5** and **7** with 2-bromo-1-fluoro-4-nitrobenzene **4** as starting reagent. **6** (yield 73%): ^{1}H NMR (400 MHz, $CDCl_3$): δ (ppm) = 7.46 (dd, J = 8.6, 6.0 Hz, 1H), 7.35 (dd, J = 8.2, 2.5 Hz, 1H), 7.07 (dt, J = 8.1, 4.4 Hz, 1H); ^{13}C NMR (100 MHz, $CDCl_3$): δ (ppm) = 161.7, 151.8, 132.6 (d, J = 8.8 Hz), 120.7 (d, J = 24.7 Hz), 115.1 (d, J = 19.1 Hz), 114.9 (d, J = 19.0 Hz); ^{19}F NMR (376 MHz, $CDCl_3$): δ (ppm) = −109.3 (dd, J = 14.1, 7.9 Hz); MS (ESI+): m/z (%) = 233/235 (100/100) $[M+H]^+$. **8** (yield 5%): ^{1}H NMR (400 MHz, $CDCl_3$): δ (ppm) = 7.49 (dd, J = 8.6, 5.9 Hz, 1H), 7.27 (dd, J = 8.4, 2.3 Hz, 1H), 7.00 (td, J = 8.2, 2.4 Hz, 1H), 3.44 (s, 2H); ^{13}C NMR (100 MHz, $CDCl_3$): δ (ppm) = 169.7 (d, J = 5.6 Hz), 164.2, 161.7, 133.2, 130.9 (d, J = 9.0 Hz), 120.7 (d, J = 24.7 Hz), 119.9 (d, J = 9.8 Hz), 114.7 (d, J = 21.4 Hz); MS (ESI+): m/z (%) = 218/212 (100/100) $[M+H]^+$.

3-(3-(2-Bromo-4-nitrophenyl)-1,2,4-oxadiazol-5-yl)propanoic acid (9)

The (Z)-2-bromo-N'-hydroxy-4-nitrobenzene-1-carboximidamide **5** (100 mg, 0.38 mmol, 1 eq.) was dissolved in 1 mL of dimethylformamide (DMF) under inert atmosphere. Succinic anhydride (95 mg, 0.95 mmol, 2.5 eq.) and KF (6.7 mg, 0.11 mmol, 0.3 eq.) were added, and the reaction mixture was warmed up to 130°C for 30 min. Upon cooling, 20 mL of H_2O was added and the solid was collected by filtration, washed with H_2O, and dried to give **9** as a colorless solid (123 mg, 0.36 mmol, 95%) with a melting point (mp) = 127°C. ^{1}H NMR (400 MHz, DMSO-d_6): δ (ppm) = 8.57 (d, J = 2.3 Hz, 1H), 8.36 (dd, J = 8.6, 2.3 Hz, 1H), 8.07 (d, J = 8.6 Hz, 1H), 3.23 (t, J = 6.9 Hz, 2H), 2.83 (t, J = 6.9 Hz, 2H); ^{13}C NMR (100 MHz, DMSO-d_6): δ (ppm) = 178.8, 173.2, 166.0, 148.4, 133.4, 132.3, 128.5, 122.0, 121.7, 29.5, 21.3; MS (ESI+): m/z (%) = 342/344 (100/100) $[M+H]^+$.

3-(3-(2-Bromo-4-fluorophenyl)-1,2,4-oxadiazol-5-yl) propanoic acid (10)

Compound **10** (colorless solid) was obtained under the same synthetic procedure described for compound **9** with (Z)-2-bromo-4-fluoro-N'-hydroxybenzen-1-carboximidamide **6** as starting reagent (yield 95%, mp = 104°C). ^{1}H NMR (400 MHz, DMSO-d_6): δ (ppm) = 7.86 (dd, J = 8.7, 6.1 Hz, 1H), 7.82 (dd, J = 8.6, 2.6 Hz, 1H), 7.50 to 7.41 (m, 1H), 3.20 (t, J = 6.9 Hz, 2H), 2.81 (t, J = 6.9 Hz, 2H); ^{13}C NMR (100 MHz, DMSO-d_6): δ (ppm) = 179.2, 172.7, 164.1, 161.6, 133.6 (d, J = 9.4 Hz), 124.3 (d, J = 3.5 Hz), 122.1 (d, J = 10.1 Hz), 121.4 (d, J = 25.1 Hz), 115.5 (d, J = 21.6 Hz), 29.9, 21.64; MS (ESI+): m/z (%) = 315/317 (100/100) $[M+H]^+$.

3-(3-(2-Bromo-4-nitrophenyl)-1,2,4-oxadiazol-5-yl)-N-(9-ethyl-9H-carbazol-3-yl)propanamide (11)

To a solution of acid **9** (50 mg, 0.14 mmol, 1 eq.) and 9-ethyl-9H-carbazol-3-amine **12** (30.9 mg, 0.14 mmol, 1 eq.) in 5 mL dichloromethane (DCM), N,N'-diisopropylcarbodiimide (45 μL, 0.21 mmol, 1.5 eq.) was added at 0°C, and the reaction was stirred at rt until **9** and **12** were not visible by TLC control (silica, EtOAc/IH 1:1) (2 h). The reaction was diluted with 5 mL of DCM and washed once with 10 mL 0.5 M aq. HCl, 10 mL 0.5 N aq. NaOH and 10 mL aq. NaCl saturated solution. The organic phase was dried over sodium sulfate and filtered. Evaporation of the solvent afforded a brown solid which was recrystallized from THF to give **11** (63 mg, 0.11 mmol, 85%) as a white solid. ^{1}H NMR (400 MHz, $CDCl_3$): δ (ppm) = 8.57 (d, J = 2.0 Hz, 1H), 8.36 to 8.14 (m, 2H), 8.03 (d, J = 8 Hz, 2H), 7.62 to 7.13 (m, 4H), 4.35 (q, J = 7.3 Hz, 2H), 3.49 (t, J = 7.4 Hz, 2H), 3.04 (t, J = 7.4 Hz, 2H), 1.43 (t, J = 7.2 Hz, 3H); MS (ESI+): m/z (%) = 556/558 (100/100) $[M+Na]^+$.

3-(3-(4-Amino-2-bromophenyl)-1,2,4-oxadiazol-5-yl)-N-(9-ethyl-9H-carbazol-3-yl)propanamide (19)

To a solution of oxadiazole **11** (30 mg, 0.05 mmol, 1 eq.) and $SnCl_2$-$2H_2O$ (63 mg, 0.28 mmol, 5 eq.) in 2 mL of EtOH, concentrated aq. HCl (37%) was added at rt. Upon completion (TLC, silica, EtOAc/IH 1:1), 10 mL of saturated aq. $NaHCO_3$ solution was added, and the mixture was extracted three times with 10 mL of EtOAc. The combined organic extracts were dried over sodium sulfate and filtered. Evaporation of the solvent afforded **19** (17.6 mg, 0.04 mmol, 70%) as a brown solid which was used in the next step without further purification. ^{1}H NMR (300 MHz, $CDCl_3$): δ (ppm) = 8.17 (d, J = 1.9 Hz, 1H), 7.89 (d, J = 7.8 Hz, 1H), 7.47 (d, J = 8.4 Hz, 1H), 7.37 (dt, J = 9.1, 4.6 Hz, 1H), 7.34 to 7.14 (m, 3H), 7.09 to 6.99 (m, 1H), 6.94 (d, J = 2.2 Hz, 1H), 6.61 (dd, J = 8.4, 2.3 Hz, 1H), 4.19 (q, J = 7.2 Hz, 2H), 3.24 (t, J = 7.4 Hz, 2H), 2.86 (t, J = 7.4 Hz, 2H), 1.25 (t, J = 7.2 Hz, 3H); ^{13}C NMR (75 MHz, $CDCl_3$): δ (ppm) = 178.2, 170.6, 169.2, 167.5, 157.9, 140.4, 137.2, 133.0, 132.7, 129.7, 125.7, 122.8, 122.7, 120.5, 120.4, 119.4, 118.6, 114.5, 112.7, 108.5, 108.4, 37.5, 32.6, 22.4, 13.6; MS (ESI+): m/z (%) = 528/526 (100/100) $[M+Na]^+$.

3-(3-(2-Bromo-4-(dimethylamino)phenyl)-1,2,4-oxadiazol-5-yl)-N-(9-ethyl-9H-carbazol-3-yl)propanamide (20)

To a solution of paraformaldehyde (PFA) (7.2 mg, 0.24 mmol, 6 eq.) in 90 µL of H_2O, concentrated H_2SO_4 (13 µL, 0.24 mmol, 6 eq.) was added, and the reaction was cooled in an ice bath. To the resulting solution, **19** (20 mg, 0.04 mmol, 1 eq.) in 1 mL THF was added, and the reaction mixture was stirred for 30 min at 0°C. Next, $NaBH_4$ (granules, 9.1 mg, 0.24 mmol, 6 eq.) was added in one portion, and the reaction was stirred for a further 18 h at rt. The reaction was quenched by addition of a concentrated aqueous NaOH solution (pH = 10 to 12), and the resulting aqueous phase was washed with EtOAc. The organic phase was dried over sodium sulfate and filtered. Upon purification by column chromatography (silica, EtOAc/IH 3/7) a yellow-brown solid was obtained which was further purified by recrystallization from THF to give **20** as a colorless solid (11 mg, 0.12 mmol, 53%) with mp = 125°C. ^{1}H NMR (400 MHz, DMSO-d_6): δ (ppm) = 10.11 (s, 1H), 8.39 (s, 1H), 8.02 (d, J = 7.6 Hz, 1H), 7.66 (d, J = 8.9 Hz, 1H), 7.57 to 7.45 (m, 3H), 7.48 to 7.32 (m, 1H), 7.20 to 7.07 (m, 1H), 6.95 (d, J = 2.6 Hz, 1H), 6.77 (dd, J = 8.9, 2.6 Hz, 1H), 4.38 (q, J = 7.0 Hz, 2H), 3.28 (t, J = 7.0 Hz, 2H), 2.96 (t, J = 7.1 Hz, 2H), 2.95 (s, 6H), 1.27 (t, J = 7.1 Hz, 3H); ^{13}C NMR (100 MHz, DMSO-d_6): δ (ppm) = 178.4, 168.6, 167.0, 156.7, 152.1, 139.9, 136.1, 132.2, 131.1, 125.7, 122.0, 121.8, 120.1, 118.8, 118.5, 116.0, 113.4, 111.1, 110.7, 109.1, 108.9, 40.6, 36.9, 32.0, 21.7, 13.6; MS (ESI+): m/z (%) = 556/554 (100/100) [M+Na]$^+$.

3-Bromo-4-(5-(3-((9-ethyl-9H-carbazol-3-yl)amino)-3-oxopropyl)-1,2,4-oxadiazol-3-yl)-N,N,N-trimethylbenzenaminium iodide (13)

To a solution of dimethylamine **20** (53 mg, 0.1 mmol, 1 eq.) in 1 mL of dry DMF under argon, MeI (124 µL, 20 mmol, 20 eq.) was added at rt. The reaction was sealed and warmed up to 35°C. Additional MeI (124 µL, 20 mmol, 20 eq.) was added after 2 and 5 days, while the reaction temperature was maintained at 35°C. Upon solvent evaporation, the resulting thick mass was washed three times with 4 mL of EtOAc to remove trace impurities and unreacted starting material (**20**). Upon drying, 4 mL of H_2O was added. The mixture was sonicated and placed in a fridge (+4°C) for 1 h. The solid was filtrated and rewashed with 4 mL of ice-cold H_2O. The trimethylammonium salt **13** was obtained as a light brown solid (57 mg, 0.85 mmol, 85%) with mp = 109°C. ^{1}H NMR (400 MHz,CD_3CN): δ (ppm) = 8.71 (s, 1H), 8.41 (d, J = 1.9 Hz, 1H), 8.25 (d, J = 2.7 Hz, 1H), 8.08 (d, J = 7.8 Hz, 1H), 8.05 (d, J = 8.8 Hz, 1H), 7.93 (dd, J = 8.9, 2.8 Hz, 1H), 7.57 (dd, J = 8.7, 2.1 Hz, 1H), 7.49 (dt, J = 15.4, 8.2 Hz, 3H), 7.20 (ddd, J = 7.9, 6.9, 1.2 Hz, 1H), 4.40 (q, J = 7.2 Hz, 2H), 3.59 (s, 9H), 3.39 (t, J = 6.9 Hz, 2H), 3.05 (t, J = 6.9 Hz, 2H), 1.37 (t, J = 7.2 Hz, 3H); ^{13}C NMR (101 MHz, CD_3CN): δ (ppm) = 181.1, 169.8, 167.4, 149.2, 141.3, 137.7, 134.1, 131.7, 131.6, 127.5, 126.8, 123.9, 123.4, 121.2, 121.0, 120.0, 119.5, 112.6, 109.9, 109.8, 58.1 (3C), 38.2, 33.2, 22.9, 14.0; HRMS (ESI+): m/z (%) = 546.1531/548.1436 (100/100) [M]$^+$.

2-(9H-Carbazol-9-yl)ethanol (25)

Under N_2, 9*H*-carbazole (**23**, 5.43 g, 32.5 mmol, 1.0 eq.) was dissolved in THF (55 mL) and cooled down to −78°C. *n*-Butyllithium (1.2 M in *n*-hexane, 32.4 mL, 38.9 mmol, 1.2 eq.) was added dropwise, and the mixture was stirred for 30 min at −78°C. Then, a solution of ethylene sulfate (4.51 g, 36.3 mmol, 1.1 eq.) in THF (15 mL) was added, and the mixture was stirred for 1 h at −78°C and 24 h at rt. H_2O was added and the mixture was acidified to pH 1 with concentrated $H_2SO_4$and heated to reflux for 24 h. Afterwards, the solution was neutralized with 5 M NaOH, brine was added and the mixture was extracted with CH_2Cl_2. The organic layers were dried (Na_2SO_4) and concentrated under reduced pressure, and the residue was purified by fc (d = 8 cm, l = 12 cm, cyclohexane/EtOAc 65:35, R_f 0.42). Pale yellow solid, mp = 80°C, yield 4.66 g (68%). Purity (HPLC): 98.1% (t_R = 19.28 min). ^{1}H NMR (400 MHz, DMSO-d_6): δ (ppm) = 3.86 (quart, J = 5.9 Hz, 2H), 4.47 (t, J = 5.5 Hz, 2H), 4.99 (t, J = 5.0 Hz, 1H), 7.24 (t, J = 7.4 Hz, 2H), 7.48 (t, J = 7.6 Hz, 2H), 8.18 (d, J = 7.8 Hz, 2H); ^{13}C NMR ($CDCl_3$): δ (ppm) = 45.3, 59.6, 109.6 (2C), 118.6 (2C), 120.2 (2C), 122.2 (2C), 125.0 (2C), 140.5 (2C); exact mass (APCI): m/z = calculated for $C_{14}H_{13}NOH$ 212.1069, found 212.1060.

2-(3-Nitro-9H-carbazol-9-yl)ethanol (24)

9-(Hydroxyethyl)carbazole**25** (5.11 g, 24.2 mmol, 1 eq.) was dissolved in CH_2Cl_2 (100 mL) and cooled down to 5°C to10°C. Concentrated nitric acid (density 1.5 g/mL, 1.7 mL, 36.3 mmol, 1.5 eq.) was added dropwise under vigorous stirring. Stirring was continued at <10°C until the starting material was transformed completely. H_2O (25 mL) was added and the reaction mixture was neutralized with $NaHCO_3$. Subsequently, brine was added and the mixture was extracted with $CHCl_3$. The organic layer was dried (Na_2SO_4) and concentrated under reduced pressure; the residue was supported on silica and purified by fc (d = 8 cm, l = 12 cm, cyclohexane/EtOAc 50:50, R_f 0.27). Pale yellow solid, mp = 230°C, yield 3.34 g (54%). ^{1}H NMR ($CDCl_3$): δ (ppm) = 4.13 (t, J = 5.3 Hz, 2H), 4.55 (t, J = 5,3 Hz, 2H), 7.38 (t, J = 8.0 Hz, 1H), 7.51 to 7.60 (m, 3H), 8.13 (d, J = 7.5 Hz, 1H), 8.39 (dd, J = 8.9/2.0 Hz, 1H), 9.03 (d, J = 2.2 Hz, 1H); ^{13}C NMR (DMSO-d_6): δ (ppm) = 39.4, 59.6, 110.2, 110.9, 117.3 (2C), 120.7, 121.3, 122.0, 122.3, 127.4, 139.9, 141.8, 144.1; exact mass (APCI): m/z = calculated for $C_{14}H_{12}N_2O_3Na$ 279.0740, found 279.0740.

2-(3-Amino-9H-carbazol-9-yl)ethanol-hydrochloride (26-HCl)

3-Nitro-9-(hydroxyethyl)carbazole (**24**, 500 mg, 1.95 mmol, 1.0 eq.) was dissolved in THF (10 mL/100 mg) and Pd/C (100 mg) was added. The reaction mixture was stirred for 24 h at rt under H_2 (balloon). The catalyst was removed by filtration over Celite® and the filtrate was concentrated under reduced pressure. The residue was dissolved in diethyl ether. Under N_2, HCl-Et_2O (2 mol/L, 2 mL, 4 mmol, 2.0 eq.) was added drop wise under vigorous stirring to produce the respective HCl salt. The precipitate was filtered, washed with cold MeOH, and used without further purification. R_f 0.35 (cyclohexane/ethyl acetate 30:70). Colorless solid with mp = 230°C, yield 492 mg (96%). ^{1}H NMR (**26**-HCl, DMSO-d_6): δ (ppm) = 3.78 (t, J = 5.5 Hz, 2H), 4.47 (t, J = 5.5 Hz, 2H), 7.24 (t, J = 7.4 Hz, 1H), 7.45 (dd, J = 8.7/2.1 Hz, 1H), 7.50 (t, J = 7,7 Hz, 1H), 7.66 (d, J = 8.3 Hz, 1H), 7.74 (d, J = 8.7 Hz, 1H), 8.12 (d, J = 2.1 Hz, 1H), 8.18 (d, J = 7.7 Hz, 1H), 10.4 (s, 3H); ^{13}C NMR (**26**-HCl, DMSO-d_6): δ (ppm) = 45.5, 59.7, 110.2, 110.8, 114.8, 119.3, 120.6, 121.5, 122.3, 122.8, 126.7 (2C), 139.7, 141.2; exact mass (APCI): m/z = calculated for $C_{14}H_{15}N_2O$ 217.1179, found 217.1179.

3-[3-(2-Bromo-4-fluorophenyl)-1,2,4-oxadiazol-5-yl]-N-[9-(2-hydroxyethyl)-9H-carbazol-3-yl]propanamide (14)

Compound **10** (400 mg, 1.3 mmol 1 eq.) was treated with COMU® (652 mg, 1.5 mmol 1.2 eq.) and triethylamine (0.54 mL, 3.9 mmol, 3.3 eq.) in DMF (15 mL) for 30 min at rt. The reaction mixture was cooled down to 0°C, and a solution of the 3-aminocarbazole hydrochloride **26** (222 mg, 0.9 mmol, 1.0 eq.) in DMF was added dropwise. The mixture was stirred for 24 h at <10°C. Then, H_2O and brine were added, the mixture was extracted with $CHCl_3$, the combined organic layers were dried (Na_2SO_4) and concentrated *in vacuo*, and the residue was purified by fc (d = 5 cm, l = 15 cm, cyclohexane/EtOAc 15:85, R_f 0.51 (EtOAc)). Colorless solid, mp = 164°C, yield 368 mg (80%). Purity (HPLC), 97.7% (t_R = 20.24 min). ^{1}H NMR (DMSO-d_6): δ (ppm) = 2.99 (t, J = 7.0 Hz, 2H), 3.35 (t, J = 7.1 Hz, 2H), 3.76 (q, J = 5.6 Hz, 2H), 4.40 (t, J = 5.5 Hz, 2H), 4.86 (t, J = 5.4 Hz, 1H), 7.15 (t, J = 7.4 Hz, 1H), 7.41 (t, J = 6.5 Hz, 1H), 7.46 (td, J = 8.5/2.6 Hz, 1H), 7.51 (dd, J = 8.8/1.7 Hz, 1H), 7.54 (d, J = 8.8 Hz, 1H,), 7.57 (d, J = 8.3 Hz, 1H), 7.83 (dd, J = 8.6/2.6 Hz, 1H), 7.89 (dd, J = 8.7/6.1 Hz, 1H), 8.02 (d, J = 7.8 Hz, 1H), 8.39 (s, 1H), 10.13 (s, 1H); ^{13}C NMR (DMSO-d_6): δ (ppm) = 21, 32.0, 45.3, 59.6, 109.5, 109.7, 110.9, 115.5 (d, J = 21.6 Hz,1C), 118.5, 118.7, 120.0, 121.4 (d, J = 24.9 Hz, 1C), 121.7, 122.0, 122.2 (d, J = 10.1 Hz, 1C), 124.5 (d, J = 3.4 Hz,1C), 125.6, 131.0, 133.6 (d, J = 9.3 Hz, 1C), 137.0, 140.9, 162.9 (d, J = 253.4 Hz, 1C), 166.4, 168.5, 179.6; exact mass (ESI): m/z = calculated for $C_{25}H_{20}{}^{79}BrFN_4O_3H$ 523.0776, found 523.0783.

3-[3-(2-Bromo-4-fluorophenyl)-1,2,4-oxadiazol-5-yl]-N-(9-ethyl-9H-carbazol-3-yl)propanamide (2)

The synthesis of **2** is described in [29].

3-[3-(2-Bromo-4-fluorophenyl)-1,2,4-oxadiazol-5-yl]-N-[9-(2-fluoroethyl)-9H-carbazol-3-yl]propanamide (1)

Under N_2, XtalFluor-E® (263 mg, 1.2 mmol, 1.5 eq.) was suspended in CH_2Cl_2 (15 mL). Triethylamine trihydrofluoride (NEt_3-3HF) (0.2 mL, 1.2 mmol, 1.5 eq.) and a solution of **14** (400 mg, 0.8 mmol, 1 eq.) in CH_2Cl_2 (20 mL) were added to the suspension via cannula at −78°C. The resulting mixture was warmed up to rt within 3 h. An aqueous solution of Na_2CO_3 (5% m/m) was added, and the reaction mixture was stirred for 15 min at rt. After the addition of brine, the mixture was extracted with CH_2Cl_2, the organic layer was dried (Na_2SO_4) and concentrated *in vacuo*, and the residue was purified by fc (d = 6 cm, l = 15 cm, cyclohexane/EtOAc 20:80, R_f = 0.53 (EtOAc)). The product (**1**) was recrystallized from ethyl acetate yielding 82 mg of colorless solid (yield 20%) with mp of 201°C. Purity (HPLC), 96.7% (t_R = 21.46 min). ^{1}H NMR ($CDCl_3$): δ (ppm) = 2.97 (t, J = 7.0 Hz, 2H), 3.39 (t, J = 7.0 Hz, 2H), 4.51 (dt, J = 24.2/5.1 Hz, 2H), 4.72 (dt, J = 46.8/5.1 Hz, 2H), 7.03 to 7.09 (m, 1H), 7.16 (t, J = 7.0 Hz, 1H), 7.27 (d, J = 8.6 Hz, 1H), 7.32 (d, J = 8.2 Hz, 2H), 7.36 to 7.43 (m, 3H), 7.56 (s, 1H), 7.76 (dd, J = 8.7/6.0 Hz, 1H), 7.97 (d, J = 7.8 Hz, 1H), 8.41 (d, J = 1.8 Hz); ^{13}C NMR (DMSO-d_6): δ (ppm) = 21.8, 32.0, 42.9 (d, J = 19.7 Hz), 82.6 (d, J = 167.9 Hz), 109.5, 109.6, 110.9, 115.5 (d, J = 21.7 Hz), 118.8, 118.9, 120.0, 121.4 (d, J = 25.1 Hz), 121.9, 122.1, 122.2 (d, J = 9.9 Hz), 124.5 (d, J = 3.4 Hz), 125.8, 131.4, 133.6 (d, J = 9.3 Hz), 136.7, 140.6, 162.9 (d, J = 253.2 Hz), 166.4, 168.5, 179.6; HRMS (APCI): m/z = calculated for $C_{25}H_{19}{}^{79}BrF_2N_4O_2H$ 525.0732, found 525.0757.

[2-(3-{3-[3-(2-Bromo-4-fluorophenyl)-1,2,4-oxadiazol-5-yl] propanamido}-9H-carbazol-9-yl)ethyl] 4-methylbenzenesulfonate (15)

Under N_2, compound **14** (250 mg, 0.5 mmol, 1 eq.), 4-dimethylaminopyridine (17.5 mg, 0.15 mmol, 0.3 eq.), and triethylamine (0.25 mL, 1.8 mmol, 3.6 eq.) were dissolved in THF (20 mL) and cooled down to 0°C. A solution of p-toluenesulfonyl chloride (183 mg, 1.0 mmol, 2 eq.) in THF (10 mL) was added dropwise. After 20 min, the mixture was warmed up to rt and stirred for 48 h. Subsequently, 1 M aq. NaOH (3 mL) was added and the layers were separated. The aqueous layer was extracted with CH_2Cl_2 and the organic layer was washed with brine. The combined organic layers were dried (Na_2SO_4) and concentrated *in vacuo*, and the residue was purified by fc (d = 5 cm, l = 10 cm, cyclohexane/EtOAc 40:60, R_f = 0.34 (cyclohexane/EtOAc 50:50)). The product (**15**) was recrystallized from CH_2Cl_2 yielding 197 mg (colorless solid, mp = 136°C, yield 61%). Purity

(HPLC), 96.2% (t_R = 22.85 min). ^{1}H NMR ($CDCl_3$): δ (ppm) = 2.24 (s, 3H), 3.04 (t, J = 7.0 Hz, 2H), 3.47 (t, J = 7.0 Hz, 2H), 4.38 (t, J = 5.4 Hz, 2H), 4.49 (t, J = 5.3 Hz, 2H), 6.85 (d, J = 8.0 Hz, 2H), 7.15 (t, J = 7.4 Hz, 1H), 7.17 to 7.23 (m, 5H), 7.33 (dd, J = 8.7/1.9 Hz, 1H), 7.39 (t, J = 8.1 Hz, 1H), 7.46 (dd, J = 8.2/2.4 Hz, 1H), 7.74 (s, 1H), 7.83 (dd, J = 8.7/6.0 Hz, 1H), 7.94 (d, J = 7.8 Hz, 1H), 8.31 (d, J = 1.7 Hz, 1H); ^{13}C NMR (DMSO-d_6): δ (ppm) = 21.0, 21.8, 32.0, 41.3, 68.8, 109.2, 109.3, 110.8, 115.5 (d, J = 21.1 Hz, 1C), 118.5, 118.8, 119.9, 121.4 (d, J = 24.9 Hz, 1C), 122.0, 122.1 (d, J = 9.9 Hz, 1C), 122.2, 124.5 (d, J = 3.3 Hz, 1C), 125.7, 126.6 (2C), 129.5 (2C), 131.0, 131.3, 133.6 (d, J = 9.2 Hz, 1C), 136.3, 140.3, 144.4, 162.9 (d, J = 253.5 Hz, 1C), 166.6, 168.5, 179.7; HRMS (APCI): m/z = calculated for $C_{32}H_{26}^{79}BrFN_4O_5SH$ 677.0864, found 677.0858.

Methyl-3-(3-(2-bromo-4-nitrophenyl)-1,2,4-oxadiazol-5-yl) propanoate (21)

At −10°C, $SOCl_2$ (71 µL, 0.77 mmol, 3.3 eq.) was dissolved in 0.5 mL MeOH and stirred for 10 min. Acid **9** (100 mg, 0.29 mmol, 1 eq.) was then added and the reaction was allowed to reach room temperature within 1 h. The reaction was stirred further for 1 h at rt and quenched by the addition of 5 mL saturated aq. $NaHCO_3$ solution, and the product was extracted with EtOAc (three times with 5 mL). Evaporation of the solvent afforded **21** in a quantitative manner (104 mg, 0.29 mmol). ^{1}H NMR (400 MHz, $CDCl_3$): δ (ppm) = 8.59 (d, J = 2.2 Hz, 1H), 8.26 (dd, J = 8.6, 2.2 Hz, 1H), 8.06 (d, J = 8.6 Hz, 1H), 3.73 (s, 3H), 3.32 (t, J = 7.2 Hz, 2H), 2.97 (t, J = 7.2 Hz, 2H); ^{13}C NMR (100 MHz, $CDCl_3$): δ (ppm) = 178.8, 171.6, 166.7, 149.0, 134.1, 132.8, 129.4, 122.8, 122.2, 52.3, 30.2, 22.1; MS (ESI+): m/z (%) = 356/358 (100/100) [M+H]$^+$.

Methyl-3-(3-(4-amino-2-bromophenyl)-1,2,4-oxadiazol-5-yl) propanoate (16)

To a solution of **21** (50 mg, 0.13 mmol, 1 eq.) in 2 mL EtOH, $SnCl_2$-$2H_2O$ (149 mg, 0.66 mmol, 5 eq.) was added and the reaction was stirred for 2 h at rt. Saturated aq. $NaHCO_3$ solution (5 mL) was added, and the mixture was extracted with EtOAc. The organic phase was dried over sodium sulfate and filtered. Upon solvent evaporation under reduced pressure, amine **16** was obtained as a brown solid (45 mg, 0.13 mmol, quant). ^{1}H NMR (400 MHz, DMSO-d_6): δ (ppm) = 7.45 (d, J = 8.5 Hz, 1H), 6.92 (d, J = 2.2 Hz, 1H), 6.64 (dd, J = 8.5, 2.2 Hz, 1H), 3.55 (s, 4H), 3.13 (dd, J = 7.6, 5.9 Hz, 2H), 2.93 – 2.74 (m, 2H); ^{13}C NMR (100 MHz, DMSO-d_6): δ (ppm) = 178.6, 172.8, 167.7, 152.5, 133.2, 122.4, 118.7, 114.1, 113.6, 52.4, 30.2, 22.0; MS (ESI+): m/z (%) = 348/350 (100/100) [M+Na]$^+$.

Methyl-3-(3-(2-bromo-4-(dimethylamino)phenyl)-1,2,4-oxadiazol-5-yl)propanoate (22)

Compound **22** was synthesized as described for **20** from **16** in 52% yield as a brown solid. ^{1}H NMR (300 MHz, $CDCl_3$): δ (ppm) = 7.75 (d, J = 8.8 Hz, 1H), 7.00 (d, J = 2.6 Hz, 1H), 6.70 (dd, J = 8.9, 2.6 Hz, 1H), 3.72 (s, 3H), 3.25 (t, J = 7.4 Hz, 2H), 3.01 (s, 6H), 2.93 (t, J = 7.4 Hz, 2H); ^{13}C NMR (75 MHz, $CDCl_3$): δ (ppm) = 177.2, 171.9, 168.0, 152.0, 132.7, 123.1, 117.2, 115.2, 111.0, 52.3 (2C), 40.4, 30.5, 22.2; MS (ESI+): m/z (%) = 360/362 (100/100) [M+Na]$^+$.

3-Bromo-4-(5-(3-methoxy-3-oxopropyl)-1,2,4-oxadiazol-3-yl)-N,N,N-trimethylbenzenaminium iodide (18)

Compound **18** was synthesized as described for **13** from **22** in 90% yield as a brown solid (mp = 119°C). ^{1}H NMR (300 MHz, CD_3CN): δ (ppm) = 8.29 (d, J = 2.6 Hz, 1H), 8.04 (d, J = 8.8 Hz, 1H), 7.98 (dd, J = 8.9, 2.7 Hz, 1H), 3.68 (s, 3H), 3.63 (s, 9H), 3.29 (t, J = 6.9 Hz, 2H), 2.94 (t, J = 6.9 Hz, 2H); ^{13}C NMR (75 MHz, CD_3CN): δ (ppm) = 181.1, 173.4, 168.0, 134.7, 132.1, 128.2, 124.4, 121.8, 118.8, 58.8 (3C), 53.1, 31.3, 23.3; HRMS (ESI+): m/z (%) = 368.0616/370.0615 (100/100) [M]$^+$.

Methyl-3-(3-(2-bromo-4-fluorophenyl)-1,2,4-oxadiazol-5-yl) propanoate (17)

Compound **17** was synthesized as described for **21** from **10** in a quantitative manner as a colorless solid (mp = 39°C). ^{1}H NMR (400 MHz, $CDCl_3$): δ (ppm) = 7.84 (dd, J = 8.7, 6.0 Hz, 1H), 7.47 (dd, J = 8.3, 2.5 Hz, 1H), 7.14 (ddd, J = 8.7, 7.7, 2.6 Hz, 1H), 3.73 (s, 3H), 3.29 (t, J = 7.3 Hz, 2H), 2.94 (t, J = 7.3 Hz, 2H); ^{13}C NMR (100 MHz, $CDCl_3$): δ (ppm) = 178.1, 171.7, 167.3, 164.7, 162.2, 133.4 (d, J = 9.1 Hz), 122.9 (d, J = 9.9 Hz), 121.7 (d, J = 24.7 Hz), 115.0 (d, J = 21.4 Hz), 52.2, 30.3, 22.1; ^{19}F NMR (376 MHz, $CDCl_3$): δ (ppm) = −108.0 (dd, J = 14.1, 7.9 Hz); MS (ESI+): m/z (%) = 351/353 (100/100) [M+Na]$^+$.

Radiochemistry

No-carrier-added [^{18}F]fluoride ($t_{1/2}$ = 109.8 min) was produced via the [^{18}O(p,n)^{18}F] nuclear reaction by irradiation of a [^{18}O]H_2O target (Hyox 18 enriched water, Rotem Industries Ltd, Israel) on a Cyclone®18/9 (iba RadioPharma Solutions, Belgium) with a fixed energy proton beam using Nirta® [^{18}F]fluoride XL target. Aqueous [^{18}F]fluoride was dried by azeotropic distillation using MeCN in the presence of K_2CO_3 (1.78 mg, 12.9 mmol) and Kryptofix 2.2.2 ($K_{2.2.2}$, 11.2 mg, 29.7 mmol), resulting in the reactive anhydrous K[^{18}F]F-$K_{2.2.2}$-carbonate complex. Optimization of the aliphatic and aromatic radiolabellings of tosylate **15** and trimethylammonium salt **13**, respectively, were performed by varying the amount of precursor for radiolabelling and reaction time under thermal heating

(82°C) in MeCN (Scheme 1). Under optimized conditions, the reaction mixtures of [^{18}F]**1** and [^{18}F]**2** were diluted with water and directly applied to an isocratic semi-preparative RP-HPLC for isolation of the desired radiotracers (see 'Experimental' section). The collected fractions were analyzed by radio-TLC, and those with the highest radiochemical purity were combined, diluted with water, passed through a Sep-Pak C18 light cartridge (Waters, Milford, MA, USA), and eluted with 0.6 mL of diethyl ether (DEE). The elution of [^{18}F]**1** and [^{18}F]**2** was performed in polypropylene vials containing 75 to 100 μL of EtOH. For biological investigations, the solvent was evaporated to dryness under a gentle argon stream, and the desired radiotracers were formulated in a sterile isotonic solution containing 10% EtOH (*v*/*v*). The identities of [^{18}F]**1** and [^{18}F]**2** were verified by radio-HPLC of samples of the respective radiotracer spiked with the non-radioactive reference compound. Radiochemical and chemical purities were assessed by radio-TLC and analytical HPLC. Specific activities were calculated using the HPLC method described in [43]. For evaluation of radiometabolites, the radiosynthesis of the trimethylammonium salt **18** to afford [^{18}F]**17** was performed following the same conditions as above stated for [^{18}F]**1** and [^{18}F]**2** (Scheme 5).

Determination of lipophilicity (logD) and stability

The distribution coefficients of [^{18}F]**1** and [^{18}F]**2** were also calculated from RP-HPLC retention times in three different systems: (1) isocratic elution (60% MeCN/20 mM NH_4OAc at a flow rate of 1 mL/min) and (2) gradient elution (starting from 10% MeCN/20 mM NH_4OAc aq. for 10 min with a gradient to 90% MeCN/20 mM NH_4OAc aq. over 30 min at a flow rate of 1 mL/min) on a Reprosil-Pur C18-AQ column (5 μm, 250 × 4.6 mm, Dr. Maisch HPLC GmbH, Ammerbruch-Entringen, Germany), and (3) isocratic elution (52.5% MeCN/20 mM NH_4OAc at a flow rate of 1 mL/min) on a Prodigy 5 μm C8 (250 × 4 mm; Phenomenex Ltd, Aschaffenburg, Germany) using the reference compounds following the protocol according to the EU guideline 67/548/EWG [44].

In vitro radiochemical stabilities of [^{18}F]**1** and [^{18}F]**2** were investigated in 0.9% NaCl solution, Dulbecco's phosphate buffer, 0.01 M Tris–HCl (pH 7.4 at 21°C), and EtOH at 40°C for 90 min. Samples were taken at 15, 30, 60, and 90 min after incubation and analyzed by radio-TLC and radio-HPLC.

In vitro CB receptor affinity assay

For binding experiments, Chinese hamster ovary (CHO) cell lines stably transfected with human CB_1R human and CB_2R were used according to the procedures previously described [29]. Briefly, displacement of CB_1R/CB_2R-specific radioligand [^{3}H]CP55,940 (6,438 GBq/mmol; PerkinElmer Life and Analytical Sciences GmbH, Rodgau, Germany; working concentration, 0.2 to 0.5 nM) by test compounds in the range of 0.1 nM to 10 μ was assessed, and IC_{50} values were estimated by non-linear regression (GraphPad Prism; version 3.0, GraphPad Software, Inc., San Diego, CA, USA). K_D values of 2.4 and 1.5 nM were previously determined for [^{3}H]CP55,940 binding to hCB_1R and hCB_2R, respectively, and used for calculation of K_i values of the test compounds according to Cheng et al. [45]. The binding experiments were performed in triplicates, and data were given as mean values from independent experiments.

Ex vivo biodistribution studies

Animals for *in vivo* studies were obtained from the Medizinisch-Experimentelles Zentrum, Universität Leipzig. All procedures that include animals were approved by the respective State Animal Care and Use Committee and conducted in accordance with the German Law for the Protection of Animal.

Female CD1 mice (10 to 12 weeks old, 20 to 25 g) received an injection of 300 to 400 kBq of [^{18}F]**1** or [^{18}F]**2** with specific activities of >450 GBq/μmol in 200 μL of 0.9% NaCl/10% EtOH into the tail vein. The animals were anesthetized (CO_2/O_2 mixture) for blood and urine sampling and euthanized by luxation of the cervical spine at 5, 30, and 60 min after injection (p.i.) (n = 2 to 5 per time). The organs of interest were removed and weighed, and the activities were measured by γ counting using a calibrated γ counter Wallac Wizard 1470 (Perkin Elmer Inc., Waltham, MA, USA). The percentage of injected dose per gram of wet tissue (% ID/g wet weight) was calculated.

To verify the specificity of [^{18}F]**1** and [^{18}F]**2** towards CB_2R, blocking experiments were performed with pre-administration of the highly selective CB_2R inverse agonist SR144528 [46] (3 mg/kg i.p. in 0.9% saline, 10 min before the injection of the radiotracer) at 60 min p.i. (n = 2 to 5). The unpaired two-tailed t test was used to compare the results between the groups. We considered differences to be significant at a p value <0.05.

Ex vivo metabolite studies

[^{18}F]**1** and [^{18}F]**2** (100 to 150 MBq, 250 to 450 GBq/μmol in 150 μL NaCl 0.9%/10% EtOH) were injected via the tail vein in CD1 male mice (10 to 12 weeks old, 20 to 25 g). Blood and urine samples were obtained at 30 and 60 min p.i. (n = 3 per time point). Twofold extractions of plasma and brain samples (n = 3) were performed using ice-cold MeCN according to the standard protocol established in our group (see [47,48]). Briefly, plasma samples were obtained by centrifugation of the blood at 4,000×g at 4°C for 10 min, and brain samples were homogenized in ice-cold 50 mM Tris–HCl (pH = 7.4). The samples were vortexed, incubated on ice, and centrifuged at 10,000×*g* for 3 min. Supernatants were collected, and the precipitates were re-dissolved in ice-cold MeCN for the second extraction. The supernatants from the two extractions were combined, concentrated under a gentle argon stream at 65°C, and analyzed by radio-TLC and gradient analytical HPLC (see 'Radiochemistry' section). Aliquots from each extraction supernatant and the precipitates were also taken and quantified by γ counting (Wallac Wizard 1470, Perkin Elmer Inc., Waltham, MA, USA) along with the respective aliquots of intact plasma samples and brain homogenates. A moderate recovery of radioactivity was obtained from plasma samples and brain homogenates (60% to 70%). Radiometabolites of $[^{18}F]$**17** in the plasma, spleen, and brain were assessed at 30 and 60 min p.i.

Conclusions

In conclusion, *N*-aryl-oxadiazolyl-propionamides were successfully radiolabelled with ^{18}F at different positions. Fluorine substitution at these positions did not affect affinity and specificity towards CB_2R. However, the radiotracers investigated in this study undergo a fast metabolism *in vivo* with the main radiometabolites crossing the blood–brain barrier. Therefore, structural changes in the enzymatic cleavage sites of the evaluated candidates have to be performed to enhance their potential as CB_2R PET imaging agents for the brain.

Abbreviations

ALS: Amyotrophic lateral sclerosis; CB_1R: Cannabinoid receptor type 1; CB_2R: Cannabinoid receptor type 2; CHO: Chinese hamster ovary; COMU: (1-Cyano-2-ethoxy-2-oxoethylidenaminooxy)dimethylamino-morpholino-carbenium hexafluorophosphate; DCM: Dichloromethane; DEE: Diethyl ether; DIC: *N,N'*-diisopropylcarbodiimide; DMF: Dimethylformamide; EtOAc: Ethyl acetate; fc: Flash chromatography; GPCR: G protein-coupled receptors; ID: Injected dose; IH: Isohexane; MeI: Methyl iodide; mp: Melting point; NCA: No-carrier added; p.i.: Post injection; PET: Positron emission tomography; PFA: Paraformaldehyde; RCY: Radiochemical yields; Succ anh: Succinic anhydride; THF: Tetrahydrofuran; TLC: Thin-layer chromatography; XtalFluor-E: Diethylaminodifluorosulfonium tetrafluoroborate; 4-DMAP: 4-dimethylaminopyridine.

Competing interests

The authors declare that they have no competing interests.

Acknowledgements

This work has been supported by the DFG (project BR 1360/12-1). The authors wish to thank the Institute of Analytical Chemistry of Universität Leipzig, Faculty of Chemistry and Mineralogy for the NMR spectra as well as Juliane Schaller for the technical assistance.

Author details

[1]Department of Neuroradiopharmaceuticals, Institute of Radiopharmaceutical Cancer Research, Research Site Leipzig, Helmholtz-Zentrum Dresden-Rossendorf e.V., Permoserstr 15, 04318 Leipzig, Germany. [2]Department of Pharmaceutical and Medicinal Chemistry, University of Münster, Correnssstraße 58-62, 48149 Münster, Germany.

References

1. Matsuda LA, Lolait SJ, Brownstein MJ, Young AC, Bonner TI (1990) Structure of a cannabinoid receptor and functional expression of the cloned cDNA. Nature 346(6284):561–564
2. Munro S, Thomas KL, Abu-Shaar M (1993) Molecular characterization of a peripheral receptor for cannabinoids. Nature 365(6441):61–65
3. Ryberg E, Larsson N, Sjögren S, Hjorth S, Hermansson N-O, Leonova J, Elebring T, Nilsson K, Drmota T, Greasley PJ (2007) The orphan receptor GPR55 is a novel cannabinoid receptor. Br J Pharmacol 152(7):1092–1101
4. Ross RA (2009) The enigmatic pharmacology of GPR55. Trends Pharmacol Sci 30(3):156–163
5. Basu S, Dittel BN (2011) Unraveling the complexities of cannabinoid receptor 2 (CB_2) immune regulation in health and disease. Immunol Res 51(1):26–38
6. Fernández-Ruiz J, Romero J, Velasco G, Tolón RM, Ramos JA, Guzmán M (2007) Cannabinoid CB_2 receptor: a new target for controlling neural cell survival? Trends Pharmacol Sci 28(1):39–45
7. Jhaveri MD, Sagar DR, Elmes SJR, Kendall DA, Chapman V (2007) Cannabinoid CB_2 receptor-mediated anti-nociception in models of acute and chronic pain. Mol Neurobiol 36(1):26–35
8. Cheng Y, Hitchcock SA (2007) Targeting cannabinoid agonists for inflammatory and neuropathic pain. Expert Opin Invest Drugs 16(7):951–965
9. Pertwee RG (2009) Emerging strategies for exploiting cannabinoid receptor agonists as medicines. Br J Pharmacol 156(3):397–411
10. Roche M, Finn DP (2010) Brain CB_2 receptors: implications for neuropsychiatric disorders. Pharmaceuticals 3(8):2517–2553
11. Scotter EL, Abood ME, Glass M (2010) The endocannabinoid system as a target for the treatment of neurodegenerative disease. Br J Pharmacol 160(3):480–498
12. Zhang H, Hilton DA, Hanemann CO, Zajicek J (2011) Cannabinoid receptor and N-acyl phosphatidylethanolamine phospholipase D—evidence for altered expression in multiple sclerosis. Brain Pathol 21(5):544–557
13. Yiangou Y, Facer P, Durrenberger P, Chessell IP, Naylor A, Bountra C, Banati RR, Anand P (2006) COX-2, CB_2 and P2X7-immunoreactivities are increased in activated microglial cells/macrophages of multiple sclerosis and amyotrophic lateral sclerosis spinal cord. BMC Neurol 6:12
14. Velasco G, Carracedo A, Blázquez C, Lorente M, Aguado T, Haro A, Sánchez C, Galve-Roperh I, Guzmán M (2007) Cannabinoids and gliomas. Mol Neurobiol 36(1):60–67
15. Hermanson DJ, Marnett LJ (2011) Cannabinoids, endocannabinoids, and cancer. Cancer Metast Rev 30(3–4):599–612
16. Alexander A, Smith PF, Rosengren RJ (2009) Cannabinoids in the treatment of cancer. Cancer Lett 285(1):6–12
17. Cudaback E, Marrs W, Moeller T, Stella N (2010) The expression level of CB_1 and CB_2 receptors determines their efficacy at inducing apoptosis in astrocytomas. PLoS ONE 5(1):e8702
18. Atwood BK, Mackie K (2010) CB_2: a cannabinoid receptor with an identity crisis. Br J Pharmacol 160(3):467–479
19. Onaivi ES, Ishiguro H, Gu S, Liu QR (2012) CNS effects of CB_2 cannabinoid receptors: beyond neuro-immuno-cannabinoid activity. J Psychopharmacol 26(1):92–103
20. Evens N, Bormans GM (2010) Non-invasive imaging of the type 2 cannabinoid receptor, focus on positron emission tomography. Curr Top Med Chem 10(15):1527–1543
21. Thakur GA, Tichkule R, Bajaj S, Makriyannis A (2009) Latest advances in cannabinoid receptor agonists. Expert Opin Ther Pat 19(12):1647–1673
22. Pertwee RG, Howlett AC, Abood ME, Alexander SPH, Di Marzo V, Elphick MR, Greasley PJ, Hans-Jürgen KG, Mackie K, Mechoulam R, Ross RA (2010) International union of basic and clinical pharmacology. LXXIX. Cannabinoid receptors and their ligands: beyond CB_1 and CB_2. Pharmacol Rev 62(4):588–631

23. Turkman N, Shavrin A, Paolillo V, Yeh HH, Flores L, Soghomonian S, Rabinovich B, Volgin A, Gelovani J, Alauddin M (2012) Synthesis and preliminary evaluation of [^{18}F]-labeled 2-oxoquinoline derivatives for PET imaging of cannabinoid CB_2 receptor. Nucl Med Biol 39(4):593–600
24. Horti AG, Fan H, Kuwabara H, Hilton J, Ravert HT, Holt DP, Alexander M, Kumar A, Rahmim A, Scheffel U, Wong DF, Dannals RF (2006) ^{11}C-JHU75528: a radiotracer for PET imaging of CB1 cannabinoid receptors. J Nucl Med 47(10):1689–1696
25. Horti AG, Gao Y, Ravert HT, Finley P, Valentine H, Wong DF, Endres CJ, Savonenko AV, Dannals RF (2010) Synthesis and biodistribution of [^{11}C]A-836339, a new potential radioligand for PET imaging of cannabinoid type 2 receptors (CB_2). Bioorg Med Chem 18(14):5202–5207
26. Gao M, Wang M, Miller KD, Hutchins GD, Zheng Q-H (2010) Synthesis and in vitro biological evaluation of carbon-11-labeled quinoline derivatives as new candidate PET radioligands for cannabinoid CB_2 receptor imaging. Bioorg Med Chem 18(6):2099–2106
27. Evens N, Bosier B, Lavey BJ, Kozlowski JA, Vermaelen P, Baudemprez L, Busson R, Lambert DM, Van Laere K, Verbruggen AM, Bormans GM (2008) Labelling and biological evaluation of [^{11}C]methoxy-Sch225336: a radioligand for the cannabinoid-type 2 receptor. Nucl Med Biol 35(7):793–800
28. Schou M, Varnäs K, Jucaite A, Gulyás B, Halldin C, Farde L (2013) Radiolabeling of the cannabinoid receptor agonist AZD1940 with carbon-11 and PET microdosing in non-human primate. Nucl Med Biol 40(3):410–414
29. Rühl T, Deuther-Conrad W, Fischer S, Günther R, Hennig L, Krautscheid H, Brust P (2012) Cannabinoid receptor type 2 (CB2)-selective *N*-aryl-oxadiazolyl-propionamides: synthesis, radiolabelling, molecular modelling and biological evaluation. Org Med Chem Lett 2(1):32
30. Mu L, Bieri D, Slavik R, Drandarov K, Müller A, Čermak S, Weber M, Schibli R, Krämer SD, Ametamey SM (2013) Radiolabeling and *in vitro/in vivo* evaluation of *N*-(1-adamantyl)-8-methoxy-4-oxo-1-phenyl-1,4-dihydroquinoline-3-carboxamide as a PET probe for imaging cannabinoid type 2 receptor. J Neurochem 126(5):616–624
31. Ahmad R, Koole M, Evens N, Serdons K, Verbruggen AM, Bormans GM, Laere K (2013) Whole-body biodistribution and radiation dosimetry of the cannabinoid type 2 receptor ligand [^{11}C]-NE40 in healthy subjects. Mol Imaging Biol 15(4):384–390
32. Pike VW (2009) PET radiotracers: crossing the blood–brain barrier and surviving metabolism. Trends Pharmacol Sci 30(8):431–440
33. Monagle JJ (1962) Carbodiimides. III. Conversion of isocyanates to carbodiimides. Catalyst studies. J Org Chem 27(11):3851–3855
34. Fischer S, Hiller A, Smits R, Hoepping A, Funke U, Wenzel B, Cumming P, Sabri O, Steinbach J, Brust P (2013) Radiosynthesis of racemic and enantiomerically pure (−)-[^{18}F]flubatine—a promising PET radiotracer for neuroimaging of $\alpha_4\beta_2$ nicotinic acetylcholine receptors. Appl Radiat Isot 74:128–136
35. Abdel-Magid AF, Carson KG, Harris BD, Maryanoff CA, Shah RD (1996) Reductive amination of aldehydes and ketones with sodium triacetoxyborohydride. Studies on direct and indirect reductive amination procedures. J Org Chem 61(11):3849–3862
36. Löhr H-G, Josel H-P, Engel A, Vögtle F, Schuh W, Puff H (1984) Inclusion compounds of organic onium salts, IV: organyl ammonium hosts as versatile clathrate formers. Ber Dtsch Chem Ges 117(4):1487–1496
37. Shufen Z, Danhong Z, Jinzong Y (1995) Nitration of carbazole and *N*-alkylcarbazoles. Dyes Pigments 27(4):287–296
38. Sandmeyer T (1884) Ueber die ersetzung der amid-gruppe durch chlor, brom und cyan in den aromatischen substanzen. Ber Dtsch Chem Ges 17(2):2650–2653
39. Nolting DD, Nickels ML, Guo N, Pham W (2012) Molecular imaging probe development: a chemistry perspective. Am J Nucl Med Mol Imaging 2 (3):273–306
40. Cheng Y, Albrecht BK, Brown J, Buchanan JL, Buckner WH, DiMauro EF, Emkey R, Fremeau RT, Harmange J-C, Hoffman BJ, Huang L, Huang M, Lee JH, Lin F-F, Martin MW, Nguyen HQ, Patel VF, Tomlinson SA, White RD, Xia X, Hitchcock SA (2008) Discovery and optimization of a novel series of *N*-arylamide oxadiazoles as potent, highly selective and orally bioavailable cannabinoid receptor 2 (CB_2) agonists. J Med Chem 51(16):5019–5034
41. Lin JH, Lu AY (1997) Role of pharmacokinetics and metabolism in drug discovery and development. Pharmacol Rev 49(4):403–449
42. Huttunen KM, Raunio H, Rautio J (2011) Prodrugs—from serendipity to rational design. Pharmacol Rev 63(3):750–771
43. Wester H-J (2011) Pharmaceutical radiochemistry (I). SCINTOMICS, Fürstenfeldbruck
44. OECD (2004) Test No. 117: partition coefficient (n-octanol/water), HPLC method. OECD guidelines for the testing of chemicals, section 1: physical-chemical properties. doi: 10.1787/9789264069824-en
45. Cheng Y, Prusoff WH (1973) Relationship between the inhibition constant (K_i) and the concentration of inhibitor which causes 50 per cent inhibition (IC_{50}) of an enzymatic reaction. Biochem Pharmacol 22(23):3099–3108
46. Rinaldi-Carmona M, Barth F, Millan J, Derocq JM, Casellas P, Congy C, Oustric D, Sarran M, Bouaboula M, Calandra B, Portier M, Shire D, Brelière JC, Le Fur GL (1998) SR 144528, the first potent and selective antagonist of the CB_2 cannabinoid receptor. J Pharmacol Exp Ther 284(2):644–650
47. Fischer S, Wiese C, Maestrup EG, Hiller A, Deuther-Conrad W, Scheunemann M, Schepmann D, Steinbach J, Wuensch B, Brust P (2011) Molecular imaging of σ receptors: synthesis and evaluation of the potent σ_1 selective radioligand [^{18}F]fluspidine. Eur J Nucl Med Mol Imaging 38(3):540–551
48. Rötering S, Scheunemann M, Fischer S, Hiller A, Peters D, Deuther-Conrad W, Brust P (2013) Radiosynthesis and first evaluation in mice of [^{18}F] NS14490 for molecular imaging of a7 nicotinic acetylcholine receptors. Bioorg Med Chem 21(9):2635–2642

Discovery of indole tetrafluorophenoxymethylketone-based potent novel small molecule inhibitors of caspase-3

Dodheri Syed Samiulla[1*], Andra Naidu[2], Gummadi Venkateshwar Rao[1] and Murali Ramachandra[1]

Abstract

Background: Caspase-3 inhibition has been demonstrated to be therapeutically effective in moderating excessive programmed cell death. Interest in caspase-3 as a therapeutic target has led many to pursue the development of inhibitors. To date, only a few series of non-peptide inhibitors have been described, and these have limitations on their drug-like properties.

Methods: Here, we report the screening of 70 novel small molecules against the caspase-3 enzyme which belongs to four different series (indole fluoromethylketone, indole difluoro and tetrafluorophenoxymethylketone, and oxalamide). Selected molecules were subjected for counter-screening, cell-based, ADME/PK assays in order to understand the potency and drug-like properties.

Results: The screening yielded series of hits with IC_{50} values ranging from 0.11 to 10 μM with reasonable SAR, irreversible mode of inhibition, and reasonable selectivity against other proteases including caspase-1, cathepsin B and D, and thrombin. On the basis of *in vitro* profile, the selected molecules were evaluated for their drug-like properties. Among the compounds evaluated, compound **3D** exhibited good solubility, low permeability, interaction with efflux pump, and low potential for CYP450 drug-drug interaction. After intravenous administration, compound *3D* showed low clearance (588 ml/hr/kg), medium volume of distribution, and good oral bioavailability (90%).

Conclusions: These results support further advancement of compound **3D** in different apoptotic models to develop as a new anti-apoptotic agent in relevant disease conditions.

Keywords: Caspase-3, Small molecule, Apoptosis, Inhibition

Background

Apoptosis or programmed cell death is a critical cellular process in normal development and homeostasis of multicellular organisms. Cells undergo apoptosis in response to a variety of stimuli, and during apoptosis, they do so in a controlled, regulated fashion [1]. A major biochemical pathway involved in the apoptosis includes a family of proteases, known as caspases, which act in a cascade to activate downstream caspases responsible for breakdown or cleavage of key cellular substrates required for normal cellular fashion, including structural proteins in the cytoskeleton and nuclear proteins such as DNA repair enzymes [2,3].

Caspases are found practically in all organisms from *Caenorhabditis elegans* to humans. At least 12 of the caspases have been identified (caspases 1 through 10, 13, and 14). Caspases share similarities in amino acid sequence, structure, and substrate specificity, and are subdivided in to two subfamilies based on their functionality: caspases involved in inflammation (caspases 1, 4, 5, 11, 12, 13, and 14) and apoptosis-related caspases (caspases 2, 3, 6, 7, 8, 9, and 10). Among the identified caspases, activation of caspase-3 is a key event integrating upstream signals into final execution of cell death [4].

Abnormally high amounts of apoptosis have been reported in several liver diseases, including alcoholic hepatitis, transplantation, Wilson's disease, and viral

* Correspondence: samiulla_d@aurigene.com
[1]DMPK Department, Aurigene Discovery Technologies Limited, Electronic City Phase 2, Hosur Road, Bangalore 560100, India
Full list of author information is available at the end of the article

hepatitis [5,6]. Several reports demonstrated that inhibition of caspases protect the liver from apoptosis-associated liver injury in preclinical models. Prototypical caspase inhibitors such as ZVAD-FMK have been shown to be efficacious in many animal models, including α-Fas- and TNF-mediated liver injury [7]. More recently, other caspase inhibitors have been shown to be efficacious in rodent models of liver disease [6] (Figure 1). Efficacy with the broad-spectrum caspase inhibitors in preclinical models suggests that they have potential for the treatment of liver diseases in humans. In addition, procaspase-3 concentration is elevated in certain neuroblastomas, lymphomas, leukemias, melanomas, and liver cancer [4]. This makes caspase-3 an interesting therapeutic target, and the search for caspase-3 inhibitors has been an ongoing endeavor by many pharmaceutical companies.

The objective of the present study is to characterize novel small molecule caspase-3 inhibitors with an emphasis on understanding absorption, distribution, metabolism, and excretion (*in vitro* ADME), and *in vivo* pharmacokinetic properties towards achieving desired pharmacodynamic effects and efficacy in preclinical *in vivo* models.

Methods

Reagents

Caspase-3 (C1224), *N*-Acetyl-Asp-Glu-Val-Asp-7-amido-4-methylcoumarin (A1086), cathepsin B (C0150), Boc-Gln-Ala-Arg-7-amido-4-methylcoumarin hydrochloride (B4153), *N*-Acetyl-Tyr-Val-Ala-Asp-7-amido-4-methylcoumarin (A2452), *N*-Acetyl-Tyr-Val-Lys (biotinyl)-Asp 2,6-dimethylbenzoyl-oxymethyl ketone (A4339) were procured from Sigma-Aldrich (St. Louis, MO). Caspase-1 enzyme (BML-AK701) was from Enzo Life Sciences, Inc. (NY, USA). Thrombin enzyme (HT1002a) was procured from Enzyme Research Laboratories (IN, USA). Cathepsin B substrate (Z-Phe-Arg-AMC HCl) was from Bachem AG (Bubendorf, Switzerland) (cat. no.: I-1160). Cathepsin inhibitor II-ALLN (cat. no.: 219426) was from Calbiochem AG (EMD Millipore Corporation, MA, USA). All other reagents were of research grade. IDN6556 was synthesized at Aurigene Discovery Technologies Ltd. (Karnataka, India). Selectivity against caspase-7, 8, and 9, and cathepsin-D were performed using Biomol kit (Enzo Life Sciences, Inc.).

General analytical methods

Fluorescence measurements were done using VICTOR2V 96/384 multilabel plate reader (PerkinElmer Life Sciences, MA, USA) at $\lambda_{ex} = 360$ nm and $\lambda_{em} = 460$ nm top readout (ex, excitation; em, emission) in Corning black 96-well flat bottom plates. The enzyme activity was measured at 30°C after 30 min. Trans-epithelial resistance (TEER) measurements (for monolayer integrity) were made using instrument from World Precision Instrument (Florida, USA). HPLC (1100 series, Agilent Technologies Inc., CA, USA) was performed on reverse phase column (Zorbax Eclipse XDB C18, 150 × 4.6 mm, 5 μm). LC-MS/MS was performed in multiple reaction monitoring mode using Applied Biosystems API 3200 (Chromos, Singapore) coupled to Agilent Technologies 1100 series HPLC on a reverse phase column (Zorbax Eclipse XDB C18, 50 × 4.6 mm, 5 μm).

Compound selection and screening

Focused diversity approach was employed for the synthesis of compounds at Aurigene Discovery Technologies

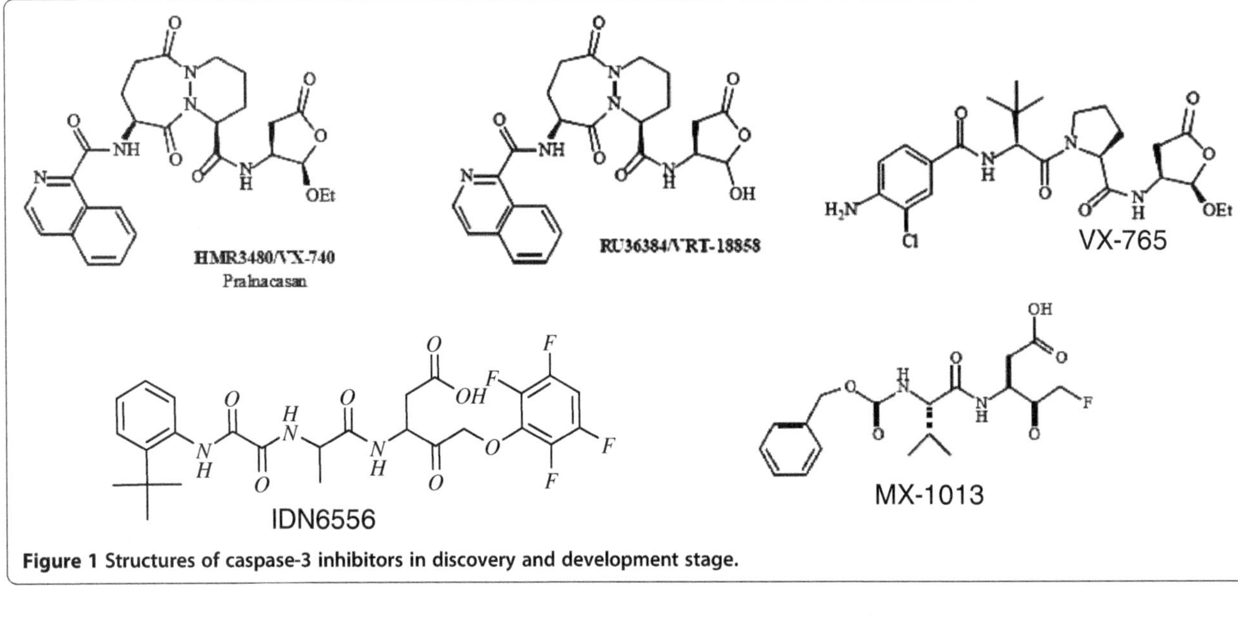

Figure 1 Structures of caspase-3 inhibitors in discovery and development stage.

Ltd., and the detailed chemistry has been reported earlier [8,9]. As the active site of caspase-3 contains a sulfhydryl moiety necessary for its catalytic activity, we focused on molecules with the warheads (electrophilic moiety: carbonyl group of fluoromethylketone) capable of reacting with the cysteinyl thiols. We selected 70 novel small molecules (NCEs) with sufficient chemical diversity belonging to four different series (indole fluoromethylketone, indole difluoro and tetrafluorophenoxymethylketone and oxalamide) and purity more than 95%.

Screening of compounds was carried out at two different concentrations (1 and 10 μM). Selected compounds were subjected to dose response determination in semi-log concentration (serial threefold dilutions) at constant DMSO concentration of 1% with highest compound concentration at 100 μM. Counterscreening against some of proteases, permeability, and CYP450 inhibition studies was carried out for few selected compounds at 10 μM concentration.

Protease inhibition assays

The ability of NCEs to inhibit the activity of human recombinant caspases as well as other proteases was determined using a standard fluorometric microplate assay as described in [1,10]. The assay buffer contained 25 mM sodium HEPES, 50 mM KCl, 0.1% CHAPS, and 1 mM β-mercaptoethanol, pH7.4. To a reaction mixture (100 μL) containing the above buffer, 10 μM AC-DEVD-AMC and 10 U caspase-3 were added in a black 96-well microplate. Activities of the other caspases were determined similarly using the corresponding fluorogenic substrates: 50 U of caspase-1 and 10 μM N-acetyl-Tyr-Val-Ala-Asp-7-amido-4-methylcoumarin.

Thrombin assay reaction mixture (100 μl) contained 140 ng of enzyme and 100 μM of substrate (Boc-Glu-Ala-Arg-AMC) in Tris–HCl buffer pH 8.5. Cathepsin-B assay buffer contained 50 mM MES, 0.01% CHAPS, 100 μM of substrate (Z-Phe-Arg-AMC HCl), and 0.1 U of enzyme. The selectivity profile of **3D** against caspase-7, 8, and 9, and cathepsin-D was performed using Biomol kit (Enzo Life Sciences, Inc.). The enzyme activities were monitored (ex/em 355/460) as a time-course measurement of the increase in fluorescence signal from fluorescently labeled peptide substrate for 120 min at room temperature. Percent inhibition calculation was calculated using following equation:

$$\text{Percent inhibition} = 100 - [(\text{RFU in test wells}/\text{RFU in basal control wells}) \times 100]$$

Mechanistic analysis of caspase-3 inhibition

Thirty microliters of caspase-3 (200 U) in assay buffer containing 30 μL of 20× NCE (the final compound concentration is approximately tenfold higher than respective IC_{50s}). The mixture was incubated for 30 and 60 min at 30°C and then diluted 100-fold with assay buffer containing 10 μM AC-DEVD-AMC. The enzyme activity was measured at 30°C after 30 min. As a control, a mixture of 1× caspase-3 and 1× NCE was prepared and incubated for the same time duration before the addition of the substrate.

Anti-apoptotic assay using Jurkat T-cells

The anti-apototic assay was done as described in [10]. Briefly, Jurkat (human T-cell leukemia) cell line (ATCC) was cultured in RPMI-1640 medium with L-glutamine and supplemented with 10% fetal bovine serum and antibiotic solution. Cells were grown at 37°C in 5% CO_2 and 95% air environment at 100% humidity. Cells were plated in 45 μL/well of serum-free medium at 2.5×10^5 cells/mL and incubated for 1 h before compound addition. Compound stock solutions were diluted with growth medium and added to the cells to obtain desired concentration. One percent DMSO was used for control wells (without the addition of compounds). Cells were incubated for 30 min before the addition of 5 μL of the apoptosis-inducer staurosporine (final concentration of 100 nM). After 24 or 48 h of incubation, resazurin reagent was added at 5.5 μL/well. Cells were further incubated for 120 min, and the fluorescence was measured using the Wallac Victor2V plate reader (PerkinElmer Life Sciences) at 531/589 nm ex/em wavelengths. The percent protection from induced apoptosis was calculated using the following equation:

$$\text{Percent protection} = (\Delta Fl_t - \Delta Fl_s)/(\Delta Fl_n - \Delta Fl_s) \times 100,$$

where ΔFl denotes the difference in resazurin fluorescence measured at point 0 and after 120-min incubation with the cells; subscripts t, s, and n are fluorescence in the presence of a test compound + staurosporine, staurosporine alone, and no staurosporine, respectively.

ADME assays

Aqueous solubility

A high throughput kinetic solubility profiling was carried out by shake flask method in 96-well format at pH 7.4 and 5.4 with theoretical test concentration of 200 μM. After 16 h of incubation, the supernatant was subjected for analysis.

Permeability

PAMPA assay was carried out using PION kit at 10-μM test concentration according to the instructions provided by the manufacturer. Permeability assay using Caco-2 cell monolayer.

Briefly, Caco-2 cells (ATCC) were grown in DMEM supplemented with 10% fetal bovine serum, 1 mM non-essential amino acids, 1 mM sodium pyruvate, and gentamicin sulfate (50 μg/ml) to 70% to 80% confluency prior to seeding in 24-well plates loaded with polycarbonate Millicell inserts (12-mm diameter, 0.4 μm, 40,000 cells/insert; Millipore Co., MA, USA) at 37°C, 5% CO_2 for 21 days. Cell monolayer integrity was assessed by measuring TEER. Drugs were applied at 10 μM in Hank's buffered salt solution to the apical or basal chamber, and transport assay was carried out for 2 h at 37°C in presence and absence of cyclosporin A. At the end of the assay, samples from both apical and basal chambers were collected for analysis, and the monolayer integrity was re-assessed by dye rejection using Lucifer yellow. Apparent permeability (P_{app}) was calculated using the equation:

$$P_{app}(\text{cm/sec}) = \text{dQ/dt} \times 1/\text{C}_o \times 1/\text{A},$$

where dQ/dt is the amount of drug transported within a given time period (μmol/sec); C_0 is the initial concentration in the donor solution (μM); A is the surface area of insert filter membrane (cm^2); and t is the incubation time (sec).

$$\text{Efflux ratio (ER)} = P_{app\ \text{B to A}}/P_{app\ \text{A to B}},$$

where $P_{app\ \text{B to A}}$ is the P_{app} value measured in the B to A direction; $P_{app\ \text{A to B}}$ is the P_{app} value measured in the A to B direction. Note that efflux ratios greater than 2 (or 3) are generally considered to be evidence for transport. Follow-up studies using inhibitors of drug transporters (e.g., cyclosporin A) was done to develop further evidence.

Microsomal stability

Mouse liver microsomes (in-house prepared) and pooled human liver microsomes (BD Gentest, CA, USA) were incubated with 1-μM test compounds at 37°C for 15 and 60 min using NADPH and UDPGA as co-factors. The reaction was stopped by the addition of cold acetonitrile, precipitated protein was removed, and the supernatants were analyzed.

Cytochrome P450 inhibition

Human recombinant CYP450 isozymes 1A2, 2 C9, 2 C19, 2D6, and 3A4 (BD Gentest) were incubated with 10 μM of test compound in buffer containing 0.1% DMSO for 10 min at 37°C, and the residual enzyme activity was measured using fluorogenic substrates as per BD Gentest protocol.

Animals

Animal experimental procedures used in this study were approved by the Institutional Animal Ethical Committee based on the Committee for the Purpose of Control and Supervision on Experiments on Animals guidelines. Mice were used for the experiment after one-week acclimatization to standard laboratory conditions. Mice were fed with standard diet and water *ad libitum*.

In vivo pharmacokinetic experiment in mice

Pharmacokinetic profiling was carried out using oral and intravenous route (IV) dosing in male NMRI mice. Three animals per route were administered test substance (1 mg/kg IV, 5 mg/kg PO) dissolved in vehicle containing 2% ethanol, 10% hydroxypropyl-β-cyclodextrin (HP-b-CD) and/or 1% Poloxamer 188 and quantity sufficient amount of 0.9% normal saline given at 10 ml/kg. The plasma samples were collected at different time points until 8 hr and were stored frozen at −80°C until analysis. Quantitative bio-analysis of the drugs in the plasma samples was done using an LC-MS/MS. Plasma samples were analyzed following protein precipitation of plasma with acetonitrile containing internal standards.

Data fitting and statistical analysis

Curve fitting was performed with Prism 5.1 software (GraphPad Software Inc., San Diego, CA) using built-in equation describing corresponding data models. All the other data were mentioned as mean ± standard deviation of triplicates values. PK parameters were determined using WinNonlin 5.2 software.

Results and discussion

Biochemical screening

For screening of the compound library, the caspase-3 biochemical assay was first optimized. The fluorescence signal as well as signal to noise ratio was optimal at 10 U of caspase-3 and 10-μM substrate. Substrate exhibited Michaelis-Menten constant of 11.7 μM and was comparable to the published data [10]. The caspase-3 assay was validated using reference inhibitor (IDN6556) across all plates and different experiments [10-12].

The primary screen of the 70 compounds at concentration of 1 and 10 μM revealed 22 hits (higher than 50% inhibition threshold at 10 μM) with dose-dependent inhibition (data not shown). The hits belong to all the four series, and most potent molecule is from indole chemotype, a chemotype previously reported to show good inhibition of cysteine proteases [4]. There was a clear trend in dose dependent inhibition of caspase-3 activity for all tested compounds from all four chemotypes (Figure 2A). It was observed that fluoromethylketone as a warhead is more potent than other substitutions like oxalamide. More bulky lipophilic groups substantially reduced the potency, and more polar and hydrophilic groups increased the potency. Electrophilic carbonyl from fluoromethylketone group might serve as sites of nucleophilic attack by cysteine thiolates in the caspase-3

A

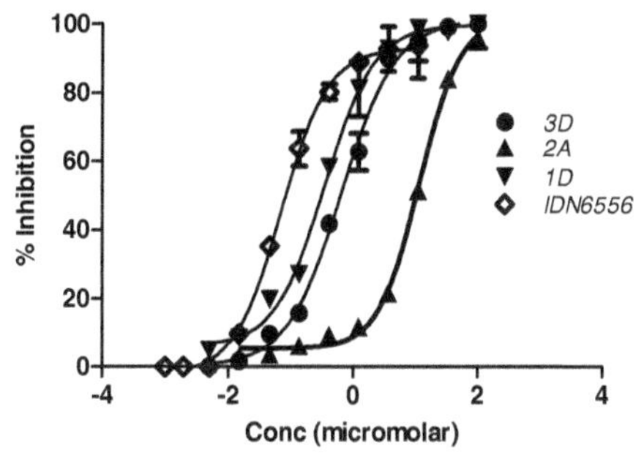

B

Target	IC50 (μM)	Fold selectivity
Caspase 3	0.11	-
Caspase 7	0.197	1.8
Caspase 8	0.182	1.7
Caspase 9	0.067	0.6
Caspase 1	>10	>100
Cathepsin D	>10	>100
Cathepsin B	>10	>100
Thrombin	>10	>100

Figure 2 Concentration-dependent inhibition and selectivity profile of NCEs. (**A**) Concentration-dependent inhibition of caspase-3 with NCEs measured in presence of substrate (AC-DEVD-AMC) at 10 μM. The percentage of inhibition was calculated relative to the enzyme activity with no inhibitor present. (**B**) Selectivity profile of **3D** using Biomol kit (Enzo Life Sciences, Inc.). The enzyme activities were monitored (ex/em 355/460) as a time-course measurement of the increase in fluorescence signal from fluorescently labeled peptide substrate for 120 min at room temperature.

catalytic domain. Few of these compounds were further characterized in the follow-up mechanistic assays, counterscreening assays against other proteases including caspase-1, 3, 7, 8, and 9, cathepsin-B and D, and thrombin.

Time-dependent inhibition of caspase-3 activity

Reversibility assessment of the caspase-3 activity with selected compounds was determined in the dilution experiment as described in the 'Methods' section. From the data shown in Figure 3, time-dependent inhibition of caspase-3 activity suggests irreversible interaction of compounds with caspase-3 enzyme and is similar to the reported caspase inhibitor IDN6556 [6,10,13].

Counterscreen profile

The selectivity profile of selected compounds was assessed using a panel of proteases including cysteine proteases. The substrate concentration as well as other reaction conditions used for each assay is described in the 'Methods' section. The selectivity studies (refer to Figure 2B) indicated that compound **3D** was not selective towards caspases 7, 8, and 9 but good selectivity

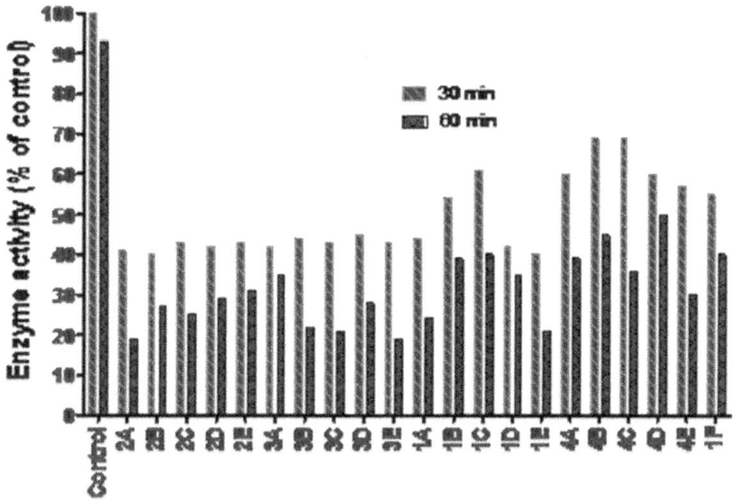

Figure 3 Time-dependent inhibition of caspase-3 activity with NCEs. Caspase-3 at a 20× concentration, as specified in the 'Methods' section, was pre-incubated with 20× NCE (the final compound concentration is approximately tenfold higher than respective IC_{50s}). The mixture was pre-incubated for 30 and 60 min at 30°C and then diluted 100-folds with assay buffer containing 10-μM AC-DEVD-AMC. The enzyme activity was measured at 30°C after 30 min. As a control, a mixture of 1× caspase-3 and 1× NCE was prepared and incubated for the same time duration before addition of the substrate. The percentage inhibition was calculated relative to the activity of caspase-3, which went through all the procedures for concentrated or control samples but without the inhibitor. Note that compounds 1A to 3E are from indole, and 4A to 4F from oxalamide series.

(>100-fold) over proteases including caspase-1, thrombin, cathepsin-B, and cathepsin D.

Evaluation of anti-apoptotic activity

Protection against cellular apoptosis was determined using staurosporine as apoptotic inducer in Jurkat cells (human T-cell leukemia), as described in the 'Methods' section. Apoptosis in cells was measured as the suppression of resazurin reduction rate after 48-h incubation with staurosporine and in the presence and absence of compounds. Most of the compounds, with the exception of compound **3D**, showed minimal protection or no effect on staurosporine-induced apoptosis likely due to low permeability as observed in PAMPA assay (data not shown).

Evaluation of compounds in *in vitro* ADME assay panel

The ADME profile for the selected set of compounds was determined using standard battery of assays including aqueous apparent solubility, microsomal metabolic stability, Caco-2 permeability, and drug-drug interaction studies using recombinant CYP450 enzymes. It is observed that the presence of polar group (such as acidic moiety) may help in good solubility and lack of transport of compound across the cell membrane in order to reach the target. Substitution of tetrafluorophenoxy showed interaction with efflux pump. Most of the compounds from fluoromethyl substitution on indole moiety and oxalamide showed relatively high microsomal stability compare to other substitutions. The optimal microsomal stability was found with substitution (Cl or OMe) on 5th position of indole with either difluoro and tetrafluorophenoxymethylketone substitution [see Table S1B in Additional file 1].

Inhibition of cytochrome P450 (CYP450) drug metabolizing enzymes may alter the metabolism of co-administered compounds, leading to a change in exposure and possible toxicity. Thus, the potential for the drug-drug interaction of NCEs was assessed by monitoring their impact on the metabolic activity of a panel of five major human CYP450 isoforms (3A4, 2 C9, 2 C19, 2D6, and 1A2) in the presence of a known fluorescent substrate for each of the isoform. CYP3A4 inhibition was determined in three assays using three distinct fluorescent substrates to account for the existence of two substrate binding sites. The results of these six assays are reported in Table S3 in Additional file 1. All the tested compounds showed no significant CYP450 inhibition under tested conditions, indicating no major alerts in drug-drug interactions.

Pharmacokinetic profile of compounds in rodents

Compounds were administered to male NMRI mice either as 1 mg/kg intravenous bolus in 1% (*v*/*v*) DMA, 10% (*w*/*v*) HP-b-CD in normal saline, or orally by gavage at 5 mg/kg in 1% (*v*/*v*) DMA, 1% (*w*/*v*) Poloxamer 147, and 10% (*w*/*v*) HP-b-CD in saline. The relevant pharmacokinetic parameters reported in Table S4 in Additional file 1 indicate that the oral bioavailability of compound 3D (having tetrafluoro substitution) in this study was 90%, which was more when compared other compounds (such as series 1 and 4). A relatively high volume of distribution observed after IV dosing indicates that the compound gets distributed rapidly from the vascular compartment into the peripheral tissues. The plasma clearance was high (greater than hepatic blood flow) for most of the compounds tested except for compound **3D** with clearance value of 588 ml/h/kg (15% of hepatic blood flow).

Caspases play an important role in different pathophysiological conditions, and specific inhibition is expected to be therapeutically valuable. Towards identifying novel inhibitors of caspases with desirable selectivity, ADME and efficacy profile, we screened a focused library of compounds and identified inhibitors from four chemical series that are distinct from other known small molecule caspase-3 inhibitors. Among the hits identified with potency ranging from 0.11 to 50 μM IC_{50}, compounds from two series that displayed potent caspase-3 inhibition were analyzed for reversibility. All the tested compounds from four series were found to be highly irreversible for their inhibition of caspase activity. Caspase-3 possess a total of seven cysteinyls, out of which three (excluding one in the active site) are readily accessible to water and, hence, to potential oxidation. It is well known in the literature that the compounds with warhead possess the irreversible type of caspase inhibition [13].

ADME properties including the permeability of the compounds with an objective of selecting the compounds with greater potential for cellular activity were analyzed. Although permeability of all the tested compounds were low, modest cellular activity suggested that compounds **3D** and **1D** were more potent than other compounds and may be because of marginally better permeability. Halogen (Cl) substitution on 5th position along with tetrafluorophenoxymethylketone substituent on right-hand side of molecule (as in compound **3D**) resulted in greater stability in liver microsomes [see Table S1A in Additional file 1] and higher interaction with efflux pump as indicated by higher efflux ratio in the Caco-2 permeability assays [see Table S3 in Additional file 1]. It also shows advantages in lowering the plasma clearance to about 10% of hepatic blood flow and increase in the oral bioavailability, which led to a good oral exposure. The interesting *in vitro* as well *in vivo* profile of compound ***3D*** supports further evaluation in efficacy models. However, such potential advantages need to be confirmed by additional characterization of compound **3D** in different pharmacological studies as well as *in vivo* toxicity evaluation.

Conclusions

In summary, this study supports the hypothesis that caspase inhibition may protect cells from abnormal amount of apoptosis seen in a number of disease states. Continual treatment with a caspase inhibitor may preserve the loss of critical numbers of cells responsible for the development of caspase-mediated cell death. These results support further analysis of compound **3D** as a potential anti-apoptotic agent in pre-clinical models of apoptosis.

Additional file

Additional file 1: Title. Structure-activity relationship analysis and pharmacokinetic properties of NCEs. **Description:** Table S1 (A and B), structure-activity relationship analysis of hits around chemotype I, II and III derived from compound template; Table S2, structure-activity relationship analysis of hits around chemotype IV derived from compound template; Table S3, structure-activity relationship analysis of hits around chemotype I, III and IV derived from compound template; and S4, pharmacokinetic properties of NCEs.

Competing interests

The authors declare that they have no competing interests.

Acknowledgments

We gratefully acknowledge our collaborators Professor Saumitra Sengupta and Subhendu Mukherjee for providing the NCEs and molecular modeling support. The authors also would like to thank Biochemistry, ADME and Analytical Departments for their assistance.

Author details

[1]DMPK Department, Aurigene Discovery Technologies Limited, Electronic City Phase 2, Hosur Road, Bangalore 560100, India. [2]Department of Chemistry, Jawaharlal Nehru Technological University Hyderabad, Kukatpally, Hyderabad 500085, India.

References

1. Kerr JF, Wyllie AH, Currie AR (1972) Apoptosis: a basic biological phenomenon with wide-ranging implications in tissue kinetics. Br J Cancer 26:239–257
2. Linton SD (2005) Caspase inhibitors: a pharmaceutical industry perspective. Current Topics Med Chem 49:7636–7645
3. Slee EA, Adrain C, Martin SJ (1999) Serial killers: ordering caspase activation events in apoptosis. Cell Death Differ 6:1067–1074
4. Nuttall ME, Lee D, McLaughlin B, Erhardt JA (2001) Selective inhibitors of apoptotic caspases: implications for novel therapeutic strategies. Drug Discov Today 6(2):110–121
5. Linton SD, Aja T, Allegrini PR, Deckwerth TL, Diaz JL, Hengerer B, Herrmann J, Jahangiri KG, Kallen J, Karanewsky DS, Meduna SP, Nalley K, Robinson ED, Roggo S, Rovelli G, Sauter A, Sayers RO, Schmitz A, Smidt R, Ternansky RJ, Tomaselli KJ, Ullman BR, Wiessner C, Wu JC (2004) Oxamyl dipeptide caspase inhibitors developed for the treatment of stroke. Bioorg Med Chem Lett 14(10):2685–91
6. Hoglen NC, Long-Shiuh C, Fisher CD, Hirakawa BP, Groessl T, Contreras PC (2004) Characterization of IDN-6556: a liver-targeted caspase inhibitor. J Pharmaco Exp Ther 309:634–640
7. Imao M, Nagaki M, Imose M, Moriwaki H (2006) Differential caspase-9-dependent signaling pathway between tumor necrosis factor receptor- and Fas-mediated hepatocyte apoptosis in mice. Liver Int 26:137–146
8. Sengupta S, Rao GV, Dubey PK (2011) Synthesis and evaluation of novel oxalamide derivatives as caspase-3 inhibitors. Indian J Chem 50B:901–905
9. Sengupta S, Rao GV, Dubey PK (2011) Synthesis and evaluation of indole aspartyl ketones as novel caspase-3 inhibitors. Asian J Chem 23(12): 5517–5520
10. Okun I, Malarchuk S, Dubrovskaya E, Khvat A, Tkachenko S, Kysil V, Ilyn A, Kravchenko D, Prossnitz ER, Sklar L, Ivachtchenko A (2006) Screening for caspase-3 inhibitors: a new class of potent small-molecule inhibitors of caspase-3. J Biomol Screening 11(3):277–285
11. Scot CW, SObotka-Briner C, Wilkins DE, Jacobs RT, Folmer JJ, Frazee WJ, Bhat RV, Ghanekar SV, Aharony D (2003) Novel small molecule inhibitors of caspase-3 block cellular and biochemical features of apoptosis. J Pharmacol Exp Ther 304:433–440
12. Galle PR (1997) Apoptosis in liver disease. J Hepatol 27(2):405–412
13. Wu JC, Fritz LC (1999) Irreversible caspase inhibitors: tools for studying apoptosis. Methods in Enzymology 17:320–328

An efficient heterogeneous catalyst (CuO@ARF) for on-water C-S coupling reaction: an application to the synthesis of phenothiazine structural scaffold

Debasish Sengupta and Basudeb Basu*

Abstract

Background: Aryl sulfides have significant importance from biological and pharmaceutical aspects. Transition metal-catalyzed carbon-sulfur cross-coupling reaction represents an important tool for the synthesis of sulfides. Among various transition metals, copper salts or oxides have found vast applicability.

Results: A simple procedure for the preparation of poly-ionic amberlite resins embedded with copper oxide nanoparticles (CuO NPs) (denoted as CuO@ARF) has been developed, characterized, and employed for the first time as a heterogeneous ligand-free catalyst for 'on-water' C-S cross-coupling reaction. The NPs of CuO with an average size (approximately 2.6 nm), as determined from high resolution transmission electron microscopy (HRTEM) images, are found to be a potentially active, chemoselective, and recyclable catalyst for the preparation of symmetrical and unsymmetrical aryl sulfides. Recycling of the catalyst was performed successfully for five consecutive runs, and apparently no leaching was observed in a hot filtration test. Excellent chemoselectivity between iodo- and bromo-arene has been exploited in step-wise C-S and C-N couplings to synthesize bioactive heterocyclic scaffold phenothiazine.

Conclusions: An efficient method is established for the C-S cross-coupling reaction using heterogeneous catalyst CuO@ARF under ligand-free on-water condition. The catalyst is highly chemoselective among different aryl halides, which has been demonstrated in the synthesis heterocyclic scaffold phenothiazine. Furthermore, it is recyclable for five consecutive runs examined.

Keywords: C-S cross-coupling; CuO NPs; Heterogeneous catalyst; On-water reaction; Phenothiazine

Background

The carbon-sulfur bonds are prevalent present in numerous medicinally important natural products [1-3]. Indeed, a number of drugs in various therapeutic uses such as HIV, cancer, diabetes, inflammatory, Alzheimer's, and Parkinson's diseases contain the aryl sulfide functional group [4-7]. A few biologically active compounds possessing a C-S bond are represented in Figure 1. For example, phenothiazines are an important class of organic compounds finding wide applications as drugs, insecticides, inhibitors of polymerization, antioxidants, paints, spectroscopic probes, etc. [8]. Therefore, in the recent era, the sp^2C-S bond formation has been the subject of intense study in organic synthesis and medicinal chemistry, and researchers develop diverse mild cross-coupling methodologies for these pharmaceuticals.

The conventional methods for the C-S bond formation involve reduction of aryl sulfones or aryl sulfoxides using strong reducing agents like DIBAL-H or $LiAlH_4$ [9]. Besides, on-water C-S bond formation has been reported via thiol addition to α,β-unsaturated carbonyl compounds at room temperature [10]. In 1980, Migita et al. first showed the Pd-catalyzed thiation of aryl bromides using $Pd(PPh_3)_4$ [11]. Subsequently, other metals like nickel [12,13], copper [12,14], cobalt [15], iron [16], rhodium [17], manganese [18], and indium [19] have also been employed, though in much less extent, as compared to other C-X (X = C, O, N, P) coupling reactions. This is possibly due to the notion that sulfur might act as the poison to suppress

* Correspondence: basu_nbu@hotmail.com
Department of Chemistry, North Bengal University, Darjeeling 734013, India

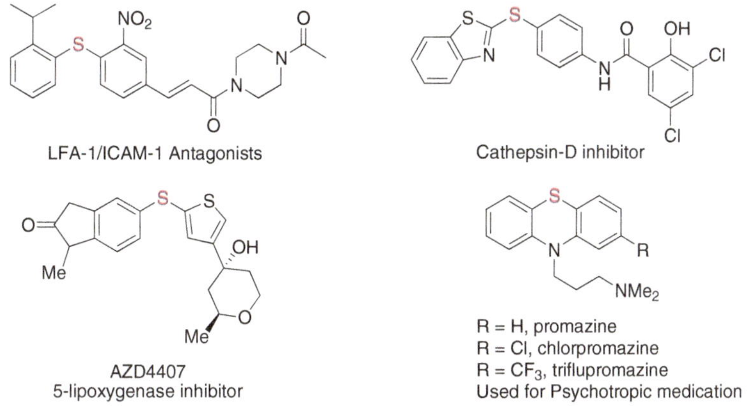

Figure 1 Some biologically active compounds bearing C-S bond.

the catalytic activity through strong coordinating and adsorptive properties [20]. However, the last two decades have witnessed several new transition metal-based catalytic systems for the C-S coupling reactions between aryl halides and thiols. Amongst various transition metals, copper has been considered as the most useful for the C-S coupling reactions due to its special redox properties and cost-effectiveness. Many strategies have been successful by using homogeneous copper salts in the presence of suitable electron-rich and precious ligands for the C-S coupling reactions [21,22].

On the other hand, nano-structured materials with high surface areas have been investigated as effective catalysts for various organic coupling reactions [23]. Catalysis of organic reactions by metal NPs supported on a suitable polymeric matrix offers the advantages of high catalytic activity, simplified isolation of the product, easy recovery, and recycling of the catalyst. Copper oxide nanoparticles (CuO NPs) are a good choice and indeed useful catalyst in the C-S coupling reaction between aryl halide and thiols [24-26]. However, previous on-water C-S coupling reactions involving copper species like CuI-TBAB [27], CuCl [28], or other metal species like Bi_2O_3 [29], $CoCl_2 6H_2O$ [30], or $FeCl_3 6H_2O$-bipyridyl complexes [31], etc. afford thioethers without easy recovery of the catalyst and recyclability. Direct use of CuO either in bulk or NPs requires organic solvents other than water and gave relatively poor yields in C-S coupling reaction. Considering our experience in the field of developing polymer-supported metal NPs as the heterogeneous catalyst in various coupling reactions, [32,33] and in conjunction with our interest in the synthesis of various biologically important heterocyclic scaffolds mediated over solid supports, [34,35] we were interested to develop polymer-supported CuO NPs and to use it as the catalyst in 'on-water' C-S coupling reaction between aryl halide and thiols.

We report herein our studies that constitute simple preparation and characterization of poly-ionic amberlite resins embedded with CuO NPs (CuO@ARF), which efficiently catalyze the C-S cross-coupling reaction under on-water and ligand-free conditions. Further application of this catalyst has been demonstrated in the synthesis of phenothiazine - an important structural motif of several potentially useful drugs and also used as chemosensors [36].

Methods

Amberlite resin formate (ARF) was prepared from commercially available inexpensive amberlite resin chloride by an ion-exchange process as reported from this laboratory [37]. A mixture of ARF resin beads and $Cu(OAc)_2$ H_2O in DMF (50 mg g^{-1} of ARF) was heated at 110°C in a Teflon capped sealed tube for 30 min with occasional gentle shaking. White ARF beads turned brownish in color during the process. Finally, these resin beads were filtered off, washed with water and acetone, dried, and characterized by Fourier transform infrared spectroscopy (FT-IR), X-ray diffraction (XRD), and transmission electron microscopy (TEM) analysis, and the copper content of the composite was estimated by atomic absorption spectroscopy (AAS). The XRD and TEM analyses suggested the presence of CuO NPs distributed on the surface of ARF, and we referred the as-synthesized nanocomposite material as CuO@ARF.

Results and discussion

At first, the presence of copper in the resin composite was measured by the AAS study. For this purpose, the sample (100 mg) was digested with concentrated HNO_3 (1 mL) and Cu content was estimated to be 0.145 mmol g^{-1} of the resin-copper nanocomposite. The FT-IR spectra of CuO@ARF were recorded and compared with those of ARF (Figure 2). In the case of a similar heterogeneous Pd or

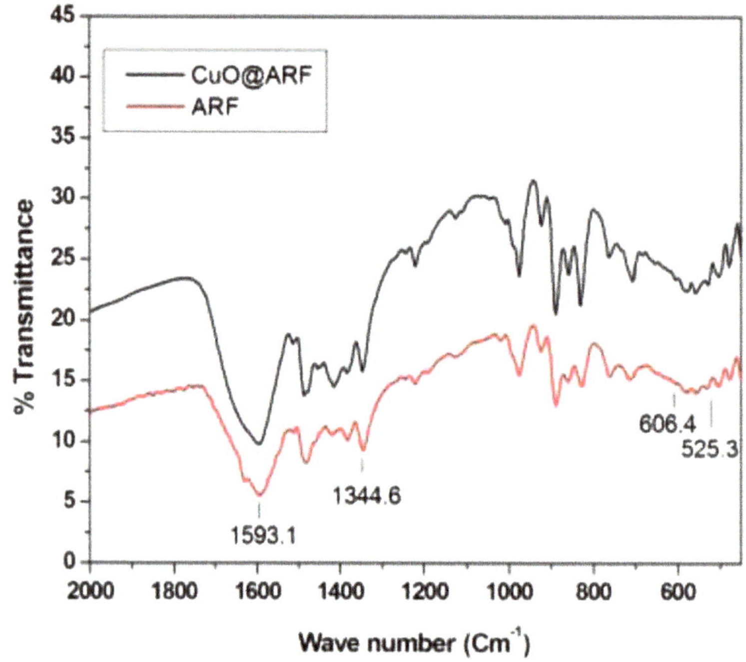

Figure 2 FT-IR spectra of the ARF and CuO@ARF.

bimetallic Pd/Cu nanocomposites, as developed from this laboratory, a significant increase in the stretching frequency of the carboxylate anion ($HCOO^-$) was observed [32,33]. Here, apparently no change of symmetric and anti-symmetric stretching vibrations (for the $HCOO^-$) was observed and appeared respectively at about 1,345 and 1,593 cm^{-1} for both ARF and CuO@ARF species (Figure 2). However, the specific IR absorption bands of CuO at 606 and 525 cm^{-1} might overlap with those of ARF in the similar region [38].

We therefore examined the powder XRD patterns of ARF and those of CuO@ARF, as shown in Figure 3. The ARF resins are amorphous in nature, and the Bragg diffraction patterns of CuO@ARF indicate the presence of cupric oxide (CuO). The JCPDS peak positions of the CuO@ARF nanocomposite with relative intensities are in good agreement (Figure 3b). The presence of XRD peaks at 2θ of 35.39°, 38.29°, 38.99°, 57.91°, and 61.64° suggested the presence of CuO ($\bar{1}11$), (111), (200), (202), and ($\bar{1}13$) planes, respectively (JCPDS#01-089-2531). Further examination of high resolution TEM (HRTEM) images of the CuO@ARF at different magnifications (Figure 4a,b) suggested that the CuO NPs are embedded on the resin polymeric matrices with an average size around 2.6 nm (Figure 4c).

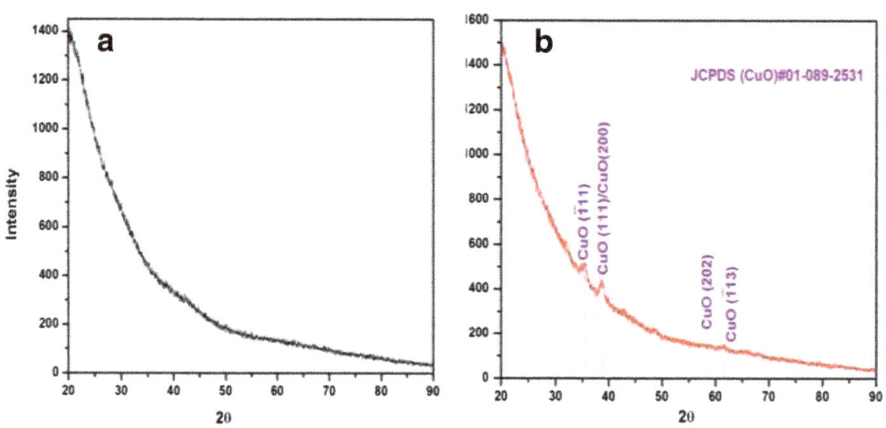

Figure 3 XRD patterns of (a) ARF and (b) CuO embedded on the surface of amberlite resin formate (CuO@ARF).

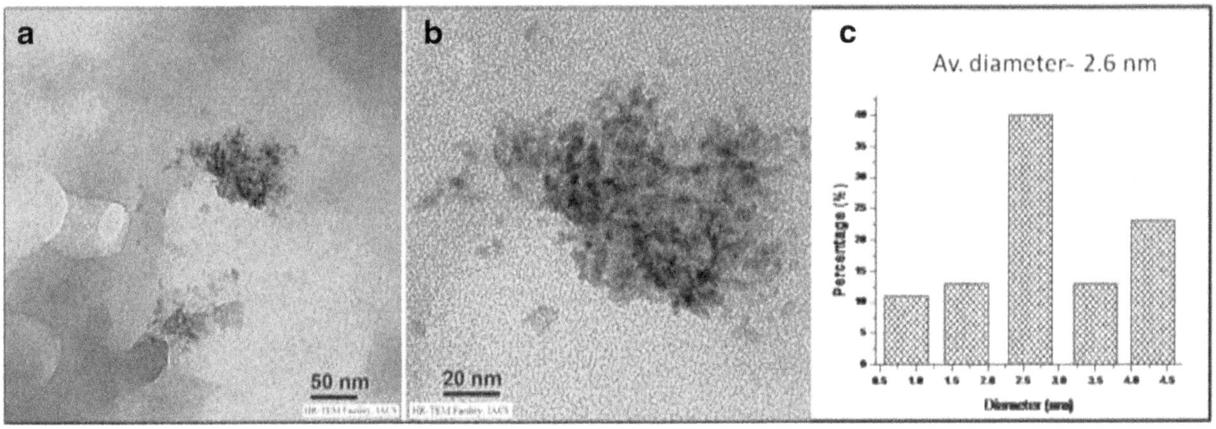

Figure 4 TEM images of CuO@ARF. (a) Scale bar 50 nm; **(b)** 20 nm; **(c)** average particle size from **(b)**.

Catalytic activity of CuO@ARF

In order to evaluate the catalytic activity of this newly developed nanocomposite (CuO@ARF) in C-S cross-coupling reaction between aryl halide and thiol, we performed a model study by taking a mixture of 4-iodoanisole and benzenethiol (in 1:1.2 ratios) and the catalyst (200 mg $mmol^{-1}$ of aryl iodide) in water (Table 1). The first reaction in the presence of a base (K_2CO_3) at 100°C did afford the desired unsymmetrical sulfane but with a modest yield (62%) (Table 1, entry 1). Considering that the modest conversion might be due to the poor solubility of aryl iodide in water, we used an additive - tetrabutylammonium bromide (TBAB), in equimolar quantity. This afforded the corresponding thioether in fairly good yield (83%; entry 2). Further improvement was achieved by using the catalytic amount of sodium dodecyl sulfate (SDS; 10 mol%), [39] which furnished the desired product in 90% isolated yield (entry 3). While there was no cross-coupling observed at room temperature, reaction carried out at 60°C or in the absence of the base produced the sulfane in 56% to 68% isolated yields (entries 4 to 6). We also tried the reaction in DMF at 100°C, which did not produce the desired sulfane in very good yield (entry 7). In each case, a small quantity of the diphenylsulfide (≤5%) as the side product was also formed.

Table 1 Optimization of reaction condition for the C-S cross-coupling using CuO@ARF[a]

Entry	Solvent	Base	Additive	Temperature/time	Yield (%)[b,c]
1	Water	K_2CO_3	-	100°C/24 h	62
2[d]	Water	K_2CO_3	TBAB	100°C/8 h	83
3[e]	*Water*	*K_2CO_3*	*SDS*	*100°C/8 h*	*90*
4[e]	Water	K_2CO_3	SDS	RT/24 h	00
5[e]	Water	K_2CO_3	SDS	60°C/24 h	68
6[e]	Water	-	SDS	100°C/24 h	56
7	DMF	K_2CO_3	-	100°C/24 h	67

[a]4-Iodoanisole (1 mmol), benzenethiol (1.2 mmol), CuO@ARF (200 mg), K_2CO_3 (1.1 mmol), and solvent (3 mL). [b]Isolated yield. [c]Small quantity of diphenyl disulfide was formed (≤5%). [d]TBAB (1 eqv) was used. [e]SDS (10 mol%) was used.

Minimum loading of the catalyst

After optimizing the reaction conditions, we examined the minimum amount of the catalyst loading that is required to obtain effective conversion to sulfane. Experiments were performed with 4-iodoanisole (1 mmol) in the presence of varying quantities of CuO@ARF (from 50 mg to 250 mg; i.e., 0.46 mg to 2.30 mg of copper $mmol^{-1}$ of iodoarene) and the results are shown in Figure 5. Conversions to the thioether at different time intervals were measured by high-performance liquid chromatography (HPLC) and the plot of percent conversion (±2%) versus time (h) revealed that minimum 200 mg of the catalyst (approximately 1.8 mg of copper) $mmol^{-1}$ of iodoarene can give rise to the best result. In each case, reaction was continued up to 24 h and HPLC analysis showed no appreciable changes in the conversion (Figure 5 was plotted up to 12 h).

The optimized reaction conditions were then employed with different iodoarenes and other aromatic halides to couple with variety of aryl thiols to examine the scope and limitations of our catalyst for on-water C-S cross-coupling reaction. In general, it was observed that the cross-coupling reaction was successful producing corresponding diaryl sulfide in good to excellent yields. The results are presented in Table 2. Iodoarenes with both activated (methoxy, methyl) and deactivated functional groups (nitro or acetyl) effectively underwent C-S cross-coupling with different aryl thiols (entries 1 to 5). On the other hand, similar coupling reactions with bromo- and chlorobenzenes, including *p*-chloroacetophenone were not successful (entries 6 and 7). Increasing the catalyst loading and changing the base did not facilitate the C-S cross-coupling of *p*-bromotoluene (entry 8). The selectivity however might be useful for substrates bearing different halides. Thus, iodobromoarenes and

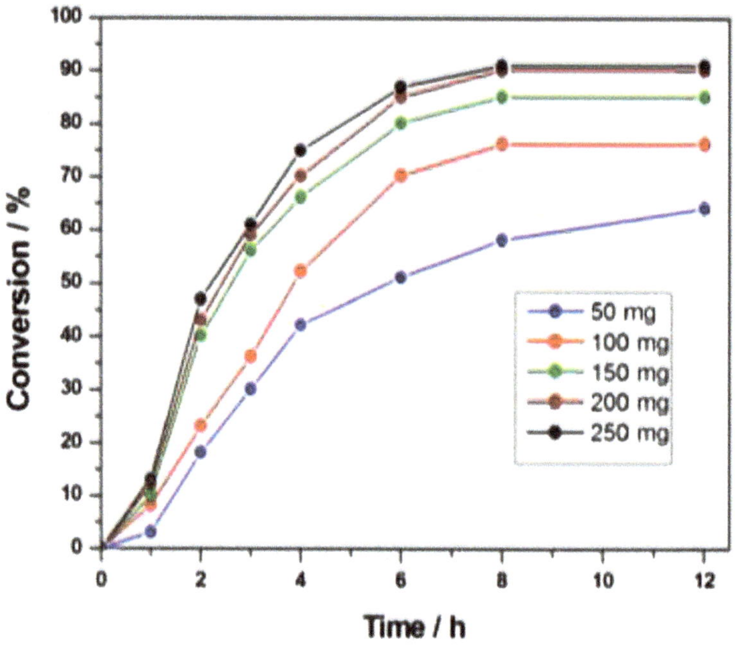

Figure 5 Time conversion plots for the C-S cross-coupling between 4-iodoanisole and thiophenol.

iodochloroarene were subjected to coupling with aryl thiols in the presence of this heterogeneous catalyst affording highly chemoselective iodo-coupled product only (entries 9 to 11). Substituted thiophenol like 2,5-dimethylbenzenethiol underwent smooth reactions giving the corresponding unsymmetrical diarylsulfide in 89% isolated yield (entry 12). Aliphatic thiols also gave cross-coupling products without any difficulty but relatively in lower yields as compared to aromatic thiols (entries 13 to 15), which might be attributable to the fact that aliphatic thiols are less reactive than aromatic thiols [40]. Bis-couplings were performed equally efficiently starting from 1,3-diiodobenzene and *p*-tolylthiol

Table 2 CuO@ARF-catalyzed C-S cross-coupling reactions between haloarenes and thiol[a]

Entry	Aryl halide	Thiol	Time (h)	Product	Yield (%)[b]
1	$(4\text{-}H_3CO)C_6H_4I$	C_6H_5SH	8	$(4\text{-}H_3CO)H_4C_6$ - S - C_6H_5	90
2	$(3\text{-}H_3CO)C_6H_4I$	$(4\text{-}C1)C_6H_4SH$	12	$(3\text{-}H_3CO)H_4C_6$ - S - $C_6H_4(4\text{-}C1)$	85
3	$(2\text{-}H_3CO)C_6H_4I$	$(4\text{-}CH_3)C_6H_4SH$	18	$(2\text{-}H_3CO)H_4C_6$ - S - $C_6H_4(4\text{-}CH_3)$	75
4	$(3\text{-}NO_2)C_6H_4I$	$(4\text{-}CH_3)C_6H_4SH$	11	$(3\text{-}NO_2)H_4C_6$ - S - $C_6H_4(4\text{-}CH_3)$	78
5	$(4\text{-}H_3CO)C_6H_4I$	$(4\text{-}CH_3)C_6H_4SH$	10	$(4\text{-}H_3CO)H_4C_6$ - S - $C_6H_4(4'\text{-}CH_3)$	75
6	$(4\text{-}H_3C)C_6H_4Br$	C_6H_5SH	24	No reaction	-
7	$(4\text{-}CH_3CO)C_6H_4C1$	C_6H_5SH	24	No reaction	-
8[c]	$(4\text{-}H_3C)C_6H_4Br$	C_6H_5SH	24	No reaction	-
9	$(5\text{-}Br)(2\text{-}H_3CO)C_6H_3I$	C_6H_5SH	8	$(5\text{-}Br)(2\text{-}H_3CO)H_3C_6$ - S - C_6H_5	90
10	$(3\text{-}Br)C_6H_4I$	$(4\text{-}CH_3)C_6H_4SH$	16	$(3\text{-}Br)H_4C_6$ - S - $C_6H_4(4\text{-}CH_3)$	79
11	$(3\text{-}C1)C_6H_4I$	$(4\text{-}CH_3)C_6H_4SH$	16	$(3\text{-}C1)H_4C_6$ - S - $C_6H_4(4\text{-}CH_3)$	79
12	$(4\text{-}H_3CO)C_6H_4I$	$(2,5\text{-}(CH_3)_2)C_6H_4SH$	7	$(4\text{-}H_3CO)H_4C_6$ - S - $C_6H_3(2,5\text{-}(CH_3)_2)$	89
13	$(4\text{-}H_3CO)C_6H_4I$	CySH	16	$(4\text{-}H_3CO)H_4C_6$ - S - Cy	70
14	$(4\text{-}H_3CO)C_6H_4I$	$n\text{-}C_5H_{11}SH$	16	$(4\text{-}H_3CO)H_4C_6$ - S - $C_5H_{11}\text{-}n$	73
15	$(3\text{-}H_3CO)C_6H_4I$	$n\text{-}C_7H_{11}SH$	16	$(4\text{-}H_3CO)H_4C_6$ - S - $C_7H_{15}\text{-}n$	76
16[d]	$1,3\text{-}C_6H_4I_2$	$(4\text{-}CH_3)C_6H_4SH$	14	$1,3\text{-}((4\text{-}CH_3)C_6H_4S)_2$ - C_6H_4	79
17	$(2\text{-}Br)C_6H_4I$	$(2\text{-}NH_2)C_6H_4SH$	8	$(2\text{-}Br)H_4C_6$ - S - $C_6H_4(2\text{-}NH_2)$	82

[a]Aryl halide: thiol: catalyst (1 mmol: 1.2 mmol: 200 mg), SDS (10 mol%), and K_2CO_3 (1.1 mmol) were taken in water (3 mL) and heated at 100°C. [b]Yield refers to pure isolated products characterized by spectroscopic (^1H and ^{13}C NMR) data. [c]Catalyst (300 mg $mmol^{-1}$ of aryl bromide), SDS (10 mol%), and Cs_2CO_3 (1.1 mmol). [d]Aryl halide: thiol: catalyst (0.5 mmol: 1.2 mmol: 200 mg), SDS (10 mol%), and K_2CO_3 (1.1 mmol) were taken in water (3 mL).

and affording the desired 1,3-bis(*p*-tolylthio)benzene as the only product in 79% isolated yield (entry 16). It may be mentioned that only benzenethiol and 4-tolylthiol gave a minor quantity of corresponding disulfides during the reaction (≤5%), while in other cases, no disulfide was detected on thin-layer chromatography (TLC) or by HPLC analysis.

As reported previously [26], the mechanism of the resin embedded CuO-catalyzed C-S coupling reaction is believed to proceed through the oxidative addition followed by reaction with thiol and then reductive elimination steps ($Cu^{II} \rightarrow Cu^{III} \rightarrow Cu^{II}$). The role of the additive SDS is presumably to solubilize the organic substrates in an aqueous medium [41,42]. Further beneficial assistance of the 'microreactors' formed by the surfactant like SDS in water medium organic reactions, as observed in other cases, cannot be ruled out [43]. In addition, the role of water might be attributed to the H-bonding (HB) effect, as reported previously on other occasions [44], has also been noticed in our cases. Thus, we isolated the cross-coupled product in higher yield performing the reaction in an aqueous medium as compared to in DMF (Table 1, entries 3 and 7).

Leaching of any metallic species from the amberlite resin polymeric matrices during or after the reaction was tested following the literature procedure [33,45]. Accordingly, the reaction mixture of the C-S cross-coupling between 4-iodoanisole and thiophenol is filtered off to separate out the solid catalysts after 2 h in hot condition, and the filtrate was analyzed by HPLC (approximately 43% conversion). The AAS analysis of the filtrate solution did not show the presence of any copper species. Moreover, further continuing the reaction by heating the liquid phase at 100°C for another 6 h in the absence of any added catalyst (CuO@ARF) did not afford any appreciable conversion (HPLC analysis). These observations signify that any copper species might not be leached out from the heterogeneous support during the initial 2 h of the reaction (Figure 6).

One of the important factors for a heterogeneous catalyst lies in its efficiency for recycling. We investigated the reusability of CuO@ARF in the reaction between 4-iodoanisole and thiophenol again as the model case. After completion of the reaction, resin beads were filtered off from the reaction mixture, washed thoroughly with water followed by acetone (two times), and then dried under vacuum. The catalyst was reused in five consecutive runs including the first run. Gratifyingly, there was no considerable loss of the catalytic efficiency observed (Figure 7).

Since the present catalytic system is highly selective to aryl iodides only (i.e., the first oxidative addition to the sp^2C-I bond), we decided to utilize this chemoselectivity between iodo- and bromo-substituents attached to the aryl moiety. Thus, a reaction of 1,2-bromoiodobenzene with 2-aminothiophenol in the presence of the catalyst CuO@ARF under similar conditions in water was performed. The C-S coupling occurred selectively at the sp^2C-I bond, and we obtained 2-(2-bromophenylthio) benzene in 82% yield (Scheme 1). Further intramolecular Buchwald-Hartwig type coupling between amino-and

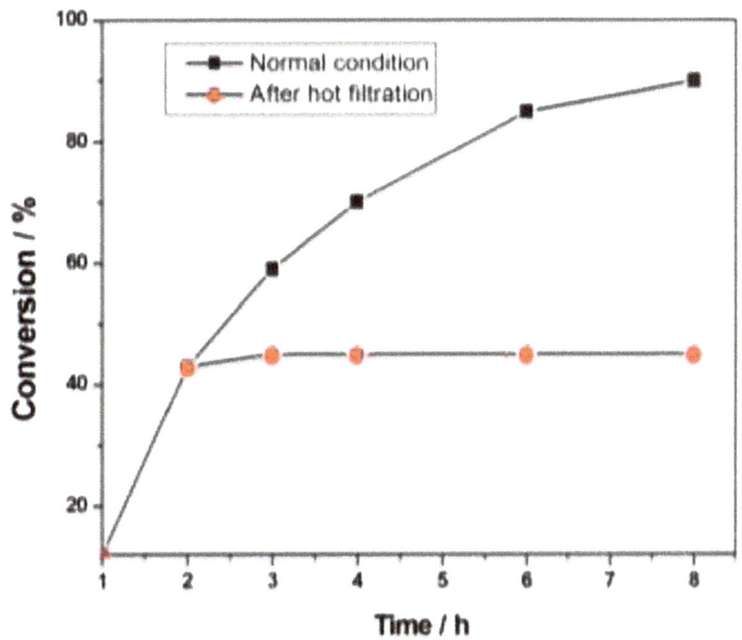

Figure 6 Comparison of normal time profile with that of hot filtration test. Conversions (±2%) at different time intervals for each plot were measured by HPLC.

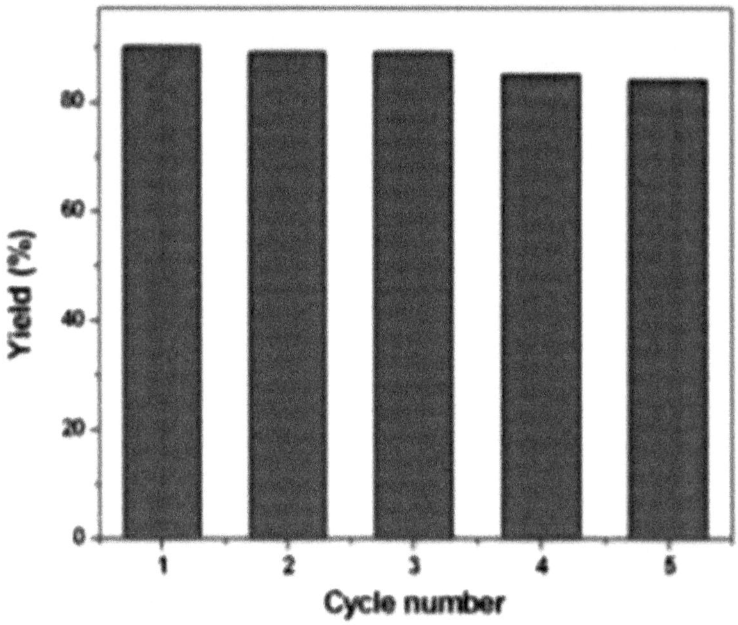

Figure 7 Recycling experiments using CuO@ARF in the C-S cross-coupling reaction between 4-iodoanisole and thiophenol.

bromo-substituents attached with two aromatic rings under Pd-BINAP catalyzed condition was carried out to afford phenothiazine in 84% isolated yield. The C-N coupling can also be accomplished by using the new catalyst (CuO@ARF) in the presence of L-proline as the ligand (Scheme 1) [46]. The ^{1}H nuclear magnetic resonance (NMR) spectra run in DMSO-D6 and DMSO-D6-D_2O confirmed formation of phenothiazine with the labile NH proton appeared at δ 8.5 ppm (see Additional file 1). We also performed the intramolecular Buchwald coupling in a water medium using both catalytic systems. Although the reaction works well with comparative yield of the phenothiazine in the case of using $Pd_2(dba)_3$, the use of CuO@ARF as the catalyst however does not give a satisfactory yield of the desired cyclic product.

A comparison chart of the efficiency of the present catalytic system with other metal-based 'on-water' catalytic systems reported in the literature showing advantages in terms of low loading, high efficiency, stability of the catalyst, recyclability, etc. has been presented in Table 3.

Conclusions

Our studies established that poly-ionic resin-supported CuO NPs (CuO@ARF) are an efficient catalyst in the C-S coupling reaction under ligand-free 'on-water' conditions. Low loading of the catalyst, recyclability without leaching, and chemoselectivity amongst aromatic halides are notable features. Further application of the chemoselectivity has been demonstrated in the synthesis of bioactive heterocyclic scaffold phenothiazine. Considering the inexpensive catalytic system along with the application to the synthesis of medicinally important structural scaffold, this heterogeneous catalyst and greener method can find wider applications in organic synthesis.

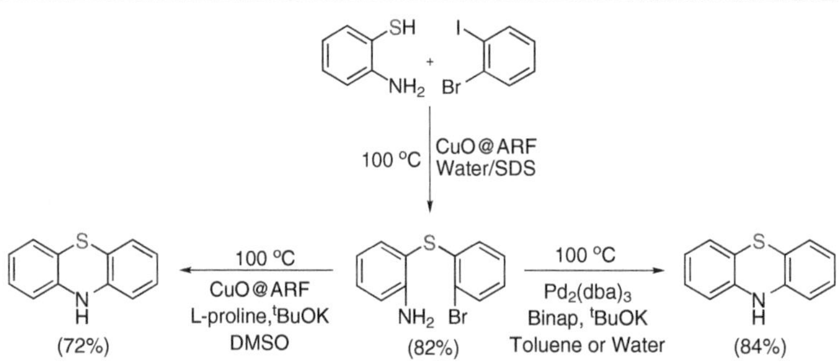

Scheme 1 Synthesis of phenothiazine.

Table 3 Comparison of various metal-based catalytic 'on-water' C-S coupling reactions with the present system CuO@ARF

Entry	Catalytic system	Applicability	Remarks	Reference
01	CuI (1 mol%) 1.5 eqv TBAB (1 eqv); base KOH (1.5 eqv); 80°C, 10 h	With aryl iodide; bromo- and chloroarenes gave poor yields even using 5 mol% CuI	Excess strong base, not recyclable; CuI is poorly soluble in water, TBAB is moisture sensitive.	[27]
02	CuCl and 1,2-diamine as ligand (>2 eqv); 120°C overnight heating	With iodo- and bromoarenes. No selectivity was examined	Precious 1,2-diamines in >2, equivalents, long reaction time, recyclable using the recovered solution - catalyst was not separated.	[28]
03	Bi_2O_3/Diamine ligand; (each 10 mol%); 1 eqv KOH at 100°C	With aryl iodide	Presence of a ligand, high loading of the metal catalyst, long reaction time; recyclable using the recovered solution - catalyst was not separated.	[29]
04	$CoCl_2 \cdot 6H_2O$/cationic 2,2'-bipyridyl system, 1 eqv KOH; excess zinc, 100°C	With aryl halides (iodide, bromide, and chloride).	Presence of cationic 2,2'-bipyridyl; excess Zn; long reaction time; recyclable using the recovered solution - catalyst was not separated.	[30]
05	$FeCl_3 \cdot 6H_2O$ (10 mol%) - bipyridyl complexes (10 mol%) ; KOH (4 eqv); 100°C, 24 h	With aryl iodide	Excess base, long reaction time; recyclable using the recovered solution - catalyst was not separated.	[31]
06	CuO@ARF; copper oxide (2.8 mol%); base K_2CO_3 (1.1 eqv); 100°C, 8 h	With aryl iodide	Mild base - nearly equivalent (1: 1.1); shorter reaction time; chemoselectivity between iodo and bromo has been utilized in the synthesis of medicinally important phenothiazine scaffold, easy separation of heterogeneous catalyst (by simple filtration of resin beads), recyclable for five runs without loss of activity; catalytic amount of SDS, ligand-free.	

Experimental

Amberlite IRA 900 (chloride form) was purchased from Acros Organics, Geel, Belgium, and used after washing with water and acetone followed by drying under vacuum. Cupric acetate was purchased from S.D. Fine Chem. Limited, Mumbai, India, and other chemicals were purchased and used directly. For column chromatography, silica (60 to 200 μm) (Sisco Research Laboratories, Mumbai, India), and for TLC, Merck plates coated with silica gel 60, F254 were used (Merck & Co., Inc., Whitehouse Station, USA). FT-IR spectra were recorded in FT-IR-8300 Shimadzu spectrophotometer (Shimadzu, Kyoto, Japan). NMR spectra were taken in $CDCl_3$ using Bruker Avance AV-300 spectrometer (Bruker AXS, Inc., Yokohama-shi, Japan) operating for ^1H at 300 MHz and for ^{13}C at 75 MHz. The spectral data were measured using TMS as the internal standard (for ^1H) and $CDCl_3$ (for ^{13}C). AAS measurements were made using Varian SpectrAA 50B instrument (Varian Medical Systems, Melbourne, Australia). Progress of the reaction was monitored by HPLC (1260 Infinity, Agilent Technologies, Santa Clara, USA), column: ZORBAX Rx-SIL (4.6 × 150 mm, 5 μm), eluent: n-hexane (flow rate 2 mL min^{-1}). The XRD studies of the powder samples were done using the Rigaku SmartLab (Shibuya-ku, Japan) (9 kW) diffractometer using CuKα radiation. HRTEM of the samples was recorded with JEOL JEM-2100 F (FEG) (JEOL Ltd., Akishima-shi, Japan) operating at 200 kV.

Preparation of CuO@ARF

To a solution of $Cu(OAc)_2 \cdot H_2O$ (50 mg, 0.25 mmol) in DMF (5 mL) was added ARF (1 g), and the mixture taken in a Teflon-capped sealed tube was heated at 110°C for 30 min with occasional gentle shaking. The supernatant liquid became completely colorless by this time, and the greyish beads of ARF visibly turned brownish. The mixture was cooled to room temperature, and the resin beads were filtered off and washed repeatedly with water (3 × 5 mL) and acetone (2 × 5 mL). Resulting brown beads were dried under vacuum and used for analyses and evaluation of catalytic activity.

General conditions for C-S cross-coupling reaction

To a suspension of CuO@ARF (200 mg) in water (3 mL) were added aryl halide (1 mmol), thiol (1.2 mmol), K_2CO_3 (1.1 mmol), and SDS (10 mol%), and the reaction mixture was heated in a screw-capped sealed tube at 100°C for several hours as mention in Table 2. Proceeding of the reaction was monitored by TLC at time intervals. After completion, the mixture was cooled, diluted with water (5 mL), and then filtered through a cotton bed to separate out the resin beads. The resin beads were washed with ethyl acetate (2 mL), and the filtrate was extracted with ethyl acetate (3 × 10 mL). The combined organic layer was dried over anhydrous Na_2SO_4 and concentrated under vacuum. The residue obtained was purified by column chromatography using light petroleum as the eluent. All products were identified on the basis of spectral data (^{1}H and ^{13}C NMR) and also compared with reported melting point (for solid compounds and as available) (see Additional file 1).

The resin beads separated out from the reaction mixture were successively washed with water (3 × 5 mL) and acetone (2 × 5 mL) and then dried under vacuum for use in the next batch of recycle run.

Preparation of phenothiazine from selective iodo-coupled product (Table 2, entry 17) using Pd-BINAP catalyst

To a mixture of 2-(2-bromophenylthio)benzeneamine (1 mmol, 280 mg) in toluene were added ^{t}BuOK (1.5 mmol, 168 mg), $Pd_2(dba)_3$ (2 mol%), and BINAP (4 mol%). The reaction mixture taken in a screw-capped sealed tube was heated at 100°C for 4 h. After cooling, the reaction mixture was diluted with water (5 mL) and extracted with ethyl acetate (3 × 10 mL). The combined extracts were washed with brine, dried (Na_2SO_4), and evaporated. The residue was purified over a silica gel column to obtain white crystals of phenothiazine (167 mg, 84%), characterized by ^{1}H and ^{13}C NMR, and compared with literature data (see Additional file 1).

10*H*-phenothiazine [46], m.p. 185°C to 186°C (Lit. m.p. 186°C to 187°C). ^{1}H NMR (DMSO-d6, 300 MHz): δ/ppm 6.72 to 6.77 (*m*, 4H, ArH), 6.89 to 7.01 (*m*, 4H, ArH), 8.58 (*s*, 1H, NH) ^{13}C NMR (DMSO-d6, 75 MHz): δ/ppm 114.4, 116.4, 121.8, 126.3, 127.5, and 142.1.

Preparation of phenothiazine from selective iodo-coupled product (Table 2, entry 17) using CuO@ARF catalyst

To a mixture of 2-(2-bromophenylthio)benzeneamine (1 mmol, 280 mg) in dimethyl sulfoxide were added ^{t}BuOK (1.5 mmol, 168 mg), CuO@ARF (200 mg, 1.8 mg of copper, 2.83 mol% Cu) and L-proline (5.66 mol%). The reaction mixture taken in a screw-capped sealed tube was heated at 100°C for 48 h. After cooling, the reaction mixture was diluted with water (5 mL) and extracted with ethyl acetate (3 × 10 mL). The combined extracts were washed with brine, dried (Na_2SO_4), and evaporated. The residue was purified over a silica gel column to obtain white crystals of phenothiazine (143 mg, 72%), characterized by ^{1}H and ^{13}C NMR and compared with literature data (see Additional file 1).

Additional file

Additional file 1: Supporting data. ^{1}H and ^{13}C NMR spectral data for sulfanes and scanned spectra and a comparative ^{1}H-NMR spectra of Phenothiazine.

Competing interests

The authors declare that they have no competing interests.

Authors' contributions

DS carried out the whole work and drafted the manuscript. BB conceived the study, followed the development, and finalized the manuscript. Both authors read and approved the final manuscript.

Acknowledgements

We thank DST, New Delhi, for financial support [Grant No. SR/S1/OC- 86/ 2010 (G)], and DS thanks CSIR, New Delhi, for awarding research fellowship. We thank Dr. G. De, CSIR-CGCRI, Kolkata for Powder XRD measurements and Prof. A. K. Nandy, I.A.C.S., Kolkata for HRTEM analysis.

References

1. Procter DJ (2000) The synthesis of thiols, selenols, sulfides, selenides, sulfoxides, selenoxides, sulfones and selenones. J Chem Soc Perkin Trans 1:835–871
2. Liu L, Stelmach JE, Natarajan SR, Chen M-H, Singh SB, Schwartz CD, Fitzgerald CE, O'Keefe SJ, Zaller DM, Schmatz DM, Doherty JB (2003) SAR of 3,4-dihydropyrido[3,2-d]pyrimidone p38 inhibitors. Bioorg Med Chem Lett 13:3979–3982
3. Jones DN (1979) 3. In: Barton DH, Ollis DW (ed) Comprehensive Organic Chemistry, vol 3. Pergamon, New York
4. Kaldor SW, Kalish VJ, Davies JF, II, Shetty BV, Fritz JE, Appelt K, Burgess JA, Campanal KM, Chirgadze NY, Clawson DK, Dressman BA, Hatch SD, Khalil DA, Kosa MB, Lubbehusen PP, Muesing MA, Patick AK, Reich SH, Su KS, Tatlock JH (1997) Viracept (nelfinavir mesylate, AG1343): a potent, orally bioavailable inhibitor of HIV-1 protease. J Med Chem 40:3979–3985
5. De Martino G, Edler MC, La Regina G, Cosuccia A, Barbera MC, Barrow D, Nicholson RI, Chiosis G, Brancale A, Hamel E, Artico M, Silvestri R (2006) New arylthioindoles: potent inhibitors of tubulin polymerization. 2. Structure-activity relationships and molecular modeling studies. J Med Chem 49:947–954
6. Liu G, Huth JR, Olejniczak ET, Mendoza F, Fesik SW, von Geldern TW (2001) Novel *p*-arylthio cinnamides as antagonists of leukocyte function-associated antigen-1/intracellular adhesion molecule-1 interaction. 2. Mechanism of inhibition and structure-based improvement of pharmaceutical properties. J Med Chem 44:1202–1210
7. Nielsen SF, Nielsen EØ, Olsen GM, Liljefors T, Peters D (2000) Novel potent ligands for the central nicotinic acetylcholine receptor: synthesis, receptor binding, and 3D-QSAR analysis. J Med Chem 43:2217–2226
8. Korth C, May BCH, Cohen FE, Prusiner SB (2001) Acridine and phenothiazine derivatives as pharmacotherapeutics for prion disease. Proc Natl Acad Sci U S A 98:9836–9841
9. Hickman RJS, Christie BJ, Guy RW, White T (1985) Synthesis of aromatic S-substituted derivatives of *N*-acetyl-L-cysteine. Aust J Chem 38:899–904
10. Khatik GL, Kumar R, Chakraborti AK (2006) Catalyst-free conjugated addition of thiols to α, β-unsaturated carbonyl compounds in water. Org Lett 8:2433–2436
11. Migita T, Shimizu T, Asami Y, Shiobara J, Kato Y, Kosugi M (1980) The palladium catalyzed nucleophilic substitution of aryl halides by thiolate anions. Bull Chem Soc Jpn 53:1385–1389
12. Eichman CC, Stambuli JP (2011) Transition metal catalyzed synthesis of aryl sulfides. Molecules 16:590–608
13. Guan P, Cao C, Liu Y, Li Y, He P, Chen Q, Liu G, Shi Y (2012) Efficient nickel/ N-heterocyclic carbene catalyzed C–S cross-coupling. Tetrahedron Lett 53:5987–5992
14. Chen C-K, Chen Y-W, Lin C-H, Lin H-P, Lee C-F (2010) Synthesis of CuO on mesoporous silica and its applications for coupling reactions of thiols with aryl iodides. Chem Commun 46:282–284
15. Wong YC, Jayanth TT, Cheng CH (2006) Cobalt-catalyzed aryl-sulfur bond formation. Org Lett 8:5613–5616
16. Correa A, Carril M, Bolm C (2008) Iron-catalyzed S-arylation of thiols with aryl iodides. Angew Chem Int Ed 47:2880–2883
17. Lai CS, Kao HL, Wang YJ, Lee CF (2012) A general rhodium-catalyzed cross-coupling reaction of thiols with aryl iodides. Tetrahedron Lett 53:4365–4367
18. Liu T-J, Yi C-L, Chan C-C, Lee C-F (2013) Manganese-catalyzed cross-coupling of thiols with aryl iodides. Chem Asian J 8:1029–1034
19. Reddy VP, Kumar AV, Swapna K, Rao KP (2009) Nano indium oxide as a recyclable Catalyst for C-S cross-coupling of thiols with aryl halides under ligand free conditions. Org Lett 11:1697–1700

20. Hegedus LL, McCabe RW (1984). In: Catalysis Poisoning. Marcel Dekker, New York
21. Chen YJ, Chen HH (2006) 1,1,1-Tris(hydroxymethyl)ethane as a new, efficient, and versatile tripod ligand for copper-catalyzed cross-coupling reactions of aryl iodides with amides, thiols, and phenols. Org Lett 8:5609–5612
22. Bates CG, Gujadhur RK, Venkataraman D (2002) A general method for the formation of aryl-sulfur bonds using copper(I) catalysts. Org Lett 4:2803–2806
23. Heiz U (2007) Landman U Nanocatalysis. Springer–Verlag, Springer Berlin
24. Kamal A, Srinivasulu V, Murty JNSRC, Shankaraiah N, Nagesh N, Reddy TS, Rao AVS (2013) Copper oxide NPs supported on graphene oxide- catalyzed S-arylation: an efficient and ligand-free synthesis of aryl sulfides. Adv Synth Catal 355:2297–2307
25. Schwab RS, Singh D, Alberto EE, Piquini P, Rodrigues OED, Braga AL (2011) C–S cross-coupling of thiols with aryl iodides under ligand-free conditions using nano copper oxide as a recyclable catalyst in ionic liquid. Catal Sci Technol 1:569–573
26. Rout L, Sen TK, Punniyamurthy T (2007) Efficient CuO-nanoparticle-catalyzed C-S cross-coupling of thiols with iodobenzene. Angew Chem Int Ed 46:5583–5586
27. Rout L, Saha P, Jammi S, Punniyamurthy T (2008) Efficient copper(I)-catalyzed C–S cross coupling of thiols with aryl halides in water. Eur J Org Chem 2008:640–643
28. Carril M, SanMartin R, Dominguez E, Tellitu I (2007) Simple and efficient recyclable catalytic system for performing copper-catalysed S-arylation reactions in the presence of water. Chem Eur J 13:5100–5105
29. Malik P, Chakraborty D (2012) Bi(III)-catalyzed C-S cross-coupling reaction. Appl Organomet Chem 26:557–561
30. Lan M-T, Wu W-Y, Huang S-H, Luo K-L, Tsai F-Y (2011) Reusable and efficient $CoCl_26H_2O$/cationic 2,2'-bipyridyl system-catalyzed S-arylation of aryl halides with thiols in water under air. RSC Adv 1:1751–1755
31. Wu WY, Wang JC, Tsai FY (2009) A reusable $FeCl_3 \cdot 6H_2O$/cationic 2,2'-bipyridyl catalytic system for the coupling of aryl iodides with thiols in water under aerobic conditions. Green Chem 11:326–329
32. Basu B, Das S, Das P, Mandal B, Banerjee D, Almqvist F (2009) Palladium supported on a polyionic resin as an efficient, ligand-free, and recyclable catalyst for Heck, Suzuki-Miyaura, and Sonogashira reaction. Synthesis :1137–1146
33. Sengupta D, Saha J, De G, Basu B (2014) Pd/Cu bimetallic NPs embedded in macroporous ion-exchange resins: an excellent heterogeneous catalyst for the Sonogashira reaction. J Mater Chem A 2:3986–3992
34. Paul S, Basu B (2011) Synthesis of libraries of quinoxalines through eco-friendly tandem oxidation–condensation or condensation reactions. Tetrahedron Lett 52:6597–6602
35. Paul S, Basu B (2012) Highly selective synthesis of libraries of 1,2-disubstituted benzimidazoles using silica gel soaked with ferric sulfate. Tetrahedron Lett 53:4130–4133
36. Rhee H-W, Choi SJ, Yoo SH, Jang YO, Park HH, Pinto RM, Cameselle JC, Sandoval FJ, Roje S, Han K, Chung DS, Suh J, Hong J-I (2009) A bifunctional molecule as an artificial flavin mononucleotide cyclase and a chemosensor for selective fluorescent detection of flavins. J Am Chem Soc 131:10107–10112
37. Basu B, Bhuiyan MMH, Das P, Hossain I (2003) Catalytic transfer reduction of conjugated alkenes and an imine using polymer-supported formates. Tetrahedron Lett 44:8931–8934
38. Dar MA, Nam SH, Youn SK, Kim WB (2010) Synthesis, characterization, and electrochemical properties of self-assembled leaf-like CuO nanostructures. J Solid State Electrochem 14:1719–1726
39. Bahrami K, Khodaei MM, Nejati A (2010) Synthesis of 1,2-disubstituted benzimidazoles, 2-substituted benzimidazoles and 2-substituted benzothiazoles in SDS micelles. Green Chem 12:1237–1241
40. Jammi S, Barua P, Rout L, Saha P, Punniyamurthy T (2008) Efficient ligand-free nickel-catalyzed C–S cross-coupling of thiols with aryl iodides. Tetrahedron Lett 49:1484–1487
41. Cramer CJ, Truhlar DG ACS (eds) (1994) Structure and Reactivity in Aqueous Solution. Washington, DC
42. Sharma G, Kumar R, Chakraborti AK (2008) 'On water' synthesis of 2,4-diaryl-2,3-dihydro-1,5-benzothiazepines catalysed by sodium dodecyl sulfate (SDS). Tetrahedron Lett 49:4269–4271
43. Kumar D, Seth K, Kommi DN, Bhagat S, Chakraborti AK (2013) Surfactant micelles as microreactors for the synthesis of quinoxalines in water: scope and limitations of surfactant catalysis. RSC Adv 3:15157–15168
44. Seth K, Roy SR, Pipaliya BV, Chakraborti AK (2013) Synergistic dual activation catalysis by palladium nanoparticles for epoxide ring opening with phenols. Chem Commun 49:5886–5888. and references cited therein
45. Jana S, Dutta B, Bera R, Koner S (2008) Immobilization of palladium in mesoporous silica matrix: preparation, characterization, and its catalytic efficacy in carbon-carbon coupling reactions. Inorg Chem 47:5512–5520
46. Ma D, Geng Q, Zhang H, Jiang Y (2010) Assembly of substituted phenothiazines by a sequentially controlled CuI/l-proline-catalyzed cascade C–S and C–N bond formation. Angew Chem Int Ed 49:1291–1294

Synthesis of 2-cyclopropyl-3-(5-aryl-1*H*-pyrazol-3-yl)-1,8-naphthyridine

Mallaiah Bucha[1], Laxminarayana Eppakayala[1], Thirumala Chary Maringanti[2*], Giri Tharikoppula[1] and Shashikala Kethireddy[2]

Abstract

Background: 1,8-Naphthyridine derivatives have attracted considerable attention because the 1,8-naphthyridine skeleton is present in many compounds that have been isolated from natural substances, with various biological activities.

Findings: *N,N*-dimethoxy-*N*-methyl-1,8-naphthyridine-3-carboxamide (1) on reaction with Grignard reagent forms 2-methoxy-1,8-naphthyridine-3-carbaldehyde (2). Compound 2 on reaction with different aromatic aldehydes provided 1-(2-cyclopropyl-1,8-naphthyridin-3-yl)-3-arylprop-2-en-1-ones (3a-e) and these compounds on cyclisation with hydrazine hydrate 99% yielded 2-cyclopropyl-3-(5-aryl-1*H*-pyrazol-3-yl)-1,8-naphthyridines (4-a-e).
Synthesis of the target compounds involved the formation of 4a-e. It was accomplished using Grignard reaction, condensation reaction, and cyclisation reactions. All the synthesized compounds were readily soluble in DMSO. Spectral data of the synthesized compounds were in full agreement with the proposed structures.

Conclusions: In conclusion, we have developed a simple and an efficient Synthesis of 2-cyclopropyl-3-(5-aryl-1*H*-pyrazol-3-yl)-1,8-naphthyridine.

Keywords: Grignard reagent; Cyclisation; 1,8-naphthyridine

Findings

Background

Among the wide variety of heterocycles that have been explored for developing pharmaceutically important molecules, such as chalcones, pyrazolines and amino pyrimidines have played an important role in medicinal chemistry. The presence of reactive α,β-unsaturated carbonyl function in chalcones is found to be responsible for their antibacterial and antifungal activity. Nitrogen containing heterocyclic compounds find extensive pharmaceutical applications and possess biologically activity. Many of the naphthyridines have shown bacterial, fungicidal and carcinogenic activity [1-3]. As a step in this direction and in continuation of our work on 1, 8-naphthyridines [4-7], synthesis of the title compounds was carried out. The general synthetic procedures used in the preparation of these compounds involved the cyclisation of Schiff's bases [8-12].

* Correspondence: mtcharya@yahoo.com
[2]Jawaharlal Nehru Technological University Hyderabad College of Engineering, Nachupally, Karimnagar 505 501 Telangana, India
Full list of author information is available at the end of the article

The structure of the compounds were confirmed on the basis of their spectral (^{1}H NMR and mass) data. The synthetic approach is outlined in Scheme 1.

Methods

A simple conventional method is followed to prepare all the title compounds.

Results and discussion

Compound (1), when reacted with Grignard reagent and gave 2-methoxy-1,8-naphthyridine-3-carbaldehyde (2) which was reacted with different aldehydes to form arylidene derivatives (3a-e), which on treatment with hydrazine hydrate afforded compound (4a-e).

Experimental

Melting points were determined in open capillaries and are uncorrected. ^{1}H NMR spectrum is taken on a Varian 500 MHz instrument with TMS as an internal standard. The chemical shifts are expressed δ ppm, and the solvent used is DMSO-d_6. Mass spectrum is taken on Hewlett-Packard mass spectrometer operating at 70 eV. All the compounds are recrystalised from ethanol.

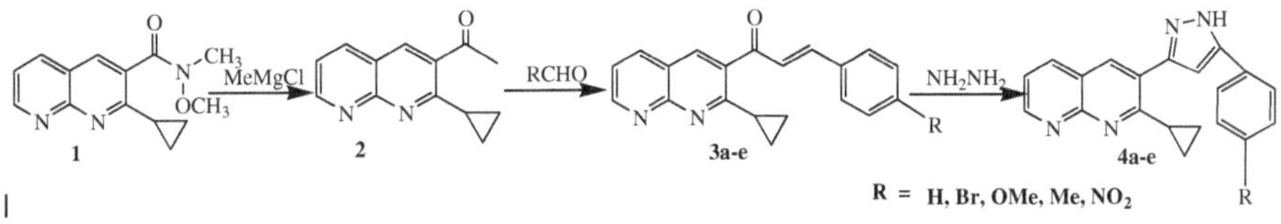

Scheme 1 Synthesis of 1,8-naphthyridines.

1-(2-cyclopropyl-1,8-naphthyridin-3-yl)ethanone (2)

To a solution of 2-cyclopropyl-*N*-methoxy-*N*-methyl-1,8-naphthyridine-3-carboxamide (1) (1.01 mmol) in THF (10 mL), MeMgCl (3.03 mmol) was added drop wise at −30°C and stirred for about 2 h at −30°C. The resulting solution is quenched with a saturated NH_4Cl solution (30 mL), filtered, extracted with EtOAc (3 × 30 mL) and dried over Na_2SO_4. The resulting crude compound was purified by a column chromatography by eluting 20% to 40% ethyl acetate in hexane to obtain the light yellow colour solid.

^1H NMR (DMSO-d_6, 500 MHz): δ 1.06-1.21 (m, 4H, 2CH2), 2.24 (s, 3H, CH_3), 2.57 (m, 1H, CH), 7.57 (t, 1H, *J* = 12Hz CH), 8.31 (s, 1H, *J* = 12Hz CH), 8.42, (d, 1H, CH), 9.02 (d, 1H, *J* = 10Hz CH). Mass [M + 1] peak at *m*/*z* 213.

1-(2-cyclopropyl-1,8-naphthyridin-3-yl)-3-phenylprop-2-en-1-one (3a)

To a solution of 1-(2-cyclopropyl-1,8-naphthyridin-3-yl) ethanone (2) (0.53 mmol) in DMF, NaOH (0.79 mmol) and aldehyde (0.63 mmol) were added at 0°C and stirred for about 1 h. Then water was added and extracted with DCM (2 × 15 mL), dried over Na_2SO_4 and evaporated under reduced pressure. The resulting crude compound was purified by a column chromatography by eluting 20% to 40% ethyl acetate in hexane to obtain the light yellow colour solid.

^1H NMR (DMSO-d_6, 500 MHz): δ 1.12-1.28 (m, 4H, $2CH_2$), 2.61 (m, 1H, CH), 7.62 (m, 2H, *J* = 14Hz 2CH), 7.81 (dd, 2H, *J* = 18Hz 2CH), 8.23, (m, 3H, 3CH), 8.51-8.61 (m, 4H, *J* = 18Hz 4CH), 9.12 (s, 1H, CH). Mass [M + 1] peak at *m*/*z* 301.

Other compounds in the series were prepared similarly and their characterization data are recorded below.

3-(4-bromophenyl)-1-(2-cyclopropyl-1,8-naphthyridin-3-yl) prop-2-en-1-one (3b)

^1H NMR (DMSO-d_6, 500 MHz): δ 1.14-1.29 (m, 4H, $2CH_2$), 2.52,(m, 1H, CH), 7.62 (m, 4H, 4CH), 7.71 (d, 2H, *J* = 12Hz 2CH), 8.23, (d, 1H, 1CH), 8.69 (s, 1H, 1CH), 9.22 (s, 1H, CH).Mass [M + 1] *m*/*z* 380.

1-(2-cyclopropyl-1,8-naphthyridin-3-yl)-3-(4-methoxyphenyl) prop-2-en-1-one (3c)

^1H NMR (DMSO-d_6, 500 MHz): δ 1.16-1.27 (m, 4H, 2CH2), 2.48 (m, 1H, CH), 7.62 (m, 4H, 4CH), 7.69 (d, 2H, *J* = 12Hz 2CH), 8.33 (d, 1H, , *J* = 12Hz, 1CH), 8.71 (s, 1H, 1CH), 9.24 (s, 1H, CH). Mass [M + 1] peak at *m*/*z* 331.

1-(2-cyclopropyl-1,8-naphthyridin-3-yl)-3-p-tolylprop-2-en-1-one (3d)

^1H NMR (DMSO-d_6, 500 MHz): δ 1.19-1.28 (m, 4H, $2CH_2$), 2.53 (m, 1H, CH), 7.63 (m, 4H, 4CH), 7.72 (d, 2H, *J* = 14Hz 2CH), 8.42 (d, 1H, *J* = 14Hz, 1CH), 8.78 (s, 1H, 1CH), 9.28 (s, 1H, CH).Mass [M + 1] peak at *m*/*z* 315.

1-(2-cyclopropyl-1,8-naphthyridin-3-yl)-3-(4-nitrophenyl) prop-2-en-1-one (3e)

^1H NMR (DMSO-d_6, 500 MHz): δ 1.23-1.31 (m, 4H, $2CH_2$), 2.62 (m, 1H, CH), 7.73 (m, 4H, 4CH), 7.81 (d, 2H, *J* = 18Hz 2CH), 8.56 (d, 1H, *J* = 16Hz, 1CH), 8.64 (s, 1H, 1CH), 9.32 (s, 1H, CH).Mass [M + 1] peak at *m*/*z* 346.

2-cyclopropyl-3-(5-phenyl-1H-pyrazol-3-yl)-1,8-naphthyridine (4a)

To a solution of 1-(2-cyclopropyl-1,8-naphthyridin-3-yl)-3-phenylprop-2-en-1-one (3a) (0.31 mmol) in ethanol (5 mL), hydrazine hydrate 99%(2 mL) was added. The resulting solution was refluxed for about 12 h. After completion of a starting material, the ethanol was evaporated completely under a reduced pressure then the title compound was recrystalised from diethyl ether to obtain the brown colour solid.

^1H NMR (DMSO-d_6, 500 MHz): δ 1.16(m, 2H, CH_2), 1.22 (m, 2H, CH_2), 2.21 (m, 1H, CH), 5.21(s, 1H, *J* = 12Hz CH), 5.41(s, 1H, *J* = 12Hz CH), 6.31 (m, 1H, *J* = 12Hz CH), 6.59, (m, 2H, 2CH), 7.19 (d, 1H, *J* = 10Hz CH), 7.69 (m, 4H, 4CH), 8.42 (m, 2H, 2CH), 9.11 (s, 1H, CH), 10.81 (s, 1H, NH). Mass [M + 1] peak at *m*/*z* 313.

Other compounds in the series were prepared similarly and their characterization data are recorded below.

3-(5-(4-bromophenyl)-1H-pyrazol-3-yl)-2-cyclopropyl-1,8-naphthyridine (4b)

^1H NMR (DMSO-d_6, 500 MHz): δ 1.21(m, 2H, CH_2), 1.28 (m, 2H, CH_2), 2.37 (m, 1H, CH), 6.21 (s, 1H, *J* = 12Hz CH), 7.32(s, 1H, CH), 7.41 (m, 4H, *J* = 12Hz 4CH), 8.19 (m, 2H, 2CH), 8.39 (d, 1H, CH), 10.69 (s, 1H, NH). Mass [M + 2] peak at *m*/*z* 392.

2-cyclopropyl-3-(5-(4-methoxyphenyl)-1H-pyrazol-3-yl)-1,8-naphthyridine (4c)

^{1}H NMR (DMSO-d_6, 500 MHz): δ 1.24 (m, 2H, CH_2), 1.29 (m, 2H, CH_2), 2.28 (m, 1H, CH), 4.12 (s, 3H, CH_3), 6.23 (s, 1H, CH), 7.35 (s, 1H, CH), 7.29 (m, 4H, J = 12Hz 4CH), 8.03, (m, 2H, 2CH), 8.42 (d, 1H, CH), 10.46 (s, 1H, NH). Mass [M + 1] peak at m/z 343.

2-cyclopropyl-3-(5-p-tolyl-1H-pyrazol-3-yl)-1,8-naphthyridine (4d)

^{1}H NMR (DMSO-d_6, 500 MHz): δ 1.18 (m, 2H, CH_2), 1.31 (m, 2H, CH_2), 2.20 (m, 1H, CH), 2.39 (s, 3H, CH_3), 6.28 (s, 1H, CH), 7.25 (s, 1H, CH), 7.39 (m, 4H, 4CH), 8.23, (m, 2H, 2CH), 8.44 (d, 1H, J = 12Hz, CH), 10.59 (s, 1H, NH). Mass [M + 1] peak at m/z 327.

2-cyclopropyl-3-(5-(4-nitrophenyl)-1H-pyrazol-3-yl)-1,8-naphthyridine (4e)

^{1}H NMR (DMSO-d_6, 500 MHz): δ 1.18 (m, 2H, CH_2), 1.31 (m, 2H, CH_2), 2.20 (m, 1H, CH), 6.18 (s, 1H, CH), 7.15 (s, 1H, CH), 7.27 (m, 4H, 4CH), 8.12, (m, 2H, 2CH), 8.24 (d, 1H, J = 12Hz, CH), 11.19 (s, 1H, NH). Mass [M + 1] peak at m/z 358.

Conclusions

We have presented simple, cost effective, and practical method for preparation of some 1,8-naphthyridines. This methodology provides an efficient alternative to existing methods for the synthesis of 2-cyclopropyl-3-(5-aryl-1*H*-pyrazol-3-yl)-1,8-naphthyridine. Here in step-1, we observed the formation of Grignard product which on condensation of aldehydes Schiff's base is formed. Further reaction Schiff's base with hydrazine we obtained the pyrazoles.

Competing interests

The authors declare that they have no competing interests.

Author details

[1]Mahatma Gandhi Institute of Technology, Gandipet, Hyderabad 50075 Telangana, India. [2]Jawaharlal Nehru Technological University Hyderabad College of Engineering, Nachupally, Karimnagar 505 501 Telangana, India.

References

1. Nezval J, Halocka J (1967) The enhancing effect on the antibacterial activity of nalidixix acid against Pseudomonas aeruginosa. Experientia 23:1043
2. Egawa H, Miyamido A, Nishimra Y, Okada H, Uno H, Matsumato J (1984) Pyridonecarboxylic acids as antibacterial agents. J Med Chem 27:1543
3. Suzuki N, Dohmori R (1979) The chemistry of heterocyclic compounds: the naphthyridines. Chem Pharma Bull 27:410
4. Shiva Shankar S, Laxminarayana E, Haripriya V, Thirumala Chary M (2011) Synthesis of 5-(2-methoxy-1,8-naphthyridin-3-yl)-4-aryl-4H-1,2,4-triazole-3-thiols and 5-(2-methoxy-1,8-naphthyridin-3-yl)-n-aryl-1,3,4-thiadiazol-2-amines. Indian J Heterocycl Chem 21:101
5. Narender A, Thirumala Chary M, Laxminarayana E, Haripriya V (2013) Synthesis and antimicrobial activity of 2-cyclopropyl [1,8]naphthyridine-3-carboxylic acid (4-phenyl-2-thioxo-thiazol-3-yl)-amides, [1,3,5]triazine, [1,3,4] thiadiazole-2-thiol, [1,2,4]triazole-3-thiol and coumarine derivatives. Indian J Chem 52B:440
6. Mallaiah B, Shiva Shankar S, Laxminarayana E, Thirumala Chary M (2013) Synthesis of 2-(5-(2-methoxy-1,8-naphthyridin-3-yl)-1,3,4-oxadiazol/triazol-2-ylthio)-1-(4-alkylbenzofuran-2-yl)ethanones and 2-methoxy-3-(5-(4-alkylbenzofuran-2-yl)-7aH-thiazolo[2,3-b][1,3,4]oxadiazol/triazol-2-yl)-1,8-naphthyridines by conventional and eco-friendly methods and evaluation of their antibacterial activity. Indian J Heterocycl Chem 22(2):333
7. Shiva Shankar E, Laxminarayana M, Thirumala C (2013) Synthesis of 5-(2-methoxy-1,8-naphthyridin-3-yl)-1,3,4-oxadiazole-2(3H)-thione and 1-(2-methoxy-1,8-naphthyridin-3-acetyl)-4-arylthiosemicarbazides. Indian J Heterocycl Chem 23(2):139
8. Vadim A, Soloshonok CC, Yamada T, Hisanori U, Ohfune Y, Hruby VJ (2005) Michael addition reactions between chiral equivalents of a nucleophilic glycine and (*S*)- or (*R*)-3-[(*E*)-Enoyl]-4-phenyl-1,3-oxazolidin-2-ones as a general method for efficient preparation of β-substituted pyroglutamic acids: case of topographically controlled stereoselectivity. J Am Chem Soc 43:127
9. Reddy KR, Kumar NS (2006) Cellulose-supported copper(0) catalyst for Aza-Michael addition. Synlett 6:224
10. Wu F, Li L, Hong R, Deng L (2006) Construction of quaternary stereocenters via efficient and practical conjugate additions to α, β-unsaturated ketones with a chiral organic catalyst. Angew Chem Int 45:947
11. Bensa D, Constantieux T, Rodriguez J (2004) A new efficient and commercially available user-friendly and recyclable heterogeneous organocatalyst for the Michael addition of 1,3-dicarbonyl compounds. Synthesis 06:923
12. Ooi T, Ohara D, Fukumoto K, Maruoka K (2005) Importance of chiral phase-transfer catalysts with dual functions in obtaining high enantioselectivity in the Michael reaction of malonates and chalcone derivatives. Org Lett 7:3195

Method development and validation of potent pyrimidine derivative by UV-VIS spectrophotometer

Anshu Chaudhary[1,2*], Anoop Singh[1] and Prabhakar Kumar Verma[3]

Abstract

Background: A rapid and sensitive ultraviolet-visible (UV-VIS) spectroscopic method was developed for the estimation of pyrimidine derivative 6-Bromo-3-(6-(2,6-dichlorophenyl)-2-(morpolinomethylamino) pyrimidine4-yl) -2H-chromen-2-one ($BT_{10}M$) in bulk form.

Results: Pyrimidine derivative was monitored at 275 nm with UV detection, and there is no interference of diluents at 275 nm. The method was found to be linear in the range of 50 to 150 µg/ml. The accuracy and precision were determined and validated statistically. The method was validated as a guideline.

Conclusions: The results showed that the proposed method is suitable for the accurate, precise, and rapid determination of pyrimidine derivative.

Keywords: Pyrimidine; Derivative; UV-VIS spectroscopy; Validation

Background

Nitrogen containing heterocyclic ring such as pyrimidine is a promising structural moiety for drug design. Pyrimidine derivatives form a component in various useful drugs and are associated with many biological and therapeutic activities. Condensed pyrimidines have been reported as antimicrobial [1-3], anti-inflammatory [4,5], analgesic [6,7], anticancer [8-10], anti-HIV [11], antitubercular, antimalarial, diuretic, and cardiovascular disease [12] (Scheme 1).

The present work is a synthesis, a biological evaluation and validation of novel pyrimidine derivatives. Research workers have synthesized 50 pyrimidine derivatives (T_1M-$T_{10}M$, T_1P-$T_{10}P$, BT_1M-$BT_{10}M$, BT_1P-$BT_{10}P$, CT_1M-CT_5M, and CT_1P-CT_5P). Among them, $BT_{10}M$ exhibited maximum antimicrobial, anti-inflammatory, and analgesic activity. Hence, a validation study was done on $BT_{10}M$. $BT_{10}M$ is chemically [6-Bromo-3-(6-(2,6-dichlorophenyl)-2-(morpolinomethylamino) pyrimidine4-yl) -2H-chromen-2-one]. It is a yellow crystalline powder with a molecular formula of $C_{24}H_{19}BrCl_2N_4O_3$ and a molecular weight of 562.24. It is a potent antimicrobial, analgesic and anti-inflammatory agent among all the synthesized derivatives. Hence, the aim of present investigation is to develop a simpler, rapid, and cost-effective analytical method for the determination of pyrimidine derivative ($BT_{10}M$) in bulk dosage form suitable for routine quality control analysis.

Method validation is the process used to confirm that analytical procedure employed for a specific test is suitable for its intended use. It is an integral part of any good analytical practice. Methods need to be validated or revalidated [13].

* Correspondence: anshu_17oct@yahoo.co.in
[1]NIMS University, Shobha Nagar, Jaipur 303001, Rajasthan, India
[2]Vishveshwarya Institute of Medical Science, Gautambudh Nagar 203207, Uttar Pradesh, India
Full list of author information is available at the end of the article

Methods

Chemical and reagent

$BT_{10}M$ was synthesized by research workers and then validated. Methanol and acetonitrile (1:1) were used throughout spectrophotometric method development and validation.

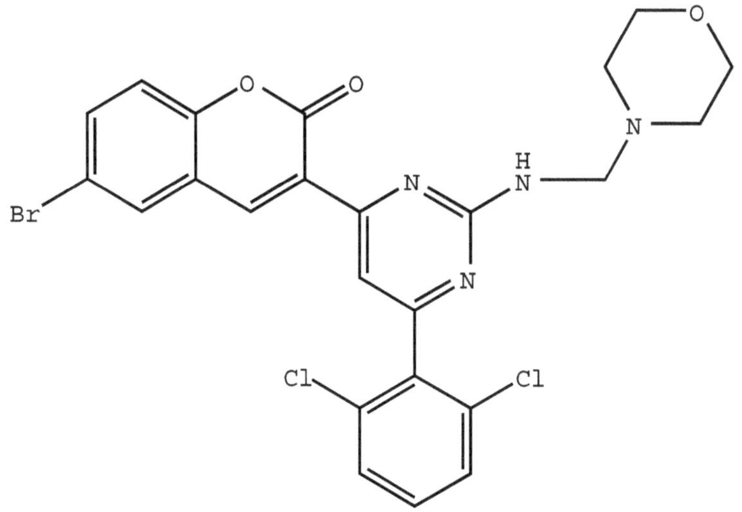

Scheme 1 Chemical structure of $BT_{10}M$.

Instrumentation

The method was performed on a double-beam ultraviolet-visible (UV-VIS) spectrophotometer (Shimadzu model 1700 (Shimadzu, Kyoto, Japan)) having two matched quartz cells with a 1-cm light path.

Determination of maximum wavelength (λ_{max}), methodology, and sample preparation

About 50 mg of $BT_{10}M$ was weighed accurately and transferred into a 50-ml volumetric flask and dissolved in 25 ml of methanol and acetonitrile (1:1) and made up to the volume with the same solvent mixture to give a standard concentration of 1,000 μg/ml. Transfer 5 ml of above solution into the 50-ml volumetric flask, dilute, and made up to the volume with the same solvent mixture to get a standard concentration of 100 μg/ml. This solution was scanned against a blank over the entire UV-VIS wavelength of 200 to 400. Based on the spectrum, a λ_{max} of 275 nm was selected for further analysis.

Table 1 Validation summary

Serial number	Parameters	Acceptance criteria	Observation
01	Precision		
	(a) System precision %RSD	NMT 1.5%	0.0968
	(b) Method precision %RSD	NMT 1.5%	0.27995
02	Specificity	No considerable absorbance of any other component of formulation at λ_{max} of analyte or at detection wavelength	No absorbance observed at 275 nm
03	Accuracy (by recovery)		
	% Recovery	100% ± 2%	100.12%
	%RSD	NMT 1.5%	1.1777%
	% Deviation from accuracy	±1.5%	080%: +01.46
			100%: −00.77
			120%: −00.32
04	Linearity	Coefficient of correlation	r^2: 0.997
		(r^2) NLT 0.998	
05	Ruggedness	%RSD: NMT 1.5%	%RSD: 0.1572
06	Robustness	%RSD: NMT 1.5%	Original condition: +0.72
			Changed condition: −0.82
07	Limit of detection and limit of quantitation	LOD	145.2 mg
		LOQ	440.00 mg

NMT, not more than; NLT, not less than.

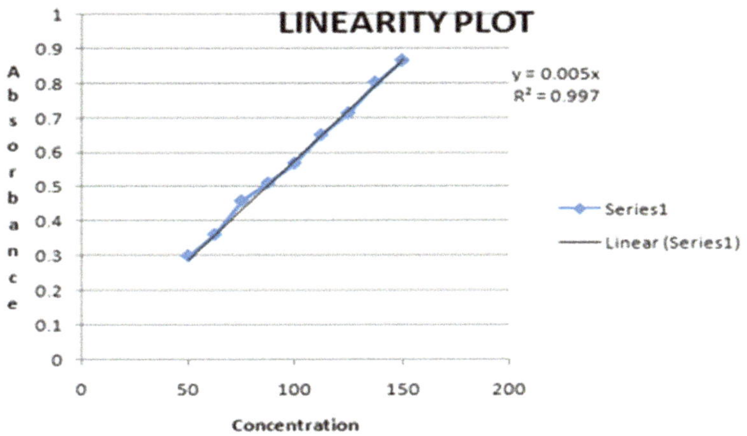

Figure 1 Linearity plot. The BT10M absorbance response in the concentration range of about 50 mcg/ml to 150 mcg/ml was found to be linear to the analyte concentration in the solution with a correlation coefficient (r2) of 0.997.

Results

The method was validated with respect to linearity, accuracy, precision, specificity, robustness, ruggedness, LOD, and LOQ in Table 1.

Discussion

The method was validated with respect to linearity, accuracy, precision, specificity, robustness, ruggedness, LOD, and LOQ. The method was established according to the International Conference on Harmonisation of Technical Requirements for Registration of Pharmaceuticals for Human Use (ICH) guidelines. $BT_{10}M$ exhibited maximum absorption at 275 nm and obeyed Beer's law in the concentration range of 50 to 150 μg/ml. The proposed method for the determination of $BT_{10}M$ showed linear regression $y = 0.005x + 0.025$ with a coefficient correlation (r^2) of 0.997 (Figure 1). The precision was determined by the relative standard deviation of the six-assay sample of $BT_{10}M$, and the assay of each was calculated and the obtained relative standard deviation of % assay was less than 1.5%. The percentage recovery for $BT_{10}M$ was found in the range of 98.97% to 99.83% which indicates that the developed method was simple, rapid, and precise. LOD was found to be 145.2 and limit of quantitation to be 440.0. The proposed method will be suitable for the analysis of newly synthesized pyrimidine derivative ($BT_{10}M$) in bulk dosage form.

Experimental

Validation

The methods were validated with respect to linearity, accuracy, precision, specificity, ruggedness, robustness, limit of detection (LOD), and limit of quantitation (LOQ).

Linearity

The linearity of an analytical method is its ability to elicit test results that are directly, or by a well-defined mathematical transformation, proportional to the concentration of analyte in the samples within a given range. For assay determination, the concentration of $BT_{10}M$ is 100 μg/ml. So the working range of analyte was set between 50, 62.5, 75, 87.5, 100, 112.5, 125, 137.5 and 150 μg/ml to show the linearity of the curve obtained. The observations and calibration curve are shown in Table 2 and Figure 1.

Accuracy (by recovery test)

Accuracy of method is by shown by recovery study and spiking working standard in the placebo at levels 80%, 100%, and 120% of the working standard. Recovery study was performed by spiking in $BT_{10}M$ to the placebo at levels 80%, 100%, and 120% of working standard. The samples were prepared according to the assay procedure. The results are shown in Tables 3 and 4.

Table 2 Linearity table of $BT_{10}M$ in working standard

Serial number	Approximate concentration (μg/ml)	Average absorbance at 275 nm
1	50.0	0.299
2	62.5	0.361
3	75.0	0.458
4	87.5	0.511
5	100.0	0.569
6	112.5	0.651
7	125.0	0.714
8	137.5	0.803
9	150.0	0.866

Table 3 Accuracy reading

Level (Approximate)	Standard added (mg)	Absorbance at 275 nm	Standard recovered (mg)	%Recovery	Mean recovery	%RSD
80%	40.5	0.458	40.43	99.83	99.37%	0.4366
		0.451				
		0.459				
100%	50.8	0.567	50.28	098.97		
		0.561				
		0.574				
120%	60.1	0.670	59.68	099.30		
		0.676				
		0.673				

The percentage recovery for $BT_{10}M$ was found in the range of 98.97% to 99.83% with an overall relative standard deviation (%RSD) of 0.4366. From the data obtained which was given in Table 3, the method was found to be accurate. Formula of standard deviation was SD = (xi − x/n − 1)1/2 if n is very large. In case of very small data, SD = (xi − x/n)1/2.

Precision

The precision of an analytical method is the degree of agreement among individual test results when the method is applied repeatedly to multiple sampling of homogenous sample. The precision of an analytical method is usually expressed as the standard deviation or relative standard of a series of measurements. Assay preparation and standard preparation were prepared as per method of analysis of six $BT_{10}M$ assay sample preparations as per the experimental conditions in method of analysis. Calculated percent of $BT_{10}M$ in each assay sample percent by spectrophotometry and the results and observation are summarized in Tables 5 and 6.

Assay

$$\%\,\textbf{Assay} = \frac{\text{Abs. of Smp.}}{\text{Abs. of standard}} \times \frac{\text{Wt. of standard}}{\text{Dil. factor}} \times \frac{\text{Dil. factor}}{\text{Wt. of Smp}} \times 100$$

Table 4 Deviation from recovery

Level (Approximate)	Actual concentration (μg/ml)	Concentration calculated (mg/ml)	Accuracy (%)	% Deviation
80%	080.75	081.9289	101.46	+01.46
100%	100.40	099.6269	099.23	−00.77
120%	121.05	120.6626	099.68	−00.32

The precision will be determined by the relative standard deviation of the six-assay sample of $BT_{10}M$, and the assay of each is calculated and the obtained relative standard deviation of % assay should be less than 1.5%. The %RSD shows that precision of the method was satisfactory.

Specificity

Specificity study is designed to prove that the $BT_{10}M$ in the solution gives maximum absorbance at wavelength 275 nm, and there is no interference from the solvent. The purpose of this study is to establish the fact that inherent chemical stability of the molecule remains intact during its existence. If any degradation product formed, it can be monitored and resolved to quantify the nature and extent of degradation. For this, the spectrum of $BT_{10}M$, placebos are studied. The sample preparation is as per methodology. The spectrum of $BT_{10}M$ is shown in Figure 2.

For the spectrophotometric method, no other component of formulation shows considerable absorbance at the λ_{max} of the analyte or at the detection wavelength of the subject analyte. In this case of $BT_{10}M$, the detection wavelength is 275 nm. The placebo solution under the same condition does not show any absorbance at 275 nm.

Table 5 System precision data of $BT_{10}M$ working standard solution

Serial number	Absorbance at 275 nm
1	0.566
2	0.565
3	0.565
4	0.566
5	0.566
6	0.565
Average	0.565
%RSD	0.0968

Weight of $BT_{10}M$ WS = 50.0 mg.

Table 6 Method precision data for estimation of $BT_{10}M$

Assay	Sample weight (mg)	Absorbance	% Assay
1	50.2	0.576	101.75
2	50.4	0.576	101.29
3	50.2	0.572	101.02
4	50.8	0.580	101.22
5	50.0	0.569	100.96
6	50.7	0.579	101.37
	Average		101.2683
	%RSD		0.27995

Ruggedness

The ruggedness of the analytical method is the degree of reproducibility of test results obtained by the analysis of the sample on different days, by different chemist using different instruments. In this study, two individual assay sample preparations of $BT_{10}M$ drug product were prepared by different chemists for analysis. Six (6) replicate observations of the same standard solution were obtained as well as six observations of different sample solution were recorded. The assay percentage of each sample was calculated in each case. The results are summarized in Tables 5, 6, 7, 8, 9.

The ruggedness (inter-day precision) will be determined by the relative standard deviation of the results of assay of two different chemists on different days.

Robustness

The robustness of an analytical method is a measure of its capacity to remain unaffected by small but deliberate variations in method parameters and provides an indication of its reliability under normal usage. Method robustness was determined by analyzing the same sample at normal operating conditions and also by changing some operating analytical conditions. The result and observation are summarized in Table 10.

The robustness will be determined by the relative standard deviation of the results of assay of two different conditions by a change in original parameter.

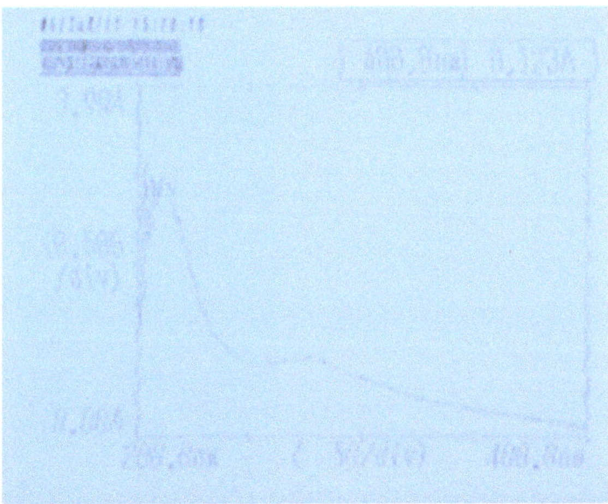

Figure 2 Spectrum of $BT_{10}M$.

Table 7 System precision data of $BT_{10}M$ working standard solution

Serial number	Absorbance at 275 nm
1	0.559
2	0.561
3	0.560
4	0.561
5	0.560
6	0.561
Average	0.560
%RSD	0.14571

Weight of $BT_{10}M$: 49.8 mg.

Limit of detection and limit of quantitation

Limit of detection LOD is defined as the lowest concentration of an analyte in a sample that can be detected, not quantified.

Limit of quantitation The lowest concentration of an analyte in a sample that can be determined with acceptable precision and accuracy under the stated operational conditions of the method.

$$\begin{aligned}\mathbf{LOD : 3.3(SD)/Slope} \\ \mathbf{3.3(0.200)/0.005\ [SD = 0.2200]} \\ \mathbf{= 145.2\,mg}\end{aligned}$$

$$\begin{aligned}\mathbf{2. LOQ : 10(SD)/Slope} \\ \mathbf{10(0.2200)/0.005} \\ \mathbf{= 440.00\,mg}\end{aligned}$$

Conclusions

All the validation parameters for all the developed methods were studied as per ICH guidelines. All the

Table 8 Method precision data for $BT_{10}M$

Assay	Sample weight (mg)	Absorbance	% Assay
1	50.2	0.566	100.27
2	50.5	0.572	100.73
3	50.8	0.582	101.94
4	50.7	0.578	101.45
5	50.2	0.568	100.64
6	50.9	0.579	101.23
		Average	101.0433
		%RSD	0.6041

Table 9 Mean % assay and %RSD

Chemist A	Chemist B	Average	%RSD
101.2683	101.0433	101.1558	0.1572

Table 10 Percentage deviation for sample under both conditions

Parameter	Original condition	Changed conditions
Dilution medium	Acetonitrile:methanol	Acetonirile:methanol
	1:1	1:2
Assay in %	101.98	100.44
% Deviation from mean assay value obtained in precision studies	+00.72	−00.82

methods were found to be accurate, simple, specific, selective, precise, and reproducible. Hence, the method can be used for routine analysis of $BT_{10}M$ in bulk dosage form.

Competing interests

The authors declare that they have no competing interests.

Acknowledgement

Thank to Mr. Rupesh Dudhe, Department of pharmacy, SMAS, Galgotias University, Greater Noida, U. P. India for kind support for validation.

Author details

[1]NIMS University, Shobha Nagar, Jaipur 303001, Rajasthan, India. [2]Vishveshwarya Institute of Medical Science, Gautambudh Nagar 203207, Uttar Pradesh, India. [3]Department of Pharmaceutical Sciences, M.D. University, Rohtak 124001, Haryana, India.

References

1. Mohmed MS, Awad SM, Sayed IA (2010) Synthesis of certain pyrimidine derivatives as antimicrobial agents and anti-inflammatory agents. Molecules 15:1882–1890
2. Munawar AM, Azad M, Siddiqui L (2008) Synthesis & antimicrobial study of some quinolinyl pyrimidine derivatives. J Chin Chem Soc 55:394–400
3. Ashraf HF, Abd EIW (2012) Synthesis, reactions and evaluation of the antimicrobial activity of some 4-(p-Halophenyl)-4H-naphthopyran, pyranopyrimidine and pyranotriazolopyrimidine derivatives. Pharmaceuticals 5:745–757
4. Nofal MZ, Emans Z, Wafaa EE (2011) Synthesis of pyrimidines and fused pyrimidines and their evaluation of antimicrobial activity. Acta Polnniae Pharmaceutica-Drug Res 68(4):507–517
5. Kota RK, Kompelly KK, Surampudi R, Kulkarni R (2011) Synthesis and anti-inflammatory activity of novel pyrazolo [3,4-d] pyrimidines. J Chem Pharm Res 3(4):848–853
6. Gupta JK, Sharma PK, Dudhe R, Chaudhary A (2011) Synthesis and analgesic activity of novel pyrimidine derivatives of coumarin moiety. Acta Polnniae Pharmaceutica-Drug Res 68(5):785–793
7. Sondhi SM, Dinodia M, Shukla R (2009) Synthesis, anti-inflammatory and analgesic activity evaluation of some pyrimidine derivatives. Indian J Chem 49B:273–281
8. Sharma S, Sharma PK, Kumar N, Dudhe R (2011) A review on various heterocyclic moieties and their antitubercular activity. Biomed Pharmacother 65:244–251
9. Al-abdullah ES (2011) Synthesis and anticancer activity of some novel tetralin-6-yl-pyrazoline, 2-thioxopyrimidine, 2-oxopyridine, 2-thioxo-pyridine and 2-iminopyridine derivatives. Molecules 16:3410–3419
10. EL-Zahar MI, Adb El-Karim SS, Haiba ME, Khedr MA (2011) Synthesis, antitumor activity and molecular docking study of novel benzofuran-2-yl pyrazole pyrimidine derivatives. Acta Polnniae Pharmaceutica-Drug Res 68(3):357–373
11. Mohamed YA, Mohamed SF, Abdullah MM (2012) Cytotoxicity and anti-HIV evaluations of some new synthesized quinazoline and thioxopyrimidine derivatives using 4-(thiophen-2-yl)-3,4,5,6-tetrahydrobenzo[h]quinazoline-2 (1H)-thione as synthon. J Chem Sci 124(3):693–702
12. Chaudhary A, Sharma PK, Verma PK, Kumar N, Dudhe R (2012) Microwave assisted synthesis of novel pyrimidine derivatives and investigation of their analgesic and ulcerogenic activity. Med Chem Res 21(11):3629–3645
13. Chaudhary A, Verma PK, Dudhe R (2012) Significant anti-microbial activity of novel pyrimidine derivatives. Elixir Pharmacy 45:7956–7963

Permissions

All chapters in this book were first published in OMCL, by Springer; hereby published with permission under the Creative Commons Attribution License or equivalent. Every chapter published in this book has been scrutinized by our experts. Their significance has been extensively debated. The topics covered herein carry significant findings which will fuel the growth of the discipline. They may even be implemented as practical applications or may be referred to as a beginning point for another development.

The contributors of this book come from diverse backgrounds, making this book a truly international effort. This book will bring forth new frontiers with its revolutionizing research information and detailed analysis of the nascent developments around the world.

We would like to thank all the contributing authors for lending their expertise to make the book truly unique. They have played a crucial role in the development of this book. Without their invaluable contributions this book wouldn't have been possible. They have made vital efforts to compile up to date information on the varied aspects of this subject to make this book a valuable addition to the collection of many professionals and students.

This book was conceptualized with the vision of imparting up-to-date information and advanced data in this field. To ensure the same, a matchless editorial board was set up. Every individual on the board went through rigorous rounds of assessment to prove their worth. After which they invested a large part of their time researching and compiling the most relevant data for our readers.

The editorial board has been involved in producing this book since its inception. They have spent rigorous hours researching and exploring the diverse topics which have resulted in the successful publishing of this book. They have passed on their knowledge of decades through this book. To expedite this challenging task, the publisher supported the team at every step. A small team of assistant editors was also appointed to further simplify the editing procedure and attain best results for the readers.

Apart from the editorial board, the designing team has also invested a significant amount of their time in understanding the subject and creating the most relevant covers. They scrutinized every image to scout for the most suitable representation of the subject and create an appropriate cover for the book.

The publishing team has been an ardent support to the editorial, designing and production team. Their endless efforts to recruit the best for this project, has resulted in the accomplishment of this book. They are a veteran in the field of academics and their pool of knowledge is as vast as their experience in printing. Their expertise and guidance has proved useful at every step. Their uncompromising quality standards have made this book an exceptional effort. Their encouragement from time to time has been an inspiration for everyone.

The publisher and the editorial board hope that this book will prove to be a valuable piece of knowledge for researchers, students, practitioners and scholars across the globe.

List of Contributors

Alice MR Bernardino
Departamento de Química Orgânica, Instituto de Química, Programa de Pós-Graduação em Química, Universidade Federal Fluminense, Campus do Valonguinho, 24020-150, Niterói, RJ, Brazil

Alexandre R Azevedo
Departamento de Química Orgânica, Instituto de Química, Programa de Pós-Graduação em Química, Universidade Federal Fluminense, Campus do Valonguinho, 24020-150, Niterói, RJ, Brazil

Luiz CS Pinheiro
Departamento de Química Orgânica, Instituto de Química, Programa de Pós-Graduação em Química, Universidade Federal Fluminense, Campus do Valonguinho, 24020-150, Niterói, RJ, Brazil

Júlio C Borges
Departamento de Química Orgânica, Instituto de Química, Programa de Pós-Graduação em Química, Universidade Federal Fluminense, Campus do Valonguinho, 24020-150, Niterói, RJ, Brazil

Izabel CP Paixão
Departamento de Biologia Celular e Molecular, Instituto de Biologia, Universidade Federal Fluminense, Campus do Valonguinho, 24020-150, Niterói, RJ, Brazil

Milene Mesquita
Departamento de Biologia Celular e Molecular, Instituto de Biologia, Universidade Federal Fluminense, Campus do Valonguinho, 24020-150, Niterói, RJ, Brazil
Programa de Pós-Graduação em Biologia Celular e Molecular, Fundação Oswaldo Cruz, Instituto Oswaldo Cruz, 21040-900, Rio de Janeiro, RJ, Brazil

Thiago ML Souza
Departamento de Biologia Celular e Molecular, Instituto de Biologia, Universidade Federal Fluminense, Campus do Valonguinho, 24020-150, Niterói, RJ, Brazil
Programa de Pós-Graduação em Biologia Celular e Molecular, Fundação Oswaldo Cruz, Instituto Oswaldo Cruz, 21040-900, Rio de Janeiro, RJ, Brazil

Maurício S dos Santos
Departamento de Física e Química, Instituto de Ciências Exatas, Universidade Federal de Itajubá, 37500- 903, Itajubá, MG, Brazil

Abid H Banday
Department of Chemistry, Islamia College of Science and Commerce, Srinagar 190009, J&K, India

Shameem A Shameem
Department of Chemistry, Islamia College of Science and Commerce, Srinagar 190009, J&K, India

Bashir A Ganai
Department of Biochemistry, University of Kashmir, Srinagar 190009, J&K, India

Rosario Astrid Vargas Cárdenas
Department of Chemistry, The University of Texas-Pan American, 1201 West University Drive, Edinburg, TX 78539, USA

Blanca Olinda Quintanilla Leal
Department of Chemistry, The University of Texas-Pan American, 1201 West University Drive, Edinburg, TX 78539, USA

Ashwini Reddy
Department of Chemistry, The University of Texas-Pan American, 1201 West University Drive, Edinburg, TX 78539, USA

Debasish Bandyopadhyay
Department of Chemistry, The University of Texas-Pan American, 1201 West University Drive, Edinburg, TX 78539, USA

Bimal K Banik
Department of Chemistry, The University of Texas-Pan American, 1201 West University Drive, Edinburg, TX 78539, USA

Mahendra Kumar
Department of Chemistry, University of Rajasthan, Jaipur 302 055, India

Kailash Sharma
Department of Chemistry, University of Rajasthan, Jaipur 302 055, India

Dinesh Kumar Sharma
Department of Chemistry, University of Rajasthan, Jaipur 302 055, India

Yekkirala Venkateswarlu
Department of Chemistry, Osmania University College for Women, Koti, Hyderabad 500095, India

Sudhagani Ramesh Kumar
Department of Chemistry, Osmania University College for Women, Koti, Hyderabad 500095, India

Panuganti Leelavathi
Department of Chemistry, Osmania University College for Women, Koti, Hyderabad 500095, India

Suresh
Department of Chemistry, Punjabi University, Patiala, Punjab 147 002, India

Jagir Singh Sandhu
Department of Chemistry, Punjabi University, Patiala, Punjab 147 002, India

Xiang Li
Key Laboratory of Energy Sources & Chemical Engineering, Development Center of Natural Products and Medication and School of Chemistry and Chemical Engineering, Ningxia University, Yinchuan 750021, China
Key Laboratory of Medicinal Chemistry for Natural Resource (Yunnan University), Ministry of Education, Yunnan University, Kunming 650091, China

Xue-Qiang Li
Key Laboratory of Energy Sources & Chemical Engineering, Development Center of Natural Products and Medication and School of Chemistry and Chemical Engineering, Ningxia University, Yinchuan 750021, China

He-Mei Liu
Key Laboratory of Energy Sources & Chemical Engineering, Development Center of Natural Products and Medication and School of Chemistry and Chemical Engineering, Ningxia University, Yinchuan 750021, China

Xue-Zhang Zhou
Key Lab of Ministry of Education for Protection and Utilization of Special Biological Resources in Western China, School of Life Science, Ningxia University, Yinchuan 750021, China

Zhi-Hui Shao
Key Laboratory of Medicinal Chemistry for Natural Resource (Yunnan University), Ministry of Education, Yunnan University, Kunming 650091, China

Mahesh Kumar Teli
School of Biotechnology, National Institute of Technology Calicut, Calicut, 673601 Kerala, India

Rajanikant G K
School of Biotechnology, National Institute of Technology Calicut, Calicut, 673601 Kerala, India

Ashok Penta
Department of Pharmacy, Birla Institute of Technology & Science, Pilani Rajasthan 333031, India

Swastika Ganguly
Department of Pharmaceutical Sciences, Birla Institute of Technology, Mesra-Jharkhand 835215, India

Sankaran Murugesan
Department of Pharmacy, Birla Institute of Technology & Science, Pilani Rajasthan 333031, India

Sunil Kumar
Laboratory for Drug Design and Synthesis, Department of Pharmaceutical Chemistry, Indo-Soviet Friendship (ISF) College of Pharmacy, Moga, Punjab 142 001, India

Samir Mehndiratta
Laboratory for Drug Design and Synthesis, Department of Pharmaceutical Chemistry, Indo-Soviet Friendship (ISF) College of Pharmacy, Moga, Punjab 142 001, India

Kunal Nepali
Laboratory for Drug Design and Synthesis, Department of Pharmaceutical Chemistry, Indo-Soviet Friendship (ISF) College of Pharmacy, Moga, Punjab 142 001, India

Manish K Gupta
Laboratory for Drug Design and Synthesis, Department of Pharmaceutical Chemistry, Indo-Soviet Friendship (ISF) College of Pharmacy, Moga, Punjab 142 001, India

Surrinder Koul
Division of Bio-Organic Chemistry and Pharmacology, Indian Institute of Integrative Medicine (IIIM), CSIR, Jammu Tawi 180 001, India

Parduman R Sharma
Division of Bio-Organic Chemistry and Pharmacology, Indian Institute of Integrative Medicine (IIIM), CSIR, Jammu Tawi 180 001, India

Ajit K Saxena
Division of Bio-Organic Chemistry and Pharmacology, Indian Institute of Integrative Medicine (IIIM), CSIR, Jammu Tawi 180 001, India

Kanaya L Dhar
Laboratory for Drug Design and Synthesis, Department of Pharmaceutical Chemistry, Indo-Soviet Friendship (ISF) College of Pharmacy, Moga, Punjab 142 001, India

Uttara Soumyanarayanan
Department of Pharmaceutical Chemistry, Manipal College of Pharmaceutical Sciences, Manipal University, Manipal, Karnataka 576104, India

Varadaraj G Bhat
Department of Pharmaceutical Chemistry, Manipal College of Pharmaceutical Sciences, Manipal University, Manipal, Karnataka 576104, India

Sidhartha S Kar
Department of Pharmaceutical Chemistry, Manipal College of Pharmaceutical Sciences, Manipal University, Manipal, Karnataka 576104, India

Jesil A Mathew
Department of Pharmaceutical Biotechnology, Manipal College of Pharmaceutical Sciences, Manipal University, Manipal, Karnataka 576104, India

Sneha Das
Department of Pharmaceutical Sciences, Guru Jambheshwar University of Science and Technology, Hisar, Haryana 125001, India

Neeru Vasudeva
Department of Pharmaceutical Sciences, Guru Jambheshwar University of Science and Technology, Hisar, Haryana 125001, India

Sunil Sharma
Department of Pharmaceutical Sciences, Guru Jambheshwar University of Science and Technology, Hisar, Haryana 125001, India

Pascal Amoa Onguéné
Department of Chemistry, Faculty of Science, University of Douala, 00237, P. O. Box 24157 Douala, Cameroon

Fidele Ntie-Kang
Department of Chemistry, Faculty of Science, Chemical and Bioactivity Information Centre, University of Buea, 00237, P. O. Box 63 Buea, Cameroon
Department of Pharmaceutical Sciences, Martin-Luther University of Halle-Wittenberg, Wolfgang-Langenbeck Str. 4, Halle (Saale) 06120, Germany

James Ajeck Mbah
Department of Chemistry, Faculty of Science, Chemical and Bioactivity Information Centre, University of Buea, 00237, P. O. Box 63 Buea, Cameroon

Lydia Likowo Lifongo
Department of Chemistry, Faculty of Science, Chemical and Bioactivity Information Centre, University of Buea, 00237, P. O. Box 63 Buea, Cameroon

Jean Claude Ndom
Department of Chemistry, Faculty of Science, University of Douala, 00237, P. O. Box 24157 Douala, Cameroon

Wolfgang Sippl
Department of Pharmaceutical Sciences, Martin-Luther University of Halle-Wittenberg, Wolfgang-Langenbeck Str. 4, Halle (Saale) 06120, Germany

Luc Meva'a Mbaze
Department of Chemistry, Faculty of Science, University of Douala, 00237, P. O. Box 24157 Douala, Cameroon

Rupesh Dudhe
Uttarakhand Technical University, Dehradun, Uttarakhand 284007, India
Department of Pharmacy, SMAS, Galgotias University, Greater Noida, Uttar Pradesh 201306, India

Pramod Kumar Sharma
Department of Pharmacy, SMAS, Galgotias University, Greater Noida, Uttar Pradesh 201306, India

Prabhakar Kumar Verma
Department of Pharmaceutical Sciences, M. D. University, Rohtak, Haryana 124001, India

Yihenew Simegniew Birhan
Department of Chemistry, Natural and Computational Science College, Debre Markos University, Debre Markos, Ethiopia

Adnan Ahmed Bekhit
Department of Pharmaceutical Chemistry, Alexandria University, Alexandria 21215, Egypt

Ariaya Hymete
Department of Pharmaceutical Chemistry and Pharmacognosy, School of Pharmacy, Addis Ababa University, Addis Ababa, Ethiopia

Poonam Singh
Department of Pharmaceutical Technology, Meerut Institute of Engineering & Technology, NH-58, Baghpat By-pass Crossing, Delhi-Haridwar Highway, Meerut-250005, India

Pramod Kumar Sharma
Department of Pharmaceutical Technology, Meerut Institute of Engineering & Technology, NH-58, Baghpat By-pass Crossing, Delhi-Haridwar Highway, Meerut-250005, India

Jitendra Kumar Sharma
Faculty of Pharmacy, Dehradun Institute of Technology, Dehradun, Uttarakhand, India

Anshu Upadhyay
Department of Pharmaceutical Technology, Meerut Institute of Engineering & Technology, NH-58, Baghpat By-pass Crossing, Delhi-Haridwar Highway, Meerut-250005, India

Nitin Kumar
Department of Pharmaceutical Technology, Meerut Institute of Engineering & Technology, NH-58, Baghpat By-pass Crossing, Delhi-Haridwar Highway, Meerut-250005, India

Nadezhda E Shchepina
Laboratory of Radiochemistry, Natural Sciences Institute of Perm State University, 4 Genkel St, Perm 614990, Russia

Viktor V Avrorin
Chemistry Department, St-Petersburg State University, 26 Universitetsky Pr, St-Petersburg, Petrodvorets 198504, Russia

Gennady A Badun
Radiochemistry Department, M. V. Lomonosov Moscow State University, Leninskie Gory, Moscow 119992, Russia

Nikolay A Bumagin
Department of Organic Chemistry, M. V. Lomonosov Moscow State University, Leninskie Gory, Moscow 119992, Russia

Scott B Lewis
Department of Chemistry, James Madison University, Harrisonburg, VA 22807, USA

Sergey N Shurov
Department of Organic Chemistry, Perm State University, 15 Bukirev St, Perm 614990, Russia

Shailesh V Jain
Institute of pharmacy, Nirma University, Ahmedabad, Gujarat 382481, India

Manjunath Ghate
Institute of pharmacy, Nirma University, Ahmedabad, Gujarat 382481, India

Kamlendra S Bhadoriya
R. C. Patel Institute of Pharmaceutical Education and Research, Shirpur, Dhule District, Maharashtra 425405, India

Sanjaykumar B Bari
R. C. Patel Institute of Pharmaceutical Education and Research, Shirpur, Dhule District, Maharashtra 425405, India

Amar Chaudhari
R. C. Patel Institute of Pharmaceutical Education and Research, Shirpur, Dhule District, Maharashtra 425405, India

Jayshri S Borse
R. C. Patel Institute of Pharmaceutical Education and Research, Shirpur, Dhule District, Maharashtra 425405, India

Thomas Rühl
Department of Neuroradiopharmaceuticals, Institute of Radiopharmacy, Research Site Leipzig, Helmholtz-Zentrum Dresden-Rossendorf e.V., Permoserstr. 15, Leipzig 04318, Germany

Winnie Deuther-Conrad
Department of Neuroradiopharmaceuticals, Institute of Radiopharmacy, Research Site Leipzig, Helmholtz-Zentrum Dresden-Rossendorf e.V., Permoserstr. 15, Leipzig 04318, Germany

Steffen Fischer
Department of Neuroradiopharmaceuticals, Institute of Radiopharmacy, Research Site Leipzig, Helmholtz-Zentrum Dresden-Rossendorf e.V., Permoserstr. 15, Leipzig 04318, Germany

Robert Günther
Department of Neuroradiopharmaceuticals, Institute of Radiopharmacy, Research Site Leipzig, Helmholtz-Zentrum Dresden-Rossendorf e.V., Permoserstr. 15, Leipzig 04318, Germany

Lothar Hennig
Institute of Organic Chemistry, Faculty of Chemistry and Mineralogy, Universität Leipzig, Johannisallee 29, Leipzig 04103, Germany

Harald Krautscheid
Institute of Inorganic Chemistry, Faculty of Chemistry and Mineralogy, Universität Leipzig, Johannisallee 29, Leipzig 04103, Germany

Peter Brust
Department of Neuroradiopharmaceuticals, Institute of Radiopharmacy, Research Site Leipzig, Helmholtz-Zentrum Dresden-Rossendorf e.V., Permoserstr. 15, Leipzig 04318, Germany

Luciana MR Antinarelli
Departamento de Parasitologia, Microbiologia e Imunologia, I.C.B, Universidade Federal de Juiz de Fora, Campus Universitário, Juiz de Fora, MG 36036-900, Brazil

Arturene ML Carmo
Departamento de Química, I.C.E., Universidade Federal de Juiz de Fora, Campus Universitário, Juiz de Fora, MG 36036-900, Brazil

Fernando R Pavan
Departamento de Ciências Biológicas, F.C. F., Universidade Estadual Paulista "Júlio de Mesquita Filho", Rod. Araraquara-Jaú Km.01 s/n, Campus, 14801-902, Araraquara, SP, Brazil

Clarice Queico F Leite
Departamento de Ciências Biológicas, F.C. F., Universidade Estadual Paulista "Júlio de Mesquita Filho", Rod. Araraquara-Jaú Km.01 s/n, Campus, 14801-902, Araraquara, SP, Brazil

Adilson D Da Silva
Departamento de Química, I.C.E., Universidade Federal de Juiz de Fora, Campus Universitário, Juiz de Fora, MG 36036-900, Brazil

Elaine S Coimbra
Departamento de Parasitologia, Microbiologia e Imunologia, I.C.B, Universidade Federal de Juiz de Fora, Campus Universitário, Juiz de Fora, MG 36036-900, Brazil

Deepak B Salunke
Centre National de la Recherche Scientifique, Institut de Chimie des Substances Naturelles, UPR 2301 CNRS, Avenue de la Terrasse, 91198, Gif-sur-Yvette, France

Zainab Hussain
Department of Chemistry, College of Science for Women, Baghdad University, Baghdad, Iraq

Emad Yousif
Department of Chemistry, College of Science, Al-Nahrain University, Baghdad, Iraq

Ahmed Ahmed
Department of Chemistry, College of Science, Al-Nahrain University, Baghdad, Iraq

Ali Altaie
Department of Chemistry, College of Science for Women, Baghdad University, Baghdad, Iraq

Fidele Ntie-Kang
CEPAMOQ, Faculty of Science, University of Douala, P.O. Box 8580, Douala, Cameroon
Chemical and Bioactivity Information Centre, Department of Chemistry, Faculty of Science, University of Buea, P.O. Box 63, Buea, Cameroon
Department of Pharmaceutical Sciences, Martin Luther University of Halle-Wittenberg, Wolfgang-Langenbeck Str. 4, Halle (Saale) 06120, Germany

James A Mbah
Department of Chemistry, Faculty of Science, University of Buea, P.O. Box 63, Buea, Cameroon

Lydia L Lifongo
Chemical and Bioactivity Information Centre, Department of Chemistry, Faculty of Science, University of Buea, P.O. Box 63, Buea, Cameroon

Luc C Owono Owono
CEPAMOQ, Faculty of Science, University of Douala, P.O. Box 8580, Douala, Cameroon
Laboratory for Simulations and Biomolecular Physics, Advanced Teachers Training College, University of Yaoundé I, P.O. Box 47, Yaoundé, Cameroon

Eugene Megnassan
Laboratory of Fundamental and Applied Physics, University of Abobo-Adjame, Abidjan 02 BP 801, Cote d'Ivoire, Africa

Luc Meva'a Mbaze
Department of Chemistry, Faculty of Science, University of Douala, P.O. Box 24157, Douala, Cameroon

Philip N Judson
Chemical and Bioactivity Information Centre, 22-23 Blenheim Terrace, Woodhouse Lane, Leeds LS2 9HD, UK

Wolfgang Sippl
Department of Pharmaceutical Sciences, Martin Luther University of Halle-Wittenberg, Wolfgang-Langenbeck Str. 4, Halle (Saale) 06120, Germany

Simon MN Efange
Department of Chemistry, Faculty of Science, University of Buea, P.O. Box 63, Buea, Cameroon

Goutam Brahmachari
Laboratory of Natural Products and Organic Synthesis, Department of Chemistry, Visva-Bharati University, Santiniketan, West Bengal 731 235, India

Bubun Banerjee
Laboratory of Natural Products and Organic Synthesis, Department of Chemistry, Visva-Bharati University, Santiniketan, West Bengal 731 235, India

Tabassum Bano
Department of Pharmaceutical Technology, Meerut Institute of Engineering and Technology, Baghpat Bypass Crossing, NH-58, Delhi-Roorkee Highway, Meerut, Uttar Pradesh 250005, India

Nitin Kumar
Department of Pharmacy, Galgotias University, Yamuna Expressway, Greater Noida, Uttar Pradesh 201306, India

Marco Brito-Arias
Unidad Profesional Interdisciplinaria de Biotecnología del Instituto Politécnico Nacional, Avenida Acueducto s/n La Laguna Ticomán DF cp 07340, Mexico

Carlos Aguilar-Lemus
Unidad Profesional Interdisciplinaria de Biotecnología del Instituto Politécnico Nacional, Avenida Acueducto s/n La Laguna Ticomán DF cp 07340, Mexico

Pamela B Hurtado-Ponce
Unidad Profesional Interdisciplinaria de Biotecnología del Instituto Politécnico Nacional, Avenida Acueducto s/n La Laguna Ticomán DF cp 07340, Mexico

Guadalupe Martínez-Barrón
Escuela Nacional de Ciencias Biológicas del Instituto Politécnico Nacional, Carpio y Plan de Ayala Colonia Santo Tomas DF cp11340, Mexico.

Miguel Ibañez-Hernandez
Escuela Nacional de Ciencias Biológicas del Instituto Politécnico Nacional, Carpio y Plan de Ayala Colonia Santo Tomas DF cp11340, Mexico.

Rodrigo Teodoro
Department of Neuroradiopharmaceuticals, Institute of Radiopharmaceutical Cancer Research, Research Site Leipzig, Helmholtz-Zentrum Dresden- Rossendorf e.V., Permoserstr 15, 04318 Leipzig, Germany

Rareş-Petru Moldovan
Department of Neuroradiopharmaceuticals, Institute of Radiopharmaceutical Cancer Research, Research Site Leipzig, Helmholtz-Zentrum Dresden- Rossendorf e.V., Permoserstr 15, 04318 Leipzig, Germany

Corinna Lueg
Department of Pharmaceutical and Medicinal Chemistry, University of Münster, Correnssstraße 58-62, 48149 Münster, Germany

Robert Günther
Department of Neuroradiopharmaceuticals, Institute of Radiopharmaceutical Cancer Research, Research Site Leipzig, Helmholtz-Zentrum Dresden- Rossendorf e.V., Permoserstr 15, 04318 Leipzig, Germany

Cornelius K Donat
Department of Neuroradiopharmaceuticals, Institute of Radiopharmaceutical Cancer Research, Research Site Leipzig, Helmholtz-Zentrum Dresden- Rossendorf e.V., Permoserstr 15, 04318 Leipzig, Germany

Friedrich-Alexander Ludwig
Department of Neuroradiopharmaceuticals, Institute of Radiopharmaceutical Cancer Research, Research Site Leipzig, Helmholtz-Zentrum Dresden- Rossendorf e.V., Permoserstr 15, 04318 Leipzig, Germany

Steffen Fischer
Department of Neuroradiopharmaceuticals, Institute of Radiopharmaceutical Cancer Research, Research Site Leipzig, Helmholtz-Zentrum Dresden- Rossendorf e.V., Permoserstr 15, 04318 Leipzig, Germany

Winnie Deuther-Conrad
Department of Neuroradiopharmaceuticals, Institute of Radiopharmaceutical Cancer Research, Research Site Leipzig, Helmholtz-Zentrum Dresden- Rossendorf e.V., Permoserstr 15, 04318 Leipzig, Germany

Bernhard Wünsch
Department of Pharmaceutical and Medicinal Chemistry, University of Münster, Correnssstraße 58-62, 48149 Münster, Germany

Peter Brust
Department of Pharmaceutical and Medicinal Chemistry, University of Münster, Correnssstraße 58-62, 48149 Münster, Germany

Dodheri Syed Samiulla
DMPK Department, Aurigene Discovery Technologies Limited, Electronic City Phase 2, Hosur Road, Bangalore 560100, India

Andra Naidu
Department of Chemistry, Jawaharlal Nehru Technological University Hyderabad, Kukatpally, Hyderabad 500085, India

Gummadi Venkateshwar Rao
DMPK Department, Aurigene Discovery Technologies Limited, Electronic City Phase 2, Hosur Road, Bangalore 560100, India

Murali Ramachandra
DMPK Department, Aurigene Discovery Technologies Limited, Electronic City Phase 2, Hosur Road, Bangalore 560100, India

Debasish Sengupta
Department of Chemistry, North Bengal University, Darjeeling 734013, India

Basudeb Basu
Department of Chemistry, North Bengal University, Darjeeling 734013, India

Mallaiah Bucha
Mahatma Gandhi Institute of Technology, Gandipet, Hyderabad 50075 Telangana, India

Laxminarayana Eppakayala
Mahatma Gandhi Institute of Technology, Gandipet, Hyderabad 50075 Telangana, India

Thirumala Chary Maringanti
Jawaharlal Nehru Technological University Hyderabad College of Engineering, Nachupally, Karimnagar 505 501 Telangana, India

Giri Tharikoppula
Mahatma Gandhi Institute of Technology, Gandipet, Hyderabad 50075 Telangana, India

Shashikala Kethireddy
Jawaharlal Nehru Technological University Hyderabad College of Engineering, Nachupally, Karimnagar 505 501 Telangana, India

Anshu Chaudhary
NIMS University, Shobha Nagar, Jaipur 303001, Rajasthan, India
Vishveshwarya Institute of Medical Science, Gautambudh Nagar 203207, Uttar Pradesh, India

Anoop Singh
NIMS University, Shobha Nagar, Jaipur 303001, Rajasthan, India

Prabhakar Kumar Verma
Department of Pharmaceutical Sciences, M.D. University, Rohtak 124001, Haryana, India